CLINICAL PRACTICE IN

CORRECTIONAL MEDICINE

CLINICAL PRACTICE IN
CORRECTIONAL MEDICINE

EDITOR-IN-CHIEF
MICHAEL PUISIS, D.O.

Regional Medical Director,
New Mexico State Prison System,
Albuquerque, New Mexico

ASSOCIATE EDITORS ────────────

B. JAYE ANNO, PH.D., C.C.H.P.-A.
Consultants in Correctional Care,
Santa Fe, New Mexico

ROBERT L. COHEN, M.D.
Assistant Professor, Social Medicine and Clinical
   Epidemiology,
Albert Einstein College of Medicine,
New York, New York
Board member, National Commission for Correctional
   Health Care

BUDD HEYMAN, M.D.
Director of Prison Health Services, Bellevue Hospital Center;
Clinical Instructor, Department of Medicine,
New York University School of Medicine,
New York, New York

LAMBERT N. KING, M.D., PH.D.
Senior Vice President for Medical and Academic Affairs,
Saint Vincents Hospital and Medical Center of New York;
Professor of Clinical Community and Preventive Medicine,
New York Medical College,
Valhalla, New York

JOHN P. MAY, M.D.
Assistant Medical Director,
Central Detention Facility Health Services,
Washington, D.C.

JACK RABA, M.D.
Medical Director, Fantus Health Center,
Cook County Hospital,
Chicago, Illinois

RONALD SHANSKY, M.D.
Correctional Health Consultant,
Chicago, Illinois

ARMOND START, M.D., M.P.H.
Associate Professor (CHS), Department of Family Medicine,
University of Wisconsin-Madison School of Medicine,
Madison, Wisconsin

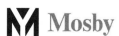 Mosby

St. Louis Baltimore Boston Carlsbad Chicago Minneapolis New York Philadelphia Portland
London Milan Sydney Tokyo Toronto

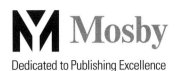

Dedicated to Publishing Excellence

A Times Mirror
Company

Publisher: Laura DeYoung
Managing Editor: Gina Byrd
Senior Development Editor: Kris Horeis
Designer: Jennifer Marmarinos
Manager, Periodical Editing: Kirk Swearingen
Manuscript Editor: Amanda Maguire
Project Supervisor, Production: Joy Moore
Project Assistant, Production: Laura Bayless
Electronic Layout: Lara Gniadek

Printed in the United States of America
Printing/binding by Maple-Vail Book Mfg. Group

Mosby, Inc.
11830 Westline Industrial Drive
St. Louis, Missouri 63146

International Standard Book Number: 0–8151–2704–9

Contributors

Carl Alaimo, Psy.D.
Cermak Health Services of Cook County,
Chicago, Illinois

Frederick L. Altice, M.D.
Assistant Professor of Medicine,
Yale University AIDS Program,
New Haven, Connecticut

Eran Y. Bellin, M.D.
Program Director, Montefiore-Rikers Island Health Services;
Assistant Professor of Epidemiology and Social Medicine,
Montefiore Medical Center and The Albert Einstein College of
    Medicine;
Assistant Professor of Medicine,
Department of Medicine, Division of Infectious Diseases,
Montefiore Medical Center and The Albert Einstein College of
    Medicine,
New York, New York

H. Blair Carlson, M.D., M.S.P.H.
Clinical Professor of Medicine,
University of Colorado School of Medicine;
Chair, Committee on Addiction Medicine,
American Society of Addiction Medicine,
Denver, Colorado

Michael D. Cohen, M.D., F.A.A.P.
Medical Director,
Division of Rehabilitative Services,
New York State Office of Children and Family Services,
Rensselaer, New York

Nancy Neveloff Dubler, LL.B.
Director, Division of Bioethics,
Montefiore Medical Center and Professor of Bioethics,
Albert Einstein College of Medicine,
Bronx, New York

Anderson Freeman, Ph.D.
Cermak Health Services of Cook County,
Chicago, Illinois

Jordan B. Glaser, M.D.
Director of Infectious Diseases,
Staten Island University Hospital,
Staten Island, New York

Laurie Goldman, M.D.
Cermak Health Services of Cook County,
Chicago, Illinois

Robert B. Greifinger, M.D.
Chief Executive Officer,
The Bromeen Group,
Dobbs Ferry, New York

Lindsay M. Hayes, M.S.
Assistant Director,
National Center on Institutions and Alternatives,
Mansfield, Massachusetts

Martin Horn, M.A., B.A.
The Secretary of the Pennsylvania Department of Corrections,
Camp Hill, Pennsylvania

Lisa Keamy, M.D.
Helixcare Medical Group,
Baltimore, Maryland;
Former Associate Director, Cermak Health Services,
Cook County Department of Correction,
Chicago, Illinois

Jane A. Kennedy, D.O.
Assistant Clinical Professor of Psychiatry,
University of Colorado School of Medicine, Diplomate;
American Board of Neurology and Psychiatry with added
    Qualification in Addiction Psychiatry
Denver, Colorado

William E. Lambert, Ph.D.
Environmental Epidemiologist,
The University of New Mexico Health Sciences Center,
Cancer Research and Treatment Center, NM Tumor
    Registry/CRTC,
Albuquerque, New Mexico

William C. Levine, M.D.
Division of STD Prevention,
National Center for HIV, STD, and TB Prevention,
Centers for Disease Control and Prevention,
Atlanta, Georgia

Kristen J. Mertz, M.D.
Division of STD Prevention,
National Center for HIV, STD, and TB Prevention,
Centers for Disease Control and Prevention,
Atlanta, Georgia

Joseph E. Paris, M.D., Ph.D., C.C.H.P.
Medical Director,
Georgia Department of Corrections,
Atlanta, Georgia

Stamatia Z. Richardson, M.D.
Senior Physician, Women's Health Care,
Cermak Health Services,
Cook County Bureau of Health,
Chicago, Illinois

John M. Robertson, M.D., M.P.H.
Medical Director, New Mexico Correctional Department,
Santa Fe, New Mexico;
Clinical Associate Professor of Medicine, University of New
    Mexico,
Albuquerque, New Mexico

William J. Rold, J.D., C.C.H.P.-A.
Attorney at Law,
New York, New York

Roxane Sanders, M.D.
Cermak Health Services of Cook County,
Chicago, Illinois

Gordon Schiff, M.D.
Director, Clinical Quality Research Unit,
Department of Medicine, Cook County Hospital,
Chicago, Illinois

Jonathan Shuter, M.D.
Director of Infectious Diseases, Montefiore-Rikers Island Health
    Services;
Assistant Professor of Medicine,
Department of Medicine, Division of Infectious Diseases,
    Montefiore Medical Center and the Albert Einstein College of
    Medicine,
New York, New York

Patricia M. Simone, M.D.
Division of Tuberculosis Elimination,
Centers for Disease Control and Prevention,
Atlanta, Georgia

Steven S. Spencer, M.D., F.A.C.P., C.C.H.P.
Consultant, Correctional Health Care,
Santa Fe, New Mexico

Leslie Stein, Psy.D., R.N.
Cermak Health Services of Cook County,
Chicago, Illinois

David Vlahov, Ph.D.
Professor of Epidemiology, Joint Appointment in Medicine,
The Johns Hopkins School of Hygiene and Public Health,
    Baltimore, Maryland

Andrea Weisman, Ph.D.
Director, Mental Health Services,
District of Columbia Central Detention Facility,
Washington, D.C.

To Coral and Sam.

Preface

This first textbook of Correctional Medicine is intended to provide guidance to clinical staff working in correctional facilities. Existing standards provide minimum requirements necessary to operate a medical service, but they are more administrative than clinical in nature. We hope that this text fills a void by providing physicians and other clinical staff with information on how to practice medicine in a correctional environment.

Lack of controlled studies and other data on practice methods in correctional facilities makes definitive practice recommendations difficult. Therefore, authors have been chosen who are experts in their field and/or who have experience in correctional medicine. Some chapters, especially those dealing with the unique environment of correctional facilities, are authoritative to the extent that they represent the opinions of experts in the field. Other chapters giving practice recommendations are based on current clinical consensus guidelines.

The first section provides a historical, moral, and ethical perspective for physicians entering into this practice. The challenge of maintaining professional demeanor and providing patient-centered medical care to people who are generally despised and placed in restricted facilities as punishment is daunting. Continuous quality improvement is discussed in this section because those techniques give physicians the tools to change their environment and should form the basis for our practice.

The next section covers processes which are unique to correctional medicine: intake screening, chronic clinics, sick call, infirmary care, and secure hospital units. Physicians realize in these settings that process, teamwork, and management skills are as important as clinical skills in caring for inmates. Even though jails and prisons are "houses of correction," physicians who work in these facilities must be guided by good public health knowledge and sound clinical guidelines. Medical staff working in a correctional facility can be co-opted into acting like corrections officers. These chapters guide clinicians into developing clinical programs that remain medically based despite being within a correctional facility.

Contagious diseases have always been a significant problem in jails and prisons. Section three focuses on current contagious disease issues in correctional facilities: tuberculosis, sexually transmitted diseases, and HIV management. Particularly in jails, it is imperative that tuberculosis screening and treatment be performed appropriately if this country is to eliminate the threat of tuberculosis. Likewise, given the large numbers of people entering jails in our country, correctional

facilities which do not adequately screen for and treat sexually transmitted diseases are failing in their public health responsibility as members of their communities. In a different vein, the treatment of HIV is now expected to prolong life. It is therefore the responsibility of physicians working in correctional facilities to understand this dramatic and everchanging specialty area of practice. While these chapters provide sufficient clinical guidance, physicians must understand the limits of their abilities and refer to and collaborate with public health departments and HIV specialists if they are to provide sound care for their patients.

Though the absolute numbers of females in correctional facilities are small, the number of females behind bars is the fastest-growing of any segment of the population. Physicians working in male dominated facilities must understand the unique problems affecting female patients. Section Four helps the reader understand some basic principles in caring for the pregnant patient and in providing routine care for female patients.

The deinstitutionalization of patients with mental illness over the past few decades has resulted in the incarceration of large numbers of mentally ill patients. Jails and prisons have become de facto housing for the mentally ill, in particular the mentally ill homeless. The moral strength of our nation is measured by how we care for people like this. Because mental illness is often not life threatening (with the exception of suicide), it may be tempting to avoid treatment or to make it less of a priority. Section Five provides recommendations on treatment of these vulnerable patients.

Jails and prisons are most often viewed as places for punishment; the mission of health promotion and prevention of disease in correctional facilities is often forgotten. The opportunity to prevent future illness by vaccination and primary prevention is great in correctional facilities, and correctional authorities must play a part in the public's health with appropriate preventive measures. In addition, violence, drug use, alcohol use, and tobacco use plagues our patients. Section Six addresses how physicians might begin to think about promoting positive changes in inmates, and offers some practical advice on how to institute programmatic change. Special needs and unique issues are addressed in the final section of the text. Anyone may be incarcerated, including the disabled, juveniles, and individuals who are dying. Thoughtful, sympathetic leaders might find other alternatives to incarceration for these individuals. Nevertheless, physicians working in correctional facilities must help care for these individuals even when this means assisting in trying to get out of prison. This series of chapters gives guidance on these unique subpopulations and, additionally, offers a history of how the practice of medicine in correctional facilities has been changed by litigation.

Finally, I would like to thank every author for their time and patience in seeing this project through. It is only because of the dedication of people like them that the practice of medicine in correctional facilities has advanced as it has. In addition, I would like to thank Mosby for giving us the opportunity to provide this service for our readers. Time constraints have limited the number of chapters which have been included. Others were planned but could not be included. Emergency care and annual health maintenance examinations are two areas which need to be addressed. Hopefully, though, readers will find this book useful. The editorial staff would appreciate any comments or suggestions you may have on how to improve our work.

Michael Puisis, D.O.

Contents

Section One

The Correctional Physician

1

Doctors, Patients, and the History of Correctional Medicine

Lambert N. King, M.D., Ph.D.

The prison should, were the world not full of paradox, be a very paradigm of the rule of law.

Norval Morris, The Future of Imprisonment, *1974*

INTRODUCTION

For physicians practicing medicine today, it is the best of times and the worst of times. Biomedical research is ascendant, producing magnificent advances in the diagnosis and treatment of heart disease, cancer, and HIV infection. At the same time, however, many physicians are demoralized by what they perceive as the transformation of the profession and art of medicine into an industrial and bureaucratic model, symbolized by managed care organizations.

Long before managed care organizations began to transform medical practice, small numbers of doctors cared for patients within bureaucratic structures such as the military, Veterans Administration hospitals, and public health clin-

ics. However, the practice of medicine in prisons and jails is probably the most enduring example of how the doctor–patient relationship may be affected by a bureaucracy whose mission and priorities subordinate those of the medical profession. Thus, the history and nature of correctional medicine are of special interest today as growing numbers of physicians are employed and compensated by entities whose priorities compete with those of the doctor–patient relationship.

Before 1775, imprisonment was rarely used as a punishment for crime. Since that time, however, the use of prisons and jails has grown dramatically, and physicians working in correctional institutions have long struggled with conflicts between professional covenants and the purposes and conditions of confinement. Like the history of public health, with which correctional medicine is intertwined, the development of correctional medicine can be understood as a series of evolving perceptions of acceptable conditions. This chapter will describe some of the history of correctional medicine, summarize progressive advances that have been made, and suggest salient lessons for physicians committed to correctional medicine today.

This chapter suggests that much remains to be done to improve the quality of correctional medicine and doctor–patient relationships in prisons and jails. As the number of incarcerated in the United States continues to increase, correctional medicine will have greater importance for both the public health and the well-being of many individual citizens. Perhaps an understanding of the history of correctional medicine will assist those concerned about the health of confined individuals as they continue to push back walls of inevitability and transform stringent limitations into humane possibilities.

A book, rather than a chapter, would be required to document the complete history of correctional medicine. In deference to space limitations, I have chosen to present four "case studies" that are representative of the history of correctional medicine. These four case studies carry us from 1775 to 1975, and from England to France to the United States. Each demonstrates characteristics, perspectives, and principles relevant to current conditions and issues in correctional medicine. In particular, I have selected subjects that involve the doctor–patient relationship in prisons and jails, the need for correctional medicine physicians to conduct epidemiologic and clinical investigations that may improve the health of prisoners, and the responsibility of the correctional medicine physician to foster more humane, lawful, and constructive institutions.

The last historical case study in this chapter addresses issues in correctional medicine, circa 1975. Since that time, many important developments and changes affecting correctional medicine have occurred. Among these developments are the extraordinary impact of federal court decisions and consent agreements in class action suits concerning prison conditions in more than 30 state prison systems; comprehensive studies and recommendations by the American Medical Association concerning deficiencies in health care programs in jails and prisons; and the promulgation of detailed standards for correctional health services by the American Public Health Association, American Correctional Association, and the National Commission on Correctional Health Care. These and many other crucial developments in the history of correctional medicine have already been thoroughly and perceptively summarized.[1]

Case Study 1: The Medical Officer in Victorian Prisons

Because of the growth in the use of prisons after 1775, hygiene problems became readily apparent throughout England and in var-

ious other settings and institutions in which the poor were congregated. Among those seeking reform was a wealthy philanthropist and devout ascetic, John Howard, who in 1773 at the age of 47 years left his country estate and began a career of prison and hospital reform throughout Europe. His quest cost him his fortune and, finally, his life in a typhus ward in Russia in 1791. Among John Howard's closest collaborators was a well-to-do Quaker physician, John Fothergill, whose involvement with prison reform was an outgrowth of his interest in improving urban and institutional sanitation. Like Howard, Fothergill was very interested in science, subsidizing Joseph Priestley's experiments and writing treatises on hygienic burial practices.

As Michael Ignatieff documented in his book, *A Just Measure of Pain*, hygienic reform was both a moral and a medical crusade because disease was seen as an outcome of vice to which the poor were susceptible. Jail fever was attributed to improper discipline as well as poor hygiene. Moreover, typhus and other forms of jail fever were spreading to outside communities. Prison magistrate supervisors became convinced that some form of hygiene and medical supervision was needed to contain diseases. The problem was to convince colleagues and government authorities that the introduction of basic hygiene, uniforms, clean clothing, regular medical attention, and regimented diets would not compromise the pain and humiliation for which penitentiaries were intended.[2]

Physicians involved in the hygienic reform movement viewed the sicknesses of the poor as manifestations of their lack of character and worthiness. In 1795, John Mason Good, a physician at Cold Bath Fields prison, wrote, "The poor are in general but little habituated to cleanliness" and "feel not, from want of education, the same happy exertion of delicacy, honour and moral sentiment which everywhere else is to be met with." Ignatieff observes that Good and other 18th-century doctors were inclined to view physical illnesses as having "moral causes." One early hospital reformer, Jonas Hanway, described immorality as an "epidemical disorder which diffuses its morbid qualities."[3]

As judgmental as the views of the hygienic reformers were toward the poor, John Howard's famous account of the *State of the Prisons* is a prototype for approaching social evils in terms of their consequences for the community's health. For every prison in the country, Howard recorded details about buildings, diet, inmate population, and even the weight of the chains used. Through his revelations of the relations between jails and jail fever, Howard aroused and galvanized public opinion and made improved conditions possible.[4]

In his book, *Victorian Prison Lives—English Prison Biography*, Philip Priestley writes about the role of the Victorian prison medical officer in performing the medical examination and making decisions concerning special diets and admission to the prison hospital.[5] There is deep ambiguity, both professionally and ethically, in the work of the early English prison medical officer. The paradoxical duties of physicians caring for individuals in 19th-century English prisons were welcomed and emulated in early prisons in the United States, where they persisted in whole or in part well into the 20th century. Aspects of this ambiguity persist today, posing continuing questions about what organizational structures and reporting relationships are most appropriate for physicians working in correctional institutions.

In early English prisons like Cold Bath Fields and Pentonville, the customary entrance medical examination consisted of weighing and measuring, followed by a doctor's examination and a rapid determination of prisoners' fitness to be assigned to labor, light labor, the hospital, or an observational cell. The doctor's examinations were cursory, sometimes performed with the prisoner fully clothed. However, on entry into the Gloucester prison, convicts were stripped naked, probed and examined by a doctor, and then bathed, shaved, and uniformed. Ignatieff writes that this purification rite cleansed inmates of vermin, but also stripped them of defining marks of identity.

Victorian prison officials sought to avoid providing food that would be criticized as luxurious, while, at the same time, attempting to avoid severe malnutrition in those in their charge. An English public committee studying this issue in 1864 recommended that the existing dietary scales be reduced, but added the caveat that the prison medical officer see every prisoner on admission to certify his fitness for placement on the various diets. Priestley observes that the discretion placed in the doctor's hands raised tantalizing visions of better food in the eyes of hungry prisoners and helped turn the practice of prison medicine into a battleground between desperate and cunning convicts and suspicious and resentful physicians.

The English prison medical officer also was responsible for admissions to the prison hospital, which were much sought after by inmates, because the food there was more abundant and palatable. One inmate wrote when he was at last admitted to the hospital, "Now that I lay stretched helpless on my back everyone was gruffly kind to me, so kind indeed, that in my weakness I often cried softly into my pillow with gratitude."[6]

Inmates incarcerated in Victorian prisons wrote many accounts of their experiences, some terrible and some laudatory, with prison medical officers. Priestley synthesizes these experiences in an eloquent fashion:

> *These touching and sentimental scenes from institutional life do nothing to rescue the practice of Victorian prison medicine from the consequences of its appointment to fundamentally disciplinary tasks. The doctors patrolled the narrow straits that separate hunger from starvation and punishment from outright cruelty, hauling aboard the life raft of their dispensations this drowning soul or that, and repelling, with brute force if necessary, the efforts of others to climb to safety. In doing so, they lent to the work of preserving their employer's reputations whatever dignity and authority their emerging profession possessed–and lost it.*[7]

Some Victorian physicians did, however, become strong advocates for the powerless individuals in their charge. Charles Short was the visiting surgeon at Bedford Prison from 1810 until 1844. In 1836, he drew public attention to the increasing cases of petechial disease, which he thought was caused by exposure to cold, poor living, silence, and solitary confinement. In 1838, he told court justices that an improved diet was needed to correct the poor state of the prisoners' health. In response to Dr. Short's advocacy, the home secretary issued minimum standards for prison diets. The minimum diet was to include animal food for prisoners employed at hard labor, a considerable portion of the food was to be solid, and there was to be variety in the kinds of food provided. In 1845, however, inspectors found that Bedford prisoners were not getting the recommended minimums.[8]

CONTEMPORARY IMPLICATIONS OF VICTORIAN PRISON MEDICINE

Many physicians familiar with correctional medicine in the United States today will see parallels between the roles of medical officers in Victorian prisons and the dilemmas that doctors working in jails and prisons must face on a daily basis. To be sure, institutional conditions, the quality of nutrition, and the professionalism of the security staff are far better today than in 19th-century England or the United States, but the physician working in correctional medicine is still vested with the authority to influence the confinement conditions and must constantly seek to balance the primacy of the doctor–patient relationship with the imperatives of security and institutional policies. In many jails and prisons today, physicians still face conditions and deficiencies that compromise the health of their patients, just as Dr. Short did in Bedford Prison in 1838. These dynamics continue to raise questions about whether physicians working in correctional medicine are best employed under the aegis of the correctional authority or should preferably be deployed at "arms length" through a health care agency or independent contractor.

Case Study 2: Louis René Villermé, Public Health and Prisons in Early Industrial France

Among other early developments in the history of correctional medicine was the work of Louis René Villermé (1782–1863), a physician and pioneering hygienist, whose study, *Des Prisons*, was published in 1820. The work of Villermé and other French hygienists was an inspiration to German, American, and British public health leaders, who fostered large-scale achievements in England after the passage of the General Health Act of 1848.[9] Villermé's accomplishments have been chronicled and examined in detail by William Coleman in his book, *Death is a Social Disease*, from which much of the material in this second case study is derived. In a chapter titled "The Prison and Social Inquiry," Coleman describes how the vital conditions of people in French penitentiaries provided problems and data that induced Villermé to pursue a career in sociomedical investigation.[10]

In his studies of prison populations, Villermé employed inchoate numerical methods to investigate how the health and social conditions of prison inmates affected mortality. Among the principal purposes of these investigations was to assure health during incarceration, while contributing to the moral regeneration of the inmates, through just and fair treatment, proper housing, discipline, education, and labor. Accomplishing these objectives was a formidable task because Villermé found that virtually no aspect of the prisons proved satisfactory. As Coleman indicates, "To the ideal of security had been sacrificed all concern for salubrity." There was inveterate filth, poor access to light and air, absence of appropriate exercise areas, and severe overcrowding.

Villermé worked closely with Etienne Pariset, a medical jack-of-all-trades and publicist, who insisted that systematic and continuous collection of vital statistics within the prisons was essential to their improvement and correct administration. Establishing systems to collect such data was arduous, but eventually Villermé and Pariset were able to ascertain annual mortality rates per 1,000 inmates in several Parisian prisons, based on data collected between 1815 and 1827. Extraordinary differences were revealed; the worst-case institution exhibited ten times the mortality of the best. For the years 1815–1818, mortality in the Grande Force was 24.5 per 1,000 compared with 251.9 in an infamous prison at Saint Denis. Villermé further observed that these huge differences in mortality were explainable, in large part, by differences in the health status of the inmates, the length of incarceration, the prison location, and the conduct of affairs in the various institutions. Villermé later extended his investigations to include analysis of mortality rates in The Netherlands and Belgium, where at no time did workhouse mortality reach the dismally high levels of France.

Another major aspect of Villermé's investigations was a comparison of French prison mortality rates between 1815 and 1818 with those for 1819–1827, wherein data showed marked reductions in mortality rates after improvements had been made in food, bedding, clothing, and administrative practices. These two time periods were divided by what Villermé considered a critical event in the history of the French prison system, namely, the founding of the Societe royale des prisons, which effectively advocated prison and public health reforms.

CONTEMPORARY IMPLICATIONS OF VILLERMÉ'S WORK

Fortunately, mortality rates in U.S. prisons and jails today are a small fraction of those that Villermé observed and worked to improve in early 19th-century Paris. We have far greater capabilities to capture and analyze measures of health status and outcomes in different populations, but the systems and procedures in place to collect and compare health-related data concerning prisoners are fragmented and highly variable in nature. Although contemporary epidemiologic studies concerning morbidity and mortality among prisoners are published occasionally, it is apparent that we have not moved much beyond the level of sophistication achieved by Villermé. Except for certain communicable diseases, there are no uniform and consistent reporting requirements concerning mortality and morbidity in county and city jails or state and federal prisons, although, within particular correctional systems and jurisdictions, data allowing some institutional comparisons may be collected.

In all probability, significant differences exist among correctional institutions with respect to mortality and morbidity associated with a variety of causes, including cardiovascular and infectious diseases, accidents, and violence. Are deaths resulting from cardiovascular diseases less frequent in institutions that ban cigarettes? Are hypertension and cerebrovascular accidents more common in tense and stressful institutions? Are some state prisons and systems more effective than others in preventing violent deaths? These and many other important questions would be far easier to answer and the implications of unacceptable answers more corrigible if we had consistent and reliable systems to collect demographic and epidemiologic data concerning incarcerated populations. Working individually and together, physicians committed to improving the level

of correctional medicine should strive to establish better and more uniform information systems to collect and analyze health care and outcomes data. Organizations such as the National Commission on Correctional Health Care, American Correctional Health Services Association, and the Society for Correctional Physicians should collaborate, emulating Villermé and the Societe royale des prisons, to achieve this historic objective.

Case Study 3: Report on Health and Medical Service in American Prisons and Reformatories by the National Society for Penal Information (1929)

In 1929, long before the United States federal courts began to intervene in prisons, as a result of class action litigation, the National Society for Penal Information published a comprehensive report, prepared by Frank L. Rector, M.D., titled *Health and Medical Service in American Prisons and Reformatories*.[11] This extraordinary 282-page report was based on field surveys begun in November 1927 and completed in October 1928 of every state and federal prison. Although the survey and report were organized with the assistance of an advisory medical commission that included Dr. David Edsall, Dean of the Harvard Medical School, and Dr. George Crile of the Cleveland Clinic, Dr. Rector visited all 100 institutions and secured the data firsthand. Cooperating organizations included the American College of Surgeons, American Hospital Association, American Medical Association, American Psychiatric Association, American Public Health Association, and the U.S. Public Health Service.

The introduction to the 1929 report of the National Society of Penal Information indicates that in former surveys its representatives observed the inadequacy of hospital facilities, equipment, and personnel and that in the majority of institutions there was a lack of adequate hospital resources for "treatment of inmates as might return them to social living in better physical and mental condition than when they entered prison." Supporting the idea that rehabilitation should be a primary emphasis in prisons and correctional medicine, the introductory section of the report addresses other fundamental questions concerning society's responsibility to offer decent health care within its prisons, speaking first to the need to standardize health and hospital practices:

After careful consideration it was decided that a complete survey of the health and medical service in American prisons would serve to bring out the deficiencies and inequalities in this work in the various penal institutions of the country. It was felt that such a demonstration would furnish information respecting this special branch of institutional management which might be of material assistance to prison authorities in the improvement of such conditions, and possibly bring about a standardization of health and hospital practices in penal institutions.[11]

The report speaks further about correctional health care in the context of community and moral obligations:

In exacting the penalty which society demands for the infraction of its laws, the state removes the individual from his usual social conditions and places him under conditions which deprive him of the ability to help himself...Having assumed this guardianship, the state is under obligation to care for the needs of the individual while he is deprived of the opportunity to care for himself. It is one of the laws of civilized communities which in fact reaches back to the dawn of human civilization that the sick and the injured are entitled to the best care that the community can furnish...although the state may rightfully deprive a citizen of his usual freedom and social contacts, it is morally and traditionally obligated to care for him when, in case of illness or other forms of disability, he is unable to care for himself. This responsibility is as binding as is that of furnishing food, clothing and shelter to such individuals.[11]

Addressing the reluctance of some to accept the concept of rehabilitation as a function of prisons, the report cautions that the harsher functions and characteristics of prisons, including overcrowding, can have deleterious effects not only on inmates but also on outside communities:

While there may yet be an unwillingness in certain quarters to accept the theory that a primary function of the state in dealing with its prisoners is to refit them for acceptable living upon release, it is certainly to the interest of the state to assume this responsibility...The housing of large numbers of individuals from all walks of life in congested quarters, particularly with the serious overcrowding which prevails in practically all penal institutions in this country at the present time, makes it necessary to watch carefully over the health of these persons in order to prevent the introduction of contagious or epidemic diseases...Viewed from whatever angle, whether social, economic, administrative, or moral, it is seen that adequate provision for health supervision of the inmates of penal institutions is an obligation which the state cannot overlook without serious consequences to both the inmates and the community at large.[11]

Among the other findings in the report by the National Society of Penal Information were that existing prison conditions make the careful observation and care of inmates who may be physically or mentally ill unusually urgent. Concern was expressed about overcrowding and the responsibility it placed on the medical department to see that communicable diseases do not adversely affect the health of inmates. Among the other issues about general prison conditions that were identified were grave restrictions imposed on inmates, lack of privacy, and "all elements of the artificial environment of institutional life," that are often the cause of mental as well as physical stress.

With respect to medical administration, the report indicated that the prisons of many states were part of the political spoils system that often affects the physician in charge and interferes with the constructive programs that were part of the physician's health and hospital work. With few exceptions, the prison hospitals were found to be greatly understaffed for the work needed to be done and most physicians, even in the largest prisons, were found to be employed on a part-time basis. In very few prisons was the work so organized that the physician was the administrative head of the health and hospital activities, although such a model was believed to offer more efficiency and better coordination of services to inmates.

The report evaluated prison hospitals and expressed concern that their equipment left much to be desired when compared with modern hospital equipment. Admission physical examinations were found to vary from a casual inspection requiring but a few moments of time to a complete examination of the stripped body with such laboratory work as was indicated by the physical findings. It was found that about one in five prisons re-examined the inmate before parole or release, which was a practice that was thought to be gaining favor and possibly becoming as routine as the entrance examination. Wassermann tests for syphilis and dental examinations frequently were found to be a part of the admission process, but eye examinations usually were not.

The mental health section of the report noted that "The daily regime of prison life with its necessity of conforming to the activities of the group regardless of the inmate's individualistic tendencies and the lack of privacy increase the mental stress under which the inmate lives." Serious concern was expressed about cases of unrecognized mental illness made worse by the prison experience. Mental health evaluations were not a standard practice but were increasing in use; the care of insane prisoners was found to be addressed in a satisfactory manner in but few prisons.

The report found that, in most prisons, although not in some older and overcrowded facilities, general sanitation was satisfactory. The need for adequate ventilation was found to be neglected, especially in double-celled situations. Bathing facilities usually were insufficient to permit daily bathing of the entire population. No evidence was found that prisoners were receiving an insufficient diet, although more meat was being fed than was necessary and larger amounts of coarse vegetables (spinach, cabbage, turnips, and string beans) would be a major improvement. With respect to recreation and entertainment, the report found that such activities were not considered as coddling of the prisoners but rather as a procedure that contributes to the health of inmates and that may assist in social rehabilitation.

Furthermore, health education was found to be badly neglected because of a lack of medical personnel. The report suggested implementing formal programs, developed in cooperation with local and state health authorities, and using movies, lectures, hygiene courses, and articles in the prison newspaper to promote health education.

In response to the issues raised by its national survey, the report offered many specific recommendations, including a series of provisions related to the physicians in the prison medical service. It was recommended that the physician be appointed on merit, without political considerations, be compensated properly for the responsibilities involved, have the opportunity for continuing medical education, and have full authority in the hospital and with regard to all health activities of the prison. With respect to reporting relationships, it was recommended that the prison physician report to the executive head of the institution. Among the other remarkable recommendations was a staffing pattern for prison physicians, namely, one full-time physician for prisons with 500 or more inmates, and another physician for each additional 1,000 inmates or a substantial percentage thereof.

CONTEMPORARY IMPLICATIONS OF THE 1929 REPORT BY THE NATIONAL SOCIETY ON PENAL INFORMATION

The Great Depression shortly followed the publication of the 1929 report of the National Society on Penal Information. Many states experienced grave financial distress and had difficulty maintaining even earlier penal standards.[12] There is scant historical record of organized responses to the recommendations concerning this report on prison health and medical services. As will be seen in the next case study, many of the recommendations in the 1929 report concerning correctional medicine were visionary in that they were resurrected in the 1970s.

The most unique aspect of the 1929 report, however, was its advocacy of the prison as a rehabilitation instrument and the important role that improved prison health care could play in achieving this objective. The same year, President Herbert Hoover appointed the National Commission on Law Observance and Enforcement, popularly known as the Wickersham Commission after its chairperson, former Attorney General George Wickersham. The 14 reports published in 1931 were the first comprehensive survey of American criminal justice at the national level. Volume Nine of the Wickersham Commission unequivocally endorsed the concept of individualized correctional treatment, probation, and parole. This and other recommendations marked the stirrings of a prolonged cycle of American correctional reform that would build slowly and reach its peak in the mid-1960s.[13]

Case Study 4: Prescriptive Package—Health Care in Correctional Institutions (1975)

Forty-six years after the publication of the National Society for Penal Information report, the National Institute of Law Enforcement and Criminal Justice elevated professional awareness about key issues in correctional medicine through a publication titled *Prescriptive Package—Health Care in Correctional Institutions*.[14] The authors of this report were Mr. Edward Brecher and Dr. Richard Della Penna, both of whom were well prepared to confront what they viewed as the typical chaos of health care delivery in most prisons and jails at that time. It was a time when all aspects of correctional institutions, including medical services, were under increasing scrutiny and pressure from the courts, legal aid groups, prisoners' organizations, and, in some states, from the public and legislators.

In his forward to *Prescriptive Package*, Gerald M. Caplan, Director of the National Institute of Law Enforcement and Criminal Justice, states that the publication did not seek to set minimum standards for correctional health care and was not, "except incidentally," a plea for higher standards. This demurral by Mr. Caplan did little to obscure the fact that the report was far more than what it stated itself to be, namely, a practical "how to" guide on the organization of medical services in prisons and jails. By virtue of its publication and the careful collection of information on which it was based, *Prescriptive Package* was an ambitious and effective exhortation closing a wide gap that "exists between the quality and quantity of health care currently available to inmates" and "the care correctional officials themselves would like to see delivered."

Prescriptive Package contained several original and noteworthy aspects. First was the premise that correctional medicine must be conceived and delivered in the context of the health care and financing mainstream. It identified the continuing dilemma of how to provide, within correctional facilities, the increasingly varied and complex services available in the community or, alternatively,

how to arrange for inmate health care services outside the walls. Second, the authors acknowledged the useful synergy between class action litigation attacking prison conditions and the resultant provision of more and better health care resources for inmates. Although as a reaction to litigation concern was expressed about defensive medicine, the authors emphasized that the best defense against litigation was a system of care that offered consistent service of good quality in adequate supply.

Prescriptive Package included detailed guidance and practical administrative advice about almost every aspect of medical care in correctional institutions, with the notable exceptions of dental and mental health services. A panoply of subjects was considered, ranging from the use of physicians' assistants to the importance of sound medical record systems to the provision of secure units in community-based hospitals. The authors urged that the authority of statewide prison health service administrators be strengthened and that correctional health systems establish working relationships with outside health agencies and organizations such as county medical societies. The report also urged that better systems be developed to improve the evaluation and response to inmate complaints about inadequate medical care.

With respect to the still prevalent dilemma of recruiting, training, and retaining health care professionals to work in correctional health care, Brecher and Della Penna suggested greater attention to compensation, working conditions, academic faculty appointments, continuing education, relationships with medical and nursing schools, and improvements in secretarial and clerical assistance. Assembling resources and acquiring proper space for the provision of medical care, supply management, and medical library resources were also identified as priorities. Like its predecessor, the report of the National Society for Penal Information, *Prescriptive Package* contained assessments and recommendations about the key subjects of environmental health, nutrition, and health education in correctional institutions.

Before *Prescriptive Package*, no similar evaluation of problems in correctional medicine had explicitly suggested that it might be desirable, at least in some instances, to transfer administrative responsibility for correctional medicine from correctional agencies to outside health care agencies. In 1975, such a transfer had occurred in only a few instances, most of which were presented as positive and important models by the authors of *Prescriptive Package*. The pioneering precedents for moving leadership and authority for correctional medicine from correctional agencies to health care organizations included New York City, which, in 1971, transferred all its correctional health care from its department of corrections to its health services administration. Then, in 1973, the New York City Health Services Administration entered into a contract under which Montefiore Hospital and Medical Center agreed to provide correctional health services for inmates in the multiple, large jail facilities on Rikers Island. Dr. Della Penna, in fact, served as the first medical director of this contractual program on Rikers Island. Another example of such a transfer of authority was the responsibility assumption for Cermak Memorial Hospital at Cook County Jail by the Health and Hospitals Governing Commission of Cook County in the early 1970s. "Contracting out" the responsibility for these correctional medicine services to health care agencies or, in the case of Montefiore, a nonprofit academic medical center, represented a fundamental change in the course of correctional medicine. This change, which has since been replicated in several different forms, has important implications for relationships between physicians and correctional authorities, and also for the doctors and patients in jails and prisons.

CONTEMPORARY IMPLICATIONS OF THE PRESCRIPTIVE PACKAGE

In the majority of correctional institutions and systems, the correctional agency continues to employ physicians and provide medical care directly. However, in the past 20 years, there has been rapid growth in the use of the contractual model, especially through the use of for-profit companies, such as Correctional Medical Services and Prison Health Services. Such companies specialize in correctional health care delivery and compete avidly for such contracts. The momentum that the contractual model has acquired was stimulated by the positive review that it received in *Prescriptive Package* in 1975.

When correctional medicine services are contracted out, using one of several models that evolved, physicians and other health professionals no longer report directly to the administrative structure of the prison or jail in which they work. They are, however, directly accountable to the administrative structure of the health care agency or organization that employs them, and the nature of this new relationship determines the degree to which they exercise professional autonomy and judgment, as it would if practicing in a setting that was not correctional in nature.

As far-sighted, comprehensive, and practical as *Prescriptive Package* was, its correctional medicine consideration in relation to the criminal justice system's purposes was anemic in comparison with the National Society on Penal Information's 1929 report. The report explicitly identified correctional medicine as a critical factor in the rehabilitation and education of inmates and viewed rehabilitation as essential to the mission of correctional institutions. In contrast, *Prescriptive Package* omits any consideration of the objectives and philosophy of incarceration and the effect that the relative balance of punishment, incapacitation, and rehabilitation may have on the nature of correctional medicine. Undoubtedly, the acceptance and use of recommendations and methods found in *Prescriptive Package* contributed to safer and more humane health conditions in correctional institutions. However, unlike its predecessor report in 1929, *Prescriptive Package* begs the question of the responsibility of physicians who work in correctional facilities as advocates for basic prison and jail reforms, above and beyond competent provision and administration of medical services.

DOCTORS, PATIENTS, AND PRISONS: THE ROAD AHEAD

Some basic issues and questions concerning correctional medicine today emerge from the four historical case studies presented in this chapter. The first issue pertains to the roles and relationships among doctors, their inmate patients, and the authorities responsible for managing jails and prisons. The second issue is the need for physicians working in correctional institutions to foster and develop systems to collect organized, epidemiologic, and clinical information concerning their patients. As Villermé demonstrated, through the acquisition and use of such information, significant differences between institutions can be demonstrated, and improvements in health conditions can be achieved. The third issue concerns the responsibility of physicians working in correctional medicine to seek more general reforms in prison conditions, including programs of work, education, and rehabilitation.

Looking back at 200 years of correctional medicine history, we surely can be thankful for the greatly improved institutional conditions that have resulted in enormous mortality and morbidity reductions among incarcerated populations. Federal court intervention and the articulation of multiple sets of professionally supported standards for health services in correctional institutions have been effective in elevating the quality of care and marshaling significant financial support for the provision of inmate health care. Indeed, the growth of public funding for such services has been so robust that correctional medicine is of considerable interest to private, for-profit companies that seek to provide such services on a contractual basis or as integral participants in privately owned and administered correctional facilities. The perennial problem of recruitment of well-qualified physicians to work in prisons and jails has been somewhat alleviated by burgeoning numbers of physicians in general and their brewing discontent with the influence of managed care organizations on the autonomy and income of physicians working in the free community.

In spite of the progress in correctional medicine, especially since 1975, there remains cause for deep concern as a result of several recent developments. The growth in the number of individuals confined in prisons and jails has doubled in the past decade and tripled in the past 20 years. This growth in population and the escalating costs of caring for individuals infected with HIV have eroded some of the progress in the quality of care that was achieved with increased public funding. In 1996, Congress passed the Prison Litigation Reform Act (PLRA), which sharply curtails the authority of the federal courts to intervene in class action suits concerning prison conditions, including the delivery of medical care. The passage of the PLRA is symptomatic of prevailing political and social hostility toward prisoners and advocates of continued reform of correctional institutions. Evidence of such hostility is found in multiple media accounts of successful campaigns to remove weight-lifting equipment from prisons, restore highway chain gangs, and install tents to house inmates.

In the first case study in this chapter, Victorian medical officers sometimes emerged as advocates for their impoverished patients and sometimes emerged as both moral critics of the poor and apologists for the abuses imposed by judicial and prison authorities. The effect of this professional ambiguity has persisted in most correctional medical settings, although relationships today between doctors and security personnel and between doctors and inmates are usually civil and professional in content. The majority of physicians working in prisons and jails continue to be directly employed by correctional agencies, although a growing number are employed by private companies on a contractual basis. There remain a small number of jurisdictions in which doctors caring for patients in jails and prisons are employed independently by public health agencies or nonprofit health care organizations. Contracting out to a health care organization may clarify that the primary mission of the physician is patient care, it may perhaps strengthen some patients' trust in the relationship, and it may offer greater opportunities to merge correctional medicine with integrated health care delivery systems.

In most relationships between a doctor and a patient, there is a shared objective, namely, that the doctor will assist the patient in returning to valued tasks, relationships, and responsibilities. To the extent that incarceration conditions deplete the capacities and opportunities of inmates to aspire to valued tasks and lives that embody self-respect, the integrity of doctor–patient relationships will be affected and often diminished. Compassion, competence, collaboration, friendship, and wisdom are among the qualities that we seek in our relationships with physicians. Even the most dedicated physicians find that their ability to convey these qualities is strained and tested in the jail or prison setting. There is no easy solution to this dilemma; however, it is imperative that physicians who care about correctional medicine work with others to create correctional institutions that are what John Conrad once stated they should be, namely, "lawful, safe, industrious, and hopeful."[15]

Drawing on his unique experience as an attorney and special master for the federal courts in class action decisions affecting prisons in many states and jurisdictions throughout the nation, Vincent M. Nathan elaborated what an ideal prison should be. The ideal prison offers human services in a decent and healthful environment; it abjures idleness and the resulting deterioration; it provides constructive employment and recreational activities to the greatest extent possible. The civilized prison addresses human needs for self-expression, faith, and important ties to other human beings. Inmates should be safe from random violence, rape, and the exploitation of the weak by the strong. The ideal prison should insulate inmates from arbitrary chaos by adherence to due process of law and infuse the institution with constructive expectations through positive incentives for hard work and good behavior.

Recognizing the impediments that still preclude this ideal, Mr. Nathan spoke to health professionals working in correctional medicine at the 1984 meeting of the National Commission on Correctional Health Care:

Until the millennium arrives and prisons become the model institutions John Conrad has defined, the prison medical community must resist the efforts that are made to tailor the quality and quantity of medical treatment to the exaggerated demands of institutional security, productivity, discipline, and administrative convenience. On a daily basis, physicians must exercise their talents on behalf of every patient who presents himself with a complaint. Every invitation or temptation to define the quality of professional care by the substandard criteria that may govern other facets of the prison's operation must be eschewed. In short, health care professionals must practice medicine as well as they know how, in the setting in which they find themselves, with all the grace and good humor they have at their command.[16]

As isolated and distinctive as the practice of medicine in correctional institutions has been, correctional medicine could be a sentinel indicator of how organizational changes may affect far greater numbers of doctors and patients in the broader community. He who pays the piper may indeed call the tune, and the vitality of medicine as a profession may be threatened as much by large health care corporations as by prison administrations who see high-quality medical care as a secondary concern, if not a necessary evil. The history and experience of correctional medicine also reflect the degree to which society and its political leaders are willing to address deeply ingrained problems involving race, poverty, addiction, and mental illness. The populations of jails and prisons and those of economically depressed communities are dynamic and often confluent. Thus, the quality and strength of correctional medicine remain harbingers of the integrity of public health, as both a profession and a system within our society.

The millennium draws near, and physicians working in correctional medicine should be far from sanguine about the state of their endeavors, especially about the declining opportunity to practice medicine in institutions that help rebuild lives, not just incapacitate and punish. The history of correctional medicine teaches us that necessary changes and improvements, although sometimes painfully cyclical, can be achieved through technical competence and dedication to enduring professional covenants. If physicians and professional organizations committed to correctional medicine do not excel as advocates on behalf of both more constructive prisons and jails and alternatives to incarceration, who, if anyone, will?

REFERENCES

1. Anno BJ: *Prison Health Care: Guidelines for the Management of an Adequate Delivery System.* Chicago, National Commission on Correctional Health Care, 1991.
2. Ignatieff M: *A Just Measure of Pain—The Penitentiary in the Industrial Revolution—1759–1850.* New York, Pantheon Books, 1978.
3. Ignatieff M: *A Just Measure of Pain—The Penitentiary in the Industrial Revolution—1759–1850.* New York, Pantheon Books, 1978, pp 60–61.

4. Rosen G: *A History of Public Health*. Baltimore, Md, Johns Hopkins University, 1993.

5. Priestley P: *Victorian Prison Lives—English Prison Biography—1820–1914*. London, Methuen & Co., 1985.

6. Priestley P: *Victorian Prison Lives—English Prison Biography—1820–1914*. London, Methuen & Co., 1985, p 187.

7. Priestley P: *Victorian Prison Lives—English Prison Biography—1820–1914*. London, Methuen & Co., 1985, p 190.

8. Stockdale E: *A Study of Bedford Prison—1660–1877*. London, Phillimore & Co., 1977, pp 168–169.

9. Ackerknecht EH: *A Short History of Medicine*, ed 2. New York, The Ronald Press, 1968, p 213.

10. Coleman W: *Death Is a Social Disease—Public Health and Political Economy in Early Industrial France*. Madison, Wis, University of Wisconsin, 1982.

11. National Society for Penal Information: Rector FL (ed): *Health and Medical Service in American Prisons and Reformatories,* New York, J.J. Little and Ives, 1929.

12. McKelvey B: *American Prisons–A History of Good Intentions*. Montclaire, NJ, Patterson Smith Publishing, 1977.

13. Walker S: *Popular Justice–A History of American Criminal Justice*. London, Oxford University, 1980, pp 173-176.

14. Brecher EM, Della Penna R: *Prescriptive Package–Health Care in Correctional Institutions*. Washington, DC, National Institute of Law Enforcement and Criminal Justice, Law Enforcement Assistance Administration, US Department of Justice, 1975.

15. Conrad J: Ending the drift and returning to duty: Two scenarios for the future of corrections. Proceedings of the Congress of Corrections, Miami, Florida, 1981.

16. Nathan VM: Correctional health care: The perspective of a special master. Presented at the annual meeting of the National Commission on Correctional Health Care, Chicago, 1984.

2

Challenges of Improving Quality in the Correctional Setting

Gordon Schiff, M.D.
Ronald Shansky, M.D.

The prevailing public and managerial approaches to medical quality are based on inspection, incentive, punishment of offenders, and controlling outbreaks. These approaches are neither modern, nor scientifically grounded, nor likely to be powerful forces for improvement. They also add cost, reduce information exchange, produce fear, and cause their own hazards.

Adapted from D.M. Berwick, Taking Action: Leading the Reduction in Error in Health Care, *1996*[1]

Medicine began its modern era when the enterprises of diagnosis and treatment sank their roots into facts. Before that both depended on poorly validated theories, the lore of masters, and categories untested by clear observation. What would happen if physicians could help treat their organizations with the same scientific discipline they use in their care of patients or in their work as researchers?

Adapted from D.M. Berwick, The Clinical Process and the Quality Process, *1997*[2]

INTRODUCTION

Is improving quality inimical to or a natural for the correctional health care setting? Can health care workers who find themselves behind bars (for their working hours) find anything of relevance in Berwick's continuous quality improvement (CQI) philosophy when it appears to be so foreign to the punitive prison environment? How can our commitment to a broadened definition of clinical medicine lead us to more effective, productive, and rewarding work lives—so those hours make a difference in our patients' health and in the quality of health in our prisons?

Quality health care and jail medicine—the two phrases seem like they don't even belong in the same sentence. However, those who practice in the prison setting are reminded daily of two compelling truths: (1) the enormous, genuine, unmet medical needs for this population of individuals, and (2) the suboptimal processes of care in prison health delivery systems. These realities offer tremendous opportunities for improvement in both the care of the patients and the workings of the system.

As health providers, our commitment to addressing these needs often leads to frustration. Sorting through a myriad of symptoms and then translating them into diagnoses that we can actually do something about in order to help the patient and the system, is a challenge that often feels like an immense and futile task.

However, once we begin to look at these problems through the lens of quality improvement, what previously seemed to be a ubiquitous blur of untrustworthy prisoners, careless correctional workers, and impossible-to-fix obstacles, comes into sharp focus as processes begging for improvement. Quality improvement gives us not only new insights to better understand the quality problems we see, but also more effective tools to address them.

Efforts to review, improve, and assure quality need to move from a separate program or function, assigned to some unlucky staff member(s) for compliance with external regulatory (or legal) mandates, to an intrinsic function interwoven into the daily fabric of work—one that management supports and in which everyone participates.

Rather than resented as hassles, external requirements for increased accountability should actually be welcomed and harnessed to drive this daily activity. This is especially important in a prison setting in which one of the most important leverages for quality improvement, the voice of the customer, is muted. Because of prisoners' relative powerlessness, these external mandates become an important ally of the staff inside prisons seeking to ensure quality care.

WHY BOTHER?

It is reasonable to ask, "Why bother making the effort to implement a quality improvement program in a correctional setting?" Correctional professionals working in facilities that have implemented such programs describe at least four major benefits that they have experienced:

1. *Enhanced correctional health staff cooperation.* When correctional and health care staff participate jointly in quality improvement training and teams, cooperative working relationships flourish. Working side-by-side toward mutually agreed-on goals moves staff beyond traditional jurisdictional conflicts that plague prison work.[3]

2. *Decreased tensions or friction with inmates.* Institutions that have well-run services are easier to manage. Although bank robber Willie Sutton is oft quoted in medicine for his "go where the money is" wisdom, his perhaps more important insight was his statement that every prison riot is due, in part, to poor medical care.[4] Good medical services are important, but good meals and responsive legal services and case management all result in fewer problems with inmates at well-run facilities.

3. *Increased staff satisfaction.* When workers are able to participate in redesigning the programs in which they work, they tend to experience greater job satisfaction.[5] This both enhances the ability to recruit new staff as well as increases staff retention. Because few physicians or nurses graduate professional school with strong a priori desires to work in a correctional setting, attracting and retaining competent, talented, dedicated staff is a prerequisite for high quality and a result of meaningful quality improvement programs.

4. *Cost-effectiveness.* Quality improvement programs throughout the country have been able to demonstrate savings by improving both the processes and outcomes of care. By improving facility or patient compliance with medication regimens, there is likely to be less morbidity, less use of outside emergency departments, and less use of outside hospitals. By attending to needlessly complex or flawed processes, one can uncover an enormous amount of waste (often as much as 40% to 50% of expenditures in health facilities) and uproot it.[6, 7]

Many working in prisons are highly motivated to improve quality but are seeking a better theoretical and practical framework to guide their efforts. In this chapter, we will propose some ideas and offer some suggestions for projects. We begin with a brief overview of the history of formal efforts to improve the quality of health services. We offer a number of powerful change concepts and lessons derived from basic industrial quality improvement principles as well as from our personal experiences and efforts. We then describe the unique problems and obstacles complicating efforts to improve quality in correctional settings. Finally, we offer suggestions on how to organize and implement a quality improvement program, and we provide examples of specific quality improvement problems that have been successfully addressed.

HISTORY OF HEALTH QUALITY EFFORTS OUTSIDE PRISON

Historically, health care professionals have always been concerned with the quality of services that they provide. Until the late 1970s, however, formal efforts for improving quality focused on the review of interesting or exceptional medical patients or problems, and discussion about the issues raised was encouraged.[8] Such discussion, in venues such as clinical pathologic conferences or nursing staff case conferences, rarely went beyond the case at hand. In addition, the attempt was never made to develop a systematic understanding of the relationships between care processes and outcomes.[9]

Of course, physicians and nurses have long emphasized ongoing training. Activities such as grand rounds, continuing medical education, or in-service education reflect the professional commitment to improving quality by keeping staff knowledge up to date. In recent years, external demands for improved quality and accountability arose in a parallel but unlinked fashion from these professional efforts aimed at maintaining quality. Perceived as a series of unnecessary, poorly informed, and time-wasting mandates, efforts by the Joint Commission on Hospital Accreditation (now the Joint Commission on Accreditation of Healthcare Organizations [JCAHO]) and federal peer review organization legislation, such as the 1986 Health Care Quality Improvement Act, met with physician indifference or resistance.[8] This failure of 1970s and 1980s quality assurance (QA) efforts to optimally connect with clinicians reflected a bilateral failure on the part of both health professionals to appreciate its potential value and QA professionals to engage clinical issues in a constructive and relevant manner.

Thus, instead of broad and active physician participation, QA often devolved into a clerical function whereby simple and narrow documentation issues became the focus. This is ironic because one of the virtues of delegating reviews was to support clinicians by avoiding costly physician chart review time, thereby allowing more time for substantive physician participation. Once QA-required studies became perfunctory exercises to satisfy obligatory external mandates, an obsession with performing minimum study quantity rather than improving study quality became the goal. Even when bona fide problems were identified, they were often ignored, which further reinforced medical staff prejudices that QA was futile busywork.

However, it is QA's continuing fixation on identification of outliers (i.e., individuals with the worst performance) and report card style ranking that most bedevils the QA paradigm. As epidemiologic studies began to demonstrate wide, difficult-to-justify variations in medical practices,[10] the natural reflex was to target outliers for intervention. For example, if surgery rates for prostatic hypertrophy vary tenfold from one population to the next (as they were found to in Maine), then the "high utilizer" surgeons could be targeted to decrease the rate of "unnecessary" surgery. If one physician had a higher than average cesarean section rate, he could be similarly targeted.

What exactly *targeted* meant in practice exposed the weaknesses and often conflicting, untested assumptions in applying the QA model. Are certain surgeons operating excessively because they are greedy and are rewarded under fee-for-service plans by operating unnecessarily? Are they ill informed, needing more education about the diagnosis and indications for transurethral prostatectomy or cesarean section? Do they simply have a different mix of patients, such as more high-risk patients, that would justify performing surgery more often? Is it the surgeon who is entirely to blame, or do patient or hospital factors play a role in these decisions?

Even more fundamental questions began to be raised by health policy analysts, and surprising answers emerged. When the Rand Health Services Utilization Study looked at endoscopy, cardiac catheterization, and cholecystectomy, they found (using carefully designed review criteria) no significant difference in the percentage of appropriate vs. inappropriate procedures in the high- vs. low-use regions![11] Other studies showed that obstetricians who had high cesarean section rates were not the same physicians as those with high hysterectomy rates.[12]

So, who exactly are the bad apples, and what precisely should be done about them? These are questions that are not easily answered, and turn out to be the wrong questions to ask. Although the QA model was useful in identifying problems, it was more limited when it came to solving them. Thus, physicians would argue with administrators (and others) about who was really to blame when things went wrong or whether QA findings and conclusions were fair, accurate, or meaningful; however, little would change. Meanwhile, U.S. industry was discovering a different way to manage and improve quality.

WHAT AND WHY: CQI

Continuous quality improvement means nothing less than a total shift in management philosophy, practices, and assumptions (see Table 1[13]). This approach was first articulated by W. Edwards Deming and others shortly after World War II and was summarized by Deming in his Fourteen Principles.[7, 14–16]

Continuous quality improvement, also known as total quality management, is a systematic approach that strives to improve quality by involving staff at all levels in relentless experimentation to continuously improve quality. These ongoing scientific improvement efforts aim to improve work processes so that the public or patients (external customers) are better served, and they aim to improve the interactions among the institution's internal work areas (internal customers). In its fullest expression and application, CQI's quest for more efficient, satisfying, creative, error- and waste-free work processes breaks down the artificial

Table 2-1. Quality assurance vs. quality improvement

Old approach	Quality improvement
Meet standards	Improve continuously
Rely on inspection to ensure quality	Rely on statistical process control to ensure quality
Leaders order, exhort, and enforce	Leaders listen, enable, support, and facilitate
Defects and errors come from individuals	Defect and errors come from faulty process design
Workers don't try hard enough	Workers motivated to perform well
Quality is fine	Improvement is possible and needed
Better quality costs too much	Better quality saves money
Not enough time to improve quality	To much time wasted not to improve quality
Suppliers are problems; competitive bidding best deal	Suppliers are partners; work with one or a few continuously
Patients are problems; interruptions; unreliable	Patients are partners; face obstacles; knowledgeable
Improve within functions and departments; each responsible for own quality	Improve across functions and departments
"Gut feel" understanding	Learn from data and feedback

Modified from McEachern JE, Makens PK, Bachanan ED, et al: Quality improvement: An imperative for medical care, in Neuhauser D, McEachern JE, Headrick L (eds): *Clinical CQI: A Book of Readings*. Oakbrook Terrace, Ill, Joint Commission on Accreditation of Healthcare Organizations, 1995, pp 117–134, with permission.

boundaries between internal and external customers and between departments and disciplines.

SELECTED CQI CORRECTIONAL CHANGE CONCEPTS

What makes the following change concepts so striking and powerful is that they seem to defy our common sense reactions and expectations. Just as CQI turns our perceptions of external regulatory mandates inside out by changing them from burdens to building blocks, so do each of the following notions challenge our initial beliefs and responses.

There is nothing as practical as a good theory; it not only keeps us from spinning our wheels needlessly, but also guides us toward effective action. Here are a few of the theoretical and general lessons and ideas we've learned and relearned as students and practitioners of quality improvement.

If Not for You: Making Quality Assurance/Quality Improvement Work Double Time for You

Exploiting external QA requirements to leverage internal change is but one way an organization can constructively take advantage of regulatory mandates. Any data collected, any work processes audited, any reports prepared, when not driven by or connected to improvement efforts, are not worth the time and effort. Think about all the times you (and others in your institution) go through the motions, preparing reports to satisfy external agencies or your boss. Ask yourself: If this audit is never seen or used by someone at the review agency (as is often the case), how might the effort be worth my while anyway? Our answer and our desire should be to monitor ourselves. We should hunger for data to help us understand how we're doing and how we can do better. Here are a few simple and helpful lessons we

have learned in trying to better align these external data requirements and our own needs:

1. Data, to the greatest extent possible, should be captured routinely in the course of everyday care, rather than necessitate dedicated studies to unearth the information. Automated information systems obviously facilitate adherence to this maxim, but simple manual data sources, such as logbooks, call slips, and incident reports, shouldn't be overlooked. Instead of heroic one-shot looks, studies with routinely collected data lend themselves to the longitudinal monitoring and evaluation of progress and the success of interventions.

2. Turn daily problem solving into a quality resource. Whenever we fret over our inability to "get our QA/QI work done" because we've been busy dealing with day-to-day (hour-to-hour) crises, we realize that these are neither interruptions nor diversions from our QA work. Look at every problem as an opportunity to develop QA documentation systems that drive change. Logging and tracking inmate grievances as a reflection of customer feedback will allow the design of systematic solutions rather than patchwork responses. Collect every problem prescription. Use quarterly reports as a way to look back, so they can help you reflect, document, follow up, and assess progress. Send reports not just "up" but sideways and downward as a way to facilitate communication within your facility.

3. If you want data to be accurate and productive, use data for learning and improvement, not for making comparisons and judgments for disciplinary purposes. No quality improvement system is robust enough to withstand the opposition and sabotage of fearful workers, who perceive it as threatening and as spying on them rather than as supporting their efforts to do a better job.[15] This cen-

tral tenant of CQI is a lesson we constantly relearn. It goes against our knee-jerk reflex to pick off problem individuals; instead, it goes to the root of problems. We must work to get at the root of problems rather than try to reflexively find and punish problem employees.

4. Anything worth studying for QA/QI is worth presenting or publishing. Make QA an academic exercise, in the best sense of the word. This leads to professional growth of involved staff and the fun of sharing with and learning from others in the field.

Common Cause and Special Cause Variation: Liberated From Prison

A fascinating but little-known bit of history is that W.E. Deming, father of CQI, derived the terminology for perhaps his most important CQI concept—special cause and common cause variation—from prisons![14]

Building on the work of Walter Shewhart at Western Electric in the 1920s, statistician Deming emphasized that variation is inherent in any process.[17] This means that, whether we're attempting to manufacture products that conform to exact size requirements or screening all new inmates for tuberculosis, variations from our optimum specifications and procedures are inevitable. Purified protein derivatives of tuberculin may be placed improperly, their results may be interpreted improperly, positive results may fail to be followed up with chest x-ray films, and so on. How do we know when such variation is just random, as opposed to when it can be attributed to a special cause that we can pinpoint and correct? Furthermore, how do we decrease this "random" variation?

Deming graphed data on such processes and demonstrated that most variation cannot be blamed on a specific worker or a unique cause. He noted the temptation for prison riot commissions to direct their investigations toward identifying what was unique about that particular prison that led prisoners' frustrations to explode. Deming ran across a newspaper article about prison riots that stated that most riots are not due to "special" causes, but rather are related to problems "common" to all prisons. He seized on these terms to label his two different classes of variations: common cause and special cause. Special causes require 3 standard deviations from the norm (i.e., a worker's defect rate is 3 standards from the norm) for corrective efforts to be targeted at the individual worker. Otherwise, the errors are part of the system. Only by redesigning the system (the responsibility of management) will errors predictably decrease.

Leadership and Process Redesign

It is remarkable that, in the 1960s and 1970s, while U.S. auto manufacturers were hiring more quality inspectors to find and eliminate autoworkers' quality defects, the Japanese were hiring fewer inspectors and producing cars often with $1/10$ or $1/100$ the defect rate. It was assumed by the U.S. managers that carelessness and errors on the part of their workers were the cause of poor quality and that more inspection would lead to fewer defects. Those assumptions were wrong.

The Japanese quality improvement philosophy (actually made in America because the Japanese were relying on the ideas of Deming, who had previously been ignored in the U.S.) argued that you cannot inspect quality into a product or service. It must be engineered into the design of the production process. Because design and control of this system is the responsibility of management, it is management, not the workers, who are to blame for the vast majority of quality problems.[18]

Each complete blood cell count that is clotted because it was drawn in the wrong tube, every medical record that is lost, or every prisoner who is given another's medication, appears to be the fault of the individual who was nearest when the "crime" was committed. If an institution is serious about making improvement, however, the failure of management to design the system in a more error-proof way needs to be understood as the real cause of the problem. If managers just want to identify who is to blame and punish the employee so that they can say they've discharged their responsibility, then that's fine. However, it's unlikely to lead to significant, lasting improvement—improvement that will prevent the problem from recurring.

Commitment to process redesign is not simply a top-down or static thing. It is itself a process of continual study and improvement of how work is carried out. By implementing and testing interventions, teams of frontline workers intimately involved in carrying out an operation are empowered by managers to make changes. Process problems are not so much fixed or solved as they are continuously engaged and incrementally decreased.[18]

Multidisciplinary Teams, Suboptimization, and Improved Hand-offs

Putting teams together across disciplines is not just a matter of warm fuzzies or good vibes. The old way of management emphasizes that each individual and department had a job to do and needed to be held responsible for doing it well. When this concept is more carefully examined, it turns out that the majority of quality problems arise at the interface between different departments or disciplines.[19]

The laboratory turnaround for immediate testing of electrolytes may be less than $1/2$ an hour. However, because specimen drawing and transport and communication of results are included in the process, it is obvious that the laboratory alone cannot solve the 8-hour delay experienced by the clinician. Often errors and delays result from both "fumbles" in the hand-offs between areas or departments and needlessly complex steps in the process. For example, one effort to improve laboratory result turnaround occurred merely by simplifying the process. The number of individuals involved decreased from 14 to 2, and the interval the patient waited for results went from 4 days to 15 minutes.

The detrimental complexity and fumble-prone hand-offs often become apparent only after managers in different disciplines sit down and explicitly walk through the process.[20] When flow charts are drawn for both how the process is supposed to work in theory and what really happens in everyday practice, new understandings of the process and hypotheses for improvement experiments are generated. The exercise of cataloging possible factors contributing to problems (often usefully diagrammed using a "fish-bone" cause-and-effect diagram) enables a joint enumeration of possible candidates to target for change.[16]

Continuous Flow and Pull Systems

It seems obvious that quality means keeping a prison health service well stocked with supplies (e.g., forms, equipment, and other such items). Likewise, who would quarrel with a system that batches groups of tests and controls their use by creating barriers (i.e., approval mechanisms, waiting lists) to avoid overuse, thereby ensuring that scarce resources were used most efficiently. Again, however, common sense fails us. When matched against the paradigm of scientific quality improvement, a very different understanding emerges.

"Just-in-time" or "lean" production have become new buzzwords. They have been used to justify everything from cutting "fat" or "slack" in staffing levels so low that one worker's absence throws a service into complete havoc, to decreasing workers' training to a minimum or waiting until the very last moment (or not at all) to eliminate "waste" in staff education. Unfortunately, these crude misapplications do a disservice to a powerful quality improvement concept pioneered by the Japanese.

Picture a worker on a factory assembly line who drills holes in a component part, then hands it to the next worker who in turn uses it to assemble a product. If the holes are out of alignment, that next worker can hand it right back, with immediate feedback and minimal waste. What if the first worker had instead filled boxes and skids full of the drilled part, all of which were later found to be defective. This is how we're often doing it in health care—batching, deferring, stockpiling, and wasting.

How often do you return or discard outdated drugs, purchased in quantities and dosage strengths you end up not needing or using? How many forms do you have lying around your clinic, many of which are also out of date, never to be used, and eventually discarded. Meanwhile, the ones you use regularly are constantly running out. These are items that individuals hoard, overorder, and look for more storage space in which to house the hoards.

The same applies to bottlenecks created by barriers to access to triage, specialists, or tests. We may think we are defending the system from being overwhelmed, enforcing restrictions, and saving money, but, often, we spend more time and energy fending off the requests, managing the waiting lists, and pushing back and limiting demands.[21] At the other end, by requiring our clinicians to push, at times with near-heroic efforts, to overcome these obstacles when seeking to obtain these rationed services for their patients, yet another source of friction and frustration is introduced.

Why use our scarce energies to deny care when it can often take less energy to facilitate access. "Pull" systems, (the label the Japanese apply in contrast with our current "push" systems) anticipate need and build in continuous flow. Instead of hospital admission staff pushing and waiting for a bed to be emptied, an empty bed pulls the patient in via a process that anticipates and expedites.[22]

Of course, we want to make sure the tests, referrals, and admissions are appropriate. But one does not necessarily create appropriateness by bottlenecks in flow. More thoughtful attention to the process and to calibrating supply with demand means less hidden "pushing" waste. We, ourselves, are just beginning to grapple with the ramifications of this for prison health care. However, given the current obsession with cutting cost, we believe it will assume increasing importance if we want to seek genuine improvement rather than short-sighted dysfunctional fixes.[5, 23, 24]

WHAT'S WORKING; WORKING TOWARD WHAT

There is a small but growing body of literature and experience about what works in making change in ambulatory settings. Generalizing from this experience or selecting specific examples to apply to prisons risks loosing the rich and thoughtful diversity and does a disservice to the enormous creative local energies that have been devoted to improvement efforts. Focusing on narrower, bottom-line definitions of success likewise overlooks broader unmeasured salutary effects. Nonetheless, it is worth learning from the successes and the failures of various approaches.

For interventions targeted at improving provider performance, it is generally asked whether there have been measurable improvements in practitioners' knowledge, changes in actual practice behavior, and, finally, improved patient outcomes. Although the impact on outcomes is our ultimate goal, few quality improvement interventions have had the significant change magnitude, methodological rigor and statistical power, and sufficient long-term follow-up needed to realize this more definitive measure. This led a recent evidence-based review on helping practices reach primary care goals to conclude simply that "interventions improve primary care processes but not necessarily outcomes."[25]

The first lesson we can derive from this experience is that traditional educational efforts, in the form of either continuing medical education lectures or distribution of printed materials (memos, articles, and such), have little or no lasting impact. The most effective educational strategies are those closely intertwined with clinical practice. For example, efforts to educate physicians on how to approach a patient with chest pain or efforts to educate physicians on which preventive medicine measures are age appropriate need to be linked to a redesigned process based on this algorithm or guideline, which includes a standardized (ideally computerized) form to prompt real-time data collection and test and therapy ordering. An additional educational series at noontime, even when physicians are a captive audience, may have a complementary role (physicians will resist having checklists which they don't understand or agree with, shoved in front of them, and they will resist being turned into robots at the computer), but the data show it alone is useless in forging durable improvement.[26]

A second practical lesson is the usefulness of timely feedback. Auditing, with feedback of data, has been shown to be beneficial in changing a variety of physician ordering behaviors. Practitioners learn from holding a mirror up to their practice and comparing their ordering decisions with their peers. Although this approach resembles a punitive external review, it differs in that it presumes the physician is motivated to make changes once meaningful data are provided to guide practice change. This is consistent with Deming's view that workers improve based on internal motivation rather than external coercion.[18]

A third lesson we have learned, supported by the literature, relates to the value of changes in the microenvironment of the practice. When we redesigned a laboratory order form by selectively eliminating check boxes, we decreased inappropriate serum magnesium and phosphorus level orders by 100-fold, without adversely affecting the ordering of appropriate tests.

A powerful new tool, with great potential for real-time feedback and alteration of the practice milieu, is computerized physician (or other clinician) direct order entry.[27, 28] Guidelines, warnings, and alternative approaches can be suggested to clinicians at the moment they order tests or treatments. Thus, the computer can not only help bring order to the often geographically dispersed and dynamic prison population, which is a raison d'être favored by correctional officials, but also be a lever for standardizing and lifting the clinical care content. Many of us look to computers not to automate dysfunctional prison processes nor to replace registered nurses and physicians, but to help deliver more uniform, high-quality care, while facilitating capture and recording of data for quality studies.

LEGAL LEVERS

Having reviewed the above experience, it must be understood that no theory, tool, or technique is a panacea. There is no substitute for a long-term commitment to prisoners and improvement by those managing prisons. Without it, this year's fad becomes next year's forgotten failure.

One of the most important levers ensuring such accountability and commitment has been legal efforts for prisoner rights that centered in the mid-1970s on a series of class action lawsuits. Inmates began filing and winning class action lawsuits alleging that their eighth amendment con-

stitutional rights were being violated because of inadequate health care services. These lawsuits covered medical, mental, dietary, dental, and other health-related services. In 1981, in the case of *Lightfoot v Walker*,[29] a federal judge ordered the establishment of a QA program as part of a larger court order requiring improvements in services provided at a maximum security prison in southern Illinois.

In other cases, as a result of court orders or settlement agreements, agencies or institutions committed themselves to implementing QA programs. By the mid- to late 1980s, the National Commission on Correctional Health Care (NCCHC) included as one of its accreditation standards the implementation of a QA program in a jail or prison. It is now a requirement that any correctional facility desiring accreditation by either the NCCHC or the JCAHO must have an effective quality improvement program in place. The Illinois Department of Corrections and the Rikers Island Health Services were two of the first correctional health care programs to adopt and implement successful quality improvement programs.

UNIQUE CHALLENGES TO DELIVERING QUALITY IN THE CORRECTIONAL SETTING

Decisive factors that propel free world health care organizations to develop formal quality improvement programs do not necessarily apply to jails and prison. These absent imperatives include federal Medicare/Medicaid legislation, accrediting organization standards, and a drive to compete on a quality basis with other facilities; however, none of these factors play a similar role in promoting quality services in correctional facilities. For example:

- Title 18 and 19 Medicaid/Medicare expressly prohibit use of federal funds for inmates incarcerated in prisons because fiscal responsibility has always been seen purely as the state's obligation.
- Most hospitals seek JCAHO accreditation to receive federal (Medicare/Medicaid) reimbursement. This does not apply to correctional facilities in which there is no obligation to seek accreditation of any kind. Many systems have nonetheless voluntarily sought American Correctional Association accreditation, and a smaller number have sought NCCHC or JCAHO accreditation.
- Inmates obviously do not have the ability to "vote with their feet" when dissatisfied with the services that they receive. Prisoners in fact fear reprisals if they do complain, and their complaints (both medical and service dissatisfaction) are often taken less seriously than they would be if originating from patients who "didn't have so much time with nothing better to do."

Given the absence of these stimuli for implementing quality improvement programs, it should not be surprising that correctional settings have lagged behind facilities in the outside community. However, there are also other factors intrinsic to correctional organizations that create an even greater challenge to communication, caring, and the implementation of improvement programs.

Identification of these barriers is a key first step. By examining the following list, each institution can evaluate the extent to which these obstacles operate in their environment and attempt, via increased awareness and consciously designed programs, to offset their pernicious quality-impairing effects.

1. *Mission conflict.* The primary mission of any correctional facility is to securely house inmates or detainees and separate them from the rest of society. In the minds of many, this mission does not necessarily entail the provision of high-quality health care services.[30] In fact, some working in the correctional setting have the view that good-quality services, be they medical or others, somehow result in "coddling the inmates."

2. *Authoritarian organizational structure.* Prisons and jails have traditionally been organized with a warden or superintendent having full authority over the operations. In most instances, the management approach that was used was completely a top-down approach, which is an organizational philosophy diametrically opposed to a quality improvement management approach. Such a rigidly authoritarian structure was believed to be necessary to maintain order. Strict control by the warden or superintendent de-emphasized soliciting input from line staff, let alone inmates, with regard to their views about services.[31]

3. *Social, economic, and cultural prejudices and barriers.* The typical health care professional originates from and lives in a world very different from that of the inmates, 95% of whom are from a lower socioeconomic class. The prevailing cultural view is that people are poor not because they have no money, but rather because they have not made the necessary effort to become successful. The "American dream" is achievable by anyone willing to put forth the effort. This further generalizes into "they really don't care about themselves." When a prisoner is seen with a long-standing medical problem, it is all too easy to assume that patient neglect or carelessness is to blame. These class prejudices combine with ignorance about patients' culture, background, and environment to create barriers to high-quality interactions and communication.

4. *Racial impediments.* Incarceration is intertwined with racism in a multitude of overt and subtle ways. The majority of physicians and providers are not minorities, whereas prisoners are disproportionately black and Hispanic.[32] The same prejudices and imbalances of power and opportunity that make minority communities settings with high crime rates also produce a climate of mutual fear and distrust within the prison walls. Fear and distrust represent the antithesis of caring and quality management.[18]

5. *Criminal label and behavior.* All inmates in a prison system have been charged or convicted of a crime, and,

often, it is a serious crime. Notions of vengeance and punishment dominate official penal attitudes. Prisoners have been hardened by society's harsh treatment before and after their incarceration. Prisoners should not be subjected to the added punishment of inadequate health care services. Figuring out how to mitigate rather than succumb to the substandard quality ramifications of such attitudes becomes a major challenge for prison health care staff.[33]

6. *Drugs: theirs and ours.* In many urban areas, drug-related offenses dominate reasons for arrest. Regardless of one's views on whether locking up the participants in and the victims of drug abuse is an effective way to handle our society's vast drug problems, drugs do play an important role in the behaviors and interactions of inmates and health professionals. Failure to recognize the pervasive role that drugs and the pharmaceutical industry play in our own professional behavior, in tandem with the easy dismissal of prisoners' symptoms as merely drug-seeking manipulation, underlies many errors in judgment and treatment.

7. *Confounding of access.* In the outside world, individuals generally seek physicians only when they develop more serious symptoms or concerns. In the correctional setting, inmates not only request to see a doctor for this reason but also seek health services for a variety of other more trivial reasons because of institutional rules. Inmates often cannot keep their own supply of over-the-counter medications. Thus, every time they have a headache, a cold, or some other minor symptom, they must access the health care program. Health services often must be sought to ask a simple medical question or to address problems with one's shoes or bed. For locked-down prisoners, the only way to leave one's cell other than for a shower may be to access the medical program. The net result is that providers develop a sense of cynicism about whether inmates are requesting medical services for serious reasons.

8. *Turnover.* Inmates in detention facilities may be housed for only a few hours or a few days before they are released. Inmates in prisons are frequently transferred from prison to prison. This movement limits a providers' ability to take a longer-term view. The result may be an episodic approach, in which the sole focus is the acute symptom; no effort is made to investigate the patient's problems more comprehensively, take a full history, or review the patient's medical record. Rapid turnover, going hand in hand with inordinately high patient volume, leads to providers not feeling responsible or accountable for each patient's clinical outcome.

9. *Other practical and logistic barriers.* Medical procedures or consultations that could be easily obtained outside the prison often become expensive logistic nightmares when extrafacility transfer, transportation, and guards must be arranged. Even the simple fact that pris-

Table 2-2. Impediments and strategies

Obstacle	Opportunities to overcome
Mission conflict	• Maintain clear lines distinguishing two missions • Unequivocal primacy and authority of health mission for health services • Education of both correctional and health staff for better understanding of respective missions and constraints • Deeply involve security staff in health services process improvement activities and teams
Authoritarian organizational structure	• Flatten management layers and hierarchy • Empower frontline staff and teams to question rules to flexibly and creatively carry out and redesign functions • Replace old authoritarian management/manager style with new leadership skills/attributes stressing motivation, involvement, participation
Social, economic, and cultural prejudices/ barriers; racial impediments; criminal label/behaviors	• Acknowledge multiplicity of overt and subtle ways prejudices permeate prisons and society • Education/addressing underlying economic factors related to crime and punishment • Education on positive aspects of minority cultures for enhanced appreciation of diversities • Provide training in nonjudgmental style of patient interviewing and caring • Work on specific communication skills to facilitate active listening and nonthreatening two-way patient–provider history taking, plan negotiation, and patient education • To greatest extent possible, create humane environment for staff and inmates
Drugs: theirs and ours	• De-emphasis on criminalization of substance abuse • De-emphasis by staff and patients on drug treatment as sole mode of medical therapy • More emphasis on non-drug prescriptions such as diet, exercise, other lifestyle change; conservative prescription with reassurance and watchful waiting for self-limited illness
Confounding of access	• Identify sick calls that are required solely for nonmedical reasons • Create alternate pathways for inmate access to over-the-counter pharmaceuticals and toiletries (i.e., access via commissary, etc.) • Minimize structural platforms and opportunities for inmate manipulative behavior and staff counter-gaming • Ensure adequacy of prison diet, living conditions to minimize need for special dispensations
Staff and inmate turnover	• Create confidential databases that permit transmission/coordination/access of medical information across spectrum of jail and public health facilities • Coordinate hand-offs across agencies (i.e., ensuring assessment/treatment continuity when transfers to hospitals, jails to prisons) • Invest substantially in recruiting and retaining high-quality committed health professionals • Make prison health work professionally rewarding, arena for continuing medical education and contributing to advancement of state of the art
Other practical and logistic barriers; accountability deficits	• Customer service orientation: make pleasing patients rather than supervisors the aim of work • Use patient/staff grievance mechanisms as opportunities for increased accountability, responsiveness, source of information, learning • Lower threshold for tripping problem identification/investigation mechanisms; take complaints seriously • External oversight/review of health services

oners are cut off from their previous medical providers and medical records creates major disruptions in continuity and information access.

The fundamental challenge for a correctional quality improvement program is to develop an awareness and understanding of these quality obstacles. A good starting point for any prison QA program would be to evaluate what measures are in place and to strategically and systematically develop programs to mitigate and offset each of these fundamental barriers (Table 2).

HOW TO ORGANIZE A QUALITY IMPROVEMENT PROGRAM

The two fundamental elements of a CQI program are management commitment and staff participation. As elementary and self-evident as this may seem, with rare exceptions, these two prerequisites are either totally lacking or fulfilled only through token involvement. Genuine commitment to these two foundations is best structurally codified in the form of a management quality council and multidisciplinary teams.[20]

The quality council is an organizational structure that is responsible for developing the annual quality improvement plan and overseeing and evaluating its implementation and effectiveness. The warden, or equivalent executive leader, along with other top leaders from the health care program should sit on the quality council.[34] These are busy people, easily distracted by many other important competing demands on their time. However, unless there is active involvement and investment of time by such senior staff, it is unlikely that the quality improvement program will do more than raise expectations and frustrations and waste considerable organizational energies for minimal returns.

The council should meet on a regular basis (usually once monthly). Its oversight role includes ensuring that the quality improvement program:

1. Is in sync with the organizational mission and priorities by empowering and coordinating process teams in key strategic areas.
2. Is comprehensive in its scope, which means that it broadly addresses each of the key services (i.e., sick call, reception and transfer processes, infirmary services, dental services, medication services, chronic illness services, outside referral and specialty services, ancillary services, mental health services, and outside hospitalization).
3. Is adequately supported in terms of staff time and resources.
4. Is data driven, continuously evaluated for progress, and relentlessly striving for further improvement.

To effectively implement a quality improvement program, one must begin by training leadership staff, including both health care and correctional staff, in quality improvement principles and techniques. Some of this training may be done in lectures, seminars, or workshops. Other training can be done in a just-in-time manner when there is a need to learn how to engage a particular problem.

If the quality council is the backbone of an institution's quality efforts, then multidisciplinary teams are the real guts of the program.[20] It is in teams that problems are broken down and digested, and it is in teams that the absorbing task of understanding how work processes are actually carried out and how they can be improved occurs. Each team should have a trained leader and should consist of representative staff who provide services in a given area. Thus, physicians, nurses, clerks, and other staff who perform sick call or who provide urgent care should participate in those respective teams. One goal of the program might be that every health care staff member participates in at least one quality improvement team during the course of the year.

Through their intimate knowledge of the work processes, team members can share their understanding of how the patient is supposed to move, for example, through the system for a sick call. This understanding entails elaboration of how "on paper" the system is supposed to work, how in practice it actually occurs, and where it stumbles. Many

administrators consider the making and enforcing of rules as the sine qua non for well-run operations. What CQI teaches us is that there are much greater quality gains possible from understanding why glitches occur and how these variations from the ideal relate to the fundamental ways the processes are designed.[16] By rigidly imposing prescriptive rules to correct problems, administrators not only succumb to blinders resulting from their limited views of the process, but also frustrate or squash the creative energies and opportunities for diminishing barriers across disciplines (discussed previously).

MEASURING AND IMPROVING WHAT WE VALUE IN HEALTH CARE

Staff training should include both basic CQI tools and principles, as well as techniques for evaluating health care services. The JCAHO has articulated eight performance measures in its book, *The Measurement Mandate*.[35] These measures summarize JCAHO's more than three decades of experience through trial and error, about what are the attributes of good health care services. These concepts represent the values that are most important to the patients and the institutions dedicated to meeting the needs of these patients. They also represent the key challenges for designing reliable and valid indicators that accurately measure how well an institution is performing in each of these arenas.

The measures are:

1. *Accessibility.* The ease with which a patient may avail themselves of a particular service. In a correctional setting, this is particularly crucial because inmates may be locked down, and there are frequently rules that tend to inhibit easy access.
2. *Appropriateness.* Whether a provider makes the correct decisions regarding the diagnosis and treatment for any one patient, given the data available. Our efforts to credential and privilege licensed, independent practitioners and our continuing medical education and in-service training efforts are designed to increase the probability that providers will have the requisite knowledge to make appropriate decisions.
3. *Timeliness.* Whether a service is provided within the time frame that is optimal for the benefit of the patient. Delays in accessing sick call or the number of visits required before a correct diagnosis is reached have an impact on the timeliness of proper treatment and potentially have an impact on patient outcomes.
4. *Continuity.* Ongoing patient–provider relationships, as well as the ability of a health care program to pass on information from one provider to another. In a correctional setting, without a good transfer process tying together information from the sending institution and the receiving institution, continuity of care may suffer.
5. *Effectiveness.* This refers to whether the outcome of care provided is what was desired for the patient.

Effectiveness is sometimes differentiated from efficacy. For a medication or a test, for example, *efficacy* refers to the patient benefits under the ideal conditions of a carefully controlled research study, and *effectiveness* describes benefits under real-world conditions. The latter is often compromised by suboptimal test performance or patient selection or monitoring. One of the challenges in the correctional setting is for staff to work with patients and providers to minimize this gap. There is also a need for providers to work with their patients so that the provider's and patient's expectations regarding outcomes are in sync with each other.

6. *Efficiency.* Maximal use of resources with minimal waste or duplication. Clearly, cost efficiency is important whether in the correctional setting or in the outside world. We need to design our processes of care so that we are confident that they maximize our efficient use of resources.

7. *Safety of the environment.* Ensuring that, to the greatest extent possible, all unnecessary dangers to patients are eliminated. In a correctional setting, the safety of the environment refers not only to the usual hospital elements such as infection control and fire safety, but also to vigilance relating to security concerns and the prevention of security breaches.

8. *Quality of the patient–provider relationship.* Providing services with respect and caring conveyed to the patient. It requires the ability to listen and communicate effectively and, in a correctional setting, is a particular challenge because of the prejudices previously described in this chapter.

PERFORMING CQI USING TEAMWORK

Quality improvement teams can be organized around a specific area (e.g., sick call or radiology), a problem-prone process (e.g., timely receipt of and follow-up action on laboratory results), or the comprehensive care of a particular medical problem (e.g., diabetes or alcohol withdrawal syndrome). Each team should meet initially and brainstorm about which of these eight performance measures are most likely in need of improvement.

In this initial hypothesis-generating phase, participants should be encouraged to share their perspectives on the magnitude and causes of problems. Flow charts diagramming the process are particularly helpful in this phase. This should be rapidly followed by collection of data to test these hypotheses. The data will often give a much different picture than expected. The problem may turn out to be much worse than any single individual had realized, or the most common contributing causes will be very different than those team members attributed as the sources of problems.

Sometimes, because of prior deficits, a facility may be under a court order mandating, for example, that each inmate submitting a request for sick call must be seen by an advanced-level provider (physician, nurse practitioner, or physician's assistant) within a specified number of days. By studying slips for sick calls and the subsequent visits, one can determine whether the service is being provided according to the time frames believed to be appropriate. If the data show that performance is not acceptable, the team can investigate what factors are leading to the suboptimal results. Tools such as histograms (bar graphs of leading causal factors, a variant of which is the Pareto diagram, which illustrates that the three leading causes are usually responsible for the majority of the problems) and cause-and-effect diagrams are helpful at this stage.

Once processes are targeted for improvement and changes are implemented, the new process should be restudied to determine whether the change led to the desired improvement. This methodology allows team members to continually learn more about the services they provide and allows them to contribute to the analysis of which improvements need to be redesigned next. By repetitively running through this cycle of planning, studying, implementing, and checking impact, one can continuously improve a process.[36] Corporations find that their success in the marketplace depends on how rapidly they can repeat this cycle. Many have reduced the change cycle lengths from months or even years to days or even hours.

EXAMPLES OF CORRECTIONAL QUALITY IMPROVEMENT SUCCESSES
When Meeting 90% Threshold Isn't Good Enough

A large prison reception center decided to study its intake process. The process began with inmates being interviewed by a licensed practical nurse as they arrived from local jails. Based on this interview, it was determined which inmates had chronic illnesses, were taking medications, or had any acute medical conditions. The quality improvement team looking at the reception process determined that good-quality services required that individuals in any of these illness categories should be seen by a physician within 8 hours of their initial interview.

The team members were confident that this was being accomplished. Nonetheless, they designed a study to look at the timeliness of the process. To their surprise, the data showed that only two thirds of the individuals identified as having significant medical problems were being seen by a physician within 8 hours. The team, consisting of physicians, nurses, licensed practical nurses, the officer working in the reception area, and the lieutenant in charge of the reception area, was convened to study the causes for the roughly one third of inmates who weren't seen within the allotted 8 hours. They made a flow chart of the sequence of steps that a patient went through before being referred to the physician.

The team identified several factors that could prolong an inmate's stay in the reception area and, thus, delay the inmate getting to the physician. These factors included delays in obtaining housing assignments and time needed to complete various security processes. The team obtained approval for changes in several of these steps and implemented the changes. Three months later, they restudied the process. They found that 90% of all inmates arriving from the jails identified as having significant medical problems were now being seen within 8 hours. This dramatic improvement brought them to their original goal of ensuring that a minimum of 90% of inmates with significant problems should be seen by a physician within 8 hours.

When the team met again, the lieutenant in charge of reception suggested that the process could be further improved with additional changes in security processing. He was able to obtain permission from the administration to change the security processing, and the new system was implemented. Three months later, another study was done and showed that 97% of the inmates who were identified as having significant medical problems were seen by a physician within 8 hours. The remaining 3% were either seen within 12 hours or explained by some exceptional circumstance.

The members of this reception team were deservedly proud of their accomplishment, which would have been unikely had the warden merely sent out a memo requiring all staff to comply with the order to see patients within 8 hours. Is 97% compliance good enough, or are there further opportunities for improvement? Continuous quality improvement has been termed a race without a finish line. Certainly, 97% of jets landing crash free would not be acceptable. Each team needs to continually weigh the necessity and opportunities for further improvement, along with the marginal return of investing efforts here vs. other improvement areas.

Patients With Diabetes Running Behind

Another example of a quality improvement effort occurred at a maximum security prison in the Midwest. The quality improvement council decided that treatment outcomes for their program for diabetes were a priority. This prison housed approximately 1,800 inmates, of whom 30 were known to have diabetes. After reviewing the literature, the group decided that the definition of good control was a Hb A1c level of 8.5 or less within the last 3 months. They excluded charts of inmates who had been in the institution for less than 3 months, because it was believed that such individuals may not have had enough time within the facility for their diabetes program to have had a sufficient impact.

After review of 30 patients' records, it was found that 10 patients (33%) did not have an Hb A1c level checked. Of the 20 with values present in the chart, 13/20 (65%) had levels less than 8.5. The institution had set an initial threshold (minimum percent achieving control) of 80% as acceptable. Each of the 7 with unacceptable control was brought to the medical unit and interviewed by a physician.

Through this process, it was revealed that 3 of the 7 patients were, in fact, undertreated and were given a higher dose of medication. The remaining 4 patients did not comply with their therapeutic diets, so additional diet counseling was given.

Four months later the audit was repeated. Five of the 7 individuals whose control had been inadequate were now found to be under satisfactory control. On this re-audit, 18 of the 20 identified patients (90%) were in satisfactory control, whereas 2 still did not comply with their diets.

At this point, the team debated whether additional improvement was achievable. One group felt that the maximum improvement possible had been achieved, but the majority of the team was not satisfied. They believed that a greater understanding, from the patient's perspective, about dietary compliance was needed. By bringing patients back for lengthy interviews, the team learned that inmates on the diabetic special diet line were served at the beginning of each meal. The two inmates who were not compliant indicated that they were often unable to get to the diet line before the special diet line had been completed; the regular diet line had begun to be served. Each had vascular insufficiency in their legs requiring them to walk slower. The medical staff obtained "slow walking" passes for them, which allowed these patients to get their special diet even though the regular diet line had begun. When their blood sugar control was evaluated 3 months later, they were finally determined to be in control.

One could question whether, with such small numbers, the change was statistically significant or whether it represented merely a regression to the mean (i.e., because of random fluctuations, the high Hb A1c levels will more likely tend to normalize when checked again). Without a concurrent comparison control group, we cannot prove that the subsequent finding of *all* 20 patients' Hb A1c levels being in the desired range, less than 8.5, was entirely because of the team's interventions. Nonetheless, by approaching the problem systematically, they uncovered important issues that resulted in meaningful institutional changes. By plotting changes repeatedly over time, one can obtain a fairly accurate statistical picture.

This tension between methodological rigor and the making of change based on intimate patient and team knowledge is a recurrent theme in this field.[37] Certainly, if we wait before implementing each aircraft safety feature until it resulted in statistically significant fewer crashes, many lives would be lost before airplanes were made safer. Building bridges between the science of change and other scientific disciplines is a project to which we can all creatively contribute, beginning with the exciting cross-fertilization of prisons with quality improvement.

Back to the Basics in a Southern Illinois Prison

A quality improvement team monitored the frequency of different complaints evaluated on sick call during a

6-month period. Each month, they collected slips for sick call and tallied the frequency of presenting complaints such as a headache, chest pain, abdominal pain, a cough, or a backache. For the first 3 months, there was a consistent pattern of frequency for each of these and other common symptoms.

However, on the third and fourth months, they noted a significant increase of backache complaints. One team member suggested that this was probably a copycat effect, that is, individuals trying to acquire a backboard, which could only be provided by the medical program. Other staff questioned why this suddenly began to happen when it hadn't been a problem in the prior 3 months. Examining the data, they noticed that it was inmates from particular housing units who were disproportionately making these complaints in recent months.

When they visited these particular housing units and interviewed inmates, they discovered that the maintenance crew had recently installed a metal crossbar across each of the bed frames. It appeared that the location of these crossbars underneath the bed frames was the cause of the sudden increase in low back pain complaints.

The medical staff worked with maintenance staff to jointly correct the problem by modifying the beds. The result was that the low back pain complaints dropped dramatically to a level lower than that which had occurred before the implementation of these new bars. Thus, the monthly tracking and statistical analysis of the frequency of specific complaints, along with the persistence of the medical staff in following through with the findings from the data, allowed the group to adopt a systematic approach that led to identification of the underlying cause of the problem. Without this epidemiologic approach, each individual back pain complaint would have been treated separately, which possibly could have resulted in unnecessary workups and a series of symptomatic measures, including medications, unlikely to result in relief of the symptoms or identification of their underlying cause.

Sick Calls and Sports Falls in Oregon

In the Oregon Department of Corrections, quality improvement has been a mainstay since 1993. Studies are done at both a statewide and an institutional level. In 1993, the agency medical director established a task force of nurses to revise the nursing protocols for more effective triage assessment and treatment initiation.

Their first step was also to examine the reasons inmates were signing up for sick call. The statewide task force identified the 10 most common complaints. A major finding was that 41% of the reasons inmates were signing up for sick call could be categorized as administrative—things such as routine medication renewals and ordering of eyeglasses. Most of these visits were for issues for which a medical evaluation by a nurse or advanced-level provider was unnecessary. Another 18% were signing up for sick call

for "wellness" concerns like blood pressure or periodic weight checks. Although believing it to be desirable to continue to encourage prisoners' wellness concerns, the task force did not believe that these inmates required assessment by a nurse or physician. Each task force member engaged their colleagues in discussions about alternatives to sick call to address these administrative and wellness concerns. Various alternatives were implemented, including use of patient education handouts and videotapes about common health concerns.

When task force members returned to their respective home institutions, they shared this information gathered about the reasons inmates were coming to sick call. A system was developed whereby most medication renewals could be handled by written requests, and the availability of certain nonprescription medications was increased through a variety of strategies. By 1996, 73% of the inmates were seen at sick call for an illness-related reason, and the percentage of visits for administrative and wellness concerns had dropped to approximately 10%.

Our final example, also from the Oregon Department of Corrections, was initiated by a staff member at a 150-bed facility located in an extremely remote area. The facility consisted of a 100-bed labor camp and a 50-bed alcohol and drug inpatient treatment program.

The nurse was concerned about the number of inmates seen for sports-related injuries. She collected information on the number of such problems seen during a 5-month period. This information identified whether the injured inmate was in the treatment program or in a labor program, the type of sports activity that the inmate was involved in at the time of the injury, the type of injury, the cost of treating the injury, and the inmate's thoughts on why the injury had occurred.

She then shared this information with the institution's safety committee. One area the data clearly identified was injuries from rocks and holes in the recreation yard. Efforts were made to clear these obstacles from the yard. In addition, inmates were educated about the need and proper techniques for warm-up and conditioning exercises. A third area identified for improvement in athletic injuries was the high occurrence rates during holiday weekends. Another educational campaign addressed preventing injuries on these longer weekends.

For 3 consecutive years, the rate of athletic injuries in the months of April through September has been cut in half from the baseline levels. At an average cost of $240 for the treatment of each injury in 1996, there has been not only a significant improvement in inmate health, but also a significant cost savings.

CONCLUDING COMMENTS

What we learn from quality improvement is that, if we're just doing our jobs, then we're not doing our jobs. Just working in the same old ways is no longer sufficient. In industry, it means that we will have no job if our firm can't continuously improve so that it can keep pace with the competition. In prisons, ... well, what does it mean? If prisons are a growth industry, and it looks like they'll always be around, will there be no competition to drive us out of business?

What it means for those of us working with prisoners is that doing our jobs, or even doing our jobs better, is not enough. Privatization issues notwithstanding,[33] we have a special responsibility to the prisoners and to the larger society to draw the circles even wider. Few of us could justify our work if we were guards or doctors in a concentration camp, even an efficient, well-run camp. Continuous quality improvement's implied dissatisfaction with the status quo means that we have to more broadly challenge the status quo that we observe in prisons.[5, 18]

Making the commitment to give quality care to each prisoner and to respect the human dignity of each inmate, along with our faith in the potential of the employees, is crucial to challenging the unfair, violence-prone, and vengeful forces that are filling our jails and prisons. Shining a light on these dark problems, linking hands with others who have a basic faith in human nature and who believe in humane care, and striving to improve individuals' conditions and their lives should, in the end, be what high-quality caring means for this population.

REFERENCES

1. Berwick DM: Taking action: Leading the reduction in error in health care. *Qual Connect* 5: 1996.
2. Berwick DM: The clinical process and the quality process. *Qual Manage Health Care* 1:1–8, 1997.
3. Squires N: Promoting health in prisons. *BMJ* 313:1161, 1996.
4. Reynolds Q: *I, Willie Sutton.* Da Capo Press, 1993.
5. Goldfield N, Schiff G: Continuous quality improvement at the crossroads: Contradictions and challenges. *Managed Care Q* 5:10–18, 1997.
6. Berwick DM: Continuous improvement as an ideal in health care. *N Engl J Med* 320:53–56, 1989.
7. Berwick DM: A primer on leading the improvement of systems. *BMJ* 312:619–622, 1996.
8. Brennan TA, Berwick DM: The evolution of health care and its regulation, in Brennan TA, Berwick DM (eds): *New Rules.* San Francisco, Jossey–Bass, 1996, pp 149–225.
9. Schiff G: Cascade or facade: Focusing or obfuscating the pathogenesis of latrogenesis? *QRB* 19:196–198, 1993.
10. Wennberg JE: Dealing with medical practice variations: A proposal for action. *Health Aff* 3:6–31, 1984.
11. Chassin MR, Kosecoff J, Park RE, et al: Does inappropriate use explain geographic variations in the use of health care services? A study of three procedures. *JAMA* 258:2533–2537, 1987.
12. Sanazaro PJ, Mills DH: A critique of the use of generic screening in quality assessment (see comments). *JAMA* 265:1977–1981, 1991.
13. McEachern JE, Makens PK, Bachanan ED, et al: Quality improvement: An imperative for medical care, in Neuhauser D, McEachern JE, Headrick L (eds): *Clinical CQI: A Book of Readings.* Oakbrook Terrace, Ill, Joint Commission on Accreditation of Healthcare Organizations, 1995, pp 117–134.
14. Deming WE: *Out of the Crisis.* Cambridge, Mass, Massachusetts Institute of Technology, 1982.
15. Sim J: The prison medical service and the deviant 1895–1948. *Clin Med* 34:102–117, 1995.
16. Walton M: *The Deming Management Method.* New York, Perigee, 1986.
17. Berwick DM: Controlling variation in health care: A consultation from Walter Shewhart. *Med Care* 29:1212–1225, 1991.
18. Schiff GD, Goldfield NI: Deming meets Braverman: Toward a progressive analysis of the continuous quality improvement paradigm. *Int J Health Serv* 24:655–673, 1994.
19. Berwick DM, Nolan TW: Overview: Cooperating for improvement. *Joint Commission J Qual Improvement* 21:573–577, 1995.
20. Scholtes PR, Joiner BL, Braswell B, et al: *The Team Handbook.* Madison, Wis, Joiner Associates, 1988.
21. Berwick DM:. Eleven worthy aims for clinical leadership of health system reform. *JAMA* 272:797–802, 1994.
22. Berwick DM: The year of "how": New systems for delivering health care. *Qual Connect* 5:1–4, 1996.
23. Hart JT: Two paths for medical practice. *Lancet* 340:772–775, 1992.
24. Kassirer JP: The quality of care and the quality of measuring it. *N Engl J Med* 329:1263–1265, 1993.
25. ACP Jl Club, Jan-Feb 96.
26. Bates DW: Medication errors. How common are they and what can be done to prevent them? *Drug Saf* 15:303–310, 1996.
27. Bates DW: Computerized physician order entry and quality of care. *Qual Manage Health Care* 2:18–27, 1994.
28. Balas EA, Austin SM, Mitchell JA, et al: The clinical value of computerized information services. *Arch Fam Med* 5:271–278, 1996.
29. *Lightfoot v Walker*, 486# F. Supp. S04 (S.D. Ill. 1980).
30. Willmott Y: Prison nursing: The tension between custody and care. *Br J Nurs* 6:333–336, 1997.
31. Birmingham L: Should prisoners have a say in prison health care? *BMJ* 315:65–66, 1997.
32. Muwakkil S: My own private Alcatraz, in *These Times.* 21(3):24–25, 1996.
33. Lotke E: The prison–industrial complex. *Multinatl Monit* 17:18–21, 1996.
34. Palmer RH, Hargraves JL, Orav EJ, et al: Leadership for quality improvement in group practices. *Med Care* 34:SS40–SS51, 1996.
35. *The Measurement Mandate.* Oak Brook Terrace, Ill, Joint Commission on Accreditation of Healthcare Organizations, 1993.
36. Nolan T: Accelerating the pace of improvement: An interview with Thomas Nolan (interview by Steven Berman). *Joint Commission J Qual Improvement* 23:217–222, 1997.
37. Berwick DM: Harvesting knowledge from improvement (editorial). *JAMA* 275:877–878, 1996.

3

Interaction Between Correctional Staff and Health Care Providers in the Delivery of Medical Care

Armond Start, M.D., M.P.H.

FUNCTION OF A DETENTION FACILITY

It is essential that the health care staff understand the basic function of a detention facility before the interaction between correctional and health care staff can be understood. The residents of a detention facility, whether it be a juvenile facility, a jail, or a prison, have been separated from general society as punishment for breaking a law, or because they lack the means to post bond. It is important from the very onset that all citizens understand that in the United States the punishment for breaking the law is often separation from society for a specified time. Under the Constitution of the United States, one is sent to prison or jail as punishment, not for punishment. The function of a detention facility is to ensure that a resident is contained within the perimeter limits of the facility and under the supervision of the agency charged by the government to enforce that separation from society. The ultimate responsibility of the chief executive officer of the facility, or as he or she is frequently called, the warden, is to ensure that the perimeter security of the facility be as impenetrable as humanly possible. Only authorized individuals may enter and leave the facility, and only necessary materials and supplies may enter and leave the facility. All health care providers must understand and cooperate with this basic fundamental function of a detention facility. Depending on the perimeter security procedures, the health care provider may be subjected to searches and passage through metal detectors. Perimeter security procedures should always be honored by health care providers, unless such procedures are implemented in an arbitrary or capricious manner to harass or intimidate individual employees or a class of employees. It is important for health care providers to understand that a secure perimeter is a critical part of custody function. The atmosphere, culture, and environment of the facility inside the perimeter security is variable, depending on the custody level of the residents of that facility and the institutional management philosophy. Despite this variability, there are at least nine areas that need to be addressed and understood by the health care provider who chooses to work within a detention environment.

Anti-therapeutic Environment

Many believe the correctional environment to be anti-therapeutic to rehabilitative efforts. Some of the problems of this environment include:

1. Security precautions may interfere with the physician/patient relationship, e.g., maximum security inmates may have to be seen when officers require them to be shackled. An inmate with shoulder discomfort may lose faith in the physician who fails to examine the shoulder because the physician is unwilling to ask the correctional officer to loosen the shackles.
2. Overcrowding (multiple inmates housed in small cells) can contribute to increases in stress, anger, and hostility between inmates, inmates and correctional staff, and even, sometimes, inmates and medical staff. These problems are especially exacerbated when such crowding occurs in mental health units or disciplinary units where people may be locked down for long periods.
3. Excessive idleness, usually also found in overcrowded institutions, adds to the stress of the environment. Most therapeutic environments are ones in which patients or inmates are kept active.
4. Officers are rarely trained to be supportive of the medical care program as one of their major responsibilities. In fact, many officers resent what they see as extraordinary access to medical services that they and their families lack. This resentment can manifest in, at a minimum, lack of cooperation and, sometimes, literally subversion of the medical program's efforts to provide good quality service.

Paramilitary Organizational Structure

Most health care providers do not have experience working within an organizational structure that has a military form. Healthcare providers are always taught that they must focus on doing those things that they believe are in the best interest of their patients. This can conflict with rigid military-like rules and procedures that frequently do not take into account what may be best for an individual patient. The challenge to the health care provider is to work closely with the correctional staff so that they develop shared priorities with regard to providing the best quality of service. One of the most effective strategies to accomplish this is to involve correctional officers, both line staff and supervisory staff, in quality improvement activities; officers involved in the reception and diagnostic process included in the medical quality improvement team that aims to improve the quality and efficiency of the medical intake.

Balancing Institutional Movement Rules and Inmate Access to Services

One of the difficulties faced by all health care providers working in a correctional setting is strictly regulated inmate movement. Several times a day all inmates are locked down so that security staff conduct a count and assure that all inmates are accounted for. In many facilities, these counts disrupt the health care program from effective use of human resources. In many prisons, although a dentist may be on site 8 hours a day, both morning and afternoon counts reduce the availability of dental chair time to 3–4 hours per day. In the correctional setting, dentists and other health care providers have an obligation to work with security to devise a system that allows for counts to be conducted at the same time the inmates have access to the professional resources on site. One strategy to accomplish this is to allow for "outcounting." This means that inmates who are in the dental or medical area are counted as being in those areas rather than as being in their cells. This may seem like a simple solution, but if medical staff do not advocate the implementation of such procedure modifications, resources will not be used wisely and access will be significantly diminished.

Another problem related to inmate movement is the provision of specialty services that are not provided on site. This usually requires both officers and vehicles to transport inmates to the off-site service. Corrections administrations have the responsibility to ensure that necessary vehicles and custody staff are available to provide transportation. On the other hand, the medical staff have an equal responsibility to monitor the appropriateness of the referrals. This means that before a patient is referred to a specialist, an institution should ensure that all of the necessary diagnostic and therapeutic strategies that could be used on site have been used. The referrals should be for very specific questions to be answered or procedures to be done. It is very helpful for facilities to use commonly accepted practice guidelines such as the guideline developed by the Agency for Healthcare Policy Research regarding the management of chronic backache. Within this guideline there are a series of recommendations that should be carried out prior to the initiation of a referral to a specialist. The medical program should monitor the frequency with which outside medical trips are cancelled due to either absence of transport vehicle or officers. In general, such cancellations should occur less than 10% of the time. The medical staff should also work with custody so that when there is a shortage of either officers or vehicles, the medical staff is able to prioritize those trips that are to be made that day and make decisions in the best interests of the patients. These kinds of decisions, besides being difficult, are somewhat unique to the correctional setting and pose a challenge for many of the medical staff.

Patient Autonomy vs. Institutional Control

In the corrections setting, when inmates refuse to do what officers tell or request them to do, the inmates may be sanctioned. Such sanctions can include being locked down, losing certain privileges, and even being required to stay longer within the correctional setting. It is difficult sometimes for correctional staff to understand the very different philosophical milieu that is a necessary part of any health care environment. Health care providers are taught that each patient must have ultimate control over the health care decisions that affect their lives. Thus, refusing to take a medication or refusing to allow a laboratory test is considered a patient's right. This kind of issue becomes particularly difficult when patients refuse to eat, refuse to take medications for such things as tuberculosis, or when patients refuse to have a blood test in the context of a staff member coming into contact with the patient's blood. In many jurisdictions, medical staff are encouraged to force on inmates either blood tests or medications or food. Clearly, medical staff must work very hard to create an environment in which security staff respect their professional obligations. Ultimately, no medical staff member should work in any environment in which the leadership attempts to force them to do what they believe is professionally wrong or unethical.

Inmate Turnover and the Episodic Approach to Health Services

The rapid turnover of inmate patients is a phenomenon not well appreciated by health care staff who have not worked in a corrections environment. In a jail situation a resident may be detained for hours or a few days, and any significant health care problem cannot be evaluated well in this short time. In a prison system with different facilities and significant overcrowding, inmate patients may be moved from one institution to another, or from one level of security to another, in a rapid and often difficult to understand manner. A dentist in the process of treating and restoring

the dentition of an inmate may suddenly find that inmate has been transferred to another facility. A physician in a jail may wish to adjust the insulin dosage of a diabetic patient, only to find that the day after the new orders are written the inmate has been released from custody. This type of inmate turnover creates great stresses and challenges for any health care program. It is incumbent on the health care leadership to work very closely with the custody staff involved in movement so that, prior to movement, medical staff can be notified to review medical records and summarize recommendations for continuity to pass on to the next facility. Also, when a patient is being released, an effort should be made if enough time is provided for the medical record to be reviewed and any community linkages be made for appropriate follow-up and continuity. In a corrections environment, when an inmate is discharged or leaves the facility, the responsibility of the security staff has ended. In the health care community, all health care providers have an obligation to ensure continuity, either from one institution to another, or from release of an inmate from an institution to a health service provider in the community. These differing philosophical guidelines once again challenge the medical staff to work closely with custody to achieve the outcomes to which they are professionally committed. The potential negative consequences of inmate movement within an agency from one institution to another, and particularly within jails where stays may be short, is the episodic orientation toward health care by some of the providers. What this means is that the provider, in seeing the patient at sick call, will only focus on the immediate problem, fail to adequately review the medical record, and, therefore, miss the opportunity to address a series of underlying problems in exchange for just addressing the superficial symptom. It is important for medical leadership to stress strategies that will allow avoidance of episodically managing health care, because an episodic approach is rarely consistent with good quality care.

A Single Approach for All

Within the corrections setting, it is important that officers learn a particular set of procedures that are meant to be applied to all inmates equally. Part of the philosophy behind this is to prevent the appearance of special treatment or favoritism for any particular inmate. On the other hand, in medical settings we are always taught to customize or individualize our treatment plans so that they are tailor-made for each patient. These different approaches can result in real conflict. Medical staff may request a particular housing location or bed assignment and custody may think that this is just providing special favors for or coddling the inmates. These conflicts can be avoided only when medical staff work carefully with custody so that custody can understand the basis for their requests and what problems may be prevented by individualizing treatment plans.

The Psyche and the Soma or the Chicken and the Egg

Most correctional environments are depressing for many of the detainees. People are separated from loved ones and friends and are subjected to rules pertaining to almost every aspect of their daily lives. These rules tend to create an infantilization of some of the inmates. This type of an environment is quite conducive to the development of depression and corresponding psychosomatic symptoms. When people are forced to sit in a very confined environment and remain inactive for long periods, it is natural to focus on somatic sensations. In the process, somatic sensations become more important and to some extent exaggerated. Health care providers must understand this and also that the medical program may be used by inmates for a variety of reasons that, although reasonable, do not exist in the free world. In a prison setting, one must go to the medical unit to be released from obligations to work or school. To obtain a bed board, OTC medications, more comfortable shoes, or a special diet, one must access the medical program. Thus, for a variety of reasons, inmates use medical services far more frequently than individuals of a similar age and gender in the free world. For all of these reasons, what may appear to be patient overuse has to be understood by correctional health care providers and security staff as appropriate use in the corrections environment. Only by understanding the increase in somatic symptoms, depression, the structural rules that place greater demands on the medical unit, will health care providers allow themselves to carefully and correctly respond to inmate concerns and educate security staff.

No Divorce

In a free world setting, when a physician unsuccessfully treats a patient's symptoms, the patient may attempt to obtain services from another resource, an emergency room, a clinic, or whatever appears to be reasonable. In a correctional setting, when the strategies of a physician are unsuccessful, both the patient and the physician may face the reality that they are locked into a joint therapeutic effort with no opportunity for divorce. This particular kind of stress may result in inmates complaining to the correctional staff about the incompetence and ineffectiveness of the health care program. The untrained correctional officer may begin to lose faith in the confidence of the medical program and convey this lack of faith to the inmates, reinforcing the opinions of the inmates. It is incumbent on medical staff to work with the correctional staff so that they understand that there is not always going to be a cure for every problem and that their responsibility is to provide the best quality services given the available resources. A medical staff that works closely with the correctional staff is more likely to get support from that correctional staff. This will offset some of the cynicism that may develop in patients who think that the cure they are expecting has been either delayed or denied.

Health Care Within Corrections—Valued or a Necessary Evil?

It is important that all health care providers recognize that the number one function of detention facilities is the segregation of people from society. Many health care providers working in corrections feel like guests in the correctional environment. Patients in the free world go to clinic for health care reasons only. People are sent to correctional facilities as a form of punishment, not as a vehicle to have their health needs met. In many jurisdictions, the health care services program is regarded "as a program" with the same importance attributed to it as education, chaplain services, and inmate work programs. In fact, it is quite common for the correctional administrator in charge of overseeing the health service program to be responsible for other programs in the system and to hold the title of Deputy Director for Program Services. Not infrequently, this individual has had no expertise or training in the delivery of health care services, and in this table of organization the health care program must compete with education, inmate work programs, or chaplain services for needed resources. This arrangement may create a situation where health care administrators are supervised and evaluated by non-medically trained individuals. This reality must be understood by people entering the correctional health field.

It is likely there will always be some tension between custody staff and health care staff, which frequently results from very different goals and objectives. The important goal of health service administrators is to ensure that the tension between custody and health care staff remains a healthy tension. It is critical for collaboration to occur to optimize the smooth operation of the detention facility. The health care staff needs to be reminded periodically of the difficulties of meshing these two disparate philosophical approaches in this environment. The following recommendations are meant to mitigate some of the tension and potentially destructive divergent approaches when custody and health care staff do not work closely together.

Recruitment and pre-service programs must prepare the health care provider for the frustrations that will be experienced in working with the anti-therapeutic environment of detention facilities. In a very real sense, the health care provider must be oriented to a different kind of approach to patient care, and must be aware of the increased somatic symptoms that will be expressed because of the commonness of depression and idleness in this population. The provider must realize that access to health care services is frequently very much controlled by the custody environment and that only through working closely with custody can health care objectives be achieved.

It is recommended that all providers attend a 1-week pre-service orientation. The orientation should be conducted by health care administrators and health care providers with assistance and input from custody staff. The pre-service orientation should not be the exclusive responsibility of the custody staff. Although their participation is important, the program and content of the pre-service must be designed by health care staff. The practice of placing health care providers in exactly the same pre-service programs as correctional officers is counterproductive. While some agencies believe that all employees must first be correctional officers and second a professional service employee, this belief is likely to lead to compromising of health care provider ethics with regard to their patients. The curriculum of the pre-service program should emphasize that the role of the health care provider is to always regard the inmate as a patient and function as an advocate for what is in the patient's best interest.

The practice in some jurisdictions of placing health care providers in correctional officer uniforms with badges and handcuffs, although meant to improve security at the health care interface, has the potential to seriously compromise the effectiveness of the provider in dealing with their patients. The inmate-patient must believe that the health care provider is there for only one purpose—to evaluate health care status and to provide necessary treatment. Placing health care staff in correctional officer uniforms disturbs that perception and may interfere with the development of a therapeutic relationship between patient and provider. Custody staff may see medical staff more as an extension of security than as professionals whose responsibility is to provide a service to the patients. It is recommended that the health care staff be appropriately dressed in professional clothing that clearly identifies them as a member of the health care team. It is also recommended that name tags be worn indicating the type of professional license. In some jurisdictions, the last name of the provider is not included on the name tag for security reasons and this practice may have some merit. The issue is addressed by placing the first name and the professional title on the name tag. Stressing the differing responsibilities while emphasizing the shared goal of a safe, secure facility with custody is important. Custody should understand the role a good medical program can play in reducing inmate anger.

The health services staff should be active participants in the pre-service and continuing education program of the custody staff. It is the responsibility of the health care staff to educate, inform, and explain the health services program to the custody staff. This activity has become much more important with the challenges of managing the epidemics of HIV disease and tuberculosis. The education and training of correctional officers in the control of infectious disease and the appropriate management of blood spills and other occupationally related diseases, such as tuberculosis and hepatitis, should be taught to the custody staff in a very organized and dedicated program. It is also important for health care staff to participate in the CPR and first aid training of officers. These activities should be supported by the health care budget.

Scheduled formal meetings between administrators of health care services and correctional administrators should be a requirement and articulated in policies and procedures. Meetings between health care staff, managers, and custody managers are frequently scheduled on an as-needed basis. There are enough issues that arise on a daily and weekly basis to serve as an appropriate agenda for regularly scheduled meetings. It is strongly recommended that the chief executive officer of the health care program, who must be a member of the senior staff, report directly to the warden/superintendent of the facility. To bury the health care program far down the chain of command is to create a situation in which the health care program makes little contribution to the overall functioning of the facility and may contribute to a system that fails to recruit and retain qualified, competent, well-trained professional staff. It is not realistic to expect that well-trained and motivated medical staff will report to a non-medical administrator who is far removed from the warden of the facility.

Conflict resolution between custody staff and health care staff can be addressed in two ways:

1. A staff conference to address the problems of a particularly disruptive and uncooperative patient. It has been estimated that 5% of an incarcerated population may be individuals who have severe difficulty with authority and may be uncooperative at some point in their incarcerated life. It is the experience of well-trained professionals in both the custody and health care areas that a staffing or a meeting of key individuals who impact on the inmate's status is essential. Staffing of such an individual patient should consist of the mental health staff, medical staff, custody staff, work supervisor, and the housing supervisor. A management plan should be outlined, and the inmate should be informed of the plan in the presence of all the participants.

2. Role playing: In a situation where there is a conflict and disagreements between medical and custody staff, the mechanism of role playing can be a very effective instrument. In this situation the correctional officer role plays what he or she perceives to be the behavior of the medical staff that is unacceptable. In like manner, the health care provider role plays the disputed behavior of the correctional officer. When this is done in an atmosphere of conflict resolution, it becomes a very constructive exercise. Unfortunately, in many jurisdictions this is not done because of time constraints. It is recommended that this activity be used because it will ultimately save time while reducing conflict between the custody and health care staff. This is a situation where managers should take time to save time.

The continuous quality improvement program of the facility should include a periodic evaluation of the climate or environment of the institution. It is recommended that the CQI program ask the question, "What is the relationship between the custody staff and the health care staff, and is this relationship healthy?" More importantly, the CQI program should ask the question, "How can the relationship between custody staff and health care staff be improved?" The concept of mutual respect is critically important in the operation of a detention facility. If this is absent, the inmate population will most certainly exploit this lack of collaboration.

The task of supervising incarcerated individuals is difficult enough without the added burden of staff conflict.

Good faith efforts on the part of health care managers and correctional administrators will produce a work force that carries out its assignments in a professional and dignified manner. This must be the goal of all employees who work in the correctional environment.

4

Medical Ethics and Correctional Health Care

B. Jaye Anno, Ph.D., C.C.H.P-A.

Steven S. Spencer, M.D., F.A.C.P., C.C.H.P.

INTRODUCTION AND BACKGROUND

The need to define and enforce acceptable behavior for medical practitioners undoubtedly is as old as the profession itself. Codified principles of medical ethics date from the time of Hippocrates, in the fifth century BC. Codes of ethics are characteristic not only of medicine but also of the other two "learned professions" of law and theology. In addition, discussions of medical ethics inevitably address its interface with law and religion.

Ethics, of course, is neither law nor religion. What is legal may not be ethical for a specific profession. Law governs the behavior of society as a whole. Professional ethics govern the behavior of specific occupational components of society. Usually, there is no conflict between law and ethics. When there is, however, ethical imperatives should prevail. When the law mandates medically unethical conduct, physicians should work to change the law.

Similarly, what is ethical according to a specific profes-sion may not conform to certain religious precepts nor to an individual's sense of personal morality. The classic example of this conflict for physicians is abortion. When conflicts of this nature arise, the usual and acceptable decision is to avoid doing that which violates personal morality or religion, even though it does not violate the ethics of one's profession.

Professional codes of ethics or ethical principles are consensus statements about what is right and wrong behavior for members of a particular group. They devolve from the central mission of the profession. They usually contain obligatory language, that is, you "shall" or you "must" conform to certain precepts; however, in most cases, professional codes of ethics do not have the standing of law:

For the most part, failure to follow the ethical code of one's profession may result in disapproval or ostracism by one's peers, but seldom results in anything more dramatic. It is only in well-regulated professions such as medicine and

*law that violating the ethical precepts of the profession may
result in loss of privileges, employment or licensure.[1]*

In the case of the medical profession, enforcement of ethical codes is the responsibility of state licensing boards. These boards define unethical (unprofessional) conduct, investigate complaints against physicians, and have the power to take action against a physician's license, including revocation, if they find that an ethical violation has occurred.

Although the structure of medical ethics, or biomedical ethics, has taken on considerable complexity in the past several decades, mainly because of the enormous technological advances of this century, most of the basic principles of the Hippocratic Oath have survived and are still subscribed to as core values in the practice of medicine. They may be stated briefly as the necessity to:

1. Act only for the benefit of the patient (beneficence).
2. Abstain from whatever is deleterious to the patient (no maleficence, or *primum non nocere*, "first do no harm").
3. Abstain from abusing the doctor–patient relationship.
4. Honor the confidential nature of that relationship.

These ethical imperatives continue to be expressed in injunctive or obligatory language. They have been expanded somewhat beyond the one-to-one doctor–patient relationship to embrace a responsibility to society and to professional colleagues, as exemplified by *Principles of Medical Ethics* of the American Medical Association (AMA).[2] These AMA principles, in addition to stipulating responsibilities to patients, also mention obligations to expose incompetent or fraudulent physicians; to seek changes in laws that are contrary to the best interests of patients; to study and advance scientific knowledge; to make relevant information available to patients, colleagues, and the public; to obtain consultation when indicated; and to participate in activities contributing to an improved community.

To these core principles have been added a considerable list of ethical advisories, addressing specific questions and aspects of the current practice of medicine. The medical practice acts of some states now list 40 or 50 examples of unprofessional conduct or unethical behavior warranting disciplinary action. The AMA's Council on Ethical and Judicial Affairs publishes its *Current Opinions*,[3] addressing and discussing more than 125 specific ethical issues in medicine—and the list grows each year. In contrast to *Principles of Medical Ethics*, these *Opinions* are advisory, using the word "should" rather than "shall;" however, they are accepted as mandatory by some groups and licensing boards.

The relatively new specialty of biomedical ethics has been created to assist in the interpretation and application of ethical precepts to practical situations, and, as the field has evolved, individual medical specialties have developed and adopted their own oaths, codes of ethics, or codes of conduct.

The field of correctional health care, likewise, has been grappling with the challenging ethical issues it faces. Some of these issues obviously are common to the larger field of health care, such as those involving managed care and the allocation of limited health resources. Others are issues that have special characteristics as a result of the constraints on the delivery of health care in an environment that places extreme limitations on individual patient choice, movement, and confidentiality. Still other ethical issues are unique to the correctional setting, such as body cavity searches and involvement in executions.

Conditioning the development of medical ethics in the correctional setting has been the evolution of penal reform and human rights, in not only the United States but also the world at large. The right of prisoners to humane treatment and adequate health care is recognized in case law in this country and in international covenants such as the United Nations' *Standard Minimum Rules for the Treatment of Prisoners.*[4]

Hardly a day goes by that a clinician in a jail or prison striving to provide inmates with compassionate, quality health care does not face some ethical issue or dilemma. Budgetary restrictions, public and legislative pressures, institutional custodial requirements and influences, and the increasing health care needs of a growing and aging inmate population all conspire to produce ethical complexities and challenges unparalleled elsewhere. In the sections that follow, we explore some of the basic ethical questions that confront correctional health professionals today.

MEDICAL ETHICS IN CORRECTIONS
The Correctional Setting

The primary purpose of jails and prisons is not to provide health care. It is to protect the public by confining those accused or convicted of crimes for specified periods of time. At best, the provision of health care is a support function in most institutions, and, because of this, correctional health professionals often are faced with ethical dilemmas. They are charged with the dual responsibility of serving the needs of the institution as a whole and serving the needs of their patients. Sometimes, these dual responsibilities are at odds with one another, and correctional health professionals must seek ways to compromise with their institutional responsibilities so that the primary obligations to their patients are met.

The competing priorities of correctional needs and care needs are complicated by the absence of clear-cut guidelines governing the ethical conduct of correctional health professionals. Because correctional health care is not only a nascent specialty, but also one that involves many types of health professionals other than physicians, it has been difficult to arrive at a consensus regarding ethical precepts. Recently, the American Correctional Health Services

Association (ACHSA) adopted a code of ethics for its members, and the Society of Correctional Physicians (SCP) adopted the same code with minor changes. The problem, however, is that both organizations are quite small (ACHSA has about a thousand members from various health care disciplines and SCP has about 200 physician members), and neither can claim to speak for the correctional health profession as a whole. Furthermore, neither organization has any mechanism for disciplining violations of these codes or enforcing compliance. In addition, although these codes are helpful as general principles, they are not lengthy or detailed enough to address all the many and varied ethical dilemmas faced almost daily by caregivers working behind bars.

Another organization, the National Commission on Correctional Health Care (NCCHC), has published standards for the management of health services in correctional facilities.[5–7] The NCCHC is a nonprofit 501-c-(3) organization comprised of representatives from 37 professional associations in the fields of law, corrections, and health care. Although some of its standards do address ethical concerns, they are applicable only to those correctional facilities seeking voluntary accreditation by the NCCHC.

Absent specific guidelines for the profession as a whole, it is difficult to provide definitive statements as to what is ethical in a given situation. The best that we can do at this point is to discuss some of the ethical concerns that arise in a correctional setting and provide our opinions as to how these issues should be resolved. To the extent that these issues have been addressed by national organizations, their conclusions will be included in the discussions.

General Ethical Concerns

Some of the ethical concerns that face correctional health professionals also face their colleagues on the outside, but they take on a different twist behind bars. These include the nature of the patient–provider relationship, issues of informed consent and refusal of care, the confidentiality of the patient–provider relationship, the right to die, and implications of managed care.

The nature of the patient–provider relationship. One of the primary factors that differentiates the practice of medicine on the outside from correctional medicine is the lack of choice for either provider or patient on the inside in initiating and maintaining their relationship. Because providers are either employees of a correctional system or working under a contract to provide care, they have no choice about what patients they see.

This is particularly true for the correctional physician who often is the only physician providing care at a particular facility. Regardless of the physician's feelings about the crime committed by an inmate, or the patient's lack of compliance with a prescribed treatment regimen, or the patient's ingratitude for the care provided, or even verbal abuse by the patient toward the provider, the correctional

physician cannot refuse to treat the patient's serious medical needs. To do so would be tantamount to denying care, which is proscribed by the Eighth Amendment to the U.S. Constitution.

Similarly, correctional patients have no choice of provider. Even if they do not trust the physician, or believe that he is incompetent, or believe that he does not like them, inmates seldom are in a position other than to choose between no care or care from a provider with whom they do not have a good relationship.

Because patients and providers are "stuck" with one another, it is imperative that physicians view the individuals they serve as patients rather than inmates. They must be advocates for their patients' health needs and remain neutral in other encounters between correctional staff and inmates. They must put aside any personal prejudices regarding sex and ethnicity, as well as personal feelings regarding the crime with which the individual was charged, and deal solely with the patient's health complaints.

This is, of course, easier said than done. Because of the difficulty, in particular, of setting aside one's feelings about the crimes inmates have committed, some advocates have suggested that correctional health professionals should avoid asking their patients why they are in jail or prison.[8] We generally believe this to be sound advice, while recognizing that, for certain providers such as mental health professionals, the details surrounding an individual's crime, indeed, may be relevant to the treatment provided.

Informed consent and refusal of care. In general, national organizations have adhered to the principle that inmates retain the right to autonomy in their health care decisions. All three sets of NCCHC standards explicitly recognize the inmate's rights to consent to treatment as well as to refuse care.[5–7] Similarly, the codes of ethics of the ACHSA and the SCP also preserve the patient's autonomy regarding health care decisions.

The NCCHC's standards require inmates to consent in writing to any examination, treatment, or procedure that carries some risk to the patient. Written consent is not required for routine encounters without known risks to the patient because the patient's consent is implied when he seeks care. Even in these situations, however, it is important for the provider to explain verbally what will take place so that patients can decide whether they wish to participate.

Although the laws regarding involuntary treatment of a patient may differ among jurisdictions, patients generally cannot be treated against their will unless they are found to be incompetent to make their own decisions *and* the proposed treatment or procedure is deemed necessary to protect the patient or others from harm. Within corrections, however, there has been some case law mandating that a presumably competent inmate be treated, forcibly if necessary, because the inmate's refusal was determined to be for manipulative purposes (e.g., in one case, an inmate refused dialysis because he wanted a transfer to a different institution).[8]

Correctional health professionals also must guard against encouraging inmates to refuse care to either lessen their workload or reduce the expense associated with their services. It is useful to track refusals of care for not only more sophisticated treatments and procedures but also routine services such as intake physicals. In situations in which the number of refusals for specific services is high, it is likely that some staff may be dissuading inmates from participating under the guise of allowing inmates a choice.

Confidentiality of the patient–provider relationship. Maintaining confidentiality of health information is the keystone of the patient–provider relationship. Patients must be able to trust that their physicians will not reveal their secrets regarding health risk behaviors or their particular medical conditions. Physicians must foster their patients' trust so that they can learn the things that will help them to best treat their patients.

The right to confidentiality of one's health information is not absolute, of course, even on the outside. Other providers and third-party payers may require individuals to waive their privacy rights in exchange for a particular service. Additionally, state law may compel a physician to disclose certain information about patients with reportable infectious diseases or about a patient with a mental health condition who has threatened a third party with bodily harm. Barring exceptions such as these, however, confidentiality of health information is preserved on the outside.

On the inside, it is quite a different matter. The fact that correctional facilities are closed societies makes it very difficult to maintain confidentiality of health information. Correctional staff and other inmates alike may surmise something about an individual's health condition simply by observing or hearing which provider an inmate is going to see. An inmate scheduled to see a gynecologist has "female problems," one scheduled for the psychiatrist is "crazy," and the one visiting an infectious disease specialist has HIV. In facilities holding long-term care clinics, inmates and staff soon learn which diseases are treated on which days or which physicians treat which chronic diseases.

Additionally, correctional health professionals are continually pressed by correctional staff for information about their patients, whether it is because the correctional staff simply are curious, or because they are concerned about their own welfare and that of their families if they unknowingly come in contact with inmates with certain health conditions. To complicate matters further, most correctional facilities require health professionals to disclose information about their patients if the failure to do so "threatens the safety and security of the institution."

The problem with such a statement is that it is most often defined after the fact in its breach. Few facilities provide health professionals with specific lists of the types of information they are required to disclose. Sometimes, the choice is simple, such as when an inmate relates information regarding a planned riot or escape or threatens to harm another inmate or staff member. However, what if the individual reveals in the course of a therapeutic encounter that he got drunk or high last night or had sex with another inmate? In the latter case, what if the health professional knows that the inmate with whom the individual had sex has HIV-positive status or has some other communicable disease? What if the inmate tells the physician that he has heard there is a shipment of drugs coming in or that the individual with whom he had sex is a staff member?

Correctional physicians frequently are faced with such ethical dilemmas. On the one hand, if they reveal all the rule violations they hear, inmates will label them as "snitches" and will no longer trust the physicians. On the other hand, if they fail to reveal certain information and this comes to light after an incident, they risk administrative sanctions or, at a minimum, the contempt of their correctional colleagues.

These are not easy choices, and it is difficult to provide exact guidance regarding what is the "right" response in a given situation. For us, the rule of thumb often used is if what the inmates are doing is harming only themselves, we probably would not tell, but if their actions have the potential to harm others, we would tell. In the examples given above, we would not tell the administration that an inmate got high or had sex with another inmate. We would tell about a shipment of drugs coming in and about a staff member having sex with an inmate, because this is an abuse of power. If we knew that the individual with whom the inmate was having sex had an infectious disease, we would probably call in the other party and counsel him regarding this risky behavior or recommend more restrictive housing or both.

Another alternative used when the right path simply is not clear is to reveal the information to the appropriate correctional officials, but not reveal the source of that information.

The NCCHC's standards as well as the codes of ethics of the ACHSA and the SCP require correctional health professionals to control access to health records and health information. As noted above, however, it is not the access to health records that is the problem in prisons, but, rather, it is the access to health information. One of the most common mistakes committed by correctional health professionals is discussing their patients with other colleagues and forgetting who else may overhear. In correctional clinics, there almost always are other patients, correctional staff, or inmate porters present. In a closed society in which there is no anonymity, health professionals must be particularly vigilant in ensuring that they do not reveal patient information in front of others.

The right to die. Although the issues of whether there is a right to die and, if so, what the ethical guidelines for physician involvement should be, still are being debated in the community at large, the management of terminally ill patients poses special ethical dilemmas for the correctional physician. For one thing, correctional physicians must ensure that such patients are truly informed about the choices available to them in terms of continued aggressive treatment vs. palliative relief of symptoms and that they do not push their patients toward hospice care because it is a cheaper alternative. For another, correctional physicians must be honest with their patients regarding the extent to which palliative care truly is available. In many correctional facilities, formularies either prohibit or severely limit the availability of narcotics and other pain medication.

Additionally, correctional physicians may be reluctant to use sufficient pain medication for fear of hastening an individual's death and then being sued. This is a real concern. Inmates are notoriously litigious, as are their families when there is a death behind bars. Although many of these suits do not prevail, the sheer aggravation of litigation may be enough to prevent a physician from providing adequate pain medication for a dying patient.

The physician should discuss these issues with the patient who has an incurable illness before the terminal stage of the illness, allowing plenty of time over several visits to determine the patient's wishes regarding a living will, advance directives, life support measures, do-not-resuscitate orders, and the designation of a durable power of attorney for health care. This is now the standard of care in the outside world and should apply in prisons and jails as well. If these issues are not addressed while the patient is competent to make such decisions, then it is advisable for the physician to involve family members in the decision-making process for terminally ill patients. If there are no interested family members, a patient advocate from the outside or a court-appointed guardian may assist the correctional physician in arriving at the best course of action for preserving the patient's autonomy and dignity as well as the provider's desire to do no harm.[9]

Implications of managed care. Correctional health care programs have not been untouched by the advent of managed care. The cost of care and limited budgets always have been constraints in providing correctional health care, requiring health administrators and physicians to make difficult decisions. However, the relatively recent and steadily increasing presence of private for-profit correctional health care companies has introduced new complexities to medical decision making and new ethical challenges for the practitioner. Consultations and procedures that the practitioner believes are indicated and necessary may be denied by his corporate employers or not covered by the contract. Expensive medications may not be provided or may be contract exclusions, an important consideration in state-of-the-art treatment of HIV infection. As in managed care settings outside prisons and jails, clinical decisions are no longer the sole purview of the attending physician, and correctional health care providers working for companies whose prof-

it margin is paramount need to exercise ethical vigilance in guarding their patients' welfare.

ETHICAL DILEMMAS UNIQUE TO CORRECTIONAL SETTINGS

In addition to the general ethical issues that face all health practitioners, there are certain ethical problems faced by correctional physicians that are unique to the environment in which they work. Some of the more common ones are addressed.

Body Cavity Searches

Periodically, correctional physicians may be asked to search inmates' rectal and/or genital areas for contraband. In other words, they are asked to use their medical skills for nonmedical purposes. Most physicians are reluctant to do so because they know that their actions—should contraband be found—will result in the inmate being punished. On the other hand, they worry that if such tasks are left to correctional staff, the inmate may be seriously injured.

National standards and ethical codes for correctional practitioners generally agree that body cavity searches should not be performed by providers who are in a therapeutic relationship with the inmate. The NCCHC standards state that the services of outside providers should be obtained.[5–7] This advice may be feasible in jails because they usually are located in close proximity to the community they serve. In prisons, however, it may not be practical as a result of their remote location. Additionally, correctional administrators often have trouble understanding why the physicians whose services they pay for cannot perform this task.

In larger facilities, the solution may be to find a correctional practitioner in the same institution who is not in a therapeutic relationship with the inmate. If that is not possible, the next best solution may be to transport the inmate to a neighboring correctional facility. Correctional administrators still may not be happy having to transport the inmate, but at least they will not have to pay for the services of a community physician. The best solution for all concerned with male inmates, however, may be to place the individual in a "dry cell" and let nature take its course.[8]

Collecting Other Information for Forensic Purposes

There are other instances in which correctional providers may be asked to use their medical training for nonmedical purposes. These include performing urinalyses or blood tests to detect the use of alcohol or drugs, performing x-ray scans on inmates to detect contraband or weapons, collecting specimens from inmates for DNA analysis, and performing psychological evaluations of inmates for use in adversarial proceedings or to determine parole eligibility. Such activities are considered unethical under NCCHC standards because they are performed for forensic rather than health purposes and seldom can be said to be in the best interests of the inmate.

Although, arguably, correctional administrators may need the information that such activities produce, again, they represent a conflict of interest for the correctional health professional. In most instances, the ethical approach is to use the services of an outside provider or someone in the same facility who does not play a therapeutic role in the care of the inmate in question.

Participation in Executions

There is probably no ethical issue in correctional health care on which there is greater unanimity than that of participation in executions. Every professional organization that has considered and taken a position on this issue has pronounced such participation unethical. These include, to name a few, the AMA, The American Public Health Association, The American Nurses' Association, the World Medical Association, the SCP, and the NCCHC. Unfortunately, however, laws in almost all of the death penalty states require that a physician attend and pronounce the death. In at least two states, Arizona and Utah, physicians have been successful in amending the law to remove this requirement, but physician participation continues to be widespread, in violation of professional ethics. The issue is gaining attention and importance because of the increasing use of lethal injection as a method of execution, in what has been referred to as the medicalization of the death penalty.[10, 11] The role of the physician, whatever the method, has been to examine the victim to see if he is dead and, if not, to direct that additional lethal solution (or electric current) be administered. As the popular form of execution has shifted from hanging or firing squad to electrocution, gas, and, now, lethal injection, it has become very clear that attending and determining death is a form of participation in the execution process.

The AMA has taken the lead in articulating this issue. A 1980 AMA resolution stated, "An individual's opinion of capital punishment is the personal moral decision of the individual. A physician, as a member of a profession dedicated to preserving life when there is hope of doing so, should not be a participant in a legally authorized execution."[12]

A few years later, the American College of Physicians asked the AMA Council on Ethical and Judicial Affairs to clarify what was included in "participation." The subsequent Council on Ethical and Judicial Affairs report, adopted by the AMA House of Delegates in 1992, states that participation includes:

- Prescribing or administering tranquilizers and other psychotropic agents and medications that are part of the execution procedure.
- Monitoring vital signs on site or remotely (including monitoring electrocardiograms).
- Attending or observing an execution as a physician.

- Rendering technical advice regarding execution.

When the method is lethal injection, participation also includes:

- Selecting injection sites.
- Starting IV lines as a port for a lethal injection device.
- Prescribing, preparing, administering, or supervising injection drugs or their doses or types.
- Inspecting, testing, or maintaining lethal injection devices.
- Consulting with or supervising lethal injection personnel.

The report also specifies what actions do not constitute physician participation:

- Testifying with regard to competence to stand trial, testifying with regard to relevant medical evidence during trial, or testifying with regard to medical aspects of aggravating or mitigating circumstances during the penalty phase of a capital case.
- *Certifying* death, provided that the condemned has been declared dead by another individual.
- Witnessing an execution in a totally nonprofessional capacity.
- Witnessing an execution at the specific voluntary request of the condemned individual, provided that the physician observes the execution in a nonprofessional capacity.
- Relieving the acute suffering of a condemned individual while awaiting execution, including providing tranquilizers at the specific voluntary request of the condemned individual to help relieve pain or anxiety in anticipation of the execution.

Agreement is lacking among psychiatrists, however, regarding their ethical responsibilities to death row inmates. Many believe that treating mentally incompetent condemned inmates is ethical because the main purpose is to relieve symptoms, even though the outcome may be the restoration of competence to be executed. Likewise, testifying as to competence to be executed is a controversial issue among psychiatrists, although it seems clear that it would be unethical for such testimony to be provided by the treating psychiatrist. The mental health professional societies are grappling with these issues and may reach consensus. Addressing the ethical responsibilities of correctional psychiatrists, the NCCHC has issued the following position statement:

> … the determination of whether an inmate is "competent for execution" should be made by an independent expert and not by any health care professional regularly in the employ of, or under contract to provide health care with, the correctional institution or system holding the inmate. This requirement does not diminish the responsibility of correctional health care personnel to treat any mental illness of death row inmates.[13]

The Use of Restraints

Occasionally, a patient may require the application of therapeutic restraints to prevent harm to self or others. There is no problem with physicians ordering restraints for therapeutic purposes as long as they follow generally accepted guidelines on the type to be used, the duration of use, and the frequency of the monitoring of patients in restraints. In correctional facilities, however, restraints also are used by correctional staff. Correctional health providers should not be involved in the application of restraints for nonmedical purposes except to monitor the health status of those so confined. This is consistent with NCCHC standards, which also require health staff to notify the correctional administration if they determine that an individual is being restrained in an unnatural position or one that could jeopardize his health.

Witnessing the Use of Force

In the past, some health staff were asked to serve as witnesses when correctional staff were engaged in planned actions involving force against inmates such as cell extractions. Presumably, the reason was to have a neutral witness who could testify that the force used was necessary and not excessive. Some commentators have suggested that this presents a potential ethical conflict for correctional health professionals, although the issue was not well settled.[8] With the advent of video cameras, however, this is seldom an issue any longer. For liability purposes, most institutional rules require that use-of-force incidents be taped, which obviates the necessity for a witness not involved in security.

When there is time, we recommend that correctional staff alert medical staff regarding a planned use of force so that someone will be available to check the inmate and provide care as needed. In some cases, such as with mental patients, the health staff may be able to intervene and, thus, avert a use-of-force incident by correctional staff.

Inmate Discipline and Segregation

In the correctional setting, segregation generally refers to a situation in which inmates are confined to their cells for all but an hour or so per day and not allowed to mix with the general population of inmates. Usually, there are two types of custodial segregation: administrative segregation, which is generally a long-term stay prompted by an individual's dangerous behavior or high-custody level or by the inmate's wish to be placed in protective custody, and disciplinary segregation, which is usually of shorter duration (e.g., 30 days or less) and a consequence of an inmate's failure to follow institutional rules.

Under most circumstances, correctional health staff should refrain from participating in the disciplinary process (e.g., "writing up" inmates or testifying against them), and they should never be a part of the disciplinary committee that determines sanctions. The latter would clearly compromise their role as neutral, caring health professionals. There are a few exceptions, however, when it would be appropriate for health staff to testify in a disciplinary hearing. One is when the health provider or another individual has been

the victim of violence. The other is when the provider believes that the inmate's rule violation may have been prompted by a medical or mental condition.[14]

Once an inmate has been placed in segregation for whatever reason, national standards specify that health staff should make rounds daily for those in disciplinary segregation, and at least three times per week for those in administrative segregation.[5-7, 15] The purpose of these rounds is to ensure that the inmates' health is not deteriorating because of sensory deprivation or because of the actions of correctional staff.

Health Care Workers as Correctional Staff

There is at least one prison system (the federal system) that still requires health care workers, including physicians, to be trained as correctional officers, and this training includes participating in riot control exercises and qualifying on the firing range. In other departments of corrections, such as California's and in some jails, some health care workers are cross-trained as correctional staff and are expected to work in both capacities. The belief is that all staff are, first and foremost, correctional staff and that the best way to teach this is to have all staff share the same organizational culture.[16]

We believe this is the wrong approach. It is difficult enough in correctional facilities for health staff to resist being co-opted by security staff. Correctional health professionals constantly must balance the needs of their patients against the needs of the institution, but training them as correctional officers tips the scales too far in the direction of a correctional role. We do believe that health professionals working in the correctional setting need to be aware of security issues and need to adhere to security rules; however, in the event of a riot, an escape, or a hostage situation, we would rely on our correctional colleagues rather than health staff trained as correctional workers.

Inmates Engaging in Hunger Strikes

Although a rare event in prisons, there are probably few other situations that present such a severe ethical dilemma for correctional physicians than that of a prisoner who hunger-strikes. In most instances, such individuals are mentally competent and have undertaken such a drastic measure for political or manipulative purposes. At the core of the physician's concern is whether to respect the inmate's autonomy of decisions regarding his own body, even to the point of death, or to intercede by force-feeding the inmate. Which represents the greater good?

This is an area in which there is no clear consensus among correctional health professionals as to which is the right path, and there is no guidance from national standards. Some physicians are on the side of force-feeding inmates, which is the position recommended by the ACHSA. Others are on the side of allowing the inmate to die.[17, 18] Regardless of the ultimate outcome in such cases, most physicians would agree that the inmate's health status should be monitored daily and that the inmate should be informed continually of his health status and the impending consequences of continuing to refuse nourishment. In the absence of a consensus among correctional physicians as to the ethical management of an inmate who engages in a hunger strike, the best advice we can give at this point is to seek guidance from the courts. The court may well appoint an outside guardian to assist in determining what is best for the inmate as well as what is best for the institution and its staff.[8]

Charging Inmates Fees for Care

A relatively new phenomenon in correctional health care is to charge inmates a fee (co-pay) for health services delivered in the facility as well as by outside providers. This practice is gaining ground in both jails[19] and prisons.[20] Proponents argue that imposition of a co-pay for health care will cut down on inmates abuse of the sick call system and will make them more fiscally responsible. Those opposed to charging inmates for care believe that imposing a fee for health services in the correctional setting is tantamount to denying access to care to inmates who are basically without financial resources and that it results in a two-tier system.[21]

In its position statement, the NCCHC states that it is opposed to the establishment of fee-for-service programs in correctional facilities that restrict patients' access to care. Recognizing that many facilities already have implemented such programs, however, NCCHC has issued a series of guidelines for establishing and managing co-pay programs to ensure that access to needed care is not blocked. Among those important to correctional health care providers are the requirements that inmates be charged only for services they initiate and not those required by the institution, such as intake screening, that the assessment of a charge be made only after the care is rendered, that health professionals not be involved in collecting the fees, that inmates not be denied care because of a record of nonpayment or their current inability to pay, and that continuation of a fee-for-service program should be contingent on evidence that it does not impede inmates' access to needed care.[22]

Sharing Health Information With Correctional Staff

To make good management decisions regarding housing, work, or program assignments, our correctional colleagues often need health information about inmates. From time to time, they also need information about inmates' health status to protect their own health or that of their families. The best way to provide such information and still protect the inmate's right to confidentiality is to specify any restrictions or precautions that correctional staff should take into account but not to reveal the inmate's specific diagnosis.

For example, the physician could specify that a patient needs a lower bunk, but not that he is epileptic, or that an inmate should not work in a job involving high tempera-

tures, not that the inmate is mentally ill and receiving psychotropic medication. Similarly, correctional staff should be told that respiratory precautions should be used when handling or transporting an inmate with tuberculosis rather than that an inmate has the disease.

CONCLUSIONS

Most health professionals who work in the correctional setting believe that they are providing an important public health service to a distinctly disadvantaged group. They strive hard to balance the institution's interests with the best interests of their patients, but this is not an easy task. It is made more difficult by the lack of an agreed-on code of ethics for the profession as a whole. We urge our correctional health colleagues to work toward the establishment of such a code. Until then, each of us has to rely on our own moral compass to resolve ethical dilemmas and on the primacy of our relationship with our patients.

REFERENCES

1. Anno BJ, Dubler NN: Preface, Special forum: Ethical issues in correctional health care. *J Prison Jail Health* 11:57–59, 1992.
2. *Principles of Medical Ethics. Code of Medical Ethics, Current Opinions with Annotation.* Chicago, American Medical Association, 1996-1997.
3. Council on Ethical and Judicial Affairs: *Code of Medical Ethics, Current Opinions With Annotations.* Chicago, American Medical Association, 1994.
4. *Standard Minimum Rules for the Treatment of Prisoners.* New York, United Nations. 1995.
5. *Standards for Health Services in Jails.* Chicago, National Commission on Correctional Health Care, 1996.
6. *Standards for Health Services in Juvenile Detention and Confinement Facilities.* Chicago, National Commission on Correctional Health Care, 1995.
7. *Standards for Health Services in Prisons.* Chicago, National Commission on Correctional Health Care, 1997.
8. Dubler NN, Anno BJ: Ethical considerations and the interface with custody, in Anno BJ (ed): *Prison Health Care: Guidelines for the Management of an Adequate Delivery System.* Chicago, National Commission on Correctional Health Care, 1991, pp 53–69.
9. Ventres WB, Spencer SS: Doctor–patient communication about resuscitation: "Have you signed an advance directive?" *J Fam Pract* 33:21–23, 1991.
10. Bayer R: Lethal injections and capital punishment: Medicine in the service of the state. *J Prison Jail Health* 4:7–15, 1984.
11. The American College of Physicians, Human Rights Watch, The National Coalition to Abolish the Death Penalty, and Physicians for Human Rights: *Breach of Trust: Physician Participation in Executions in the United States.* Philadelphia, American College of Physicians, 1994.
12. American Medical Association: Physician participation in capital punishment. *JAMA* 270:365–368, 1993.
13. National Commission on Correctional Health Care: Position statement—Competency for execution. *J Correctional Health Care* 2:75, 1995.
14. Rold WJ: Consideration of mental health factors in inmate discipline. *J Prison Jail Health* 11:41–49, 1992.
15. *Standards for Adult Correctional Institutions,* ed 3. Laurel, Md, American Correctional Association, 1990.

16. Case 4: Correctional training for health professionals. *J Prison Jail Health* 11:86–97, 1992.

17. Case 1: The hunger striker. *J Prison Jail Health* 11:63–73, 1992.

18. Miller WP: The hunger-striking prisoner. *J Prison Jail Health* 6:40–61, 1986–1987.

19. Weiland C: Fee-for-service programs: A literature review and results of a national survey. *J Correctional Health Care* 3:145–158, 1996.

20. Gipson FT, Pierce EA: Current trends in state inmate user programs for health services. *J Correctional Health Care* 3:159–178, 1996.

21. Harrison BP: In the matter of correctional facilities charging prisoners for health services. *J Correctional Health Care* 3:109–125, 1996.

22. National Commission on Correctional Health Care: Position statement: Charging inmates a fee for health care services. *J Correctional Health Care* 3:179–184, 1996.

Section Two

Medical Issues
in Corrections

5

Intake Evaluation in Prisons and Jails

Robert L. Cohen, M.D.

In medical school, physicians have traditionally been taught that the initial history and physical examination are critically important in the care of the patient. This first clinical encounter sets the tone for the medical and professional relationship. A careful, sensitive, comprehensive inquiry, covering all areas, while centering on the critical issues of concern to the patient, is often the key to diagnosis. We are taught to be sensitive to a patient's perceptions, alert to their fears and anxieties, and conscious of the effects of class, cultural, and gender differences on their perception of illness and their description of symptoms.

We often learn, instead, to discount the patient's concerns and fail to understand the depths of our own prejudices. Everyone working within jails or prisons should, on a regular basis, close their eyes and imagine the cell door clanging shut, listen to the grating of metal on metal, and experience the claustrophobia and the fear.

The initial medical evaluation upon admission to a jail or a prison should similarly be sensitive to the prisoner patient's fears and anxieties, and seek to sympathetically understand the prisoner patient's health status. The tone of the initial interview and physical examination is crucial to subsequent clinical encounters. The establishment of clinical trust in the jail or prison setting begins by demonstrating, through gesture and word, by handshake and courteous introduction, that the clinician has the patient's best interests in mind.

Contrast that approach with the usual medical intake in many detention facilities. Newly arrested prisoners, hungry and tired, crammed into dirty cells (known traditionally as "bullpens") with minimal (often public) toilet facilities, wait and wait for their intake screening. Sometimes the initial medical intake is performed by security personnel. In prisons, or larger jails, a nurse's aide, LPN, or medical assistant might perform the initial intake. The first encounter with the medical system may take place in a nonmedical area, and the questioner may show little or no interest in the answers to intimate medical questions. There is a minimal physical examination, and following receiving screening the prisoner is thrown back into the bullpen.

Functionally, the initial medical encounter in a jail has some similarity to an emergency department encounter. There is an initial triage, where vital signs are assessed and acute medical problems are evaluated and treated. This should be followed by a more detailed evaluation within a reasonable time. In a prison, where intake is scheduled, occurs during weekdays, and is generally of low, or controlled volume, the initial encounter should be an initial comprehensive history and physical examination. Whether in a jail or a prison, the tone of future encounters is strongly influenced by the initial meeting of the prisoner and the medical staff. The trust necessary for an effective clinical relationship can be established or destroyed by this first meeting. The independence of the medical staff and their commitment to the prisoner's health can be clearly demonstrated at this time. Unfortunately, the subservience or collaboration of medical staff (and control of medical practice) by the prison or jail administration can also be clearly conveyed.

The purposes of the medical intake include:
* The identification of medical problems requiring urgent diagnosis and/or treatment;
* Prompt referral of prisoners with chronic diseases for treatment;
* The rapid identification of infectious diseases, especially tuberculosis, which require treatment and/or isolation;
* The identification and treatment of mental illness, particularly suicidal ideation;
* The identification of prisoners at risk for drug and/or alcohol withdrawal and the prompt initiation of detoxification for these syndromes;
* The assignment of medically appropriate housing for inmates with medical or mental health problems.

In this chapter, important elements of the intake screening and health evaluation are discussed. Common problems with medical intake are reviewed, and, where possible, solutions are suggested.

THE SETTING

The intake medical screening should take place in a medical area used only for medical purposes. The setting should be clean, quiet, and allow for confidential discussion. When this is intrinsically difficult, because the physical plant prevents visual and aural privacy, medical staff should insist that an appropriate area be established. Security staff should not be present in the room, and prisoners should not be routinely shackled. When prisoners are shackled, medical staff should request that shackles be removed for the purpose of the medical examination, including the medical history. There are, of course, exceptions to this rule, but they should be treated as exceptional. Shackling during medical evaluation should never be routine.

The prisoner and the interviewer/examiner should each be seated comfortably. Hand washing facilities must be available. A clean examination table and functioning medical equipment including thermometers, sphygmomanometer (with appropriate size cuffs), and diagnostic sets for examination of the eyes, ears, and pharynx are required. The interviewer should not know the prisoner's charge —

this information will not be helpful to the initial medical evaluation, and can be prejudicial.

Newly admitted prisoners should be kept in an isolated and designated intake housing area until the intake evaluation is finished, and especially until infectious disease screening for active tuberculosis has been completed. Efficient organization of the intake process should result in all prisoners being assigned to appropriate non-intake housing within 72 to 96 hours after admission. Significant delays beyond this time reflect problems in the intake process, which should be identified and resolved.

To assure the integrity of the medical intake process and to secure and maintain the cooperation of the security staff, no prisoner should be discharged from the intake housing area until medical screening is complete. Adherence to this principle is an essential component in any jail or prison's tuberculosis control program.

Medical Intake in Jails and Prisons

There are epidemiologic differences in the populations entering prisons and jails. Specific categories of individuals are more likely to be arrested, and are more likely to have certain kinds of acute medical problems. For example, homeless persons would have a greater incidence of mental illness, infestations, and tuberculosis, while prostitutes would have a greater incidence of venereal diseases. As a consequence, screening for mental illness, suicidality, and venereal diseases should be enhanced in the jail medical intake program.

Serious acute trauma incurred before, during, or after arrest is much more likely to be seen during jail intake, and the capacity for rapid diagnosis and treatment (or referral) of traumatic injuries should be part of the jail intake capability. Newly detained prisoners are more likely to be under the influence of alcohol or drugs, and to be at risk for drug and alcohol withdrawal. Jail intake should focus on identification of prisoners at risk for withdrawal and should initiate observation and treatment promptly.

One-third to one-half of newly sentenced prisoners arrive at prison directly from jail, where they have often had acute problems stabilized. Prisoners in state or federal prisons are somewhat older than prisoners in jails, and will, therefore, have a higher prevalence of serious chronic medical problems such as diabetes, hypertension and other cardiovascular diseases, and chronic lung disease. These kinds of chronic medical problems are, of course, present in prisoners with short stays as well as those with long stays.

Local epidemiologic factors, such as high prevalence of untreated sexually transmitted diseases, should guide local practice to assure appropriate case finding through screening. However, the presence of epidemiologic variation should not be used to decrease the scope of the intake evaluation. For sexually transmitted diseases and tuberculosis, intake screening in jails and prisons has a substantial positive public health impact. Where possible, close liaison with local public health authorities should be established. Registries for sexually transmitted diseases and tuberculosis are maintained by public health departments, and can serve to identify patients with active tuberculosis, and to interpret positive syphilis serology test results.

The National Commission on Correctional Health Care (NCCHC) has expressed concerns regarding the ability of small jails without full time medical staff to meet its health standards for receiving screening. They have codified this concern in the 1996 Jail Standards by allowing security staff to conduct "receiving screening."[1] This is unsatisfactory. Other than in emergency situations, medical information should be conveyed directly from prisoner to health professional. This is a fundamental principle of health care, and it should be respected in health care programs in jails. Should hospital security personnel make up for nursing shortages by conducting initial triage in a hospital emergency department? No more than security personnel should be conducting receiving screening in a jail.

The NCCHC allows for officer screening, thereby recognizing the serious dilemma posed by the problem of providing intake medical evaluation in small jails that do not have full time medical staff. In such cases, for jails where the population is less than 25, an alternative mechanism for medical intake must be developed. Possible approaches include:
- A contract with a nearby health care facility to provide off-site medical intake screening on a daily basis.
- A contract with a nearby county jail provide 24-hour medical coverage to perform medical intake screening.
- A contract with a nearby health provider to provide on-site on-call medical intake screening as needed.
- Regionalization of small rural jails, which permits a higher level of screening.

Initial Screening in Jails (Receiving Screening)

The medical intake procedure in prisons is often a comprehensive examination. However, the medical intake procedure in jails is usually a limited intake screening process, also known as "receiving screening." This approach delays the initial clinical evaluation (including the physical examination) by replacing it with a triage process designed to identify prisoners with urgent or emergent medical or mental health needs. By design, up to 14 days may pass in a jail before any physical examination occurs. The completed process may involve a security staff or non-registered nurse performing the screening, another nurse taking the medical history, and a different practitioner, usually a physician or a physician assistant, conducting the physical examination. The NCCHC 1996 jail standard requires that the health assessment be completed within 14 days; the NCCHC 1997 prison standards require that the health assessment be completed within 7 days. The American Public Health Association also requires that the physical examination is completed within 7 days. These encounters are each incom-

plete and inefficient. This process encourages fragmentation and discourages good medical practice. It is not possible for a physician to perform a comprehensive physical examination without the benefit of taking the medical history, yet this is normal in most jail and prison health programs.

Although receiving screening is supposed to involve some physical observation, in practice there is rarely any attempt at physical examination, except for some institutions which include vital signs (usually temperature, pulse, and blood pressure) as part of the initial receiving screening.

The receiving screening intake physical examination, must, at a minimum:
- Detect prisoners in drug withdrawal or at risk of drug withdrawal;
- Identify prisoners with painful conditions;
- Identify prisoners with chronic diseases requiring ongoing treatment;
- Identify prisoners with mental health problems, particularly severe depression and suicidal ideation, who require emergency or urgent evaluation; and
- Be conducted in a clean, private space with visual and aural privacy, and with hand washing facilities in the examination area, with appropriate equipment (light, blood pressure cuff, thermometer, clock, finger stick glucose determination) at hand.

Because of the separation of receiving screening from the health assessment, prisoners with acute or chronic medical problems may go undetected and untreated for 1 to 2 weeks.

Physical Examination

The intake physical examination must be done respectfully in a private setting. It should be conducted as soon as possible after admission, and is part of a comprehensive admission history and physical. The elements of the physical examination will not be detailed here, but the physical examination should be comprehensive, including examination of the external urogenital system.

It has been suggested that comprehensiveness is a less important criteria for physical examination than age and disease appropriateness. For example, it would not be appropriate to screen all incoming detainees, or sentenced prisoners for glaucoma, because this disease is exceedingly rare in individuals under 40 years of age. However, with regard to conducting the physical examination of a incoming prisoner, and, particularly, for a physician supervising other clinicians in this task, comprehensiveness should be stressed. I believe it is an error to "focus" on age-specific health problems determined epidemiologically to justify not examining the entire person. The complete physical examination takes only a limited amount of time, well within the amount of time allocated for intake examinations in prisons and jails. The physical examination should be done systematically, and if done routinely, regularly, and responsibly, will only require 10 to 15 minutes, particularly if vital signs have been reliably obtained by the nursing staff.

Activities Which Are Not Part of Medical Intake

Security staff commonly request their medical providers to assist in non-medical functions. It is often difficult for physicians and other staff to refuse these requests. Close relationships develop between medical and security staff and cooperation is essential to the successful operation of the medical program; refusing requests for assistance creates significant conflict.

The physical examination should not be a forensic examination, nor should it be part of the security process. The following is an incomplete list of functions which should not be performed as part of the intake evaluation:

- Body cavity searches are not part of the medical examination; medical staff should refuse to perform body cavity searches.
- Forensic examination of hair or blood, when required, should be obtained by persons who are not part of the jail or prison medical staff.
- Medical staff should not evaluate prisoners at intake for their suitability to be exposed to stun gun type weapons or noxious chemical agents like tear gas. In 1997, the New York City Health and Hospitals Corporation requested this service from bidders for a contract covering medical services for detained prisoners on Rikers Island and at the Manhattan House of Detention for Men.
- Testing for HIV infection.

Medical staff should be instructed to refuse these requests. The leadership of the medical program should educate all staff members and correctional personnel about the reasons for this refusal.

Intake Laboratory and Diagnostic Studies

Most detained prisoners remain in jail less than 2 weeks, while most prisoners in state and federal institutions are locked up for an average of 2 years. It is, therefore, reasonable to differentiate the laboratory and diagnostic studies used to screen for medical problems in these populations based on projected length of stay, as well as demographic variables, particularly age and sex.

The initial medical examination is designed to identify patients with acute and chronic medical and mental health problems that require evaluation and treatment. Laboratory evaluation of newly detained prisoners should include:

- Rapid serologic test for syphilis, with confirmation test to differentiate false-positive test results;
- PPD implantation and/or chest radiograph (see chapter on tuberculosis screening);
- PAP test (cervical cytology) and chlamydia/gonorrhea screening with gene probe for rapid detection and treatment of cervicitis;
- Urinalysis including urethral leukocyte esterase screening or urethral swabs with gene probe for urethritis in males[2] urethral swabs for chlamydia/gonorrhea screening with gene probe;
- Urine pregnancy test;
- Electrocardiogram for prisoners older than 40 (the ECG does not have a significant yield as a screening test, but is useful for comparison with later ECGs obtained because of chest pain). Blacks are incarcerated at rates far in excess of their representation in the population at large. A recent study reported that except for the 75-84 year group, black men had the highest cardiac death rates in all age groups compared to Hispanic and white men.[3]

Additional laboratory testing should be part of the intake examination for sentenced prisoners, or for detained prisoners whose stay exceeds 3 months. These tests include:

- CBC and SMA-20 or equivalent.
- Hepatitis antibody screening for Hepatitis B.
- Screening for Hepatitis C for prisoners with abnormal liver function tests.

Screening for HIV infection should not be part of the required intake examination. When HIV testing is performed in a jail or prison, results should be available anonymously if requested by the prisoner. Testing for HIV should only be performed with appropriate individual counseling and specific informed consent by the prisoner. It is particularly important that prisoners with known HIV infection not have their ongoing antiviral treatment interrupted — this may result in the development of viral resistance and treatment failure. Antiviral medications should be routinely available for prisoners receiving treatment for HIV infection. Additionally, a program of voluntary testing and counseling must be linked to prompt initiation of antiretroviral therapy.

Because of the serious sequelae of Hepatitis B infection, and because of its high prevalence among prisoners, a program of Hepatitis B screening and vaccination should be established for prisoners as well as security and medical staff in jails and prison.

Importance of Screening at Central Lockup for Large Urban Detention Systems

In certain large cities, including New York City and Philadelphia, arrested persons are kept in a pre-detention facility while bail determinations are made. In New York City this facility is called "Central Booking," in Philadelphia it is called the Police Lockup. During this period prisoners are still in the custody of the police, and have not yet been remanded to the local correction department.

Several years ago, a friend, walking in a major U.S. city, was arrested in a "sweep." Upon arrival at Central Booking, those arrested were asked if they had any medical problems. They were also advised that their medical problems would be addressed, but would result in a significant delay in their "processing." No one made anything known that day.

Other solutions could be imagined and have been implemented. In New York and Philadelphia, medical personnel screen all prisoners in the central lock-up for acute medical problems and to assure continuity of medical care for patients with significant chronic medical conditions. Prisoners with diabetes need access to insulin, and prisoners with hypertension must have their blood pressure controlled. A medical screening system in a central lockup should be based upon a medical form, and copies of this form should be forwarded to the detention facility for each prisoner who is not released directly from the lockup. Additionally, significant and/or time critical medical information should be directly conveyed from the health provider at the lockup to the health provider at the detention facility by phone and/or facsimile. Critical medical information should be relayed directly from provider to provider, with appropriate chart notation.

Recommendations for Early Comprehensive Intake Medical Evaluation

Based upon substantial experience in reviewing systems of medical care in prisons and jails, the NCCHC standards are insufficient for the prompt identification of persons with significant medical problems, including: chronic diseases requiring treatment, diagnosis of alcohol and narcotic withdrawal, and identification of prisoners with serious mental health problems requiring urgent or emergent psychiatric referral. Problems result from the fragmentation of the process. Too many different practitioners are involved in the process, and built-in delays extend a process which should be completed within twenty-four hours to one which may take two weeks by design. The following suggestions will improve the quality of the intake procedure substantially:

- In large urban jails with centralized police lock-up (central booking), a medical screening process should take place. This process should contain the elements previously recommended, in addition to the requirements identified by the NCCHC in its "Receiving Screening" standard, with the critical exception that the screening should be conducted only by health personnel, not by security staff.
- Security staff should not be part of the medical receiving or intake process in any jail or prison setting.
- The intake history and physical examination should be performed by the same individual. This will dramatically improve the quality of the physical examination. It will be more efficient by combining the three separate encounters, the receiving screening, the (traditional) nursing history, and the physical examination, into one process. Combining these medical encounters at the beginning of incarceration will prevent delays in identification of serious medical and mental health problems.
- Diagnostic testing at intake should include a screening chest radiograph in jails or prisons, unless there is a

demonstrated low incidence of tuberculosis and HIV infection.
- Sexually transmitted disease screening should make use of rapid testing methods for syphilis, gonorrhea, and chlamydia to provide early diagnosis and treatment.

Infectious Disease Screening

In practice, infectious disease screening means identification of cases of active pulmonary tuberculosis. This is critically important: tuberculosis spreads rapidly in the closed environment of a prison or jail (see chapter on tuberculosis). Recent tuberculosis epidemics in jails and prisons with multiple deaths of correctional staff and prisoners have prompted greater attention to this element of receiving screening.[4–6]

The recommendations for screening chest radiographs for incoming detainees are controversial. However, recent research has provided strong evidence that can be valuable in the identification of prisoners with active tuberculosis who would not be identified with standard PPD screening.

Studies in Chicago at the Cook County Jail,[7] and at the Manhattan House of Detention in New York City,[8] have demonstrated that case findings for active tuberculosis are significantly enhanced by routine screening chest radiographs. A study of tuberculosis transmission on Rikers Island demonstrated significant nosocomial spread of tuberculosis in a jail with a well-developed PPD testing program.[9] This study demonstrated that the incidence of new cases of active tuberculosis was directly proportional to the amount of time the individual was housed on Rikers Island. These findings are particularly important for populations at increased risk for HIV infection because:

- The risk of active tuberculosis for prisoners with HIV infection is many times greater than that for prisoners without HIV;
- The incidence of anergy and resultant false-negative PPD results is very high in patients with HIV.[10]

It is, therefore, strongly recommended that a system of PPD screening as well as a program of routine screening chest radiographs be implemented in all large and medium size jails, and in all prisons. Patients with PPD-positive results without active tuberculosis should be offered INH chemoprophylaxis unless there is a contraindication, such as diabetes, age over 35, or chronic liver disease. Prisons or jails in low tuberculosis incidence areas with low incidence of HIV infection may choose to perform PPD testing only, with screening radiographs reserved for symptomatic prisoners.

Unfortunately, neither the CDC nor the NCCHC recommend PPD screening and/or chest radiograph on intake for all prisoners admitted to all detention facilities. This is a debatable policy. Tuberculosis has been endemic in selected populations in the United States for the past 50 years, with outbreaks in selected populations. Jails and prisons are epicenters of this life-threatening infection. Fortunately, and in large measure because of the PPD test and the appropriate use of screening chest radiographs, tuberculosis is detectable, preventable, and treatable. All jails and prisons should use PPD tests on newly admitted prisoners at the time of initial intake into the facility.

Much more difficult, but, of course, much more important, is that there be a highly effective system that assures that all implanted PPDs are read appropriately, and followed up according to a carefully developed protocol (see the chapter on Tuberculosis as well as the chapter on Tuberculosis screening).

Mental Health Screening

The purpose of mental health screening is threefold:
- Identification of suicidal and psychotic prisoners in need of immediate treatment and special observation;
- Identification of prisoners with chronic mental illness in need of continuing treatment;
- Providing urgent and emergent psychiatric consultation and appropriate housing for prisoners with serious mental health problems.

Several elements are necessary for effective mental health screening. Qualified professional staff involved in receiving screening must be trained in identification of mental health problems by mental health professionals. Protocols for the identification and referral of suicidal and psychotic prisoners must be used. There must be mental health observation areas identified within the jail or prison for housing psychotic or suicidal prisoners. These areas must be suicide-proof. They must afford the possibility of continuous observation by security and/or professional staff.

Common, avoidable problems in mental health screening are:
- substantial delays for referrals to mental health staff for prisoners in need of emergent and urgent psychiatric consultation due to inadequate supply of mental health staff;
- lack of appropriate areas for mental observation;
- lack of integration of the medical and mental health record.

Women's Health

Receiving screening as well as health assessment for women require careful attention to obstetric and gynecologic history. Women prisoners must be questioned regarding their last menstrual period, methods of birth control used, and obstetrical history. Infectious disease screening for women must include a pap test, looking for early signs of cervical cancer, particularly the presence of human papilloma virus infection, as well as cervical screening for chlamydia and gonorrhea, and serum testing for syphilis. A urine screening test for pregnancy must be part of the intake examination.

There are an estimated 4 million cases of genital chlamydial infection in the United States each year; the highest rates of chlamydial cervicitis in women are among sexually active adolescents and women between the ages of 20 and 25.[11] In 1988, on Rikers Island, 27% of women entering the Correctional Institution for Women had chlamydia infection of the cervix.[12] Monitoring of chlamydia detection rates will provide an excellent quality screen for intake health assessment of women prisoners. Low rates would suggest that claimed pelvic examinations are not being done, or that cervical screening is not being done correctly.

Because of the prevalence of significant obstetric and gynecological issues for women in prison, the careful history and physical examination, including pelvic examination, pap test, and chlamydia and gonorrhea screening, at least twice the time is required for the intake evaluation of a woman, compared with a male prisoner. This increased staffing need should be included in program and in budget planning.

Detoxification

Mass incarceration has characterized the approach to illegal behavior for the past 20 years. During that period, the prison and jail population in the United States has increased more than 400%. One reason for this unprecedented increase in the number of incarcerated persons has been the ever-escalating war on drugs, wherein hundreds of addicted men and women are arrested and imprisoned each year.

The identification of prisoners who are in withdrawal from alcohol or drugs or who are at risk for withdrawal requires a sympathetic medical staff, and a commitment on the part of medical and security personnel that prisoners will not withdraw from drugs cold turkey. Carefully designed medical protocols for the identification and treatment of alcohol and drug withdrawal must be implemented in every jail and prison. Initiation of treatment, duration of treatment, and type of treatment must be medically sound and consistent. Initiation of treatment should not be based on an individual's practitioner's feelings about drugs or alcohol, or on whim.

Alcohol withdrawal can be life-threatening, and all patients at risk for alcohol withdrawal should be closely observed. Patients in minor withdrawal can be treated with observation and benzodiazepines; patients with severe alcohol withdrawal syndromes require hospitalization. Vital signs must be monitored at intake screening for all prisoners to identify prisoners in acute alcohol withdrawal. Vital signs must be monitored periodically for prisoners being treated for alcohol withdrawal or being observed for impending withdrawal.

Narcotic withdrawal is rarely life-threatening, but can be severe, especially if the prisoner has been addicted to high doses of methadone in a methadone maintenance treatment program. Withdrawal from narcotics can be accomplished, by protocol, with the judicious use of benzodiazepenes, anticholinergics, and clonidine. The use of decreasing doses of long-acting narcotics, such as methadone, is medically preferable. This may require special DEA licensure. Methadone detoxification for heroin addicts can be safely done beginning with a dose of 20 mg and gradually decreasing the dose over 7 days. Prisoners receiving methadone in methadone maintenance programs should be detoxified much more slowly. A successful regimen begins with a dose of 40 mg of methadone that is gradually decreased over 21 days. In either situation, post withdrawal treatment of insomnia is necessary. Pregnant women on methadone maintenance should be maintained on their medication.

REFUSAL OF INTAKE EXAMINATION

In rare cases, prisoners refuse to allow all or part of the intake examination. Prisoners who refuse the intake tuberculosis screening are sometimes placed in an administrative or punitive medical quarantine status. The medical staff should have a rational approach to this situation.

It is important to have policies in place that will limit the number of prisoners who refuse to allow intake medical evaluation, and that will limit the amount of time that prisoners have to spend in segregation status. All prisoners who are placed in segregation status for refusal of medical intake examination should be interviewed at least daily by a health professional, and every few days by a physician. Daily observation of the prisoner's health status, particularly the presence or absence of any signs of tuberculosis (cough, sweats, fever, appetite, weight loss, shortness of breath) should be noted in the medical chart.

Prisoners may refuse the PPD test for religious reasons; they should be given the opportunity to have a chest radiograph and allowed to refuse the PPD. Prisoners who manifest no evidence of fever, cough, or any infectious disease and who refuse PPD and chest radiograph, should be released from segregation within a reasonable time when it has been established that they pose no risk to the rest of the population. It can, of course, be extremely difficult to make this judgment. The decision to release from medical quarantine should only be made by a physician. Fortunately, enforced medical quarantine for failure to participate in medical intake is almost always a short-term issue. Because it is particularly frustrating for medical staff, extra effort should be made to assure that the quarantined prisoner is counseled and not made to feel that his health is at risk because (s)he has alienated the medical staff by refusing to cooperate.

QUALITY IMPROVEMENT IN INTAKE SCREENING

Strategies for assessment of the quality of intake screening and for improving it are essential. There are different approaches to quality improvement. The chapter by Shansky and Schiff in this volume specifically addresses these issues. In addition to the continuous quality improve-

ment approach recommended by Shansky and Schiff, the following sentinel events should be tracked closely to identify problems in the intake process:

- Active tuberculosis cases diagnosed after initial intake screening was negative;
- Prisoners being treated for narcotic or alcohol withdrawal not identified during intake screening;
- Prisoners attempting or completing suicide within 3 months of admission;
- Women prisoners who are identified as pregnant after intake examination;
- Prisoners who die while incarcerated;
- Prisoners who refuse all or part of the intake examination;
- Length of stay in medical admission area exceeding 1 week;
- Variations in incidence and prevalence rates for pregnancy, syphilis, chlamydia, and gonorrhea in women prisoners.

Forms should be developed for organization of the intake examination data. These forms should be well designed, easy to fill out, and should encourage attention to detail. They should discourage excessive use of "check offs," particularly for the physical examination. Completed forms must be legible, and should be suitable for auditing and computer-supported data collection and analysis.

CONCLUSION

This chapter has presented a physician's view of the medical intake process. It has not argued that the intake function is more important that the other components of the health care program in prisoners in jail, but it well could be. The consequences of failure in the intake process are very significant.

A successful program for medical intake is complicated, staff intensive, and requires substantial cooperation and support from the security staff. The medical intake process should be comprehensive and integrated. The complete medical intake evaluation including screening, history, physical examination, and diagnostic testing, should take place as close to intake as possible. Only professional medical staff should participate in medical intake; there is no place in this process for security staff.

Appropriate physical areas for the intake examination and for housing of newly admitted prisoners prior to completion of their medical intake must be maintained. Prisoners must not be discharged from the medical intake housing area by security staff; only medical staff can certify that a prisoner can be housed in the general population.

Prisoners experiencing, or at risk of experiencing, drug or alcohol withdrawal must be identified and treated appropriately and compassionately.

Identification of prisoners with serious mental health problems at intake is a critical element of efforts to prevent suicide in prisons and jails. Careful and sensitive interviewing by medical staff trained in this process is crucial. There must be sufficient mental health staff available to allow for emergency and urgent psychiatric referrals of suicidal and psychotic prisoners. Additionally, the medical and mental health records should be integrated.

Women's health concerns at intake require careful planning and intensive staffing. Screening at intake should identify all women who are pregnant, and must include a careful gynecologic evaluation including screening for gonorrhea, chlamydia, and syphilis. These functions are often not performed even when required by local policy. Evaluation of women prisoners takes twice as much time as evaluation of men and should be staffed accordingly.

Finally, nothing is simple when it comes to providing medical services in a jail or a prison. These institutions are designed to confine, control, and punish. They are not designed to be sensitive, sympathetic, or to facilitate minimally necessary medical services. Despite this, effective policies and procedures for medical intake evaluation can be developed and implemented. Once they are implemented, they must be monitored closely and continuously, because inevitably they will deteriorate if not vigorously and aggressively defended. This is not pessimistic. The recognition of the circumstances in which medical services are provided in jails and prisons is actually hopeful and realistic. Nobody said it was going to be easy.

REFERENCES

1. NCCHC: Standards For Health Services In Jails. Chicago, National Commission on Correctional Health Care, 1996, J-30 Receiving Screening (essential), p 41.

2. Beltrami JF, Cohen DA, et al; Rapid screening and treatment of arrestees: A feasible control measure. *Am J Pub Health* 87:1423-1426, 1997.

3. Gillum RF: Sudden cardiac death in Hispanic Americans and African Americans. *Am J Public Health* 97:1461-1466, 1997.

4. Center For Disease Control: Probable transmission of multidrug resistant TB in a correctional facility in California. *MMWR* 42:48-57, 1993.

5. Valway SE, Greifinger RB, et al: Multidrug resistant tuberculosis in the New York state prison system 1990-1991. *J Infect Dis* 170:151-156, 1994.

6. Valway SE, Richard SB, et al: Outbreak of multidrug resistant tuberculosis in a New York state prison 1991. *Am J Epidemiol* 140:113-122, 1994.

7. Puisis M, Feinglass J, Lidow E, Mansour M: Radiographic screening for tuberculosis in a large urban jail. *Public Health Rep* 111:330-334, 1996.

8. Layton MC, Henning JK, et al: Universal radiographic screening for tuberculosis among inmates upon admission to jail. *Am J Public Health* 87:1335-1337, 1997.

9. Bellin EY, et al: Association of tuberculosis infection with increased time in or admission to the New York City jail system. *AMA* 269(17):2228-2231, 1993.

10. Zoloth SR: Anergy compromises screening for tuberculosis in high-risk populations. *Am J Public Health* 83(5):749-751, 1993.

11. Hillis SD, Wasserheit JN: Screening for chlamydia — A key to the prevention of pelvic inflammatory disease. *New Engl J Med* 334:1399-1401, 1996.

12. Holmes MD, et al: Chlamydia cervical infection in jailed women. *Am J Public Health* 83:551-555, 1993.

6

Chronic Disease Management

Michael Puisis, D.O.
John M. Robertson, M.D., M.P.H.

INTRODUCTION

In response to litigation and efforts to improve quality of health care in jails and prisons, attempts have been made to improve the care of incarcerated patients with chronic disease. Chronic disease is defined as any disease or condition that affects an individual's health and well-being for an extended time (at least 6 months), and which benefits from periodic interventions by a health professional for health maintenance or prevention of disease progression. Using contemporary consensus statements and clinical guidelines[1-3,34] for common conditions, correctional physicians developed chronic care management that could be adapted to the unique conditions of the correctional environment. These chronic care programs have helped to ensure follow-up of patients with chronic disease and to encourage adoption of contemporary standards of care. These programs serve to both educate the inmate about his disease and to provide medical follow-up care to individual inmates. Chronic care programs depend on a team of physicians, midlevel providers, and nurses to collaboratively deliver care to patients over the length of their incarceration.

CHRONIC DISEASE MANAGEMENT IN JAILS

Individuals entering a jail usually have an unplanned and abrupt admission that disrupts any planned or routine medical treatment for chronic disease. They are suddenly separated from their routine care and may be separated from their medication. Also, due to socioeconomic factors, many individuals enter jails with unidentified or untreated chronic diseases. It is important for medical personnel to realize that arrest, court proceedings, booking, and admission processes in some jails may separate detainees from their required treatments anywhere from 1 to 3 days until medical contact is re-established. For these reasons, medical intake screenings and evaluations are an important first step in the management of chronic disease.

For jails, one function of intake screening is to identify patients with chronic diseases to ensure timely continuity of treatment. Intake medical screening in jails is performed by a variety of personnel, ranging from correctional officers to physician assistants. Regardless of who performs this screening, a referral process must be in place to ensure prompt physician review of existing medical treatments. A patient with chronic disease requires prompt physician attention, especially for prescribing medications required in treating the patient's chronic disease. This is particularly important for diabetics, epileptics, asthmatics, patients with HIV infection, and patients with cardiovascular disorders who may suffer harm without their routine medication. Current standards (National Commission on Correctional Health Care, NCCHC)[4, 5] refer to a 7-day health assessment for prisons and a 14-day health assessment for jails. This does not remove the need for immediate post-booking physician-directed evaluation and re-institution of therapy for patients with chronic illness.

Some smaller facilities have the on-site intake staff contact the patient's civilian physician or pharmacy and continue their verified treatment until the facility physician can evaluate the patient. For security reasons of ensuring the integrity of medication supplies, it may not be prudent to permit a patient to continue to use medication that they may have brought in with them to the facility.

Care of patients with chronic disease in jails is dominated by the short length of stays customary in such institutions. The average length of stay in many jails is easily under 1 month. Given that duration, chronic care in jails has a more episodic and temporizing nature. This is in contrast to the prison environment where the length of stay, is considerably longer. For jails, due to short length of stays some systems do not always maintain separate systems for managing ongoing chronic care needs. Because of the large volume in inmates coming into jails with urgent and episodic medical needs, chronic care follow-up is often merged into appointment scheduling for all patients. Therefore, appointment scheduling in short-term facilities serves to track follow-up care.

CHRONIC DISEASE MANAGEMENT IN PRISONS

In prisons, chronic disease management has been systematized in many state prison programs. The purpose is to ensure regular follow-up and appropriate treatment of patients with chronic disease. For long-term facilities (prisons), patients with chronic diseases are tracked differently than individuals requiring only episodic care. Patients with chronic disease are often observed in specialized chronic disease clinics. Often these clinics are subdivided into disease-specific entities (epilepsy, hypertensive, asthmatic, diabetic, cardiovascular, HIV, TB prophylaxis, etc; HIV treatment and TB treatment will be covered in separate chapters). This separation permits selected staff to focus their efforts in tracking smaller groups of patients in a more thorough manner. An example of such a team might consist of the physician, a mid-level provider, and a nurse who follow all diabetics. This concept is similar to specialty clinic arrangements in civilian settings.

Inmates with chronic illness entering prison are best identified at receiving screening. As with jails, inmates with chronic disease entering prison are best seen by a physician as soon as possible after admission. Regardless of who performs the intake evaluation, it is recommended that all initial chronic disease visits be performed by a physician. The team of individuals caring for patients with chronic disease should obtain baseline laboratory and other testing, attempt to obtain the patient's pertinent civilian medical record, and enroll the patient in the appropriate clinic.

Obviously, the concept of specialized chronic disease clinics is complicated when individuals have more than one chronic disease. In some correctional systems, the most serious chronic illness will dictate into which clinic the patient is entered, and then all other chronic diseases are followed at the same clinic appointment. In other correctional systems, a patient is seen in a separate clinic visit for each of his chronic diseases. However, scheduling a patient for multiple chronic disease clinics increases the number of physician visits and may lead to patient satisfaction problems because of redundant scheduling. Some correctional systems have facilitated tracking chronic disease using automated scheduling systems.

Some state health systems specify minimum intervals for physician visits. Hipkens and others have recommended 6-month physician visits and 3-month nursing visits at a minimum for every patient with chronic disease.[6] This plan for the Georgia Department of Corrections has been recently modified so that patients with chronic disease are examined by a physician, nurse practitioner, or a physician's assistant every 3 months, except for stable patients who are seen at 6-month intervals with a nurse visit in between physician visits. It is recommended that patients whose illness is not well controlled be seen as frequently as clinically indicated. Interval visits may need to be as frequently as weekly or daily until an acceptable degree of clinical stability is obtained. These intervals serve to prevent turning chronic disease management into episodic care.

The first step in organizing a chronic care program is for a physician to enroll the patient, thus certifying the need for chronic care follow-up. It is extremely helpful if a nurse, as well as a physician, take time to explain the program to the patient. This should include discussion of the patient's responsibility to get laboratory tests, attendance at appointments, and compliance with medication even though they may not have symptoms. This may be a dramatic change for many inmates. This educational session invested in orienting the inmate to the use of medical services is time well spent. The goal is for the patient to be knowledgeable and accept responsibility for participating actively in care decisions and strategies.

The use of a team approach enables nurses to develop expertise with specific chronic illnesses and to reinforce the physician's efforts with tailored patient education sessions. Nurses frequently accept the task of ensuring that protocols for monitoring are carried out and the results of tests are in the charts prior to the visit with the physician.

MEDICATION ADMINISTRATION

Medication administration in correctional settings is a unique process and is intimately connected to the success of chronic disease care. Inmates are responsible for taking their medication, but the facility is responsible for delivering the medication to the inmate. It has been established that inmates can reliably retain and take their own medication similar to civilians. Many correctional systems, therefore, permit "keep on person" or self-administered medication. These programs reduce the burden of having staff deliver every prescribed pill and are, therefore, more efficient. Some individuals, such as mentally impaired or psychiatrically ill patients, are usually not permitted to participate in keep on person medication programs. It is not recommended to permit patients to administer their own psychotropic medication or any medication that may have abuse potential. The Centers for Disease Control (CDC) recommends that all anti-tuberculosis medications be given under direct observation by a health care provider (directly observed therapy or DOT).[7] This means that a nurse or trained person observes the pill ingestion and inspects the oral cavity post ingestion. Recording medication administration to inmates is similar to hospital medication administration with logged entries for administration of each dose of medication. For individuals who are getting medication dose by dose, this system permits perfect auditing of compliance. Auditing medication compliance for patients participating in "keep on person" medication programs is similar to civilian audits. There are no published studies describing medication compliance rates in correctional settings, and no comparative studies using combined civilian and correctional data. Despite an absence of data, many correctional staff have a biased perception that inmates are generally non-compliant. The value of anecdotal observations and inherent biases in determining policy is questionable from a scientific point of view. Thorough studies of medication delivery systems and patient compliance are needed to assess this problem. Patients may be expected to arrive at a pill line multiple times a day. Their absence may be assumed to be non-compliance. A recent assessment of medication delivery to an AIDS patient in a civilian setting revealed that medications were to be taken seven times during the day.[8] This would be extremely difficult in a pill line system. A recent study of compliance among 244 AIDS patients at a Johns Hopkins outpatient clinic revealed that only 60% of patients were compliant 80% of the time.[8] When inmates do not arrive for medication, non-compliance cannot automatically be assumed. The patient may have been prevented from leaving their unit by security staff or may never have received a pass to leave the housing unit.

A system of medication renewal must be in place to ensure that a patient has a continuous supply of medication. For facilities with automated pharmacy service, a stop order system allows physicians to review expiring medications and to review charts of patients on medication for chronic disease. This permits the physician to not only renew medications but to review the chart and ensure that appointments have not been missed. If automated pharmacy services are not available, then notices of expiring medication must be provided through manual strategies for physicians to renew medication.

SCHEDULING CHRONIC DISEASE APPOINTMENTS

Scheduling systems for patients with chronic disease must ultimately be integrated into the correctional and security requirements of each facility. This presents a variety of problems. In both prisons and jails, inmates are not free to schedule their own appointments and, therefore, when a health care appointment is made for an inmate, there are frequently competing appointments (with lawyers, court, family, gym, commissary, etc) that reduce the chances an inmate will come to see the medical staff. In addition, correctional facilities are restrictive environments that usually require inmates be in their cell or dormitory at certain hours to be counted to ensure that no one has escaped. This reduces the time available to medical staff to see patients and increases the chance that there will not be available time to examine all patients who are scheduled. It is, therefore, imperative that inmates participate, to whatever extent possible, in the scheduling of on-site clinic appointments. Inmates should be motivated to come for care and instructed in the peculiarities of health care access that exist in their institution. Health care staff need to take security regulations into account when scheduling inmates and schedule only as many inmates as can reasonably be seen.

FLOW SHEETS

Flow sheets of laboratory and other medical data have become standard in managing patients with chronic illness. The benefit of these instruments is that they permit the rapid assessment and evaluation of the progress of a patient's treatment history. Flow sheets track important items that are ordinarily followed in managing certain chronic illnesses, such as hemoglobin A1C for diabetics. Figure 6-1 is an example of a diabetic flow sheet used to track patients in a chronic care clinic. Similar types of flow sheets can be used to track any number of important indicators used to monitor chronic care.

STANDARDS OF CARE

The management of chronic disease follows national standards of care as promulgated by consensus and expert panels which may be tailored to the unique correctional environment. Correctional standards of care, developed into practice guidelines or clinical pathways, require annual or regular review with revision if indicated. Occasionally, standards of care are modified due to the difficulty of practice in correctional settings. Physicians face difficult ethical

DIABETES FLOW SHEET

FINGER STICK BLOOD SUGARS 3-4/DAY GOAL: AM (fast) 80-120; pre-lunch 80-150; bedtime 100-150

DIABETIC TYPE _____

CLINIC DATE											
WEIGHT											
COUNSELING Smoking/Diet (q 4 months)											
HgB AJC (q 4 mos until stable then q 6 mos)											
DIALATED FUNDOSCOPIC EXAM (Annually)											
SMAC (fasting) (normally - annually) (abnormal as indicated)											
BUN/CREATININE (Baseline & as indicated)											
MICROALBUMIN* (Annually)											
FLU VACCINE											
PUNEUMOVAX											
FOOT EXAM											
INSULIN DOSE AM											
PM											
ORAL AGENT											
BLOOD PRESSURE											

NOTES:	NAME	NMCD#
*If abnormal do total protein and creatinine clearance		

SECTION 1 - MEDICAL RECORD revised 12/96

Figure 6-1. Diabetes flow sheet. (Adapted from the New Mexico Department of Corrections.)

choices when they are unable to treat a patient according to an accepted civilian standard or care. For example, multiple medication dosing may be required in some patients (e.g., multiple insulin injections or multiple dosing of anti-retroviral drugs for AIDS patients), but may be impossible to deliver within the context of the facility. In these cases, physicians need to find acceptable alternatives or discuss other housing options with the correctional authority. Also, in areas where treatment guidelines are rapidly changing, such as the care of patients with HIV, more frequent revisions may be indicated to keep abreast of current standards.

Well-managed correctional health care organizations develop systems for treating patients with chronic illness. The following sections are not meant to be a complete review of chronic disease management, but are meant to highlight some areas of concern for correctional physicians.

ASTHMA

Asthma is reversible airway obstruction characterized by inflammation and hyperresponsiveness. The rate of asthma in the United States is estimated at 4% to 5% of the population.[9] The prevalence rate of asthma in a large urban jail was 6.9%.[10] Several groups of patients are at higher risk for asthma-related death. Among blacks between ages 15 and 44, the asthma-related death rate was nearly five times the death rate for asthma for whites of the same age group.[2] Risk factors for death from asthma pertinent to this population include previous life-threatening asthma or recent emergency room visit, significant psychosocial or behavioral problems, and aspirin or non-steroidal anti-inflammatory use.[2]

The goal of asthma management in correctional settings is to monitor patients regularly, alleviate symptoms, and to provide early intervention to prevent acute and severe exacerbations. In long-term facilities, education of the patient about controlling asthma should be part of any chronic disease program. Identification of the asthmatic during intake processing or at the diagnostic reception area is crucial in maintaining continuity of care. Because of its nonspecific and intermittent symptoms, asthma is frequently underdiagnosed. Any symptoms of wheezing should strongly suggest asthma. Despite the cost constraints of managed care, it is always preferred for safety reasons to give asthmatics or those suspected of asthma an inhaler rather than wait until they are experiencing an exacerbation. The severity of a patient's asthma must be determined during receiving screening. It is also useful to identify what triggers asthma in the patient, since this may assist in preventing future exacerbations. A system should be in place to have pharmaceuticals readily accessible in the intake area if an incoming patient experiences an exacerbation. Inmates who have asthma should have their prescribed medication as soon as possible. Access to medication should not be delayed until appointments with physicians occur. In most settings, this means that an inmate should leave the intake area with an inhaler. In some jail settings, correctional officers perform reception screening. In this case, inmates identified with asthma should be referred to an advanced medical practitioner or physician so that a more detailed history can be taken. This appointment should not be extended beyond the day of intake. In small jails without medical staff on site, new patients with symptomatic asthma are best evaluated in a local area emergency room.

Peak Expiratory Flow Rate Measurements

Because patients may not recognize the severity of their asthma, follow-up of patients with asthma housed in correctional settings requires some objective measurement of lung function on which to guide therapy. Ideally, all asthmatics should have spirometry testing to characterize a baseline pulmonary function. This testing determines vital capacity, tidal volume, expiratory reserve volume, and inspiratory capacity. In short-term correctional facilities (e.g., jails), spirometry use may be impractical. At a minimum, every correctional facility should have access to peak expiratory flow rate (PEFR) measurement. This simple test is performed using office model or portable peak flow meters. It is important to remember that these tests are effort-related. Given the variability of staffing in many correctional settings, it is important that experienced trained health care staff perform the peak flow measurement. Correctional settings are often multi-site, multiple-provider arrangements with inmates moving about from facility to facility. Inter-examiner variability may exist if practitioners do not perform peak expiratory flow measurements in the same manner. Civilian asthmatics are encouraged to have their own portable peak flow meters for home use.[2, 34] In correctional settings, if this is not permitted, patients should have immediate access to nursing staff to test themselves. In situations where access to spirometry is difficult, treatment plans in chronic care clinics should include frequent peak expiratory flow measurement, especially for patients with difficult-to-control asthma. Gauging severity of asthma is made by comparing peak flow rates to standardized charts of predicted peak flow based on age and height. In addition, the personal best peak flow rate helps observe a patient's response to therapy.

The chronic care team should educate the patient about the peak flow rate in relation to the expected PEFR for his age and height. Changing therapy relative to PEFR must be communicated to the patient in an understandable manner. Contemporary standards of care[2, 11, 34] encourage patient self-monitoring and changes in treatment based on patient symptoms and PEFR readings. Unfortunately, due to the inaccessibility of personal peak flow meters to inmates who are locked in cells, it is usually not possible for inmates to frequently monitor their PEFR. There are no published data on whether there are correctional systems that permit patient self-monitoring with their own portable PEFR devices. Because these devices are hard plastic, inmates may not be permitted to keep these devices in their personal property due to the possibility of using them as weapons. In addition, inmates are usually not permitted to visit the medical area unless their symptoms are obvious to a lay correctional officer. Often, only asthmatics with exacerbations or in severe distress are permitted to make immediate visits to medical staff. For this reason, it is important to communicate to inmates, at clinic visits, an explanation of the importance of frequent PEFR measurement and how to increase medication stepwise to alleviate symptoms and maintain an acceptable peak flow rate.

It is useful at clinic visits to clarify the frequency of rescue (beta-agonist) medication, and the frequency of symptoms (cough, wheezing, etc.) to gauge the progression of the patient's disease. Clinic visits should also include PEFR measurement, which can be compared to previous values in a flow sheet arrangement. These episodic measurements are not as useful as frequent daily measurements, but may be the only practical alternative in the correctional environment.

When inmates are permitted to have their own peak flow meters, or in infirmary settings where asthma is being closely monitored, the initial PEFR reading should be in the morning before taking bronchodilators and then 12 hours later before and after using a bronchodilator. Personal best PEFRs are defined as the highest PEFR measurement in the evening after a period of maximal therapy.[11] These personal best readings are useful in educating the patient about his or her therapeutic goals. In addition, the National Asthma Education Project developed a system of zones as a mechanism to quantify treatment systems.[2] As a rough guideline, patients above 80% of predicted are considered stable and persistent readings in this range may allow for reduction in medication dosing. Patients below 50% predicted are in need of immediate treatment and may require emergent evaluation if there is no response to therapy. Patients between 50% and 80% of predicted may need evaluation and/or increased therapeutic measures. As part of chronic care management, nursing testing of PEFRs twice a day of selected individuals at risk for exacerbation may help trend response to therapy and identify deterioration early in the course of an exacerbation.

Inmate Housing for Asthmatics

Inmate housing is an important consideration for the asthmatic in correctional settings. A causative agent in asthma that is beyond the control of the inmate is the ambient air quality. The correctional setting consisting of poor ventilation and a smoke-filled environment may place asthmatic patients at risk for exacerbations. Generally, asthmatics are known to be more sensitive to sulfur dioxide, nitrogen dioxide, ozone, and mold. There are no published studies on mold formation in correctional settings, but it may be a factor in some settings, particularly where ventilation is poor. Air quality is generally poor in prison and jail cells. A recent study of a jail environment subsequent to a pneumococcal outbreak revealed that, on average, inmates in that jail shared living quarters with a median living space of 6 ft. by 6 ft. Air was 80% recirculated and outside air was delivered at less than one-third the recommended flow rate. Carbon dioxide levels ranged from 1100 to 2500 ppm (acceptable, < 1000). Measurement of this compound was done as an indicator of air quality.[12] Information from that study did not indicate whether components that affect asthmatics were present. There are no other data indicating whether there are air quality problems in jails or prisons that affect asthmatics. The exception is cigarette smoke. Few correctional facilities are smoke free. Forced living conditions often mandate that asthmatics live with someone who is smoking. Under these conditions, physicians should

be advocates for a smoke-free environment. An alternative to a smoke-free environment is for the correctional authority to designate certain living quarters as a selective smoke-free environment in which patients at risk from smoke may live.

Because housing location is intimately connected to access to medical staff (particularly for large or complex facilities), a system should be in place for special housing for at-risk asthmatics. All asthmatics should be housed in areas where they have access to medical staff in the event of an exacerbation. Asthmatics who are placed in administrative segregation should never have their medication taken from them. For stable asthmatics, general population housing (preferably smoke free) is acceptable. Symptomatic asthmatics should not be placed in general population areas unless a treatment plan with regular monitoring is in place. Inmates in the range of 50% to 80% of PEFR may need special medical housing where there is 24-hour nursing coverage capable of close observation of the inmate. Occasionally, this will consist of an infirmary unit. Symptomatic inmates whose PEFR is less than 50% of predicted should not be housed in general population. These individuals should be housed in an infirmary or a hospital, depending on the severity of their asthma.

Pharmacologic Therapy for Asthmatics

In their most recent Global Strategy for Asthma Management,[11] the National Heart Lung and Blood (Figure 6-2) Institute defines asthma medications as either controller or reliever medication. Controller medication is defined as medications, taken daily on a long-term basis that are useful in getting and keeping persistent asthma under control. Relievers or rescue medication are those short-acting medications used to act quickly to relieve bronchoconstriction and acute symptoms. Controller medications include inhaled corticosteroids, systemic corticosteroids, cromolyn sodium, sustained release theophylline, and long-acting inhaled and oral beta agonists. Reliever medications include short-acting beta agonists, systemic corticosteroids, anticholinergics, short-acting theophylline, and short-acting oral beta agonists. Figure 6-2 presents a stepwise approach to treating asthma. It is recommended by the NAEP that all asthmatics have a beta-agonist inhaler for rescue treatment of acute symptoms.[11, 34] This is a prudent practice in correctional settings. In short-term jails, where many patients are admitted and discharged within weeks, there may be a temptation to withhold beta agonist inhalers until the patient is symptomatic or until a few weeks have past and the patient has his first appointment with a physician. This is not prudent practice and places the onus of prompt and ready access to inhalers on the health authority and facility. There are also anecdotal reports of inmates using beta agonist inhalers for recreational purposes, but there are no published data describing the prevalence of this practice. Withholding metered-dosed inhalers for all

The aim of treatment is control of asthma.

Outcome: Control of Asthma
- Minimal (ideally no) chronic symptoms, including nocturnal symptoms
- Minimal (infrequent) episodes
- No emergency visits
- Minimal need for prn β_2-agonist
- No limitations on activities, including exercise
- PEF circadian variation <20%
- (Near) normal PEF
- Minimal (or no) adverse effects from medicine

Preferred treatments are in bold print.

Note:
Patients should start treatment at the step most appropriate to the initial severity of their condition. A rescue course of prednisolone may be needed at any time and at any step.

Step 4: Severe Persistent

Controller
Daily Medications
- **Inhaled corticosteroid,** 800-2,000 mcg or more, and
- Long-acting bronchodilator: either long-acting β_2-agonist, sustained-release theophylline, and/or long-acting oral β_2-agonist, and
- Oral corticosteroid long term

Reliever
- Short-acting bronchodilator: **inhaled β_2-agonist** as needed for symptoms

Avoid or Control Triggers

Step 3: Moderate Persistent

Controller
Daily Medications
- **Inhaled corticosteroid,** 800-2,000 mcg, and
- Long-acting bronchodilator, especially for nighttime symptoms: either long-acting inhaled β_2-agonist, sustained-release theophylline, or long-acting oral β_2-agonist

Reliever
- Short-acting bronchodilator: **inhaled β_2-agonist** as needed for symptoms, not to exceed 3-4 times in one day

Avoid or Control Triggers

Step 2: Mild Persistent

Controller
Daily Medication
- Either **Inhaled corticosteroid,** 200-500 mcg, **cromoglycate, nedocromil,** or sustained-release theophylline
- If needed, increase inhaled corticosteroids. If inhaled corticosteroids currently equal 500 mcg, increase the corticosteroids up to 800 mcg, or add long-acting bronchodilator (especially for nighttime symptoms): either long-acting inhaled β_2-agonist, sustained-release theophylline, or long-acting oral β_2-agonist

Reliever
- Short-acting bronchodilator: **inhaled β_2-agonist** as needed for symptoms, not to exceed 3-4 times in one day

Avoid or Control Triggers

Step 1: Intermittent

Controller
- None needed

Reliever
- Short-acting bronchodilator: **inhaled β_2-agonist** as needed for symptoms, but less than once a week
- Intensity of treatment will depend on severity of exacerbation (see chart on acute exacerbations)
- Inhaled β_2-agonist or cromolyn or nedocromil before exercise or exposure to allergen

Avoid or Control Triggers

Treatment

Stepdown
Review treatment every 3 to 6 months.

If control is sustained for at least 3 months, a gradual stepwise reduction in treatment may be possible.

Stepup
If control is not achieved, consider stepup. But first: review patient medication technique, compliance, and environmental control (avoidance of allergens or other trigger factors).

Figure 6-2. The Long-term management of asthma: treatments in the stepwise approach. (From Global Initiative for Asthma Control.)

inmates, based on the misuse of the medication by a few, is a potentially dangerous practice. Nevertheless, recreational drug seeking of metered dosed inhalers makes the diagnosis of asthma more difficult and may lead to bias against a diagnosis of asthma. Physicians must be aware of that potential.

For the stable asthmatic with intermittent exacerbations, an inhaled beta-agonist on an as-needed (prn) basis is appropriate therapy. Comparison of as-needed beta agonist medication with regularly scheduled medication for mild asthmatics has shown no advantage in using regularly scheduled medication.[13] The benefit in cost reduction can be significant in using medication on an as-needed basis. Use of as-needed medication must not, however, be construed as prohibiting an inmate from keeping a metered dose inhaler on his person. Unless immediate and ready access to nursing staff and medication is available 24 hours a day, inmates should be permitted to keep asthma medication on their person. Unless an inmate is housed in an infirmary setting, this type of access is seldom possible in any correctional facility. The nurse and physician should make certain that the patient uses the correct technique with their inhalers, or the medication is likely to be ineffective.

The NAEP recommendations call for inhaled corticosteroids for patients with mild-to-moderate persistent chronic asthma supplemented by short-acting beta agonists on an as-needed basis.[34] Regular inhaled corticosteroids have become a first line therapy for patients with mild-to-moderate persistent chronic asthma. A recent study demonstrated reduced hospitalization and significant protection against exacerbations of asthma when inhaled steroids are used by individuals who require more than occasional beta-agonist use.[14] Use of a chamber device or spacer or rinsing the mouth after use may reduce the incidence of local side effects. The treatment of acute asthma exacerbations is inhaled beta-agonist medication. Inhaled beta agonists are currently a preferred vehicle of administration because they produce more bronchodilation and fewer side effects.[2] Beta agonist inhaler medication is used for as-needed therapy for exacerbations. Regular use of beta agonist should be kept to a minimum.[11]

When a patient with moderate chronic asthma has a severe exacerbation, or when a severe asthmatic has an exacerbation, a short course of oral steroids may be necessary. These may be given, for example, at 40 mg a day for a week, to be tapered over 7 to 14 days. It is important to remember that the onset of action of oral steroids is approximately 3 hours after use and peak action occurs at about 6 hours.[11] Appropriate beta agonist therapy must be instituted in the interim. Because of the side effects of corticosteroids, upward adjustments in the dose of inhaled corticosteroids should be made so that the need for oral steroids is reduced on a maintenance basis.

The use of methylxanthines (theophylline for example) has waned. Because of the potential for adverse drug reac-

tions, serum theophylline concentrations should be monitored at baseline and every 6 to 12 months thereafter, or sooner if the patient experiences an adverse reaction on their usual dose.

Sinusitis may provoke asthma. These infections should be treated appropriately. Other conditions that may trigger asthma include viral upper respiratory syndromes, exposure to allergens, allergic and non-allergic rhinitis, and seasonal allergen exposure. Clinicians need to be vigilant during times of high pollen counts and advise patients to adhere to their treatment plan to avoid exacerbations.

Chronic care of asthmatics would include periodic PEFR measurement and assessment of symptoms. For patients who continue to have symptoms from visit to visit, a reevaluation of medication technique should be undertaken. It is important that patients know how to use their medication. Patients should be asked to bring their medication to the clinic for a demonstration. Flow sheets for asthma chronic clinics should include PEFR measurements, baseline spirometry measurements, dated exacerbations, and medication use. Patient education is crucial and every attempt must be made to involve the patient in asthma control. The number of times that a patient is using medications is also useful in evaluating their status and progress toward achieving maximal bronchodilation.

Counseling and education should be part of an asthma chronic disease program. Inmates should understand what asthma is and isn't. They should understand that this is a chronic disease with episodic acute exacerbations. Inmates should understand asthma triggers and how they might control them. Smoking cessation should be encouraged. Correct medication use should be explained. Unwarranted fears about medications should be discussed. Use of written diaries may be useful for selected patients. Use of PEFR monitoring should be explained and personal treatment goals discussed.

HYPERTENSION

Hypertension in patients in correctional facilities may have already been diagnosed prior to incarceration. An intake screening program at a large urban jail discovered that 6.1% of incoming inmates had a history of hypertension.[10] Others, however, are discovered during the intake screening, annual health assessments, and other surveillance programs. Length of incarceration, as well as crowded living space, have been associated with increased blood pressure. This reinforces the concept of annual blood pressure screening.[15–18] Intake screening in jails and prisons often includes blood pressure measurement. Because individuals entering correctional facilities, particularly jails, are often withdrawing from alcohol or other drugs, under the influence of drugs, or are anxious or tense, the blood pressure measurement is often elevated. Diagnosis of hypertension should never be made from a single reading, especially from an intake blood pressure measurement. At least three blood pressure measurements over one to several weeks apart should be taken before diagnosing hypertension. Blood pressure greater than 140 systolic and 90 diastolic qualifies as hypertension. When the diastolic pressure is below 90, a systolic value above 140 qualifies as isolated systolic hypertension. Patients should be relaxed and should avoid caffeine and smoking for about a half hour prior to blood pressure measurement. Immediate therapy based on initial blood pressure measurement may be indicated for severe blood pressure (diastolic greater than 120 mm Hg or systolic greater than 210 mm Hg) or evidence of end organ damage. Additional surveillance should include a blood pressure measurement in annual health maintenance updates.

The initial examination of hypertensives needs to be guided by clinical judgement and based on circumstances of incarceration. For purposes of physical examination, all patients with hypertension should be treated as if they were newly diagnosed, even though many hypertensive patients entering correctional facilities already know the diagnosis. The initial examination of hypertensives should include a urine analysis, complete blood cell count, blood glucose, potassium, creatinine, blood urea nitrogen (BUN), uric acid, cholesterol, high-density lipoprotein, and electrocardiogram. These tests evaluate target end organs and assess for other associated cardiovascular risk factors. The follow-up of these tests, along with history and physical examination, should include assessment for cardiovascular risk factors. These initial visits should be with a physician.

The approach for initial evaluation differs markedly for patients entering jails versus prisons. In jails, with very short length of stays it is not always practical to perform an initial battery of tests until it is known if a patient is going to be discharged from the institution after a short time. It may be appropriate to wait until after one or two chronic care visits before initiating this testing. In addition, for large jails, it is not always feasible or practical to initiate contact with the patient's civilian primary care physician to obtain treatment history. For prisons or small jails, the situation may be different. In small community jails, nurses or physicians can often contact the local doctor to obtain treatment history without difficulty. For prisons, prior medical information should be obtained on all patients and initial laboratory testing should be obtained before the patient leaves the intake facility, or within a short time after arriving at the facility.

Preventive measures are a major part of any hypertensive chronic clinic program. Often, this can be built into the education component of chronic care management. Education on smoking cessation, weight reduction and heart healthy diet, regular physical activity, and moderation of dietary sodium are all important parts of educational counseling. These items should be performed by a member of the chronic care team. For cost-efficiency reasons, this is often performed by a trained educator or a member of the nursing staff.

Unless the blood pressure is above 160 systolic or 100 diastolic, newly diagnosed patients without end organ damage or cardiovascular risk factors should undergo a trial of lifestyle changes (modifying cardiovascular risk factors) for 3 to 6 months.[1] If after this trial the blood pressure continues to be equal to or greater than 140/90, then medications should be initiated. Patients with multiple cardiovascular risk factors or cardiovascular disease should be considered for prompt pharmacologic therapy. In many correctional settings, single-dose therapy is preferred not only for patient compliance but also to reduce the amount of time staff spend in passing medications. Keep-on-person medication systems are extremely helpful in reducing the cost of medication passage systems.

Choice of medication is governed by the clinical situation of the patient, including whether the patient has other illnesses (e.g., beta blockers should be avoided in diabetics and asthmatics), the patient's race (e.g., blacks are more responsive to diuretics and calcium channel blockers), and the patient's ability to understand how to take medication (e.g., elderly patients or patients with mental deficiencies should have simplified regimens). Because diuretics and beta blockers have been shown to reduce cardiovascular morbidity and mortality in controlled trials the Joint National Committee on Detection, Evaluation and Treatment of High Blood Pressure (JNC-VI) has recommended diuretics and beta blockers as first-line therapy. In addition, a recent systematic review and meta-analysis supported diuretics and beta blockers as first line agents until long-term clinical trials evaluating the cardiovascular effects of ACE inhibitors and calcium channel blockers are completed.[19] Cost concerns also favor use of these agents.

If the initial agent is not effective in bringing the blood pressure under control, it is recommended by the JNC-VI that the dose be increased, a substitution occur, or a second drug be added. Choosing among these options will vary. Patients should be involved in making these decisions as their understanding and cooperation is imperative for adherence to therapy. Patients need to feel in control. If a second drug is added and the blood pressure is controlled, a careful trial of stopping the initial drug may be attempted to simplify therapy. If two or three drugs are being used without being able to bring diastolic blood pressure to less than 120, then consultation should be strongly considered and secondary causes of hypertension should be sought. Resistant hypertension exists when treatment fails to normalize blood pressure. Appropriate treatment for resistant hypertension is use of three drugs, including a diuretic and two additional drugs from different classes (beta blocker, direct vasodilator, calcium channel blocker, or ACE inhibitor).[1]

Follow-up visits for hypertension should occur as often as necessary to achieve blood pressure control. Too-frequent visits encourage inmate refusals for care. Patients with severely elevated blood pressure may need to be seen weekly until stabilized. Patients with moderately uncontrolled blood pressure may need to be seen monthly. Once a patient's blood pressure is controlled, many chronic disease programs schedule patients at 3-month intervals with a mid-level practitioner and at least every 6 months with a physician. In all cases, the frequency of visits must be governed by clinical judgement.

EPILEPSY

The prevalence of history of seizure disorder among inmates entering a large urban jail has been described as 4%.[10] Prevalence rates of epilepsy for men entering a state prison system have been described as 2.4%.[20] Civilian rates vary between 0.5% and 2%.[9] This increased prevalence of epilepsy in inmates has been attributed to socioeconomic factors, with almost half of cases having blunt trauma as the etiologic agent for onset of epilepsy.[20] Given these prevalence rates, epilepsy is one of the more common chronic diseases in correctional populations. Interestingly, it has been found that there is no relationship between epilepsy and ongoing violent behavior.[20]

In any correctional setting, the first step in managing an epileptic patient is to correctly classify the type of epilepsy and to rule out other primary causes for a seizure. It is crucial to accurately classify the type of seizure in order to prescribe an appropriate treatment. This is a step that is frequently missed in intake assessments and should be part of the initial examination. Drug (including alcohol) withdrawal seizures must be carefully distinguished from true epilepsy, because there is no indication for chronic treatment of drug withdrawal seizures. It is important, especially in jail settings, to identify patients at risk for withdrawal seizures and to have a protocol for treating these patients. Patients who are actively withdrawing from alcohol should not be placed in general population areas; an infirmary area is more appropriate. If alcohol withdrawal is more severe (delerium tremens), the patient should be hospitalized. Patients with new onset of seizure disorder should have an investigative workup to exclude secondary causes for the seizure.

Patients with nonepileptic events are sometimes described as having pseudoseizures. These events are not well classified. Some physicians divide pseudoseizures into factitious seizures and seizure-like phenomena, but most use terms synonymously.[21] Patients with complex partial seizures may have atypical presentations that may not appear to resemble bonafide seizure activity. There are a variety of neurologic conditions that may present with seizure-like activity and may require additional diagnosis and treatment.[22] Some patients have factitious seizures. These patients may mimic seizure activity because of psychological conflicts or for the pure secondary gain associated with being labeled with epilepsy (lower bunk status, change in work assignment, etc.). Differentiating factitious from true seizure activity can be very difficult. Experienced

neurologists identify factitious seizures only 75% of the time.[21] Observation of nonphysiologic events during these episodes is helpful in making the diagnosis, but video-EEG recording is required for accurate diagnosis.[23] Because many patients with factitious seizure disorders also have bonafide epilepsy, it becomes difficult to distinguish between the two. Neurology consultation is useful in treating these patients. In some cases, psychiatric consultation is useful.

It is also important to immediately identify epileptic patients and to begin anti-epileptic therapy for those patients on chronic therapy for epilepsy. Serum half lives of antiepilepsy drugs vary. The half life of phenytoin is 18–36 hours; phenobarbital ranges from 50 to 140 hours. Therefore, inmates, particularly in jails, who may have been held in local police lockups without medication prior to incarceration, may be susceptible to breakthrough seizures. Therefore, epilepsy must be recognized and treatment should be initiated as soon as possible after intake screening. Housing and bunk assignment may be important to address at intake in institutions where inmates may be required to sleep on top bunks. Epileptics should receive lower bunk assignment to avoid falls during nocturnal seizures.

It is preferable to treat epilepsy with a single drug and with the lowest possible dosage required. It is also preferable to attempt to convert patients on multiple therapy to single therapy, even if using a single drug requires higher than therapeutic levels.[24] Patients who have not had seizures for extended periods can be offered a trial of eliminating medication to assess whether they may stop the medication. Practice at Cook County Jail in these trials included decreasing the anti-epilepsy drug over the course of several physician visits. After the medication was discontinued, the patient was observed for several visits over the course of several months. Then the patient was observed only as needed.

Patients may require more than one drug for seizure control. Patients on polytherapy who have seizures despite adequate drug levels present management problems. Drug levels should be verified. Occasionally, drug screening for recreational drugs may be indicated. When patients have breakthrough seizures, they need to participate in discussing additional therapy. Patients should be guided through a risk assessment of treatment with multiple drugs versus the risk of breakthrough seizures. Some patients would rather not take additional medication and prefer the possibility of seizures. These patients usually need further evaluation for clarification of seizure type and consultation with a neurologist is suggested. Figure 6-3 demonstrates a flow diagram of a suggested long-term treatment strategy for patients with epilepsy.

Antiepilepsy drugs of choice are listed in Table 6-1. The choice of medication is dictated by the type of seizure disorder, side effects of medication, drug-drug interactions,

Patient With Epilepsy

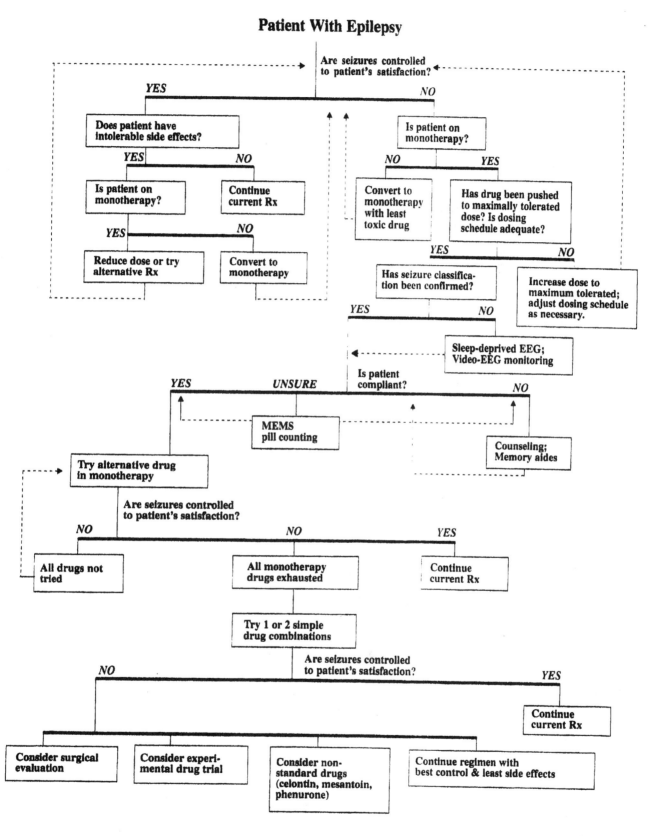

Figure 6-3. Long-term management paradigm for patients with epilepsy. Celontin = methsuximide; EEG = electroen-cephalogram; Mesantoin = mephenytoin; MEMS = Medication Event Monitoring System; Phenurone = phenacemide; and Rx = drug treatment. (From French J: The long term therapeutic management of epilepsy. *Ann Intern Med* 120:411–422, 1994.)

Table 6-1. Antiepileptic drug choices for major epilepsy syndromes and seizure types*

Syndrome	Drug[†]
Symptomatic partial epilepsy	
Complex partial seizures	cbz; pht; pb; vpa[‡]
Generalized tonic-clonic seizures	cbz; pht; pb; vpa
Idiopathic generalized epilepsy	
Absence (petit mal) seizures	esm; vpa[§]; czp
Myoclonic seizures	vpa; czp
Generalized tonic-clonic seizures	vpa; cbz' pht; bp

* See text for references.

[†]cbz = Carbamazepine; czp=clonazepate; esm = ethosuximide; pb = phenobarbital; pht = phenytoin; vpa = valproic acid.

[‡]Not as effective.

[§]Use for absence in association with other seizure types.

From Harrison's *Textbook of Medicine* 13th edition.

and, to a lesser extent, by cost. Benzodiazepines are not considered first line drugs for long-term management of epilepsy and, especially in correctional settings, the use of benzodiazepines should be discouraged because of the potential for abuse in this setting. Phenobarbital is considered a first line therapy for complex partial seizures and tonic-clonic seizures. However, in correctional settings, because of abuse potential, its use should be reserved for those patients who cannot tolerate other first line therapies. There are excellent reviews of antiepilepsy medications.[9, 24] It is important to recognize potential problems with certain medications and carefully monitor them as part of a chronic disease program. These monitored items can be charted in a flow sheet format for ease of follow-up. Patients on phenytoin should have a therapeutic drug level drawn at intervals to monitor the plasma drug level. Blood for this testing should be drawn at the same time of day for accurate comparison. The blood should be drawn just before a usual dose of medication is given (i.e., a trough level). The therapeutic levels presented by laboratory reports are ranges, which are not necessarily predictive of toxicity or of clinical efficacy. Toxicity may occur at blood levels that are sub-therapeutic or may not exist for patients whose blood levels are greater than the therapeutic range. Patients whose drug blood level is "sub-therapeutic" should not have their medication increased if they are seizure free. The therapeutic drug level should be reviewed from a perspective of other clinical correlates. It is reasonable clinically to obtain a serum drug level once every 6 months to a year for the purposes of general follow-up.

There are several items that should be tracked relative to certain medications. Patients receiving phenytoin should be checked for gum hyperplasia and referred to a dentist for evaluation and education about brushing their gums, which may reduce gum hyperplasia. Patients should be assessed at chronic clinic visits for signs of toxicity, including nystag-

mus, ataxia, dysarthria, and encephalopathy. Therapeutic drug levels with good control of seizures may produce nystagmus. Because phenytoin is teratogenic, it must be used with care in females. The lowest dose required to control seizures should be used to avoid this potential problem.

The use of carbamazepine should be monitored by regular complete blood cell counts. Carbamazepine can cause a decrease in neutrophils. Also, if the leukocytes are less than 2.5×10^9, therapy should be discontinued. In addition, carbamazepine may rarely cause bone marrow suppression with aplastic anemia. Because its side effect profile is better than phenytoin, it may make a better choice as a first line drug. Its dosing (three times a day vs. once a day to three times a day for phenytoin) and greater cost, however, make it less appealing in correctional settings. While phenobarbital is an excellent antiepilepsy drug, it presents problems when used in the correctional environment. Patients on long-term phenobarbital therapy often develop tolerance to its sedative effects. Nevertheless, resale of this drug to other inmates as well as patient drug-seeking behavior make this drug difficult to use in correctional settings. It is an inexpensive drug and has a long half-life, which permits once a day dosing. Nevertheless, because there are other acceptable medications without abuse potential problems, phenobarbital is not preferred as a first line agent in correctional settings. Many of the antiepileptics have drug-drug interactions because of induction of hepatic enzymes. Caution should be urged when using these agents in concert with other therapies, and appropriate pharmacist consultation is indicated.

DIABETES MANAGEMENT IN THE CORRECTIONAL SETTING

Diabetes, more than any other single disease, challenges correctional medical staff in its management. Review of a facility's capacity to manage diabetes is probably the single best indicator of the level of function of a medical unit. This lies in the "labor-intensive" nature of the disease and the involvement of all levels of medical providers and their interactions with security staff. Effective treatment requires input from a physician, nursing staff, a diabetes educator, dietitian, and other health professionals. Failure to diagnose and treat has potentially devastating consequences, while early recognition and management can prevent unnecessary morbidity and mortality.

Diabetes affects greater than 7 million individuals by self-reporting, a number that by conservative estimates probably doubles when taking into account those with abnormal glucose tolerance tests. Its prevalence is estimated to be approximately 3500 per 1,000,000. Currently, it is the seventh leading cause of death in the United States. These statistics are misleading however, as diabetes is underreported and, therefore, may not appear as a contributing factor on the death certificate of an individual who dies of its complications.

Diabetes is divided into two major types, insulin-dependent diabetes mellitus (IDDM) and non-insulin dependent diabetes mellitus (NIDDM). The distinction lies in that IDDM is an autoimmune disease that leads to destruction of beta cells and an insulin deficit. These individuals cannot survive without exogenous insulin. The majority of individuals have NIDDM, or "Type II" diabetes, which is a disease characterized by a relative "insulin resistance." These individuals are less prone to diabetic ketoacidosis and while a number of them may be on insulin therapy for their management, they are able to survive without exogenous insulin.

The importance of long-term management of diabetes cannot be overemphasized. The reasons for this rest with the myriad of complications encountered with the disease, including cardiac and macrovascular disease, as well as diffuse microvascular disease. Microvascular disease leads to stroke, retinopathy and blindness, and kidney failure. Diabetes is the leading cause of preventable blindness and renal failure requiring dialysis. Prior to the completion of the Diabetes Control and Complications Trial (DCCT), it was unproved if rigorous glycemic control could affect outcome in terms of reducing long-term complications in insulin-dependent individuals. Their findings, published in 1993, demonstrated that there was a significant reduction in the incidence of retinopathy, nephropathy, and neuropathy. The cost-effectiveness of tighter control has been amply demonstrated in several recent high-quality studies.

Research is currently ongoing to determine if a similar "outcome" improvement is obtainable in those with NIDDM. Based on current knowledge, it is important that one attempts to control glucose levels closer to the usual physiologic range, while recognizing that "normalization" of blood sugar may not be achievable in some individuals or desirable if the risk of hypoglycemia is too great.[25]

Diabetes is not equally distributed in the U.S. population. While type I diabetes is more common among whites, and has an earlier age of onset, type II has a higher prevalence among blacks, hispanics, and native Americans. In terms of relative risk for NIDDM, with that of whites being 1.0, the risks for minorities are: 1.3 for blacks, 3.1 for Hispanics, and 10.1 in native Americans. Given the higher incarceration rates for these minorities, it stands to reason that this disease presents a significant challenge for medical staff.

Much of what is referred to as "modifiable" factors that improve diabetic control are difficult to alter in the correctional setting. These include obesity, physical inactivity, and diet. Mass, non-selective screening of populations has not been demonstrated to be a cost-effective maneuver; however, high-risk groups for type II DM, namely native Americans, blacks, and hispanics, should be considered for screening. Because of the improved outcome with early recognition and management, correctional departments may wish to consider screening high-risk individuals. A recent study by Peters et al. demonstrated that diabetes could be effectively diagnosed using Hgb A1-C as opposed to the previous "gold standard" of the oral glucose tolerance test (GTT).[26] A random glucose level greater than 200 mg/dL confirms the diagnosis in a patient who is symptomatic.

While it is beyond the scope of this section to review the overall care of diabetes mellitus, several important goals and areas of management should be stressed. In January of 1996, the American Diabetes Association (ADA) published a consensus opinion concerning the management and treatment goals for diabetes types I and II.[27] This resource is highly recommended as it reflects the consensus opinion of a national panel of experts and clarifies the standard of care for the community. As well it identifies the key areas for intervention. Finally, the document serves as an excellent measure for the purposes of CQI and medical audits. In the New Mexico Corrections Department, a number of these parameters have been incorporated into the standards of care. Included are those entities that are most likely to result in a beneficial outcome, while recognizing the limitations of the treatment environment.

The areas that are most critical in these guidelines as a standard of care are:

Recognition of disease and documentation of diagnosis.

Screening and follow-up annual ophthalmologic examinations to diagnose and treat retinopathy.

Recognition and treatment of hypertension, using an angiotensin-converting enzyme inhibitor when microalbuminuria is present.

Immunizations as appropriate, including dT, influenza, and pneumococcal pneumonia vaccine.

Diet counseling and lifestyle counseling, including exercise and smoking cessation.

Regular podiatric care.

Baseline laboratory assessment, including Chem-20, CBC, urinalysis, and an ECG when appropriate.

Monitoring of glycemic control with every 3-6 monthly Hgb A1-C.

These items all represent readily achievable standards for correctional settings. Paramount in assuring their successful implementation is to put into place appropriate mechanisms for oversight and tracking of clinical services. One situation of particular importance in terms of recognition and management is that of gestational diabetes. This usually develops during the third trimester of pregnancy. While pregnancies tend to be more frequent and problematic in the jail setting vs. prisons, the critical point is to assure standard prenatal assessment by an appropriate practitioner. Standard prenatal care should routinely assess all patients for this complication.

The diabetic who requires insulin therapy presents a unique "problem" situation in the correctional setting. Given the "contraband" nature of needles and syringes, insulin can only be administered in a controlled setting under direct observation by medical staff with meticulous control of inventory. While a number of treatment options exist with the type II diabetic, the insulin-dependent diabetic generally requires insulin injections at least twice daily. This is highly labor-intensive for medical staff, but unavoidable given the medical need. Except in the case of particularly brittle or non-compliant diabetics, this regimen of twice-daily dosing will generally suffice for greater than 90% of diabetics. Recent data discount the practice of a "sliding insulin scale," opting instead to adjust the daily dosage rather than reacting to a single random glucose. This is clearly more practical in the correctional setting and is also safer.

Conventional insulin therapy consists of one to two insulin injections a day, along with self-monitoring of blood glucose and education about diabetes and exercise. Twice-a-day insulin therapy is the most frequently used therapy regimen.[28] Intensive insulin therapy included three or more insulin injections daily. The dosage of insulin is adjusted according to the results of self-monitoring of blood glucose (fingerstick blood glucose), anticipated amount of exercise, and dietary intake.[28] In civilian settings, patients involved in intensive therapy learn how to adjust their own insulin dosages in a comprehensive program of care. There are no studies demonstrating how this might best be done in a correctional setting. Intensive insulin therapy is the type of therapy that has been shown to reduce microvascular complications of diabetes (retinopathy, nephropathy, and neuropathy). However, intensive therapy results in a two- to threefold increase in severe hypoglycemia and significant weight gain.[29] Because inmates frequently locked in cells are not permitted to have injectable glucagon (because the needle would be a security risk), hypoglycemia is potentially dangerous in correctional settings. Nevertheless, given the results of the DCCT, the American Diabetes Association recommends that patients should aim for the best level of glucose control that they can achieve without placing themselves at undue risk for hypoglycemia.[30] The DCCT recommends glycemic control as close to normal as is safely possible.[29] The American Diabetes Association's position statement, Management of Diabetes in Correctional Institutions, recommends that people with diabetes in correctional facilities should be provided care equivalent to that provided to all patients with diabetes.[31]

While intensive therapy should be offered as an optimal goal for all patients including inmates, this presents a major challenge for correctional physicians, nurses, and security staff. The medical staff need to be familiar with monitoring patients on multiple subcutaneous insulin injections. Patients selection includes patient capabilities and understanding, site resources, personal preferences of the patient, and the presence of known risk factors. Patients must be able to understand how to adjust their insulin based on frequent self-monitored glucose values. Patients with repeated

severe hypoglycemia may not be candidates for intensive therapy. Patients with severe retinopathy may have accelerated retinopathy at initiation of intensive therapy, and patients with renal failure may not fully benefit from intensive therapy and the risks of treatment may outweigh the risks of the disease.[28] In addition, patients with sclerosed veins from intravenous drug use may be at a higher risk of sequelae from severe hypoglycemia as a result of inability to initiate intravenous therapy. Inmates should be individually evaluated for inclusion in intensive insulin therapy regimens. Results of DCCT (including benefits and risk) should be discussed with the patient. Failure to provide intensive therapy for acceptable candidates because of a lack of health care staffing or correctional obstacles or mandates results in less than optimal care. Because hypoglycemia can be dangerous, ethical issues arise when physicans are faced with the impossibility of safely providing intensive therapy because of the environment in a particular correctional facility.

Monitoring clinical response to therapy presents its own unique problems. Again, staff are faced with the issues of access and contraband. The only reliable method for monitoring response to therapy is with serial glucose levels, either by fingerstick or venous blood draws. This is much more important for the type I diabetic who requires more frequent assessment and is prone to wider shifts in glucose levels. Urine glucose levels are not considered appropriate for medical management and should not be used. This is due to the degree of variability of an individual's renal threshold for glycosuria, rendering urine glucose level a poorly correlated indicator of the plasma level. While Hgb A1-C suffices for long-term assessment, pre-prandial and pre-bedtime glucoses are most useful for adjusting insulin doses. Because of logistical difficulties, it may at times be simpler to admit individuals who are brittle to an in-patient unit (preferably within the correctional system) for insulin adjustment. It is important to note that activity and diet, as well as numerous stress factors that may differ in the cell or "pod," may subsequently affect insulin requirements. Because of this, type I diabetics require more frequent adjustments of insulin.

Type II diabetics may require large doses of insulin due to their "resistance," but are much less prone to develop hypoglycemia. Hence, once stable and satisfactory glucose levels are reached, frequent monitoring is generally not required. One exception is the patient who becomes highly compliant, loses weight, and follows a diet, thereby reducing his requirement for endogenous insulin.

The non-pharmacologic approach to management is pertinent to all diabetics. Diet is integral to this approach. For Type I diabetes, synchronizing eating with the time-action of the insulin preparation used is important.[32] This is difficult to accomplish in correctional settings. The contents of the diet are not as critical as the distribution of calories by meal and the timing of meals to insulin administration.

Meals, including evening snacks, especially for patients with Type I diabetes, should be at consistent times. When meal times vary, it becomes extremely difficult for health care staff to coordinate delivery of insulin with eating, resulting in potential hypoglycemic episodes. It may be necessary for physicians to discuss this process with the warden or correctional authority. Inmates also do not usually know what food will be offered at any given meal. For individuals who adjust their insulin dose based on the amount of food eaten, this can be problematic because there are usually few choices for meals. Individual inmates may find meals unpalatable and may not eat. To augment regular meals, inmates make frequent use of commissaries, which offer a variety of packaged, prepared food items. When commissary items are used in the inmate diet, these items should be taken into consideration in discussions about diet as well as in evaluating insulin therapy. Unless a caregiver knows what items an inmate is eating from the commissary as well as the nutritional content, it cannot be assumed that eating commissary items is detrimental.

Nutritional therapy for Type II diabetes emphasizes achieving weight loss and glucose and lipid goals.[32] The patient should consume a diet that is 40% to 50% carbohydrate. Fat should not constiue more than 30% of the toal caloric intake with less than 10% of fat as saturated fat. The cholesterol intake should be less than 300 mg. Some correctional facilities have instituted "heart healthy diets" as their facility-wide diet plan. These diets should maintain proportions of fats, carbohydrates, and protein at levels recommeded by Dietary Guidelines for Americans.[33] These types of diets benefit correctional staff by reducing the numbers of therapeutic diets that must otherwise be made available to the inmates. Patients with diabetes can manipulate the given diet to achieve their individualized needs. Despite these measures, institutional feeding with lack of food choice and inflexible meal times remain obstacles in dietary management of diabetes in correctional settings. Further study and advocacy is indicated. Knowledge of the abilities and constraints in one's particular setting is most helpful in developing a realistic approach and treatment plan. Because of the critical interface between security personnel and medical staff, it is important that correctional officers be trained to appreciate and recognize some of the risks associated with diabetes. Of particular importance is the need to consistently assure insulin administration and the recognition of the two extremes of glucose control, namely, diabetic ketoacidosis and symptomatic hypoglycemia. This is especially critical in the jail setting where rapid turnover of intakes could lead to non-recognition of a ketosis-prone individual. Additionally, knowledge of other complications of diabetes, such as myocardial ischemia, should be stressed to expedite medical evaluation of these higher-risk individuals.

Medical personnel, depending on their local situation, should become involved in officer training to assure an appropriate knowledge base to recognize and prevent potential problems. Close cooperation between security and medical staff will decrease the possibility of missed treatments and serious consequences.

Because of the greater risks found in IDDM, all individuals should be clearly identified in a separate listing for medical staff and, when appropriate, within the constraints of medical confidentiality, security should also be involved. For example, one would want to assure that a Type I diabeteic was assigned to a housing unit that was more accessible by security if a medical need arises.

SUMMARY

Care of the patient with chronic disease in a correctional setting is enhanced when it is organized rather than provided in episodic fashion. Patients with chronic disease must be identified immediately upon arrival, provided with an initial health evaluation by a physician, and enrolled in a chronic diseases program. Treatment of the patient is facilitated by standardized consensus guidelines. Physicians, nurses, and other allied health personnel working as a team use these guidelines to provide care to the patients. Unique features of the correctional environment must be addressed in ways that do not compromise the treatment plan for the patient. Under these circumstances, chronic disease management remains challenging yet rewarding for correctional health care staff.

REFERENCES

1. The Sixth Report of the Joint National Committee on Detection, Evaluation, and Treatment of High Blood Pressure (JNC–V). *Arch Intern Med* 157:2413–2446, 1997.
2. Executive Summary: Guidelines for the Diagnosis and Management of Asthma, National Asthma Education Program: Expert Panel Report: Publication No. 91-3042A. Bethesda, MD, National Asthma Education Program, Office of Prevention, Education and Control; National Heart, Lung, and Blood Institute; National Institutes of Health; 1991.
3. American Diabetes Association Position Statement: Standards of medical care for patients with diabetes mellitus. *Diabetes Care* 20: Suppl 1, 1997.
4. Standards for Health Services in Prisons. Chicago, National Commission on Correctional Health Care, 1997.
5. Standards for Health Services in Jails. Chicago, National Commission on Correctional Health Care, 1996.
6. Hipkins JH, Lamarre M, Paris JE, et al: *How To: A Manual of Essential Elements for a CQI-Driven Correctional Health Care Program.* Georgia Department of Correction, 1996.
7. Prevention and Control of Tuberculosis in Correctional Facilities: Recommendation of the Advisory Council for the Elimination of Tuberculosis. *MMWR* 45(no. RR-8), 1996.
8. Shelton DL: Hope on Hold. *American Medical News,* May 19, 1997, pp 17-19.
9. Harrison's Principles of Internal Medicine, 13th ed. New York, McGraw Hill, 1994.
10. Raba JM, Obis CB: Health status of incarcerated urban males: Results of admission screening. *J Jail Prison Health* 3:6–24, 1983.
11. Global Initiative for Asthma: Global Strategy for Asthma Management

and Prevention NHLBI/WHO Workshop Report. Bethesda, MD; National Institutes of Health, National Heart, Lung, and Blood Institute; Publication Number 95-3659, January 1995, reprinted May 1996.

12. Hoge CW, Reichler MR, et al: An epidemic of pneumococcal disease in an overcrowded, inadequately ventilated jail. *New Engl J Med* 331:643-648, 1994.

13. Drazen JM, Israel E, et al: Comparison of regularly scheduled with as-needed use of albuterol in mild asthma. *New Engl J Med* 335:841-847, 1996.

14. Donahue JG, Weiss ST, et al: Inhaled steroids and the risk of hospitalization for asthma. *JAMA* 277:887-892, 1997.

15. Olubodun J: Prison life and the blood pressure of inmates of a developing community prison. *J Human Hypertension* 10:235-238, 1996.

16. D'Atri DA, Ostfeld AM: Crowding: Its effects on the elevation of blood pressure in a prison setting. *Preventive Med* 4:550-566, 1975.

17. D'atri DA, Fitzgerald EF, Kasl SV, et al.: Crowding in prison: The relationship between changs in housing mode and blood pressure. *Psychosom Med* 43:95-108, 1981.

18. Paulus PB, McCain G, Cox VC: Death rates, psychiatric commitments, blood pressure, and perceived crowding as a function of institutional crowding. *Environ Psychol Nonverbal Behavior* 3:107-112, 1978.

19. Psaty BM, Smith NL, Siscovick DS, et al: Health outcomes associated with antihypertensive therapies used as first-line agents: A systematic review and meta-analysis. *JAMA* 277:739-745, 1997.

20. Whitman S, Coleman TE, et al: Epilepsy in prison: Elevated prevalence and no relationship to violence. *Neurology* 34:775-782, 1984.

21. Lechtenberg R: *Diagnosis and Treatment of Epilepsy.* New York, MacMillan, 1985.

22. Pellock J: The differential diagnosis of epilepsy: Nonepileptic paroxysmal disorders. In Wyllie E (ed): *The Treatment of Epilepsy.* Philadelphia, Williams and Wilkins, 1997.

23. Gumnit R: The differential diagnosis of epilepsy: Nonepileptic paroxysmal disorders. In Wyllie E (ed): *The Treatment of Epilepsy.* Philadelphia, Williams and Wilkins, 1997.

24. French J: The long-term therapeutic management of epilepsy. *Ann Intern Med* 120:411-422, 1994.

25. American College of Physicians: Risks and benefits of intensive management in non-insulin dependent diabetes mellitus. *Ann Intern Med Suppl* 124:81-186, 1996.

26. Peters AL, Davidson MB, Schriger D, et al: A clinical approach for the diagnosis of diabetes mellitus. An analysis using glycosylated hemoglobin levels. *JAMA* 276:1246-1252, 1996.

27. American Diabetes Association: Clinical practice guidelines: 1996. *Diabetes Care* 1:S1-S113, 1996.

28. Strowig S, Raskin P: Intensive management of insulin-dependent diabetes mellitus. In Ellerberg, Rifkin (eds): *Diabetes Mellitus*, 5th ed. New York, Appleton and Lange, 1997.

29. DCCT Research Group: The effect of intensive treatment of diabetes on the development and progression of long-term complications in insulin-dependent diabetes mellitus. *New Engl J Med* 3329:977-986, 1993.

30. American Diabetes Association: Position statement: Implications of the diabetes control and complications trial. *Diabetes* 42:1555-1558, 1993.

31. American Diabetes Association: Position statement: Management of diabetes in correctional institutions. *Diabetes Care* 20, 1997.

32. American Diabetes Association. Position statement: Nutrition recommendations and principles for people with diabetes mellitus. *Diabetes Care* 20, 1997.

33. U.S. Department of Agriculture, U.S. Department of Health and Human Services: *Nutrition and Your Health: Dietary Guidelines for Americans*, 4th ed. Hyattsville, MD, USDA's Human Information Service, 1995.

7

Sick Call As Medical Triage

Joseph E. Paris, M.D., Ph.D., C.C.H.P

On any given day, it is estimated that approximately 10% of inmates in prisons and jails request health care services. Some of these requests are walk-in type visits; most, however, are written requests for health care services. These written requests, called "kites" in some facilities, are the usual mechanism that inmates use to seek health care in most correctional systems. The initial evaluation of these requests consists of a paper triage and is usually performed by nurses or medics. A subsequent clinical evaluation similar to emergency room triage is performed by experienced staff who focus on the chief complaint, elicit additional medical history, and perform a complaint-directed assessment focusing on the vital signs.[1] Based on the findings, inmates may be treated with over-the-counter medication and other assessment-directed therapies or referred to a physician, physician assistant, nurse practitioner, or an emergency room as guided by protocols.

Historically, this function, as well as physician clinics and other health care encounters whereby health care personnel interact with inmates, is known as "sick call." Unfortunately, this term can be confusing and does not have a standard meaning nationwide. Were it not for the National Commission on Correctional Health Care (NCCHC) accreditation standards requiring "sick call," it might be more appropriate to separate the functions of accessing medical care into the triaging of health care requests, nursing or midlevel evaluation, and assessment and physician clinic.

MEANS OF ACCESSING SICK CALL

Mechanisms to access health care services have been formalized in most correctional settings. This process is addressed by NCCHC accreditation standards for both jails and prisons.[2, 3] NCCHC standards P-37 (for prisons) and J-34 (for jails) are essential standards dealing with non-emergency medical requests. They require a mechanism to enable all inmates, whether in general population housing units or in segregation, to request health services daily. It allows for oral requests to be entered in a log as staff make rounds in each housing area, or for written requests to be collected by health care staff or dropped by inmates into a locked box. In any case, the requests should be reviewed daily and an appropriate disposition made and recorded.

In practice, sick call access mechanisms in various correctional health care systems differ significantly. A system of written sick call requests, logged and answered timely, provides accountable access. Oral requests lend themselves to ambiguous situations where overworked nurses may downplay or postpone requests while talking to inmates, in effect conducting an undocumented screening process. In some jails and prisons, the name "sick call" is given to the process of a nurse walking through segregation units asking inmates if they have any medical needs, conducting limited assessments, and administering medications, without reviewing medical records. These activities lead to uncertain medical management, and often result in poor care and possible litigation. Instead, nursing rounds in segregation units should consist of a visual inspection of the inmates with an opportunity for all inmates to request health care services. Inmates in segregation requesting health care services should be triaged and seen in a clinic, not through iron bars.

TRIAGING WRITTEN REQUESTS

Written requests, once collected, are then triaged. Triage is defined by the NCCHC as the sorting out and classification of health complaints to determine which inmates need further clinical evaluation and in what priority. The standards recommend that triaging of written requests be accomplished within 24 hours.

The concept of triage originated in military battlefields. Triage officers would screen battle wounds and make quick medical decisions to maximize efficient use of medical resources. Under battlefield conditions, triage is performed by skilled medical officers, such as experienced surgeons. In contrast, the majority of correctional triage involves line staff, such as registered nurses (RN) or licensed practical nurses (LPN), also called licensed vocational nurses (LVN), and may even include emergency medical technicians.

The first step in triaging health care requests is to determine if an inmate has a clinical or a non-clinical problem. Care must be taken in interpreting written requests because, while some inmates cannot adequately express their problems in writing, others are illiterate or only marginally literate. Careless reviews of written requests may reward inmates with writing skills with an earlier visit, while ignoring or postponing requests from less articulate inmates. These practices may result in clinical mistakes. In Ohio, for example, a 31-year-old woman with a breast lump had to wait several months for a visit despite several written requests. At the time of her belated clinic visit, she had metastatic, advanced cancer. The Ohio Department of Corrections lost the case in litigation.[4]

Sometimes, staff can become jaded at the seemingly minor reasons for inmates' sick call request. There can even be resentment among medical and non-medical staff that some inmates have easier access to medical services than they do in the community. This perception may reflect more of a problem with health care in the community than with health care in correction facilities. Nevertheless, staff must remain professional and conscientious with each encounter. Common inmate complaints that sick call staff might consider mundane such as cough, throat irritation, earache, skin rash, and back problems, are actually five of the ten top reasons patients seek medical services in the community.[5] Inmate complaints are not much different from those in the community, and might even have more significant consequences, such as a cough heralding a contagious disease. Each complaint should be appreciated for the concern or discomfort that it is causing the patient and for its potential seriousness.

Incarcerated persons need explicit permission to do nearly everything and, therefore, rely on medical staff to

care for minor complaints and provide remedies. Presenting complaints to nursing sick call were studied systematically in a large Florida prison.[6] The study found that minor conditions, such as colds, headaches, etc., are common causes of sick call requests. About one-fifth of visits involved non-medical complaints, such as shaving exemptions, information seeking, etc. At least another one-fifth originated from policy requirements for medication refills, periodic validation of passes or exemptions, food service checks, etc. The study concluded that about 40% of nursing sick call visits were medically unnecessary or did not require a clinical examination.

Correctional health care workers should not forget that patients in the community also access health care services for non-clinical complaints, such as work absentee slips or disability claims. By carefully reviewing written requests from inmates, however, requests that do not require a clinical examination are usually apparent, because non-clinical complaints do not describe a symptom or physical ailment. Having clerical staff or case managers address non-medical information issues can be of assistance.

Some correctional systems initiated inmate co-payment methods to help cover the costs of health care services and reduce visits to health care personnel. Use of co-pay mechanisms is more of an ethical and administrative issue than a clinical one and has been demonstrated to reduce sick call numbers significantly.[7, 8] However, studies of co-pay programs have never been validated as to who is being discouraged from seeking health care. It is not known whether inmates without money or the desire to spend it or inmates without disease are not seeking care. Studies in Oregon demonstrated that by removing organizational mandated sick call visits (to renew medication, validate bunk assignment, obtain passes, etc.), sick call visits drop without charging a co-pay.[9] Further studies are necessary to determine if patients with bona fide or even serious medical conditions are discouraged from accessing health care services because of co-pay requirements. It is not known if there is any long-term increase in morbidity or mortality from the disincentive to use services. Until these questions are answered, co-pay systems cannot be unequivocally recommended.

PRESENTING COMPLAINTS TO NURSING SICK CALL AND TRIAGE

Inmates with marginal or no symptom-related complaints may have other motivations in requesting health services. Non-medical motives may include obtaining medical information, requesting changes in medical or work status, seeking an exemption or privilege, and more. Other less appropriate motives, however, might include a chance to chat with other inmates, a scheme to pass contraband, a ploy to seek out new or attractive faces, and so on. A shrewd clinician will know the difference. Usually, a frank discussion with the inmate will uncover any inappropriate motives and discourage repeat occurrences. Some inmates, particularly those new to the system, may request medical care as a means to "test" the system, seeking assurance that it is functional in case they have a true emergency. At other times, some inmates simply seek medical attention for the human connection that is often lacking in the rest of the system.

In every institution, as in the community, a few patients are perceived to overuse services. A study in the Oregon correctional system found that 25% of the inmates are responsible for 58% of the visits.[9] This is consistent with the community where 25% of the population account for more than 50% of the total office visits.[5] Instead of being frustrated or inattentive to frequent users, clinicians should try to understand the reasons for their behavior. Often such patients are found to have depression or other mental health disorders, while others are in threatening situations or experiencing abuse. Some have underlying issues that cause embarrassment or shame that they are reluctant to reveal. In a study of sick call use in a Florida federal prison, psychological and personality scales were reviewed for frequent sick call users. Such patients were found to have significantly high levels of stress-related symptoms, such as anxiety, depression, internalization of problems, and the use of somatic defenses.[10] After identifying the issues, interventions such as stress reduction through mental health counseling might be useful.

If a high volume of sick call requests is being generated, examination of the situation might reveal problems with the system rather than characteristics of the inmates. For example, in institutions where correctional case managers or social workers are in short supply, medical personnel may fulfill some of those needs indirectly. In some correctional systems, although sick call slips might be collected daily, the patients are not seen for several days. Anxious inmates may generate additional requests while waiting to be seen. By providing more timely evaluations, it is likely that the number of inmate health requests would decline. One study showed that by providing ready access to nursing staff and making nonprescription remedies easily available to inmates, the number of patients asking to see the physician decreased by 20%.[11]

CLINICAL EVALUATIONS

Health care requests that indicate a symptom or clinical condition must be referred for clinical evaluation. Requests, which in the opinion of the reviewer describe an emergency, must be appropriately referred and immediately evaluated. In most systems, non-emergency requests that are clinical in nature are referred to nurses for an evaluation. This evaluation is often referred to as nursing sick call.

Due to the large volume of requests that require clinical evaluation, RNs, LPNs, or other licensed health care providers have been used to make clinical evaluations of health care requests for cost-efficiency reasons.

Unqualified or unlicensed staff or correctional officers should not make clinical evaluations under any circumstances. An essential standard (P-18) of the NCCHC requires state licensure, certification, and registration requirements to apply to health care personnel. Nevertheless, use of unlicensed health care staff for sick call has been a recurrent issue. For instance, in 1987, the Florida DOC signed a consent decree agreeing to phase out unlicensed EMTs performing sick call or any other patient care function.

To appreciate cost-related issues, statewide use of nurse sick call in the Florida DOC in 1992 was 35.8 visits per inmate per year, versus 7.7 annual physician visits.[12] The cost of channeling all inmate visits to physicians would be prohibitive. Other states and many jails report similar figures; however, direct volume comparisons are very difficult because of the varying nature of what is being reported. In some prisons or jails, a nursing encounter for directly observed pill administration is counted as a sick call visit. It is uncertain whether midlevel (physician assistant or nurse-practitioner) sick call would reduce the numbers of inmate revisits for health services by addressing their health care needs more thoroughly. While the use of nurses may seem to be cost effective, they cannot prescribe medication or make diagnoses. Therefore, patients needing those services must be referred to physicians, physician assistants, or nurse practitioners. When midlevel providers perform this function, the numbers of re-referrals may actually be reduced. Constructing clinical protocols that define when to refer to an advanced level provider can facilitate appropriate use of staff.

CLINICAL ASSESSMENTS

The initial evaluation of a symptom or medical complaint should occur in a clinical setting. It is not appropriate to evaluate patients in cells, tiers, hallways, or other non-clinical settings. The examination room should be approximately 100 square feet, including an examination table, hand washing facilities, and other essential equipment. The medical record should be available for these encounters.

When midlevel providers perform evaluations of health care requests, the clinical encounters should use a SOAP format similar to any episodic care visit. When nurses are performing the evaluations, symptom-based protocol sheets are useful. To begin, a chief complaint is obtained followed by an assessment of objective findings. A first impression about whether or not the patient looks sick is useful in determining if the patient may need a secondary referral. The next step of the objective assessment is an accurate recording of vital signs. A frequently asked question is whether vital signs should be taken for all nursing encounters. Standard protocols use vital signs as an essential element of nursing physical assessments. Therefore, vital signs should be taken and documented for every clinical encounter. They can, however, be omitted when the patient

> **Box 7-1. The Georgia DOC 20 Nursing Protocols**
>
> | | |
> |---|---|
> | Chest pain | Musculoskeletal |
> | Facial/dental pain | complaints/pain |
> | Skin lesions/rashes | Headache |
> | Skin wounds/burns | Seizures/neurologic |
> | Ear complaints/pain | complaints |
> | Epistaxis | Cough |
> | Eye complaints/pain | Shortness of breath/ |
> | Abdominal | wheezing |
> | complaints/pain | Upper respiratory |
> | Rectal/perianal complaints | complaints |
> | Genitourinary | Miscellaneous complaints |
> | complaints/female | Multiple systems |
> | Genitourinary | complaints |
> | complaints/male | Hunger strike |

is not being examined. For example, an entry or incidental note in the medical chart indicating "Laboratory results returned, urinalysis is normal," does not require vital signs.

While normal vital signs do not exclude potentially life-threatening disease, abnormal vital signs should usually result in a consultation with a physician or mid-level provider. Vital signs outside of threshold ranges should be referred for a physician or midlevel examination on an urgent basis, or at least result in a phone consultation with a higher level provider.

After vital signs have been recorded, a more complete assessment is performed in accordance with the limits of the license of the examiner. Nursing protocols using standardized questionnaires are useful in directing the basis of the examination on the chief complaint. There are no studies in correctional facilities, however, that validate the sensitivity of nursing assessment and protocol triage in the evaluation of health complaints. Studies of community emergency rooms have found staff to be insensitive when identifying patients needing emergency room care.[1] While the initial clinical evaluation of health care requests in correctional "nursing sick call" and non-correctional emergency room nursing triage are not equivalent, there are some similarities. Ongoing refinement of nursing protocols, along with validation of triaging decisions, should be a continuous quality improvement process (CQI), intended to determine what level of provider should be performing certain triaging assessments.

Staffing recommendations for sick call have been developed by the NCCHC. For jails, it is recommended that the clinical evaluation of non-emergency requests (sick call) be conducted by any qualified health care personnel on the following schedule:
- In jails with fewer than 100 inmates, a minimum of 1 day a week.
- In jails with from 100 to 200 inmates, a minimum of 3 days times a week.

- In jails with 200 or more inmates, a minimum of 5 days a week.
- In prisons, it is recommended that nursing sick call occur 5 days a week.

Physician clinics are to be counted separately.

NURSING PROTOCOLS

Nursing protocols are complaint-specific guidelines usually developed by the nursing staff with physician input, and are approved by the medical director. A sample of protocols from the Georgia Department of Corrections are listed in Box 7-1. The protocols aim to provide nurses with reasonable boundaries for the assessment and management of common health conditions. Care must be taken to tailor the protocol to the skill level of the anticipated provider and to keep it within the limits of the applicable state practice acts. Protocols should contain a definition of the medical problem in question, a description of its causes, clinical features most commonly associated with the condition, details of the assessment process, appropriate treatment measures, patient education, and criteria for referral. Nursing protocols often use prompt-driven questionnaires and assessment sheets with written algorithms or instructions for treatment. The assessment sheets provide structure to the nursing assessment process. See Figures 7-1–7-3 for samples of the protocols from the Georgia Department of Corrections.

The patient's medical history and problem list must be reviewed prior to any nursing assessment. Nurses should make every effort to retrieve and read the health record before they see the patient. Using a complaint- or disease-specific fill-in-the-blanks form encourages compliance and reduces risk-management problems. Using complaint-specific protocol assessment sheets, the nurse will elicit a chief complaint and refer to the protocol for that complaint. The specified history is taken, vital signs are obtained, and general observations followed by specific observations are made. The assessment is then either a reiteration of the complaint (e.g., headache) or a description of the findings (e.g., abrasion on scalp). Disease-specific protocols can be used if a medical diagnosis has already been made by a physician. The nurse will follow parameters of the protocol, such as measuring blood pressure and referring if it exceeds certain limits, and providing patient education. The phrase "alteration in comfort" used by nurses as a stand-alone nursing assessment provides no useful information about the patient. In general, it should be avoided, and other, more specific nursing assessments should be used, such as fever, chest pain, or alteration in comfort secondary to postoperative pain. The key decision in a nursing protocol is whether the patient should be referred to an advanced level provider. Proper construction of the protocols will guide this decision.

Which protocols to use for patients with multiple complaints can be a difficult decision for nurses conducting sick call and triage. Patients may present with a number of prob-

GEORGIA DEPARTMENT OF CORRECTIONS

Name_____

No._____

NURSING ASSESSMENT
FOR MUSCULOSKELETAL COMPLAINTS/PAIN

Date of Birth_____

Race_____Sex _____

DATE: ___/___/___   **TIME:** _____   **FACILITY:** _____

SUBJECTIVE: This _____ year old ☐ male   ☐ female   presents with the chief complaint of _____

Has been present for: _____

Characterizes pain as: ☐ Dull   ☐ Sharp   ☐ Aching   ☐ Throbbing   ☐ Radiating (Where?) _____

What makes it better: _____   What makes it worse: _____

History of: ☐ Recent trauma   ☐ Old trauma   If yes, describe: _____

☐ Numbness   ☐ Tingling   ☐ Loss of sensation (Explain): _____

_____

Evaluate any low back pain for urinary symptoms such as: ☐ Burning   ☐ Frequency   ☐ Urgency   ☐ Pain

Allergies are: _____

_____

OBJECTIVE: Vital Signs: B/P _____/_____   T _____   P _____   R _____

Examination of affected area reveals: ☐ Swelling   ☐ Deformity   ☐ Tenderness   ☐ Heat   ☐ Crepitus with movement (explain):

_____

☐ Discoloration   ☐ Loss of motion (explain) _____

☐ Range of Motion: ☐ Full   ☐ Limited (describe) _____

_____

_____

ASSESSMENT: ☐ Joint Pain   ☐ Low back pain   ☐ Urinary Symptoms   ☐ Other (describe) _____

PLAN: ☐ Aspirin or Acetaminophen 325 mg., 1-2 tabs every 4 hours prn   ☐ Ibuprofen 200 mg., 2 tabs every 6 hours prn

☐ Analgesic cream prn   ☐ Other (describe): _____   Stat dose: _____   Amount issued: _____

_____

DISPOSITION: (All referrals must follow nursing protocol guidelines including referral for any vital signs abnormalities)

☐ REFERRAL   ☐ STAT   ☐ URGENT   ☐ ROUTINE   ☐ OTHER   ☐ Appointment made   Date: ___/___/___

EDUCATION: _____

_____

_____

_____

Signature_____

PI-2115 (REV.9/96) DO NOT WRITE ON BACK-USE BLACK INK ONLY **NURSING ASSESSMENT FOR MUSCULOSKELETAL COMPLAINTS/PAIN**

Figure 7-1. Nursing assessment for musculoskeletal complaints/pain.

GEORGIA DEPARTMENT OF CORRECTIONS

Name_____

No._____

NURSING ASSESSMENT
FOR SKIN WOUNDS/BURNS

Date of Birth_____

Race_____Sex_____

DATE: ___/___/___   **TIME:** _____   **FACILITY:** _____

SUBJECTIVE: This _____ year old ☐ male   ☐ female presents with the chief complaint of: _____

_____

States problem is due to ☐ Bite   Describe: _____   ☐ Burn   Describe: _____

☐ Trauma   Describe: _____   ☐ Other   Describe: _____

If pain present, it is described as: ☐ Mild   ☐ Severe   ☐ Burning   ☐ Aching   ☐ Throbbing   ☐ Other   Describe: _____

Other symptoms: ☐ Dizziness   ☐ Nausea   ☐ Vomiting   Date last tetanus: ___/___/___

☐ Allergies: _____

OBJECTIVE: Vital Signs: B/P ___/___   T _____   P _____   R _____

General appearance: ☐ Alert   ☐ Oriented   ☐ Any distress   Describe: _____   ☐ Any drainage   Describe: _____

☐ Bleeding   ☐ Swelling   ☐ Signs of Infection   Describe: _____

Describe areas affected, extent of involvement, depth: _____

_____

ASSESSMENT: ☐ Burn   ☐ Bite   ☐ Sunburn   ☐ Abrasion   ☐ Blister   ☐ Other (describe): _____

PLAN: Cleanse area with   ☐ Soap and water   ☐ Mild antiseptic   ☐ Apply non-adhering dressing prn   ☐ Dressing Materials issued

☐ Tetanus Toxoid   Dosage given: _____   ☐ Silvadene Cream applied as ordered

☐ Acetaminophen 325 mg., 2 Every 4-6 hours prn   ☐ Stat dose given   T____otal number issued: _____

DISPOSITION: (All referrals must follow protocol guidelines including referral for any vital signs abnormalities)

☐ REFERRAL: ☐ STAT   ☐ URGENT   ☐ ROUTINE   ☐ Return appointment for dressing change   Date: ___/___/___

☐ Other: _____

EDUCATION: _____

_____

_____

Signature_____

PI-2119 (REV.9/96)   DO NOT WRITE ON BACK - USE BLACK INK ONLY   **NURSING ASSESSMENT FOR SKIN WOUNDS/BURNS**

Figure 7-2. Nursing assessment for skin wounds/burns.

GEORGIA DEPARTMENT OF CORRECTIONS

Name_____

No._____

NURSING ASSESSMENT
FOR SKIN LESIONS/RASHES

Date of Birth_____

Race_____ Sex _____

DATE / / **TIME:** **FACILITY**:

SUBJECTIVE: This _____ year old ☐ male ☐ female presents with the chief complaint of _____

States problem has been present for: _____

Also complains of ☐ Itching ☐ Dandruff ☐ Acne ☐ Callus ☐ Other: _____

History of : ☐ Similar problem ☐ Recent contact with: ☐ Weeds ☐ Plants ☐ Bushes ☐ Sun ☐ Chemicals

Previous treatments: _____

_____

States Allergies are: _____

OBJECTIVE: Vital Signs: B/P _____/_____ T_____ P_____ R_____

Is there evidence of: ☐ Rash ☐ Callus ☐ Dandruff flakes ☐ Lice ☐ Nits ☐ Lesions ☐ Other

Location: _____

Today the lesions are: ☐ Open ☐ Closed ☐ Draining (Describe): _____

☐ Signs of infection (Describe): _____

_____

ASSESSMENT: ☐ Acne-like lesion ☐ Contact Rash ☐ Fungal Rash ☐ Pseudofollicular Rash ☐ Lice/Nits

☐ Callus ☐ Bruise ☐ Other (describe) _____

PLAN: ☐ Benzoyl Peroxide 5% gel prn ☐ Tolnaftate Cream bid to affected area ☐ Calamine Lotion prn itching ☐ Corn Pad

☐ Hydrocortisone Cream 1% prn ☐ Nix Shampoo ☐ Dandruff Shampoo ☐ Shave Pass Issue, for _____ days

☐ Acetaminophen 325mg., 2 tabs every 4-6 hours prn ☐ Stat dose given Number Issued: _____

Other items issued: _____

_____

DISPOSITION: (All referrals must follow protocol guidelines, including referral for any vital signs abnormalities)

☐ REFERRAL ☐ STAT ☐ URGENT ☐ ROUTINE ☐ OTHER ☐ Appointment given Date: / /

_____

EDUCATION: _____

_____

_____

Signature_____

PI-2118 (REV.9/96)   DO NOT WRITE ON BACK - USE BLACK INK ONL   **NURSING ASSESSMENT FOR SKIN LESIONS/RASHES**

Figure 7-3. Nursing assessment for skin lesions/rashes.

Table 7-1. Suggested values for referral of patients with abnormal vital signs to higher provider

Vital sign	High/low
Temperature	> 103 F < 96 F
Systolic blood pressure	> 170 mmHg < 90mmHg
Diastolic blood pressure	> 115 mmHg < 45 mmHg
Pulse	> 110/min < 50/min
Respirations	> 30/min < 10/min

Adapted from the Georgia DOC 20 Nursing Protocol Assessment forms.

lems which, if taken literally, may require the performance of five or more assessments. While complaints should never be taken lightly, it is possible to focus on one or two meaningful areas by asking the patient to identify the most important complaints and then assessing the relative urgency of each. If no assessment form exists for a certain patient complaint, a miscellaneous complaint form may be used, or a thorough progress note should be written.

Recently, the term nursing diagnosis has been used. It is important to make a distinction between medical and nursing diagnoses. A diagnosis is a "process of determining by examination the nature and circumstances of a disease condition."[13] State licensure laws often set limits for those who can make diagnoses. Mostly, this is an act of medical judgment made by a licensed physician, physician assistants, or nurse practitioners. Nursing diagnoses are actual or potential health problems that nurses, by virtue of their education and experience, can recognize. A nursing diagnosis is made after subjective and objective data are assessed. For example, a nurse may identify a patient complaining of a headache with a blood pressure reading of 160/110 mmHg as "elevated blood pressure reading." However, only an advanced level practitioner may make a medical diagnosis of hypertension. A problem associated with the introduction of the term nursing diagnosis into the clinical record especially on records where physicians and nurses write on the same progress notes is that readers of the record may interpret a nursing diagnosis as an actual medical diagnosis, which could lead to mistreatment of patients. For example, if a physician writes an assessment of "rule out exacerbation of chronic lung disease versus congestive heart failure," and the nurse writes a nursing diagnosis of "shortness of breath and chronic lung disease," subsequent readers may interpret the nursing note to mean that the patient does not potentially have congestive heart failure. For risk management reasons, it may be prudent not to use this term in the medical record.

REFERRAL TO PHYSICIANS OR MID-LEVEL PRACTITIONERS

Once an assessment has occurred, a disposition must be made. A decision is made whether the patient can be treat-

ed and released or needs to be referred to a physician or mid-level practitioner. The number of patients referred to physicians or mid-level practitioners will depend on the number of patients with actual serious medical need, the existing nursing protocol, and the skills of the nurse who performs the initial assessments. In one study, Florida triage nurses referred approximately half of their sick call cases to advanced level providers on the same day. An additional one-fourth were given a physician appointment. A small number was sent at once to the emergency room.[6] This referral pattern may have been a result of poor protocols, sick patients, or inadequate nursing skills or training. In systems that use nurses for this function, continuous quality improvement processes will be helpful in reducing unnecessary referrals. Studies of this type also suggest that perhaps mid-level providers should perform some of these evaluations.

On the other hand, failure to refer appropriate patients to advanced practitioners may cause more serious problems. Continuous monitoring of encounters, ongoing training, and inservice and educational lectures are essential to reducing nursing triage mistakes.

Nurses faced with referral or treatment decisions must make those decisions only if they feel certain that they are within the scope of their license and ability. Nursing protocols should not be designed to force nurses to make diagnostic decisions, but should be written so that nurses refer all patients requiring a medical diagnosis to an advanced level practitioner. Safety should guide their determinations. Decisions should be based on a judgment of the acuity of the patient combined with guidelines obtained from the nursing protocols. In general, an abnormal vital sign should be a cause for concern. Some systems provide guidelines (Table 7-1) defining vital sign abnormalities that must result in physician referral. Regardless of whether such guidelines are given, nurses should feel comfortable contacting a physician for any abnormal vital sign or other abnormality. Phone consultation for questionable concerns often prevents clinic visits. Beyond vital sign evaluation, well-designed nursing protocols will minimize over- or under-referral. Nursing protocols should provide explicit criteria for referral to the physician. These criteria, determined by a responsible physician, should include all potential medical conditions in the differential that require a physician evaluation. In addition, the judgment of the nurse as to the acuity of illness is extremely valuable in assessing whether a referral is indicated. Therefore, nurses should refer patients who may not otherwise need to be referred based on the protocol, but who appear to be "sick" in the opinion of the nurse.

Nurses conduct the bulk of sick call and triage and have become the backbone of correctional health care systems everywhere. Especially on weekends and after hours, nurses may be the only link between patients and available medical resources. As a licensed provider, the nurse is held responsible for making all appropriate referrals and initiating the chain of care to address emergencies. Therefore, nursing assertiveness may be critical. If a nurse, using a protocol to assess a patient, concludes that an emergent referral is indicated, the nurse has a duty to make all appropriate referrals. While the judgment of the nurse should be heeded and respected, the recipient of such calls sometimes minimizes or fails to appreciate the urgency of the matter. The nurse making the call should be commended for becoming more assertive or, if necessary, going higher in the chain of command to best serve the patient's interests.

TIMELINES FOR REFERRAL TO ADVANCED PROVIDER

Nursing protocols should incorporate criteria for immediate, urgent, and routine referral. Generally accepted definitions of these are:

Immediate ("stat"): A referral that must immediately result in a response or evaluation by an advanced level practitioner (M.D., D.O.). Immediate referrals are needed for all potentially life-threatening conditions.

Urgent: A referral that should result in evaluation the same day. Urgent referrals should be made for patients whose condition may deteriorate if left untreated, or for painful conditions uncontrolled with mild analgesics. At a minimum, there must be same-day phone consultation with an advanced level practitioner.

Routine: A referral that should result in a scheduled evaluation, usually within 10 days. Routine evaluations are for non-urgent conditions requiring an initial diagnosis, or diagnosed conditions not responding to treatment given per nursing protocol.

NURSING TREATMENT PROTOCOLS

Patients not requiring a referral to the physician may need treatment for minor conditions (such as abrasions), education, or provision of over-the-counter medications. Nursing protocols often detail patient education items or other therapies. Patient education should be simple and direct and instruct when follow-up should occur if symptoms worsen. Certain standards (NCCHC P-40 and J-41) recommend that nursing protocols not include instructions for using prescription medication except for life-threatening emergencies (e.g., anaphylaxis). These standards further recommend that prescription medication only be used with verbal or written orders from a physician and not in protocol fashion. This is prudent practice and is consistent with most state-licensing laws.

Instructions for treatment and provision of over-the-counter medication are generally given for minor ailments that would ordinarily be treated by the individual with self-care (NCCHC standards J-41 and P-40). Examples include giving acetaminophen for headache or dressing a minor abrasion. These treatments should be explicitly stated in the nursing protocol. Many correctional systems have developed a registry of over-the-counter (OTC) medications. These are medicines that, in civilian settings, can be obtained legally without a prescription. Common OTC medications include acetaminophen, antacids, aspirin, cough drops, and decongestants. For certain minor conditions, it is more cost effective and convenient to assess and provide immediate care with an OTC medication than to refer to an advanced level practitioner. Placement of over-the-counter medication on commissary lists permits the inmate to have access to simple medications customarily available to any person in the community. The additional benefit is a reduction in health care requests for simple remedies. If nursing sick call is the only source for OTC medication, overuse of sick call services will occur. Some correctional systems make OTC medication available from correctional officers or from nurses out of the context of a clinical evaluation. Some have argued against such access out of concerns for inmate misuse of OTC products, which can and does occur in non-incarcerated populations. Nevertheless, few would argue for eliminating over-the-counter products from public availability. Some correctional systems that have OTC medication in commissary stores have, with the advice of the responsible physician, eliminated products that have abuse potential, such as antihistamines. It is also prudent to restrict such products from patients with poorly controlled mental health problems. There are no reports or studies that demonstrate increased morbidity or mortality from the introduction of OTCs into general population commissaries.

LOGGING, TRACKING, AND REPORTING

Accurate maintenance of logs that track health care requests and clinical encounters in nursing sick call are important continuous quality improvement measures to study trends, verify that a request or encounter occurred, and to spot problem patients. For example, logs may be used to identify patients presenting to sick call three times for the same unresolved complaint. These patients should be referred to a higher-level practitioner. To monitor this requirement, a log of nursing sick call requests and visits is needed. Logs should be simple, easy to read, and maintained by reliable staff. Some systems, such as, Florida have computerized sick call logs. Other systems rely on paper logs.

In my experience, many prison/jail medical directors and administrators do not design, monitor, or manage logs. The task often is delegated to nurses or clerks who may not understand the use of these logs and, therefore, are careless in their design. Oftentimes, a change in responsible personnel results in a dislocation or interruption of the log-keeping activities, with resulting disruption of sick call care. Administrators, medical directors, and directors of nursing should take a very personal interest in sick call and related logs to discern trends, track compliance to institutional policies, monitor staff, and follow utilization patterns. For both computer- and paper-based systems, periodical reporting of key indicators will generate useful information for managers.

CONTINUOUS QUALITY IMPROVEMENT AND MONITORING OF SICK CALL AND TRIAGE

The intent of a continuous quality improvement (CQI) program is to involve institutional staff in ongoing quality measurements leading to self-improvement in performance.[14] Quality improvement control of nursing sick call and triage are strongly recommended. Fertile CQI areas are patient satisfaction surveys regarding sick call, clinic no-show studies aimed to understand why they occur, and documentation of patient education. Other useful sick call CQI indicators are: waiting time in the waiting room, presence of vital signs in every charted encounter, and appropriate use of nursing protocols and assessments. This may not be a precise or reproducible measuring tool, but because of its methods, institutional staff may acquire long-lasting educational benefits.[15]

Monitoring or auditing sick call and the triage process require a visit by central office or other health care teams from outside the institution. The auditors collect data in standardized data fields measuring specific clinical aspects of sick call and triage performance.[16] Audits are rigorous measuring tools capable of yielding reproducible, verifiable information on institutional quality. Because audits involve central office rather than institutional staff, they are of less educational benefit to line staff. Continuous quality improvement and audits complement each other and should be used jointly to monitor and improve the quality of sick call and triage in prison.

CONCLUSIONS AND RECOMMENDATIONS

Nursing sick call and triage are critical functions of correctional health care systems. Health care planners must properly design and monitor sick call and triage systems. Standards of the NCCHC should be incorporated, with particular attention to access systems and accountability of inmate requests. Other tasks in need of careful planning are: determining the number and type of providers required, choosing which OTC medication to be used, monitoring the impact of sick call co-pay fees if any, projecting costs, and aiming to avoid over- and under-use by inmates and over- and under-referral by nursing staff. Standardized nursing protocols and assessments of the type presented here may be helpful.

Sick call encounters must be conducted in privacy and in a medically equipped room with hand washing facilities, with the health record present. Nurses should work in triage and sick call areas only after suitable training and demonstrated proficiency. Training should emphasize the importance of interpreting vital signs, thorough evaluation of patients, nursing responsibility, and assertiveness. Institutional CQI and central monitoring play a significant role in the continuous improvement of correctional sick call and triage activities.

A copy of the Georgia DOC nursing protocols is available from the author on request.

REFERENCES

1. Adams SL, Fontanarosa PB: Triage of ambulatory patients. *JAMA* 276(6):493-494, 1996.
2. Standards for Health Services in Jails, Chicago, National Commission on Correctional Health Care, 1996.
3. Standards for Health Services in Prisons, Chicago, National Commission on Correctional Health Care, 1992.
4. Tomcik v. Ohio Department of Rehabilitation and Corrections. 598 NE, 900 (Ohio Court of Claims, October 7, 1991). Commented on the American Medical News, Sept 6, 1993, p 10.
5. Farley, PJ: Hospital and ambulatory services for selected illnesses. *Health Services Res* 21(5), 1986.
6. Paris JE: Inmate overutilization of health care. Is there a way out? *J Correctional Health Care* 1:73-90, 1994.
7. Annual Report of the Office of Health Services of the Florida Department of Corrections, Tallahassee, Florida 1997.
8. Jails' fee for service leads to drop in doctor visits. *American Medical News,* April 8, 1996, p 84.
9. Shelton S, Knox C: Evaluating the dynamics of sick call. Presentation to the National Commission on Correctional Health Care, Nashville, TN, Nov 1996.
10. Howe B, Froom J, Culpepper L, et al: Adoption of the sick role by prisoners: Report of a multi-functional experiment. *Social Sci Med* 11:507- 511, 1997.
11. Megaree EI, Carbonell JL: Personality factors associated with frequent sick call utilization in a federal correctional institution. *J Prison Jail Health* 10(1):19-42, 1991.
12. Annual Report of the Office of Health Services of the Florida Department of Corrections, 1992.
13. *The Random House Dictionary of the English Language,* 2nd ed, New York, Williams and Wilkins, 1993.
14. Hipkens JH, LaMarre M, Paris JE, Shansky R: "How To." A Manual of Essential Elements for a CQI-driven Correctional Health Care Program. Distributed by the Office of Health Services of the Georgia Department of Corrections, Atlanta, Georgia 1995.
15. Paris JE: The quest for quality management measurements in the correctional setting: Outpatient health care review. *J Prison Jail Health* 9(2):135-154, 1992.
16. Paris JE: Clinical Contract Monitoring of Correctional Managed Care: The Georgia Experience. Presented at the 20th National Conference on Correctional Health Care, Nashville, TN, October 30, 1996

8

Infirmary Care

Joseph E. Paris, M.D., Ph.D., C.C.H.P.

In a vintage movie, Cool Hand Luke, a rebellious state prisoner, played by Paul Newman, is subject to a vicious beating. As he lies on the ground, a correctional officer offers to take him to the local emergency room. However, a sergeant orders the officer to take Luke to the prison infirmary, where he dies later on. The message is clear: in these primitive times, correctional officers made medical decisions, and inmate patients were sometimes placed in infirmaries unable to care for them. Much progress has been made since Cool Hand Luke's times, but the medical care provided in correctional infirmaries is limited by design. Accordingly, infirmaries have the potential to do harm to patients who are beyond their medical capabilities. Still, correctional infirmaries are an opportunity for cost-effective correctional health care. The advantages of operating correctional infirmaries and how to avoid inappropriate infirmary placements is discussed.

WHAT ARE INFIRMARIES?

Infirmary care might be described as inpatient correctional facility bed care, with registered nurse (RN) supervision and regular physician rounds as appropriate for the level of illness—illness that does not require admission to a licensed hospital or nursing care facility.

In practice, correctional facility infirmaries are protected housing with a variable level of nursing staff and physician coverage. The National Commission on Correctional Health Care (NCCHC) has promulgated essential standards governing the scope of care rendered in prison and jail infirmary units.[1] The scope of care required by these standards is listed in Box 8-1. According to standards P-53 and J-50, an infirmary is an area accommodating two or more inmates for a period of 24 hours or more, expressly set up and operated for the purpose of caring for patients who are not in need of hospitalization or licensed nursing facility placement.[1]

The NCCHC infirmary standard, therefore, defines infirmary care as services that are not hospital care. The NCCHC standard does not provide guidance for the types of clinical practice that can safely be performed in such a unit. The difficulty with the NCCHC standard is the ever-changing nature of community standards regarding thresholds for hospital admissions. In the past decade, criteria for hospital admission have become very stringent. With the advent of managed care, which is changing the way medicine is practiced in this country, as well as home health care and same day surgical centers, much medical care previously delivered in hospitals today is performed on an outpatient basis. Previous practice patterns established correctional infirmaries as fillers for the gap between hospital care and return to a cell. In addition, infirmaries have treated self-limited minor illnesses, housed patients with chronic conditions precluding general population placement, and served as medical observation areas. As a result of recent secular trends in managed care, however, the expectations of correctional infirmaries are expanding.

Most state or county correctional facilities capable of housing more than 500 inmates have two or more infirmary beds. Typical correctional infirmaries are located near the institution's outpatient clinic and have 2–20 inpatient beds, and the larger units resemble small rural hospitals. Physical plants vary from institution to institution. Many infirmary facilities in old prisons or jails were built when building codes and federal regulations governing health care facilities were either not yet enacted or not strictly enforced. Cells may be single or have two, four, or more beds. Some infirmaries are of the open-bay configuration and resemble small pre-war community hospitals.

Box 8-1. Scope of Services for Infirmaries

1. Accommodates two or more inmates for 24 hours or more
2. Cares for patients not in need of hospitalization or a licensed nursing facility
3. Inpatient bed care with registered nurse supervision
4. Illness requires limited observation and/or management
5. A single physician is responsible for "advancement of quality care"

From Standards for Health Services in Prisons. Chicago, National Commission on Correctional Health Care, 1992, with permission.

Box 8-2. Requirements for an Infirmary Unit

1. Physician on call 24 hr/day
2. Daily supervision by a registered nurse
3. Sufficient staff for 24-hr coverage
4. Patients kept within sight or hearing of health care staff
5. Existent manual of nursing procedures
6. Complete inpatient record for each patient
7. Admission and discharge only by order of a physician or other health professional where permitted by state law

From Standards for Health Services in Prisons. Chicago, National Commission on Correctional Health Care, 1992, with permission.

Modern infirmaries favor very secure layouts with locked single cells.

Although there are strict codes and regulations governing hospital buildings and practice, oversight of correctional infirmaries is limited. This deficit creates the potential occurrence for a wider range of unmonitored clinical activities in facilities that are not equipped for certain clinical practices. A typical example includes housing patients with active tuberculosis (TB) in ordinary locked cells that do not have certified negative pressure venting and other appropriate ventilation controls. For large facilities, given the direction of managed care, it is prudent for new infirmaries to be constructed in accordance with all regulations and codes governing a skilled nursing facility. Otherwise, infirmary units may be ill-equipped for the use of anything other than protected housing.

NCCHC INFIRMARY STANDARDS

The NCCHC Standards P-53 and J-50 (Infirmary Care) specify that a physician is to be on call 24 hours a day. Infirmaries also must have a daily RN supervisor, and sufficient and appropriate health care personnel should be on duty 24 hours a day. All inmate patients must be within sight or hearing of a health care staff member. There should be a manual of nursing care procedures. A complete health care record must be kept for each inmate. Admission to and discharge from the infirmary should be on the order of a physician or on the order of another health professional where permitted by state law. Box 8-2 lists the infirmary requirements of the NCCHC.

The NCCHC standards define a scope of care, but do not address the types of clinical practice that would be acceptable in infirmary units similar to the way the Joint Commission on the Accreditation of Hospitals (JCAHO) regulates hospitals, nor does the NCCHC define the physical structures or processes that must be in place before certain medical practices are performed. At times, appropriate clinical care is limited by the type of physical structure, equipment, or processes in an infirmary unit. It is, therefore, recommended that the medical director or responsible

physician advise correctional authorities of appropriate codes and regulations that govern medical practices occurring in an infirmary unit. Because of the complexity of current rules and regulations, consultation with experts in these areas may be indicated before instituting a new practice or when reviewing current practices. Examples of issues that may require oversight include (1) ventilation controls for patients with TB, (2) Occupational Safety and Health Administration (OSHA) directives on infection control and ventilation control practices, (3) disposal of infectious waste, (4) safe storage and delivery of oxygen, (5) performance of medical procedures, and (6) storage and handling of pharmaceuticals. In addition, when procedures are contemplated for an infirmary unit, professional guidance should be obtained for the design and operation of any treatment facility.

INFIRMARY LEVELS OF CARE

Nationwide, the level of care in infirmary units varies substantially. Some units have virtually no staff and consist of a few observation beds to which nurses, normally assigned to other areas, make rounds a few times a day to check the patients. Other infirmaries have dozens of beds and a large professional staff and function like secondary care hospitals.

Correctional authorities must decide what level of care they desire for their facilities. This choice is based on the needs of the patient population, economic considerations, the size of the facility, and the availability of professional staff in the geographic area surrounding the prison or jail. The simplest solution for health authorities is to maintain an infirmary for protected housing only and to send any other complicated problem off site. The opposite extreme is the infirmary unit that is equivalent to a skilled nursing unit.

Generally, infirmaries lack certain types of monitoring associated with hospital care: cardiac telemetry, access to imaging services such as ultrasound, magnetic resonance imaging, or computed tomography, and access to 24-hour emergency radiology or emergency (stat) laboratory tests.

Used as an example to illustrate infirmary operations, the Georgia Department of Corrections (GDC) operates infirmaries at most of its 37 prisons. The GDC infirmary policies describe levels of care, staffing, and nursing supervision, and are very specific about the type of monitoring and nursing supervision infirmaries are authorized to perform. The GDC operates two levels of infirmaries. A level 1 or observation infirmary is protected housing, and a level 2 infirmary allows more advanced medical management. The GDC level 1 infirmaries are usually located in the smaller institutions and may have fewer beds. They include, at a minimum:

- Physician rounds 5 days a week;
- Physician phone coverage 24 hours a day;
- An RN physically present at the infirmary for no less than 16 hours a day.

An RN may be present at the institution the remaining 8 hours, make rounds at the infirmary frequently, and be available to tend to patient needs anytime. Care must be exercised to afford level 1 infirmary patients sight or sound access to medical staff after hours. This is generally accomplished by an intercom or buzzer–light system reaching the nursing area elsewhere in the clinic, where the after-hours nursing staff may be immediately alerted. Disorders appropriate for level 1 infirmary care include shingles, severe colds, healing fractures, ambulatory stability problems, hunger strikes, and similar conditions that do not result in changes of vital signs or that do not include individuals whose medical conditions require frequent monitoring. Patients not suitable for level 1 infirmary care are, for example, those who need continuous nursing supervision, vital sign monitoring around the clock, or IV or oxygen therapy. Some of these may be appropriate for placement at a level 2 infirmary; others may need hospital care.

Level 2 infirmaries are generally found in large institutions housing 1,000 inmates or more and may have six or more beds. They should include:

- Physician rounds 7 days a week;
- Physician phone coverage 24 hours a day;
- An RN physically present at the infirmary 24 hours a day.

Examples of disorders appropriate for level 2 infirmary care are any disorder appropriate for level 1 infirmary care, viral gastroenteritis, controlled seizure disorders, bronchitis, mild-to-moderately out-of-control blood pressure, influenza, malnutrition, diabetic control problems not related to ketoacidosis, hyperosmolarity states or serious infections, urinary tract infections, and similar conditions that can be monitored with simple equipment and intermittent physician supervision.

Although the examples from the GDC are illustrative, they do not constitute guidelines for individual facilities. The important point is that care in infirmaries should be limited by the availability of equipment and staff. For example, states having large numbers of inmates infected with HIV who may require intermittent IV therapy, or states having large numbers of patients with tumors, may have units with specialized nursing teams to provide chemotherapy or other

specific therapy on site. These special circumstances will be determined by the types of illnesses that need care in a specific facility. The decision to augment staffing and equipment in the infirmary to deal with these circumstances will be dependent on the cost of other arrangements.

CONDITIONS GENERALLY INAPPROPRIATE FOR INFIRMARY CARE

It is recommended that patients who are at risk for life-threatening complications, or need specialized diagnostic evaluations or monitoring, not be housed in infirmary units. A partial list would include (1) any chest pain suggestive of myocardial infarction, (2) malignant hypertension or shock, (3) any respiratory condition that requires blood gas monitoring, such as asthma or intubation, (4) potentially life-threatening cardiac arrythmias, such as paroxysmal tachycardias or ventricular tachycardia, (5) any abdominal complaint suggesting a surgical abdomen, (6) status epilepticus or patients with more than two or three seizures in a single day, (7) closed head injuries with loss of consciousness, nausea, or vomiting, (8) acute altered mental status changes, particularly with fever, (9) overdoses, whether suspected or confirmed, and (10) TB. Generally, although none of these conditions is suitable for infirmary care, they are a common problem in correctional infirmaries. Each is discussed individually.

- Patients with suspected cardiac chest pain should not be housed in the infirmary unit until hospital diagnostic workups conclude that it is safe to do so. Pain that is cardiac in origin may lead to rapid onset of arrhythmias, myocardial infarction, cardiac arrest, and death. These conditions require telemetry in a unit equipped and staffed for emergency resuscitation, endotracheal intubation, defibrillation, emergency catheterization, and beyond.
- Patients with malignant hypertension and shock should be immediately referred to a hospital. High blood pressure without end-organ damage (diastolic blood pressure, less than 120) can usually be managed in an infirmary unit; however, symptomatic low blood pressure (systolic, less than 90) or shock should be managed in a hospital.
- Patients with chronic lung disease and asthma are frequently housed in infirmary units. Any patient with asthma sick enough to be transferred to an emergency department should be considered for infirmary housing on return to the prison until deemed stable by direct physician examination. On the other hand, patients with asthma or chronic lung disease who have uncertain status should not be housed in the infirmary. One rule of thumb to follow when making this decision may be to send to the emergency department any patient with asthma or chronic lung disease whose diagnostic status requires an arterial blood gas measurement. Pulse oximeter testing is not sufficient in the evaluation of patients with acute asthma. Any patient with a new onset of shortness of breath

---

Box 8-3. Infirmary Care Services Appropriate for the Stable Patient

INTRAVENOUS THERAPY
continuous hydration, antibiotics, chemotherapy, hyperalimentation, peripheral IVs, central lines, port-a-caths, Hickman catheters, dialysis access lines

CATHETER CARE
Foleys; nasogastric, gastrostomy, nephrostomy, and T tubes

WOUND CARE
dressing changes; moist, sterile, and medicated dressings; Penrose drains

RESPIRATORY CARE
oxygen administration, aerosol treatments, intermittent positive-pressure breathing, tracheostomy care

CARE BEFORE HOSPITAL ADMISSION
preoperative preparation, testing, and education

CARE AFTER HOSPITAL DISCHARGE
postoperative monitoring, testing, and education; progressive ambulation

LONG-TERM CARE
monitoring for asthma, diabetes, hypertension, seizures, HIV, and other conditions

ORTHOPEDIC CARE
cast care, traction, circulation monitoring, progressive ambulation

LONG-TERM ANTICOAGULATION
(in institutions without capabilities for routine monitoring)

GENERAL NURSING SERVICES
vital sign monitoring, positioning and turning, oral and injectable medication administration, multiple daily complex dressing changes, bathing and toileting assistance, urine dipstick checks, accuchecks, hematocrits, specimen collection, ECG, respiratory isolation, universal isolation, patient education

---

who requires arterial blood gas measurements or immediate radiographic evaluation should generally be sent to an emergency department.

- Patients with a new onset of cardiac arrhythmias causing life-threatening consequences should be evaluated in a hospital in which appropriate telemetry, cardiac care units, and a 24-hour physician staff are available.
- Patients with any gastrointestinal symptom suggesting an acute surgical abdomen or patients with nausea and vomiting of unknown origin that require diagnostic workup should be sent to a hospital.
- Patients with seizure disorders sometimes may be cared for in an infirmary, at least until their status can be deter-

mined. Patients with two or more seizures in a given day or any patient with status epilepticus, however, should be sent to a hospital. New onset seizures should result in hospital admission.

- Patients with closed head injuries and loss of consciousness may require brain imaging, such as computed axial tomography scanning or MRI, and observation with frequent neurologic checks. These patients should not be housed in an infirmary, as they may require neurosurgical intervention.
- Patients with altered mental status, particularly when associated with a fever, require close physician involvement and an involved workup, including brain imaging and a spinal puncture. Infirmary placement would be proper only after completion of the workup.
- Patients with suspected or confirmed drug overdoses should not be placed in an infirmary until there is proof that the quantity of the drug(s) ingested does not pose a threat. This type of admission requires immediate (stat) toxicology screening. After hospitalization, mental health and suicide assessments should be included in infirmary care for patients who have overdosed.
- Patients with active TB should not be housed in an infirmary unit, unless that unit is properly equipped with negative pressure ventilation units that can pass an OSHA inspection.

TYPES OF SERVICES APPROPRIATE FOR INFIRMARY CARE

The correctional medical director needs to determine whether a particular service is appropriate for each individual infirmary, and he may decide to house additional classes of patients in an infirmary, depending on the conditions in the facility's general population. Services that are appropriate for infirmary care of stable patients, provided the medical director has concluded that sufficient staff and equipment are available for monitoring these services, are listed in Box 8-3.

Intravenous therapy generally requires 24-hour RN supervision and 24-hour on-call physician services. Depending on the type of IV therapy, it may be necessary to have immediate access to laboratory testing. Placement of peripheral IV lines and central IV lines may be beyond the expertise of the staff. It is not recommended for staff members to insert an IV line or device unless they have been trained to do so. Because an immediate chest radiograph before catheter insertion is usually required, most central line placement is performed in an outpatient surgicenter or a hospital.

Care of patients with specialized devices (central IV lines, gastrostomy tubes, nephrostomy tubes, etc.) is best detailed in a combined nursing and physician treatment plan written in the medical record.

Oxygen is frequently used in infirmary units. Practical guidelines for oxygen use in infirmaries should be based on the ability and need to monitor the patient's status. For example, some physicians routinely treat patients having asthmatic exacerbations with oxygen. Pulse oximeter testing may be used to monitor these patients; however, a complete arterial blood gas workup may be required in patients unresponsive to therapy to more accurately stage their disease and determine whether intubation is necessary. These patients should be sent to an emergency department in which arterial blood gas testing can be done immediately, and in which ventilatory support is available if necessary.

Generally, infirmary units are ideal locations to house patients who have chronic diseases and need more intensive monitoring. For example, patients with diabetes whose blood sugar levels are temporarily elevated because of minor infections can often be placed in infirmary units for management and the administration of antibiotics. Because most infirmaries do not have the appropriate support services to manage diabetic ketoacidosis, infirmary housing is appropriate for these individuals unless ketoacidosis is present.

INFIRMARY STAFFING PATTERNS

The GDC levels 1 and 2 infirmary coverage hours discussed earlier may serve as a guideline for staffing requirement patterns. Daytime staffing usually is heavier than evening or night shifts. In addition to the nursing staff, a half-time physician is needed in a typical infirmary with eight to ten beds. Insufficient physician hours is a pervasive problem that may lead to low-quality infirmary care and medical complications. Physician coverage needs to include time to examine all patients. It is recommended that the physician write daily notes on patients who have uncertain diagnoses or are acutely ill, but patients who are boarders or are being housed in the infirmary because of acute or chronic disabilities generally do not need daily notes. Infirmaries with more than 15 beds may need clerical support and additional nursing staff, such as licensed practical nurses and nurses' aids.

PHYSICIAN COVERAGE IN INFIRMARY UNITS

In addition to the physician staff on site during the day shift, infirmaries need after-hours medical coverage. Problems with a lack of physician coverage occur more frequently during the evening, night, and weekend shifts. Typically, arrangements for physician coverage include phone consultations. These arrangements are often problematic for the following reasons:
- The physician cannot be found.
- The physician would downplay the medical situation and recommend to wait until daytime.
- The physician is not certain of what clinical action to take and recommends temporary measures only.
- The physician agrees to go to the prison soon to make an evaluation, but takes several hours to do so.

- The doctor–nurse communication is imperfect, and the appropriate amount of information is unavailable for a clinical evaluation over the phone.

Phone consultation outcomes are an excellent continuous quality improvement study. Physicians taking phone calls must know that infirmary patients may be sick individuals and should be taken seriously. Physician coverage arrangements should specify who will take phone calls and who will return to the prison to see infirmary patients after hours.

SECURITY ISSUES

As in other areas of correctional care, infirmaries face the conflicting imperatives of security and medical care. Barrack-type arrangements with multiple beds lined up in a communal room are particularly difficult to secure. On the other hand, when inmates in infirmary units are locked in separate cells, routine medical monitoring may become very difficult, and identification of an emergency may be delayed. Checking vital signs, a simple undertaking in community hospitals, becomes an involved process in infirmaries with multiple gates, locked cells, and control rooms. The health care staff has to adapt to a secure environment while delivering high-quality care. It may be advisable to develop treatment plans involving correctional staff. Patients with wired and banded jaw fractures, for example, are at risk for aspiration if they vomit. Immediate access to these patients is mandatory to cut the bands and prevent aspiration. This may be difficult when single, locked rooms are used. Additionally, patients who are seriously ill may be unable, in some locked-room arrangements, to call for help because they are too ill. When these conditions exist, nursing rounds or cooperative treatment plans with correctional staff can reduce the likelihood of poor outcomes.

Some infirmaries have the problem of excessive medical–correctional staff interaction and wasted time. While watching inmates, correctional staff work long periods in apparent inactivity. Male correctional officers in close contact with female nursing staff may engage in long conversations and slow medical work. Careful layout planning separating control rooms from nursing stations may alleviate the problem. Also, it may be necessary to instruct the professional nursing staff not to discuss medical matters with correctional officers.

Inmate custody grades may introduce constraints. In some infirmaries, certain rooms are secure and others are open. Care must be exercised to ensure that patients in locked rooms receive the same care, vital sign monitoring, and nursing checks as the patients in open areas. Wardens, superintendents, or sheriffs are the maximum correctional authority in prisons, jails, detention centers, and other correctional facilities. Under their direction, specialized security functions take place, such as keeping accurate inmate counts, securing adequate transportation, assigning inmate housing, and many other functions. In many facilities, there is a bed shortage for the part of the population incarcerated for the long term. At the same time, infirmary work entails periods with high and low rates of bed occupancy. In crowded facilities, the correctional authority may be tempted to use empty infirmary beds for inmates without medical conditions. The NCCHC standard P-53 specifies admissions and discharges to be ordered by physicians or other health care professionals. Infirmary bed use for nonmedical reasons is sometimes rationalized by stating that these inmates are not admitted but merely temporarily housed in the infirmary. Such nonmedical uses should be kept to a minimum or eliminated. Nonmedical use of infirmary beds should never interfere with medical infirmary bed availability and use.

INFIRMARY RECORD KEEPING

The NCCHC standard P-53 mandates that infirmary records include admission notes, a discharge plan, and complete documentation of the care and treatment given. The NCCHC takes a neutral stand regarding the issue of whether infirmary records should be a continuation of the outpatient record or a separate record altogether. The advantages of separated infirmary records are better accountability and standardization of infirmary-specific forms, such as vital sign charts, flow sheets, and the like. A disadvantage is the need for additional paperwork. I favor separate records, which make it easier to enforce rules about prompt filing of admission histories and physicals and encourages thoroughness. Single-record systems may lead to ambiguous situations in which the reader cannot determine whether a patient was admitted. For separate record systems, the NCCHC requires that a discharge summary be placed in the outpatient record. The quality of infirmary documentation varies from system to system. The GDC mandates that all infirmary patients give a standard medical history and have a physical on the day of admission.

SHORT-STAY INFIRMARY ADMISSIONS

In a number of correctional infirmaries there are two types of infirmary admissions: formal admissions and short-stay admissions. The rationale for the short stay is that there is a number of self-limiting conditions requiring less than 24 hours to resolve. To simplify paperwork, exemptions from the complete documentation required for formal infirmary admissions are made for these patients admitted for a short stay. These abridged workups, however, may be a source of problems. Staff may overlook the development of serious medical conditions in a short-stay patient, who may become quite ill before being noticed. Ideally, there should be only one standard of documentation for all infirmary admissions. If short-stay documentation is used, close monitoring for appropriateness and management is recommended.

Examples of short-stay infirmary admissions include bowel preparation for gastrointestinal procedures, 24-hour urine collection, preoperative preparations, postoperative observation, and observation after blunt head trauma with loss of consciousness.

RESPIRATORY ISOLATION ROOMS IN THE INFIRMARY

According to the Centers for Disease Control, a respiratory isolation room is a single-patient room specifically designed with ventilation characteristics appropriate for isolation and maintaining negative air pressure. There are very specific OSHA guidelines that should be followed in the design and maintenance of negative-pressure isolation rooms. Negative-pressure ventilation usually requires not only the engineered installation of fans or vents, but also an active maintenance program that provides ongoing air pressure monitoring across the entry to the room and in the interior of the room. Any new construction for negative-pressure vented rooms usually calls for provision of an anteroom. These rooms are connected to the patient room and are often equipped with a sink for provider hand washing. These anterooms provide an air break that reduces the chance for contamination of hallways or common spaces with droplet nuclei. Retrofitting an ordinary inmate cell into an isolation room is difficult for engineering reasons. In older prisons and jails, rooms that are adjacent to day rooms or that open into common living space or hallways may have a fan installed so that they can be used for TB isolation. Caution is urged in this practice. Consultation with licensed engineers familiar with negative-pressure venting regulations is recommended. Rooms used for respiratory isolation should be equipped with a private shower and commode. Portable sputum induction units can be installed near these rooms to reduce the time out of the room, which will reduce potential exposure risk. Doors to respiratory isolation rooms should be kept closed except when patients or personnel must enter or exit the room. Respiratory isolation rooms should have six air exchanges per hour to enable a reduction in the concentration of droplet nuclei.[2, 3] Infirmaries in the larger institutions find that retrofitting one or more rooms for respiratory isolation is cost-effective because it allows the rapid isolation of patients with suspected TB and rules out TB without costly transfers to other centers. Care must be taken in placing patients with TB in isolation rooms when they have uncertain diagnoses. Patients without fevers and with few constitutional symptoms are excellent candidates for isolation in appropriately equipped infirmary isolation rooms. However, patients who are febrile, those who have radiographs that may indicate other infectious causes, those who may need bronchoscopy, or those who appear unstable, are best admitted to a hospital.

SPECIAL INFIRMARY PATIENTS: HUNGER STRIKERS, DISABLED INMATES, AND THOSE IN NEED OF TERMINAL OR HOSPICE CARE

Infirmary care for hunger strikers is cost-effective and humane, and access to physical health and mental health staff is required. Ongoing supervision should include vital sign and food intake monitoring, as well as daily weighing. An inmate with an advanced case may need fluid and electrolyte monitoring. In many instances, infirmary placement alone breaks a vicious cycle of confrontations in the general population and cell blocks and allows for the gradual return of the inmate to counseling, reasoning, and eventual resumption of feedings.

Many prisons and jails either lack or have limited special housing facilities for the disabled. Inmates needing help for activities of daily living gravitate toward infirmaries for housing. Although infirmary placement is an acceptable short-term measure, other problems are created, including the lack of available infirmary beds for short-term care and the restriction of certain activities, jobs, and programs available to the general population. Infirmary settings and rules may cause activities such as feedings and medication intake to become medical in nature and more labor intensive than in an inmate dormitory.

Terminal or hospice care may take place in infirmaries so that terminally ill patients with deteriorating conditions may end their days with dignity and peace. However, a number of terminal cases do not follow a predictable, steady course but are punctuated by crisis. Metastatic disease may cause bowel, esophageal, or urinary obstruction; pulmonary or great vessel embolization; peripheral vascular obstruction; tracheal compression; superior vena cava syndrome, etc. Patients with terminal diseases and obstructive syndromes may require short-term care for temporary relief. Infirmaries housing these patients need to have arrangements with prison hospitals or community hospitals with secure beds so that the patients can promptly receive short-term services. The relationships between correctional infirmaries and correctional hospitals are discussed elsewhere in this book and in the literature.[4]

Ill or dying infirmary patients should have an advanced directive in their medical record where it is clear for all staff to see. Advanced directives are signed by the patient and detail the extent of medical care desired in the event of a deterioration in clinical condition. The patient should be included in all decisions, not only about rescucitation but also about hospitalization, heroic measures, infection treatment, oxygen therapy, and so on. The directive provides the medical staff guidance on how the patient wishes to be treated, although patients may change these directives at any time.

INFIRMARY CRISIS AND STABILIZATION UNITS (CSUS), AND OTHER MENTAL HEALTH SERVICES

Crisis and stabilization units, described elsewhere in this book, are units for inpatients with mental health conditions.

Although some CSUs are located in dedicated buildings, they are designated physical health infirmary beds in a substantial number of systems. These are usually unacceptable arrangements, particularly when the infirmary is an open bed configuration because, for safety reasons, patients with mental health conditions should not be housed with patients with medical conditions. For example, patients with mental health conditions who may be restrained for their protection are vulnerable to assault in an open architecture room. In addition, patients with mental health conditions in medical infirmaries are cared for in a medical environment usually devoid of the day rooms, occupations, opportunities, and programs that characterize the better mental health inpatient or CSU programs. Although it is tempting to use infirmaries for both patients with mental health conditions and patients with medical conditions for cost reasons, these are not usually clinically appropriate arrangements.

INFIRMARY SANITATION AND INFECTION CONTROL

Sanitation and infection control policies are an essential ingredient of infirmary work. An infection control policy should define sanitation and sterilization practices, and should instruct in both the cleaning of biohazard spills and the disposal of infectious biohazard waste and soiled linen. Responsible personnel should be assigned to infection control coordination duties. There should be an infection control policy manual, and a log should be maintained detailing the progress of infection control activities. Periodic infection control committee meetings should be held, with minutes kept. These infirmary-specific infection control activities may be combined with other institutional infection control activities.

ROLE OF PHYSICIANS, NURSES, AND ADMINISTRATORS

Power and control struggles are negative and detract from the professional infirmary environment needed for quality health care delivery. In correctional infirmaries with an imprecise chain of command, doctors, nurses, and administrators vie for control. Correctional health authorities must understand and accept that only physicians give medical orders. It is essential to write accurate job descriptions and delineate a viable organization chart describing professional relationships carefully.

INFIRMARY INMATE WORKERS

Folklore of infirmary care tells anecdotes about convicted physicians redeeming themselves by performing heroic medical services in poorly equipped infirmaries with scant surgical facilities. These situations are rare today. Contemporary correctional infirmaries, however, may use inmate workers for janitorial work. With time, medical staff may rely on these inmate workers for broader duties and eventually breach the NCCHC standard (P-25) regarding inmate workers. The standard states that written institutional policy prohibits inmates from being used as health care workers and that actual institutional practice should reflect such policy.[1] Inmate workers often are used as janitors in infirmary units, but caution is urged so that they do not have access to medical records or equipment. Occasionally, inmate workers are assigned as helpers to debilitated inmates. Although these are worthwhile and cost-effective ideas, care must be taken so that the inmate worker does not interfere in medical work. Continuous monitoring by the health care authority is needed to avoid these situations.

CONTINUOUS QUALITY IMPROVEMENT (CQI) AUDITS

Infirmary health staff may benefit from CQI activities. Parameters worth studying include readmission to the infirmary within 2 weeks of a previous admission; inmate satisfaction with care received; compliance with deadlines for completion of admission histories, physicals, and discharge summaries; medication administration; and others.[5] These activities may complement the performance of infirmary audits by the health authority. Audits usually deal with chart review for appropriateness of admissions, length of stay at the infirmary, completeness of workups and nursing care plans, and similar areas.[6]

INMATE ATTITUDES TOWARD INFIRMARIES

There seems to be a wide spectrum of inmate attitudes toward infirmaries. Some inmates are attracted to the idea of spending time in a medical environment with attentive health care staff, a controlled temperature, and no work. Other inmates are reluctant to give up previous housing and work arrangements and may refuse infirmary admission to the detriment of their health. A third group may accept infirmary placement while distrusting the infirmary staff and doubting their professional competency. Infirmary staff need to take every opportunity to educate inmate patients about their conditions and gain their confidence and trust.

A more difficult situation arises when inmates who should be housed in infirmary units refuse to comply. This may place the inmate in jeopardy and may place additional burdens on the institution resources. Although inmates have the right to refuse medical treatment, their housing assignment is not something they can decide. In coordination with the correctional authority, it may be prudent to continue to place inmates in an infirmary when their medical condition warrants that placement, even though they may refuse care.

COST-EFFECTIVENESS OF INFIRMARIES: THE CONCEPT OF REGIONALIZATION

For appropriate conditions and diagnoses, infirmary care is very cost-effective. A typical infirmary admission may cost a few hundred dollars per day per patient, including security. If the same patient were hospitalized, expenses would rise to thousands of dollars per day per patient. Because of fixed costs, however, potential infirmary savings are heavily volume-dependent. Fixed costs, such as building and equipment amortization and minimum staffing levels, accrue whether there is one patient or one dozen patients. Predictably, high rates of infirmary bed occupancy are essential in preserving cost-effectiveness. Small, freestanding jails may not find it cost-effective to run an infirmary. Suitable arrangements can be made with community hospitals and nursing homes for the occasional medical decompensation.

In state prison systems, it may be impractical to build an infirmary at each prison. Assuming that a state system is composed of a number of institutions with 500–1,000 inmates each and that each institution runs an infirmary, one could expect that the volume of infirmary occupancy would be an average of two to four patients each. Quick calculations would favor the creation of a full-service infirmary for every other institution or even every third one. The remaining institutions would have no infirmary. Another approach would be to intersperse level 1 and level 2 infirmaries throughout the system. For these arrangements to work, there should be a sufficient number of vehicles and transportation-ready correctional officers, and the participating institutions need to be in relatively close proximity. The correctional health authority needs to define the role, mission, staffing patterns, and coverage duties of each prison involved and needs to coordinate closely with the correctional authority.

In both prisons and jails, a scarcity or an overabundance of infirmary beds would increase operating costs. An infirmary system with too few beds would fill quickly and result in patient diversion to expensive hospitals. An infirmary system with too many beds may operate infirmaries with too few patients to offset fixed costs.

The establishment of shared infirmaries and special mission institutions is sometimes referred to as regionalization. The concept entails a well-thought out redistribution of medical staff that concentrates in a few institutions the resources based on the service demands and operates other institutions with minimal medical staff and without infirmary care. Regionalization could result in substantial savings, but demands careful planning by the correctional health authority and close communication with the correctional authority. There is a consensus on the growing number of beds needed for the correctional population for the foreseeable future,[7] and the total number of infirmary beds needed is expected to rise accordingly. Therefore, expert health care planning for infirmary facilities is essential.

CONCLUSIONS

We have come a long way since Cool Hand Luke's untimely fictional death. Infirmaries today play an important role in the correctional health picture. The responsible correctional health authority needs to ensure adherence to NCCHC standards. Planning should include a determination of the level of care in the infirmary and the number of beds most appropriate for each facility. Both scarcity and overabundance of infirmary beds may lead to inordinate expenditures and should be avoided. Medical staff education is needed to ensure that patients with conditions that result in rapid changes in vital signs are only admitted to infirmaries with the appropriate medical resources. Nursing and physician coverage arrangements should be well defined. Layouts separating nursing stations and control rooms are highly desirable. Policy manuals should describe infirmary sanitation and infection control. Infirmaries need arrangements with short-term care hospitals for the occasional decompensation of previously stable patients. Both CQI and health care authority audits are essential ingredients in ensuring quality care. With proper planning, correctional infirmaries are a key component in the organization of a cost-effective health care delivery system and in the development of comprehensive medical care for correctional populations.

REFERENCES

1. *Standards for Health Services in Prisons.* Chicago, National Commission on Correctional Health Care, 1992.

2. Guidelines for preventing the transmission of *Mycobacterium tuberculosis* in Health-Care Facilities, 1994. CDC Recommendations and Reports. *MMWR* 43(RR-13): I-132, 1994.

3. Prevention and control of tuberculosis in correctional facilities. Recommendations of the advisory council for the elimination of tuberculosis. *MMWR*. 45(RR-8):1–27 1996.

4. Paris JE: Inpatients behind bars. The unique complexities of running a prison hospital. Presented at the 18th National Conference on Correctional Health Care, San Diego, Calif, September 24–28, 1994.

5. Hipkens JH, LaMarre M, Paris JE, et al: *How To: A Manual of Essential Elements for a CQI-driven Correctional Health Care Program.* Georgia Department of Corrections, Atlanta, 1995.

6. Paris JE: Clinical contract monitoring of correctional managed care: The Georgia experience. Presented at the 20th National Conference on Correctional Health Care, Nashville, Tenn, October 30, 1996.

7. Federal and State Prisons. Inmate Populations, Costs, and Projection Models. U.S. General Accounting Office. Report to the Subcommittee on Crime, Committee on the Judiciary, House of Representatives. November 25, 1996, pp 1–38.

9

The Hospital Secure Unit

Budd Heyman, M.D.

A hospital secure unit is a specially dedicated configuration of beds within a hospital that houses patients/inmates in the custody of the correctional department and separate from civilian patients. A survey performed by the National Association of Public Hospitals in 1993 revealed that 58 public hospitals provided inpatient services to inmates (personal communication, Jack Raba, M.D., Chicago, IL). Twenty-three of these hospitals had a secure unit on the premises, while 35 did not. While there are private hospitals with secure units, cumulative data are unavailable. The main reasons given for maintaining a secure unit were that it isolated inmates from civilian patients and it permitted the corrections department to reduce labor costs by employing fewer officers per patient. Those against having a secure unit asserted that tests, surgeries, and procedures performed off the unit were not consistently performed because escort officers were not available often. The potential advantages and disadvantages of a hospital secure unit are listed in Box 9-1.

When choices are available, correctional authorities should choose hospitals for secure units that are closest to the correctional facility. The level of acuity that a hospital is licensed to treat is also a consideration. Hospitals in proximity to the correctional facility may not be able to manage some of the more complex trauma, HIV care, or critical care that may arise. In this case, referral arrangements must be made that satisfy community standards of care. With the development of prisons in rural areas, there are often insufficient resources at local area hospitals to treat complex cases. In these situations, correctional

authorities have developed various strategies for moving inmates to larger referral hospitals as would otherwise occur in their communities. In large urban areas, a tertiary care hospital is a preferred site for a secure ward unless the distance to the correctional facility is greater than 15 minutes. In that case, safety considerations should determine the choice of hospitals. In any case, tertiary care must be available for inmates.

Some secure units have divisions of correctional health that function as departments or divisions of the hospital. This autonomy gives the correctional physician a means of leverage within the hospital departmental structure and facilitates inmate care. This is an especially attractive arrangement when hospitalization of inmates occurs at a local public hospital where multiple residents may be caring for the inmate population. In these types of situations, the correctional physician can ensure that what needs to get done gets done. When such a unit has its own medical director, administrator, consistent nursing and correctional staff, day-to-day management is superior to situations where transitory or coverage staff exist. This level of administrative control may not be possible, except in large urban areas or for states serving large inmate populations. For smaller jails or prisons, the on-site medical team needs to coordinate hospital care with outpatient care at their facility. In larger systems, coordination between hospitalization and correctional facility care is often standardized for the purposes of utilization.

While physicians working in correctional facilities work as guests in the house of corrections, inmates as patients in

---

Box 9-1. Advantages and Disadvantages of the Hospital Secure Unit

ADVANTAGES
1. Staff are oriented to the unique requirements of patient/inmates and the correctional system. This results in:
   a.) staff who are better suited and more willing to advocate and care for the patient/inmate
   b.) expedited delivery of care
   c.) enhanced conflict avoidance and/or resolution between hospital staff, patient/inmates, and correctional personnel
   d.) decreased delays during the admission and discharge processes
   e.) enhanced rapport between secure unit staff, correctional staff and patient/inmates
2. Decreased presence of patient/inmates and officers on civilian hospital units resulting in:
   a.) a more pleasant environment in which to attract civilian patients
   b.) reduced number of guns on civilian wards
   c.) less confusion regarding patient/inmate rights and requirements
   d.) decreased occurrence and length of delays in patient procedures
   e.) decreased lengths of stay
3. Improved therapeutic environment via:
   a.) patient support groups
   b.) group counseling sessions
   c.) dedicated social work support
   d.) an on-site law library
   e.) better patient/inmate access to the supervisory staff of the correctional health service and correctional department
   f.) the ability to intermingle in a dayroom with other patient/inmates
4. Improved oversight of inmate diagnostic work ups and treatments
5. Improved communication of medical information between the hospital and correctional facility

DISADVANTAGES
1. Correctional staff may be assigned to the unit who perceive the unit as an extension of the jail or prison. This results in:
   a.) an anti-therapeutic environment that is more like a prison than a hospital
   b.) possible hostility or even inappropriate behavior toward hospital staff and inmate/patients
   c.) behavior on the part of correctional staff that is dangerous to the health of inmates such as inappropriate shackling, non compliance with treatment plans, etc.
2. Inappropriate correctional staffing, which results in:
   a.) missed diagnostic evaluations and treatments
   b.) extended lengths of stays because of missed treatments and evaluations
   c.) single officers observing multiple inmates who then may be shackled, resulting in adverse clinical events
3. Creation of a unit that is not seen as part of the hospital resulting in:
   a.) provision of less than the full complement of hospital support services
   b.) creation of dual standard of care in the hospital
   c.) lack of customary hospital oversight (infection control or continuous quality improvement activities)

---

hospitals must be secured while maintaining the therapeutic mission of the hospital. Secure units will not function well unless correctional authorities understand and accede to the needs of medical staff to undertake expeditious diagnostic workups and treatment. If such an understanding is not in place, it is difficult to care for patients on a secure unit. When this does occur, a secure unit offers many efficiencies to the correctional authority.

THE ADMISSIONS PROCESS
Identifying Patients for Hospital Referral

For jails, patients are admitted to the secure unit emergently, electively, or as transfers from a hospital lacking a secure unit. In addition, in jail settings, patients in police custody may be remanded to correctional custody and moved to the secure unit. Occasionally, a judge may issue a court order for a patient to be admitted for medical and/or psychiatric evaluation.

Emergency admissions

Prisons. Inmate admissions to secure units from prisons are generally straightforward. Arrangements for hospitalization from prison are often similar to any managed care system. There is a gatekeeper system of triage beginning with nursing evaluation, physician consultation, and emergency room referral or elective or emergent admission. If a prison has a secure unit arrangement at a local area hospital, communication to the hospital by the correctional physician should occur for all admissions, whether they are elective or emergencies. Patients are sometimes sent to the emergency room without any endorsement to the local hospital. This is unacceptable medical practice.

Box 9-2. Emergency Response Log Items

1. When the clinic was notified of the emergency
2. When the patient arrived in the clinic (if the patient was capable of being moved)
3. When the practitioner(s) arrived at the patient's side
4. When the 911 operator was called
5. Arrival time of correction escort officers
6. Time of paramedic arrival
7. Time patient departed for hospital

Jails. Admissions to hospitals from jails is affected by the nature of the populations coming into jails. In large urban jails, inmates are delivered to the facility in their most recent civilian physical condition, which is generally poor. At Cook County Jail in Chicago, almost one-third of hospital admissions from a 1993 audit were within the first 7 days of incarceration. One-third of these admissions were for trauma (personal communication, Michael Puisis, D.O., Chicago). These individuals often arrive at the facility as recent victims of violence and have not often had good civilian medical care. Intake tuberculosis screening at a large urban jail revealed that, of patients with newly diagnosed tuberculosis, 24% were homeless.[1] Common types of hospital admissions from the jails of the New York City Department of Correction include patients with significant mental illness, AIDS-related illnesses, abnormal chest radiographs, chest pain, asthma exacerbations, and trauma. Referral patterns for hospital admission depend on the capacity of outpatient and infirmary care at the correctional facility.

There is a wide spectrum of medical capabilities in various correctional facilities throughout the country. Some institutions have outpatient units or infirmaries that are capable of providing services at a level equivalent to a skilled nursing unit, while there are other facilities that have almost no physician coverage. In addition, due to local conditions, certain facilities will use a hospital for services that cannot be provided easily at the facility. For example, until recently, for cost reasons, Cook County Jail used their secure unit for purposes of routine renal dialysis. Some correctional facilities have appropriate facilities for tuberculosis isolation; others require admission to a hospital or secure unit.

Once it is determined that an acutely ill patient requires hospital evaluation, the practitioner must decide whether the patient is in need of emergent transport to the hospital.

While the mode of transportation to the hospital is a medical decision, it requires cooperation of correctional staff. Correctional staff are notified, and either on-site ambulance services or local area emergency response ambulances are called through 911 access. A mechanism for communication with higher-level correctional staff must be in place in case of emergency transport delays. Physicians and other health care staff should not assume that line-correctional staff are aware of the emergent nature of an admission. Lack of correctional staff may result in delayed admissions. In these situations, a higher-level correctional staff must be notified.

The practitioner should provide all pertinent information to the 911 operator, including the location and condition of the patient as well as the designated entrance site for the paramedics. The patient should remain closely monitored while the practitioner completes the necessary medical documentation. To avoid unnecessary delays, the referral form should be ready before the paramedics arrive and should contain the reason for referral, vital signs, pertinent physical findings, medical history, current medications, allergies, and treatment provided prior to the arrival of the paramedics.

In some states, the Emergency Medical Response system requires emergency medical technicians to transport patients to the nearest hospital, based on an evaluation they make in conjunction with the designated area medical response physician. This process may exclude the correctional physician from decision making. If the hospital secure unit is not the closest hospital, patients can be taken to hospitals not affiliated with the correctional facility.

Log books documenting the emergency response are useful continuous quality improvement tools that assist in evaluating emergency response. Items that should be contained in the logs are listed in Box 9-2.

At the Manhattan House of Detention for Men in New York City, the most common cause of delay in transporting the acutely ill patient to the hospital is the unavailability of correction escort officers. If there is any undue delay in securing officers for escort, our practice is for the practitioner to contact the Tour Commander immediately. Once informed of the medical urgency, the Tour Commander will often locate an escort team quickly.

Elective hospital admissions. Elective admissions to the Bellevue Hospital Jail Ward occur less frequently than acute admissions. Common reasons for elective admission at Bellevue's secure unit include hernia repair, cardiac catheterization, chemotherapy administration, and diagnostic bronchoscopy.

Managed care practices for review of elective hospital admissions have helped to screen out inappropriate hospital admissions. At the Manhattan House of Detention, prospective elective admissions are reviewed daily by the chief physician of the referring jail. Those approved for admission are then prioritized on a numbered system that refers to the time limitations set upon scheduled hospitalization.

Hospital-to-hospital transfer. Occasionally, patients/ inmates are referred from hospitals without secure units. Policy and procedure should state that all potential transfers are to be screened for appropriateness by the medical director of the correctional health service. The referring physician should present the patient to the medical director of the secure unit, who then determines whether the patient is suitable for transfer. If a patient is accepted, the referring physician should be required to contact the physician who will be responsible for the patient's care upon arrival at the accepting hospital. This allows the accepting physician to ensure that all pertinent documents are sent with the patient and that special arrangements can be made, if necessary.

In our experience at Bellevue, patients who are inappropriate for transfer include:

• Anyone intubated or in a acute cardiac unit or intensive care unit.
• Septic patients.
• Patients less than 48 hours status post major surgery.
• Patients requiring less than 48 additional hours of hospitalization (loss of continuity of care and cost of transfer outweigh the benefit of transfer in our situation).
• Any other condition that is considered unstable for transportation.

When there are disagreements about whether a patient requires hospitalization, the medical director or senior physician associated with the secure unit should determine the appropriate treatment setting for the patient.

Frequently, the patient being referred to the hospital may no longer need hospitalization. Instead, the patient may be best suited for infirmary level care or possibly the general population. Since the referring physician will tend to be unaware of these options, it is the responsibility of the medical director to determine which is the most appropriate setting for the patient.

The medical director should inform the correction department promptly of all patients accepted from other hospitals. This will allow the correctional staff more time to make security preparations and adjust manpower needs.

Patients in police custody. For jails, patients in police custody may be arraigned while they are hospitalized and remanded to the correctional department. This may occur in a hospital with or without a secure unit. In the latter, the patient can be referred for transfer to a hospital with a secure unit in anticipation that, when remanded, the patient can be placed on the secure unit. In some hospitals with secure units, patients in police custody are not permitted on secure units for security reasons. However, once remanded, the patient should be transferred to the secure unit to take advantage of all of the previously cited benefits of a secure unit. For this to occur promptly, the medical director should be aware of the location of each patient scheduled for arraignment and the time it is to occur. Those patients remanded to correction custody would then be evaluated by the medical director for transfer to the secure unit. If the patient is appropriate for the secure unit, the medical director would next contact the practitioner caring for the patient and give instructions to write transfer orders to the jail ward. To expedite the transfer, the charge nurses of both

units and the admitting office should be notified of the impending transfer.

Court-ordered admissions and procedures. Infrequently, inmates are ordered to the secure unit by a judge. Often there is no medical indication for acute care hospitalization. Therefore, court orders should be read carefully by the medical director and administrator of the jail health service. The medical director determines if the request is medically appropriate while the administrator decides if the order is properly addressed. If there are questions about the appropriateness of the court order, the court and the hospital risk management department should be contacted for further evaluation and advice.

The most common reason for court-ordered hospitalization at Bellevue Hospital is for blood sampling. However, participation in collection of forensic information is prohibited by National Commission on Correctional Health Care Standards.[2, 3] It is preferable that a practitioner or technician not responsible for patient/inmate care obtain blood samples or other specimens, since it may place the practitioner in an adversarial relationship with the patient. For this reason, practitioners caring for incarcerated patients should not be involved in obtaining evidence for the court.

Hospital Evaluation

The emergency department. Hospital emergency departments are busy, chaotic, non-secured areas creating problems and concerns for correctional officers guarding inmate/patients. Correctional policies often require shackling inmates to gurneys during triage and sometimes during examinations, which may create conflict with medical staff. It is useful to encourage the heads of emergency departments to have policies in place whereby inmates receive expeditious evaluation in the emergency department. There are many reasons for this. First, the emergency room is a non-secure area with a great deal of activity, making it the most difficult area of the hospital in which to maintain security. In this hectic environment, practitioners are more likely to leave sharp objects and other equipment within the reach of patients, while officers are more likely to engage in conversation with each other and/or emergency department staff. In addition, potential distractions, such as arriving trauma cases and/or unruly patients may also divert the officers' attention. Second, the presence of loaded weapons increases the risk of gunplay in the emergency room. Third, patient/inmates may be intimidating to civilian patients, leading them to seek care at other institutions in the future. Fourth, emergency department personnel and correctional officers may disagree over security precautions. This particular scenario occurs more frequently when officers not permanently assigned to the hospital are posted in the emergency room. These officers are often less aware of the policies and procedures of the emergency department. Fifth, officers posted in the emergency department are unavailable to escort inpatients to procedures and/or clinics.

Multidisciplinary coordination in combination with oversight from the medical director of the correctional health service can ensure prompt evaluation of the patient/prisoner in the emergency department. Each morning at Bellevue Hospital, the medical director of the prison health service makes emergency department rounds to determine if there are any delays in patient evaluation, security risks, discord between the hospital and correctional staff, high profile patients, patients not expected to survive, medicolegal issues, patient requests, and whether a patient is suitable for transfer to a jail-based infirmary. These rounds help expedite patient care.

Patient evaluation. In hospitals with secure units, delayed patient evaluation in the emergency room is often due to a lack of escort officers or hospital transport personnel. The secure unit medical director can facilitate expeditious workups by acting as a liaison to correctional supervisory staff.

Security issues. Civilian emergency room staff are frequently unaware of the security requirements of correctional staff. Therefore, security issues in the emergency department should be discussed with supervisory personnel of both the emergency and correctional departments. It is preferable to err on the side of caution in matters of security unless patient care is significantly compromised. Sharps and intravenous poles should not be left unattended within reach of the patient. The staff of the emergency department should be inserviced and frequently reminded to inventory and properly dispose of sharps.

It is useful if the emergency department is alerted in advance if a patient requiring additional security is en route to the emergency department. These patients usually require heavily armed escort officers, which can be unsettling to hospital staff and civilian patients alike. On occasion, correctional staff may request that a high security patient be taken to the secure unit for emergency evaluation. Evaluation and treatment of these patients on the secure unit should be done only if it is medically safe and if appropriate diagnostic equipment is available. It is better to discourage this practice as medically unsafe.

Patients appropriate for infirmary level care. Prompt physician utilization review of hospital referrals can reduce unnecessary hospitalization. Not infrequently, patients appropriate for infirmary level care are referred to the emergency department. This may be due to lack of bedspace at the infirmary or incomplete evaluation by the referring correctional practitioner. In large correctional systems with multiple clinic sites, practitioners may be unaware of the capabilities of the infirmary, or may be unable to contact the infirmary practitioner. Correctional facilities may be unable to perform appropriate diagnostic testing on site. Well-maintained data on hospital referrals helps identify areas where on-site care can be improved. In our practice at Bellevue, it has been cost effective to have the secure unit medical director screen all admissions and to refer selected patients to the infirmary for their care. Since emergency physicians may be unaware of the existence or capabilities of the infirmaries, the secure unit medical director will need to "walk them through" the procedure in a step-by-step manner.

Medicolegal issues. At Bellevue, the most common medicolegal problem in the emergency department involving patient/inmates is the refusal of treatment. If the patient has the capacity to make decisions, any and all therapies and procedures may be refused. However, the patient cannot dictate housing assignments. Thus, physicians may choose to house patients in a secure unit rather than send a critically ill patient who refuses care back to the correctional center. If an inmate at some point agrees to treatment, they can be immediately cared for. When inmates are hospitalized in private hospitals, the cost of this strategy is prohibitive. In any case, inmates who are critically ill, refuse care, and are returned to the correctional facility should be housed in the highest level of acuity consistent with their illness. Some of these patients need hospice care if it is available. Placement of critically ill patients in a cell raises risk management and ethical issues.

Admitting the patient/inmate. Timely admission requires coordination of all medical, correctional, and transportation staff. Often, maintaining logs as continuous quality improvement vehicles helps to indicate problem areas in the admission process. Secure wards do not always offer a complete range of services, therefore, patients requiring intensive or specialized care such as isolation for tuberculosis may not be housed on the secure unit. Occasionally, in hospitals with housestaff, the physicians may not want to come to the secure unit or would prefer to have the patient in a location that is more convenient for them. Occasionally, at Bellevue, the Department of Corrections has requested that extremely violent or antisocial patients be housed off the secure unit. These situations require intensive utilization management to obtain maximum efficiency from having a secure unit. At the Bellevue secure unit, all patients housed off the secure unit are reviewed each morning by the medical director of the secure unit.

Utilization review. The purpose of a secure unit is to efficiently care for hospitalized incarcerated patients. If patients are not housed on the secure unit, the cost efficiency of the unit decreases. Poor utilization of the secure unit may result in revenue loss for the hospital (by occupying a bed off the unit that could be filled by a paying patient). When patients are not housed on the secure unit, the cost to the department of corrections is increased by the cost of 24-hour-a-day security staff for each patient not on the secure unit. At times, when a large number of patients are housed off the secure ward, correctional staffing on the secure unit is decreased to provide staffing for patients off the unit. This practice disrupts care on the secure unit, and routine diagnostic testing for inmates on the secure unit is delayed or canceled. This situation is complicated when residents or attending physicians are reluctant to care for patients on the secure unit because of difficulties in transportation or because the unit is difficult to access.

At Bellevue Hospital, these types of problems are addressed by aggressive utilization management by the medical director of the secure unit. We found that physician-directed utilization is important for success. At Bellevue, all patients (except for intensive care patients and tuberculosis patients in isolation) housed off the secure unit require approval of the medical director. The medical director performs rounds 5 days a week on all patients off the secure unit, and reviews the care of each patient with the following questions in mind:

Can this patient be moved safely to the secure unit?

Is appropriate and expeditious care being given to the inmate?

Is the civilian staff properly oriented to the care of the inmate/patient?

Is there discord between hospital and correctional personnel?

Is the inmate ready for transfer to the correctional facility or infirmary unit?

Daily rounds on patients off the secure unit also permit the medical director to assist nurses in transportation problems related to correctional officers and to orient other health care staff to security regulations. In addition, at our institution, inmates often have non-medical needs such as verification of methadone maintenance or questions regarding court appearances, which the medical director can help address. We have found that helping solve these ordinary problems increases patient compliance and reduces staff friction in caring for our patients. Attempting to get residents and attending physicians to transfer patients to the secure unit is a negotiated process. At Bellevue, patients with marginal reasons for remaining off the secure unit are generally not permitted to do so. When the secure unit medical director strongly thinks that the patient could be housed on the secure unit, the medical director has the authority to transfer the patient to the secure unit. The patient remains under the care of the same medical team.

At Bellevue, there are no negative pressure isolation rooms on the secure unit. This creates problems because patients in the hospital, to rule out tuberculosis, remain off the secure unit until 3 consecutive days of sputum sampling is done. We have found that spending time in coordinating the efforts of nursing, respiratory therapy, transportation, and the correctional staff will reduce length of hospital stay. We perform early morning sputum induction testing at a designated time when correctional staff are available. Other involved staff are informed in advance of when the correctional officer is available. For patient refusals, the medical director is notified and the patient is promptly counseled. Use of this system at Bellevue has resulted in a 95% collection rate for 3 consecutive days of sputum sampling.

Box 9-3. Medical Contraindications to Shackling a Patient/Inmate

Circulatory insufficiency (e.g., edema of extremities)

Ventilator dependency

Hypercoagulable and hypocoagulable states
   Pregnancy
   Cancer
   Post major surgery
   Severe thrombocytopenia
   Coagulation disorder

Paralysis of an extremity (e.g., post CVA, paraplegia or hemiplegia)

Seizure disorder

Dermatologic abnormalities (rash, abrasion, ulceration)

Pregnancy (because of the potential of precipitous labor and the fact that pregnancy is a hypercoagulable state, shackling should rarely if ever be used in pregnant women)

Patients in coma or imminent danger or expectation of death, under anesthesia, or unable to get out of bed without assistance

---

Shackling. Correctional staff may require that patient/inmates be shackled to a bed or other fixed object on a short- or long-term basis. This is more likely to occur if there is no secure unit or if inmates are housed off a secure unit. Regardless of the reasons of correctional staff for shackling, there are relative medical contraindications to shackling that may take precedence over the need to shackle a patient (Box 9-3).

In hospitals with secure units, attending staff and house staff may be unaware of the medical contraindications to shackling. It is good practice for the secure unit medical director to make daily rounds on each shackled patient to determine if there are instances of inappropriate shackling. At Bellevue, since most shackling occurs on patients off the secure unit, this can be accomplished in the morning when daily off-unit rounds are performed. If the patient has a relative contraindication to shackling, and there is high potential for it being detrimental to the patient's health, the medical director should inform the correctional supervisory staff of the need to promptly remove the shackles. In addition, the medical director should write a note to the correctional supervisory staff documenting the reason for shackle removal and, if necessary, a note in the patient's medical record detailing the above. Alternatively, the use of waist shackles may be an acceptable compromise in patients whose extremities cannot be shackled due to medical contraindications. Waist shackles may also allow the patient some mobility in his room. Disagreement between the correctional supervisor and the medical director over the request/order to remove or modify the shackles should be brought to the attention of the medical director of the hospital.

The secure ward. Patients housed on a secure unit should receive care identical to that given to civilian patients in that hospital. To do otherwise presents risk management and eighth amendment legal issues. This can only be achieved if the proper systems are in place and an experienced, dedicated staff is maintained and supported. A poorly operated jail ward will result in diagnostic and treatment delays, security breaches, patient dissatisfaction, interdepartmental discord, violations of patient/prisoner rights, increased outposts, staff demoralization, and loss of confidence in the supervisory staff of the jail health services.

Staffing. At Bellevue, the hospital correctional health service consists of a full-time medical director, administrator, and nursing supervisor who spend the majority of their day on the secure unit overseeing patients and staff. We have found that it is best to have consistent staffing comprising nursing staff, a social worker, an activity therapist, case manager, housekeeper, and outpatient clinic associate(s).

There may be several security posts in a hospital. Regardless of the configuration of correctional posts, consistent corrections staffing at the hospital will reduce delays in patient transport to off-unit procedures, improve security, and ultimately will result in a decreased length of stay per patient.

Recruiting and maintaining a mature and qualified staff who want to work on the secure unit may be the most vital factor in making the jail ward a worthwhile endeavor. Dedicated staff will develop strong bonds, in part due to their isolation from other hospital units and from seeing their assignment as a unique health care mission. Staff members not wishing to work on a secure unit should be counseled and, if necessary, transferred out of the secure unit, as they can have a devastating effect on staff morale and performance. It is critical to establish a good working relationship with the Department of Correction. The tone of this relationship is usually established by the supervisory personnel of the correctional department and the correctional health service. Optimally, for secure units, the correctional health service should have a horizontal working relationship with the Department of Correction.

Secure units should be integrated into the hospital structure; otherwise, a dual standard of care may develop. The secure unit hospital staff should establish open lines of communication with the hospital departments they commonly interact with, and should feel empowered to contact the appropriate supervisor(s) of any department involved in the care of their patients when the need arises. These departments may include radiology, patient transport, dietary, social work, outpatient clinics, operating room, admissions office, etc.

It is important that secure unit nursing staff work closely with the officer responsible for assigning escort personnel for off-ward tests and procedures. When there are insufficient officers available for transporting patients for their appointments, delays ensue and friction may occur. To avoid a dysfunctional system, continuous quality improvement monitoring with correctional staff involvement can be used to assess and improve this process.

Lastly, the supervisory staff of the secure unit should be strongly supported by the hospital administration when the need arises. They should also maintain open lines of communication with health providers at the referring correctional facilities.

Concerns unique to a secure unit. Unique security concerns and medicolegal issues help set the secure unit apart from the rest of the hospital. If not properly addressed, patient care can be delayed and/or compromised, staff safety may be jeopardized, and the hospital potentially liable to legal action.

Maintaining proper security is of paramount importance on the secure unit, as it is impossible to recruit and retain competent staff if the work environment is not safe. To help ensure a safe working environment, the hospital staff must be oriented to the distinctive security requisites of a secure unit and maintain open lines of communication with correctional personnel. A relationship should exist in which either discipline feels free to point out potential security lapses. The absence of such a relationship exposes staff and patients to unnecessary risks.

Security precautions must be taken with the following activities and situations: 1) sharps safety and disposal, 2) medication rounds, 3) bedside visits, 4) meal distribution, 5) on-site procedures, 6) items considered contraband on the jail ward, 7) patients prone to violence, and 8) patient discharge.

Items considered as sharps include needles, razors, nail clippers, scalpels, forks, and other spiked items that have potential use as weapons. In the secure unit, all needles and syringes should be kept under lock and key. If the unit has a treatment room, physicians should be frequently reminded and encouraged to perform patient procedures in the treatment room if the patient is stable to be transported. The advantages of this practice include privacy, the increased security of having an officer posted outside the door, more room with which to maneuver, and easier access to sharps disposal containers.

Sharps disposal containers should not be placed or brought into patient rooms. These containers are best kept secured in the nurses' station and the treatment room. This prevents practitioners from absentmindedly leaving these containers in patient rooms. Practitioners should also be oriented to bring only the equipment they need onto the jail ward and not to place equipment in loose pockets such as those seen on lab coats. Additionally, all equipment, especially sharps, should be inventoried before and after attending to a patient. Finally, all closets and drawers containing sharps should be closed promptly when no longer in use.

There are many nonmedical items that fall under the "sharps" designation. These include safety razors, nail clippers, utensils, cans, and glassware. Safety razors should be distributed only by the correction staff who keep a strict inventory of razors dispensed and returned. Recently, items with internal or external foil wrapping such as ointment and mayonnaise packets have been prohibited by the New York City Department of Correction, because it was noticed that inmates were removing the single blade from the disposable razor and replacing it with the foil from these packets. This made it appear as though the razor was being returned intact when, in fact, the inmate had removed the blade. Nail clippers should be signed out to the patient and inspected when returned. Liquids should be dispensed in paper cups, as glassware and cans may be fashioned into weapons. Metal utensils as well as plastic knives should be forbidden on the jail ward, as they can easily result in slashings and puncture wounds.

It is best to have patients confined to their rooms during medication rounds, since patients walking the hallways may remove narcotics or other medications from the medication cart while the nurse's attention is diverted. An officer should keep the hallways clear and escort the nurse throughout medication rounds to help ensure that medications are dispensed without incident. Narcotics and other abusable medications should be crushed or given in liquid form to avoid hoarding or dealing by patients.

Patient visits should occur in a designated visit area separate from the secure unit. Bedside visits are indicated if the patient is confined to the bed. Bedside visits should be minimized, since they require the presence of an officer at the bedside and raise the risk of weapons and drugs being passed from visitor to patient. For these reasons, all bedside visits should be approved by the medical director or nursing supervisor, since other physicians generally may not be aware of the disadvantages and dangers of bedside visits.

Patients prone to violence may need to be housed off the secure unit or confined to their room on the unit to minimize their contact with other patients. All personnel caring for these patients should be briefed so that all necessary security precautions can be taken. The medical director or administrator should instruct attending physicians and house staff to expedite the patient's care so that there are no unnecessary delays in diagnosis, treatment, or discharge.

Staff should be informed that they may not give any unauthorized items to patients, since this is considered contraband by the correctional department. Contraband includes food, clothing, or items of any sort not approved by the Department of Correction in conjunction with the supervisory staff of the jail health service.

Patients should not be told when they are being discharged, nor when they are to be seen in an off-ward diagnostic or consultation area. These are occasions when a patient can escape from correctional custody most easily. All secure unit staff, especially house staff, should be oriented to this rule continuously and signs should be placed in the nursing station to this effect.

The most frustrating problem encountered on the secure unit is the unavailability of officers to escort patients to off-ward procedures or clinics. It is a common cause of delayed diagnosis and care, tension between the hospital and correctional staff, and patient dissatisfaction. There are ways to maximize the number of officers available for escort. First, minimize the number of patients housed off the secure unit. This is an effective measure if it translates into additional officers available for escort duties. Second, systems should be designed to ensure expedited care in the emergency department and in other areas where patients need to go for procedures, testing, or evaluations. For example, a radiology department supervisor should instruct their personnel to evaluate patient/prisoners ahead of civilian patients. This will free-up officers more quickly for other duties and minimizes exposure of civilians to patient/inmates. Third, the secure unit medical director should organize a multidisciplinary quality improvement team to address the issue of delays in patients being produced for off-ward procedures. The team should consist of the medical director, correctional health administrator, nursing supervisor, correction supervisor, hospital transport supervisor, and other personnel as needed. It should analyze the system that is already in place for scheduling and transporting patients for off-unit procedures. A flow chart should be created and the problem areas discussed. Data are collected concerning the time needed to produce patients for off-unit procedures. Once analyzed, the data should reveal the high volume, problem-prone issues that need to be addressed to reduce cancellations or delays. For example, the data may reveal that patients awaiting non-emergent CT scans are consistently late for their appointments, resulting in frequent postponements. The medical director and/or administrator could be advised to meet with the radiology supervisor to discuss possible remedies. One possible solution may require the CT scan suite to reserve a predetermined time slot in which to perform CT scans on patient/inmates. This slot would coincide with a time when correction officers are most available. The radiology department would then agree to inform the secure unit of the patient's appointment 1 day prior to its scheduled date. To further decrease waiting time in the CT suite, the radiology department could also supply the secure unit with oral contrast material that would be administered to the patient prior to leaving the secure unit. The next step would be to have the hospital transport supervisor guarantee that a hospital transporter will be made available when given proper notice. If this solution is found to be effective, it may be extrapolated to other high-volume, problem-prone areas such as operating room procedures and routine radiographs.

Medicolegal issues. Unique medicolegal issues occur on the jail ward and may need to be addressed jointly by hospital and correctional staff. Medicolegal issues include refusal of treatment, scheduled court appearances, uses of force, patient confidentiality, visitation rights, counsel visits and access to telephones, television, newspapers, and the law library.

Like civilian patients, incarcerated patients with decisional capacity may refuse medical treatment. However, as mentioned previously, they cannot dictate where they will be housed in the correctional system. For example, a patient with unstable angina refusing treatment is best left in the hospital where he can be closely monitored. As with any patient refusing treatment, the practitioner or medical director should attempt to determine why the patient is refusing treatment. Common reasons for a patient/prisoner refusing medical treatment are varied and include concern about missing a scheduled court appearance, concern over property left at the jail facility, the potential for an altercation with another patient(s) or with officers, and distrust of hospital staff.

Once the practitioner is aware of the patient's reason(s) for refusing medical treatment, a solution may be possible that will convince the patient to agree to therapy. For example, if the patient is concerned about missing a court date, the medical director can contact the patient's lawyer to determine if and when the court appearance can be rescheduled. If the patient is worried about personal property left at the referring jail facility, correctional staff may be able to assure the patient that the property has been safely stored or, if absolutely necessary, have it shipped to the secure unit. If the patient/prisoner wishes to leave the hospital due to fear of violence from another inmate/patient(s), it may be wise to transfer one or both of these patients off the unit after notifying correctional supervisory staff. Occasionally, a patient will wish to sign out of the hospital against medical advice because there is concern that a correction officer or officers will abuse him. This concern should be promptly brought to the attention of the correctional supervisor. If necessary, the medical director should request that correctional supervisory staff interview the patient to effect a solution.

Finally, the patient/prisoner may distrust the hospital staff and believe they do not have his best interests in mind. The medical director and/or nursing supervisor should listen to the patient's concerns and see if they can be alleviated. Psychiatric counseling may be necessary.

Patient/inmates in jails may be scheduled to appear in court. While some systems have satellite courts at the hospital, the patient must be transported to the courthouse if a satellite court is not available in the hospital. It is the responsibility of the attending physician to determine whether the patient is fit to attend court. The physician must take into account the length of time the patient will spend in court; the inaccessibility to medication, observation, and treatment; the patient's condition; and the possibility of harm in traveling. The physician should state whether the patient is deemed fit to attend court on an order sheet in the patient's medical record. This should be accompanied by a daily progress note detailing the patient's current condition.

Patients may or may not wish to attend court. A common reason patients will want to attend court is the belief that they will be freed from custody. In this situation, the patient/inmate is more likely to sign out of the hospital against medical advice if the physician does not "clear" him for court. On the other hand, patients may wish to miss court if they believe it is not in their best interest to make an appearance. For example, they may believe that a hostile witness is less likely to appear if the court date keeps getting postponed. In such an instance, the patient may feign an increased level of illness to have the physician prohibit him from attending court. Since physicians tend to be naive to such a ploy, it is the responsibility of the medical director to intervene when this is suspected. The medical director would discuss these issues with the attending or resident physician and then examine the patient. If the patient is found fit to attend court, an order should be written to that extent and the correction department informed of the decision.

Occasionally, patients attending court may be released from custody. With this in mind, patients leaving for court should be advised that their condition necessitates further treatment and that, if they are released from custody, they should return to the hospital emergency department for readmission. The patient should then be given a letter summarizing his condition and the need for readmission. In some secure units, patients are simply transferred to civilian units after discharge from custody.

Occasionally, use of force by correctional personnel occurs on the secure unit. The supervisory personnel of the jail health service can attempt to ameliorate the situation. In addition, the attending physician should be summoned promptly to evaluate the patient after a use of force has occurred. The physician should fully document the patient's condition as well as any need for treatment.

The laws governing patient confidentiality on the secure unit should be no different from those on the civilian units. However, maintaining patient confidentiality on the secure unit can be difficult. If confidentiality cannot be preserved, the patient will be less likely to disclose information that may prove vital to his care.

Preserving patient confidentiality is more difficult on the secure unit for the following reasons. First, the hospital staff may become familiar with the officers assigned to the unit and be less aware of discussing restricted information in their presence. Second, physicians conducting bedside rounds may be within earshot of an officer or other patients. Third, the officer(s) assigned to transporting the patient to or from the secure unit may gain access to the medical record. Fourth, patients sent to off-ward procedures or clinics may have their confidentiality breached by hospital staff who allow an officer to remain at the patient's side during an evaluation for reasons of security.

Generally, patients with AIDS are most concerned about the loss of confidentiality. They are worried that they will receive discriminatory treatment from correction officers as well as other patients. This is the case particularly in patients with AIDS who have not significantly deteriorated and who will not require infirmary level care upon discharge from the hospital.

The preservation of patient confidentiality can be made more likely in the following manner. The staff should be inserviced periodically to the hospital policy regarding patient confidentiality and of its particular importance on the secure unit. If house staff care for patients on the unit, these issues can be brought up during their orientation. All physicians should be reminded regularly that they should discuss patient/inmate issues in privacy. Attending physicians should be informed that group discussions should not be conducted in areas where officers may overhear confidential information concerning the patient/inmate. Hospital transport personnel should be instructed not to provide correction officers access to the medical record. Upon discharge from the secure unit, all relevant medical information sent to the facility should be sealed in an envelope. It should contain information necessary for the correction department to transport the patient to the intended facility, and should be stamped "CONFIDENTIAL." Some correctional facilities have policies for automatic medical evaluation of all patients returning from hospital visits. For facilities that do not, a check-off box on the transport envelope may indicate if prompt medical attention is indicated upon return to the correctional facility.

Occasionally, visits from family or counsel will conflict with scheduled procedures or care. Since these visits can be of great importance to the patient/inmate, the physician or nurse responsible for the patient should be flexible whenever possible. In private hospital arrangements, delayed procedures may result in additional cost and should be factored into the decision. If a scheduled procedure cannot be postponed and the patient insists on meeting with the visitor(s), the physician caring for the patient should be notified. The patient should be informed of the risks of not attending the procedure and asked if it is possible for the visitor(s) to return after the procedure. If not, and the patient still wishes to attend the visit, then a refusal form should be signed and a note documenting the aforementioned events should be written in the medical record. In general, an attempt should be made not to schedule procedures during visitation times, if possible.

Ancillary Staff. Social worker services can be of great benefit to patients and staff on the secure unit.

The social worker is most helpful if the patient/prisoner is nearing release from incarceration since housing, clothing, rehabilitation, and public assistance needs may have to be addressed. The social worker can also serve as a liaison between the patient and the hospital or correctional staff and can reach out to the patient's family, particularly when they have questions regarding the patient's care.

Upon admission at Bellevue, a complete assessment of the inmate/patient is performed by the social worker. The assessment should include the patient's correct telephone number, address, and next of kin. Obtaining these data is key, since inmates incarcerated in jails often give incorrect information to the correction department upon entry to the correctional facility. If the patient deteriorates suddenly, the social worker's assessment form may be the only source of accurate information for contacting the patient's next of kin if permission is needed for procedures, when a "do not resuscitate" order is being contemplated, or if the patient dies. Finally, since the social worker addresses many problems that would otherwise be directed toward the nursing staff, it allows the nurses to allot more of their time to direct patient care. This results in a more appropriately directed nursing staff and increased patient satisfaction.

Patient advocates may play an important role on the secure unit. In the absence of a social worker, they act as liaison for the patient if there are requests or complaints involving the hospital or correctional department. They may also organize patient support group meetings on a regular basis and invite guests to speak before the group. Regular members of a support group may include the medical director or administrator, nursing supervisor, correctional supervisors, activity therapist, social worker, and the patient advocate. The group meeting permits the patients to speak about their lives, illness, or complaints they may have about their care. It also allows supervisory staff to answer questions and disseminate information pertinent to the patients.

Patients' families. The families of patient/inmates frequently request to speak to the caring physician or nurse. Prior to answering any questions, the physician should ask the patient exactly what he'd like revealed about his illness and to whom he wants the information revealed. Once this is determined, every effort should be made to communicate candidly with the patient's family. This decreases the feeling of isolation and despair the family may have when a loved one is ill and incarcerated. A caring physician, nurse, or social worker can help in assuring the patient's family that their relative is receiving appropriate medical care. Conversely, poor communication between the medical staff and the patient's family may lead the family to believe the patient is receiving inadequate care just because he is a prisoner. This can result in unnecessary complaints and a less-compliant patient.

Patient family members can also assist the medical director in securing a compassionate release for patients who are terminally ill by lobbying the assigned judge, district attorney, or parole board on the patient's behalf.

THE DISCHARGE PROCESS

Discharging a prisoner back to jail can be a problem (Box 9-4). However, discharge planning and aggressive utilization management reduces unnecessary patient length of stay, which could increase the risk of nosocomial infec-

---

Box 9-4. Problems With Discharging a Prisoner Back to Jail

1. A written discharge summary must accompany the patient
2. The patient may require specialized housing (e.g., infirmary, isolation, hospice)
3. Transfer to specialized housing may require doctor-to-doctor communication as well as approval by the doctor at the receiving facility
4. Patients accepted to specialized units may require special transport vehicles
5. Correctional transport delays may occur
6. The patient may refuse to be discharged

Box 9-5. Patients Requiring Transfer to a Specialized Unit upon Hospital Discharge

Wheelchair-bound patients or patients with significant difficulty ambulating

Postoperative patients requiring frequent wound care or other nursing attention

Patients unable to care for themselves (e.g., advanced AIDS, dementia)

Patients on medications requiring frequent monitoring (e.g., coumadin, protease inhibitors)

Patients requiring education regarding their condition (e.g., new onset diabetes mellitus)

Patients with diseases that may require close observation (e.g., congestive heart failure, poorly controlled diabetes mellitus, end stage renal disease)

Patients requiring narcotics for pain control

Patients requiring directly observed medication ingestion (e.g., anti-tuberculous medications)

Patients requiring respiratory or wound isolation

---

tions, patient unrest, staff dissatisfaction, a decreased level of security, extra costs to the hospital or referring facility, and shortage of bedspace on the secure unit. In hospitals where physicians do not understand the spectrum of services available to inmates, an experienced secure unit clerical and nursing staff can guide the physician step by step through the discharge process and work with the correctional department to ensure prompt discharge from the hospital.

Discharge: Step by Step

Physicians should not inform the patient of the planned discharge from the hospital for security reasons. After the physician has written orders for discharge, the actual discharge depends on how the correctional facility handles hospital returns. The simplest solution is for a correctional physician to evaluate the housing needs (general population, infirmary, respiratory isolation, or hospice) of inmates before the inmate leaves the hospital. In some settings, this is done by telephone between the attending or resident physician at the hospital and the correctional physician. In other settings, correctional physicians evaluate patients on the secure unit. Some systems send inmates back to correctional facilities without evaluation, or re-evaluate the patient at the correctional facility. Patients who leave the hospital without prior evaluation often have needs that the correctional facility cannot appropriately address. This results in readmissions or poor patient care.

It is best that secure unit physicians communicate with the physicians at the correctional facility and endorse the patient's needs to whomever will be caring for the patient. Physicians at the correctional facility determine where to house the patient. This should be a physician-to-physician communication because hospital physicians may not realize the extent of services provided at the correctional facility. This may cause problems for after-hours discharges. Physicians at the correctional facility should not accept patients in transfer who they think cannot be medically cared for at the facility. For example, patients with active

tuberculosis should not be accepted back into facilities that do not have negative pressure respiratory isolation.

Delays in discharge to specialized units at Bellevue Hospital occur most commonly for the following reasons: a) the accepting practitioner is lax in informing the correction department at the specialized unit of the approved admission; b) the correctional transport vehicle is unavailable or late in arriving; or c) beds are no longer available in the specialized unit.

Many similar problems occur in other systems. These types of problems are best handled as managed care problems. For systems not using a secure unit, having a utilization nurse assigned to oversee discharge planning has been extremely effective in reducing hospital stays and in returning the inmate safely to appropriate correctional housing (personal communication, Michael Puisis, D.O.). Utilization nurses assigned to the correctional medical system may be effectively used on secure units as well.

When utilization nurses are not available, the medical director or administrator should become directly involved to expedite the discharge. Because of the significant cost of hospitalization, managed discharge planning is important in reducing cost.

Occasionally, patients referred to the hospital from the general population require transfer to a specialized unit on discharge from the hospital due to changes in their condition. (Examples are listed in Box 9-5). For systems that require the inmate to return to the pre-hospital housing unit, some intervention is necessary to redirect the inmate to appropriate housing. Managed care discharge planning involving staff who understand the extent of services in the correctional facility will resolve these types of problems.

Patients inappropriately discharged to the general population can result in a number of problems, such as: they may spend hours in the correctional jail facility receiving room, awaiting transfer to specialized housing (once the correctional physician decides the patient is not fit for the general population); during this period they miss vital medications, medical care, or may not receive prescribed bedrest; they may be inappropriately accepted to the general population of the jail facility; they may be returned directly to the hospital by the jail facility health staff; or upon return to the hospital, the emergency department staff may be at a loss as to what to do with the patient.

Thus, it is vital that patients requiring specialized housing are identified by someone familiar with the services at the correctional facility so that physicians do not discharge the patient back to a general population setting, which is inappropriate.

Patients appropriate for discharge to the general population will usually require a written discharge summary. As with all discharges, the summary should include the primary and secondary diagnoses, synopsis of the patient's course, significant laboratory or procedure results, recommended follow-up care, discharge medications, and the printed name and pager number of the discharging physician. Since this may be the only communication with the jail facility, the summary should be complete and legible. If there are any outstanding laboratory or procedure results, the receiving practitioner should be informed of how to retrieve these results. Follow-up care may necessitate a return to hospital-based outpatient specialty clinics. If so, the nursing staff should inform the hospital outpatient jail health unit of the requested clinic referrals to schedule the appointments. This information is then written on the discharge summary. The patient can be informed of the need for follow-up clinic evaluation but should not be given the date of the clinic appointment, since this would be a violation of security measures.

Medications should, as a rule, not be sent from the hospital to the receiving facility. More often than not, the correctional pharmacy will be able to provide the recommended medication(s) or dispense a suitable substitute. Medication(s) may be sent to the jail facility in the following instances: a) the medication is not on the formulary and there is no suitable substitute at the correctional facility; b) missing a dose of medication can have a deleterious effect; or c) the patient would otherwise remain in the hospital unnecessarily.

Returning to the Correctional Facility

There are usually established patterns in each correctional system for bringing inmates back to the correctional facility from a hospital. However this occurs, it is important that a physician or health care staff evaluate every patient who returns from hospitalization. Policies should be encouraged so that inmates returning from the hospital do not have to undergo processing in reception areas or in the holding tank. Patient/inmates may require medication, other treatment, or specialized housing arrangements, or may be seriously ill and the time spent in processing may adversely affect their health. If processing is required, it should be performed expeditiously and, once completed, the patient should be medically evaluated. In facilities with round-the-clock physician coverage, this is best performed by physicians. In facilities without physicians, the receiving health care staff should contact the correctional physician on call and clarify physician orders. In very small jails or prisons without health care staff on site, the correctional staff should assure that the inmate can safely be housed in the facility. This may need to be done in consultation with the discharging physician.

Given the current managed care environment, patients are being discharged earlier in the course of their disease process. In addition, patients are occasionally discharged with significant medical problems because of medical error on the part of the hospital. Therefore, it is important to evaluate patients returning from hospitalization to ensure that they can safely recuperate or be housed in the correctional facility. These post-hospitalization evaluations should include a directed history and physical examination that addresses the following: a) is the patient stable? b) is the patient appropriate for housing at this facility? c) does this patient require specialized housing (e.g., infirmary, hospice etc.)?

If it is thought that the patient was inappropriately released from the hospital, the practitioner should attempt to contact the physician who discharged the patient. Patients may need to be readmitted if the correctional facility cannot care for them. If it is decided to readmit the patient to the hospital, the correctional physician should contact the discharge physician and discuss readmission. In some systems, especially public hospital systems, patients are simply returned to the emergency room. In this case, the emergency room attending physician should be contacted. This physician-to-physician communication is necessary to avoid further misunderstanding and to explain why the patient is returning to the hospital.

On some occasions, the patient is stable but inappropriate for housing at a particular facility (e.g., the patient may require infirmary level care). In these instances, arrangements should be made to transfer the patient to the appropriate facility promptly. However, transferring a patient to a specialized unit can be quite difficult during off-hours. If it is not possible to re-route the patient to the specialized unit, then the practitioner will need to decide if the patient can remain housed in general population until a transfer can be arranged. If this translates to a significant threat to the patient's well-being, then the patient should be returned to the hospital with an explanatory note accompanying a copy of the hospital's discharge summary. In addition, the correctional physician should make every effort to contact the attending physician in charge of the emergency department so that the patient can be readmitted to the hospital pending acceptance to a jail-based infirmary.

If a patient is appropriate for housing in the general population, the evaluating practitioner then orders all indicated medications and treatments; submits consultation requests for the recommended follow-up visits; re-orients the patient to the ABCs of medication rounds, sick call, etc.; and informs the patient of the need for follow-up clinics, if any, without revealing the dates of these appointments.

Logs of patients returning from hospitalization are useful for data tracking and quality improvement monitoring. A system of notifying the correctional physician at the site that a patient has returned from the hospital must be in place to ensure continuity of care. Patients should be seen in follow-up as soon as is clinically indicated.

REFERENCES

1. Puisis M, Feinglass J, Lidow E: Radiographic Screening for Tuberculosis in a Large Urban County Jail. *Public Health Rep* 111:330-334, 1996.
2. J-66: Standards for Health Services in Jails. National Commission on Correctional Health Care, 1996.
3. P-10: Standards for Health Services in Prisons. National Commission on Correctional Health Care, 1992.

Section Three

Infectious Disease

10

Tuberculosis Screening

Patricia M. Simone, M.D.

Michael Puisis, D.O.

OVERVIEW OF TUBERCULOSIS IN CORRECTIONAL FACILITIES

Tuberculosis (TB) is a significant problem in correctional facilities in the United States. The rates of TB cases in prison populations are substantially higher than the rates in the general population. For example, the incidence of TB among inmates in New Jersey during 1994 was 91.2 cases per 100,000 inmates, compared with 11.0 cases per 100,000 persons in the state.[1,2] A TB case rate of 184 cases per 100,000 inmates was reported from one state prison in California in 1991, which is ten times greater that the statewide rate.[3] Transmission of *Mycobacterium* also was documented in this prison. In addition, increases in TB cases have been reported from correctional facilities in some areas of the country. In the New York State correctional system, for example, the incidence of TB disease increased from 15.4 cases per 100,000 inmates during 1976–1978 to 105.5 cases per 100,000 inmates during 1986,[4] and reached 139.3 cases per 100,000 by 1993 (unpublished data, New York State Department of Health).

In 1993, state health departments began reporting newly diagnosed TB cases to the CDC that occurred in persons who were incarcerated at the time of diagnosis. In 1993, 48 areas (47 states and New York City) provided this information on ≥ 75% of their cases. In these areas, 3.8% of TB patients resided in a correctional facility at the time of diagnosis.[5, 6] During 1994, 4.6% of TB-infected patients in 50 areas (48 states, New York City, and the District of Columbia), and in 1995, 4.1% of TB-infected patients in 51 areas were reported as residents of correctional facilities at the time of diagnosis.[7–10]

Some studies found TB infection among inmates at a prevalence of 14% to 25%.[11–14] Other studies found a correlation between tuberculin skin test positivity and length of incarceration, indicating that transmission may have occurred in these facilities.[15, 16]

An important reason for the high rates of TB infection and disease in correctional facilities is the disproportionate number of inmates who have risk factors for TB, including infection with human immunodeficiency virus (HIV), substance abuse, and being a member of a lower socioeconomic population having poor access to health care. In addition, many correctional facilities have overcrowded environments that are conducive to transmission of *M. tuberculosis*.[16, 17]

GENERAL PRINCIPLES OF TUBERCULOSIS SCREENING

There are two types of screening activities that may be carried out in correctional facilities: 1) screening to identify persons who may have infectious TB disease so they can be isolated immediately and started on appropriate therapy, and 2) screening to identify persons with TB infection who are at high risk for the development of TB disease and who would benefit from preventive therapy.

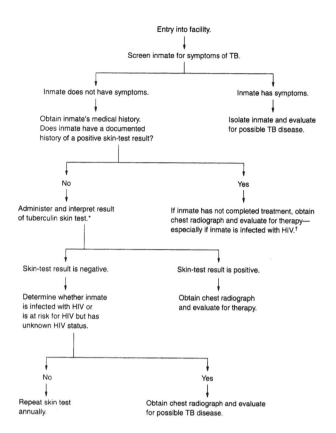

Figure 10-1. Protocol for screening inmates for TB in long-term correctional facilities. (From CDC: Prevention and control of tuberculosis in correctional facilities: Recommendations of the advisory council for the elimination of tuberculosis. *MMWR* 1996; 45:10.)

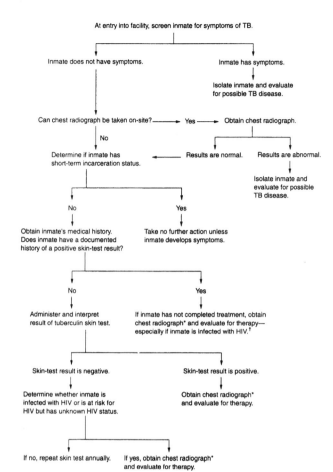

Figure 10-2. Protocol for screening inmates for TB in short-term correctional facilities that provide service to high-risk populations. (From CDC: Prevention and control of tuberculosis in correctional facilities: Recommendations of the advisory council for the elimination of tuberculosis. *MMWR* 1996; 45:12.)

How these screening activities should be implemented depends on several factors such as the type of facility, the prevalence of TB infection and disease in the facility, the prevalence of other risk factors for TB in the inmate population, and the length of stay of inmates in the facility. Recommendations for screening for tuberculosis in correctional facilities from the Advisory Council for the Elimination of Tuberculosis and the Centers for Disease Control and Prevention have been published recently[18] (Figures 10-1–10-3).

When developing and implementing a screening program in a correctional facility, it is important to determine whether the primary purpose of screening is screening for 1) TB disease (e.g., active pulmonary tuberculosis), 2) TB infection (positive tuberculin skin test but no symptoms of active TB), or 3) both. Screening for TB disease can prevent the transmission of *M. tuberculosis* in the facility and should be done in all correctional settings. In general, screening for TB infection, for the purpose of initiating preventive therapy, should be done only for groups at high risk for tuberculosis and should not be undertaken unless the necessary resources for patient evaluation and treatment are available and unless patients who are found to have positive tuberculin skin test results are likely to complete preventive

therapy. While inmates of jails and prisons are considered a high-risk group for TB, the potential for completion of therapy will vary between jails and prisons, and even different populations within jail systems. Screening for TB infection should be done in all prisons and in those populations of jail inmates who are likely to be in the facility on a long-term basis. The success of any screening activity depends on effectively identifying persons who have TB infection or disease, providing them with the appropriate follow-up and treatment, and ensuring that they complete a full course of recommended therapy.

There are three methods that are commonly used to screen for TB infection or disease: symptom screening, chest radiograph screening, and tuberculin skin test screening.

Symptom Screening

All incoming inmates in any size jail or prison should be screened for symptoms of tuberculosis by asking if the inmate has prolonged productive cough, hemoptysis, chest pain, weight loss, loss of appetite, fever, or night sweats. Persons with symptoms suggestive of TB should be evaluated immediately with a chest radiograph. These patients should also be placed in appropriate respiratory isolation until they are evaluated and infectious tuberculosis is ruled out.

The administration of health intake questionnaires by correctional officers is a common practice, particularly in small jails. The accuracy of health assessment by lay correctional officers has not been studied. Trained health care staff should perform this function because lay officers may not understand the medical concepts involved in the questionnaire. However, currently there are no data supporting officer screening for tuberculosis. The effectiveness of intake questionnaires in screening for TB and who should administer these questionnaires needs to be studied further.

During their initial medical evaluations, inmates should be asked if they have a history of active TB or if they have been treated for TB infection or disease in the past. Any inmate who has a history of inadequate treatment for TB should undergo a thorough medical evaluation.

Symptom screening alone is an unsatisfactory screening mechanism for tuberculosis, except for facilities that do not house tuberculosis patients, are located in communities without tuberculosis patients, and do not house inmates from communities with tuberculosis.[19] The use of symptom screening alone at intake fails to detect active pulmonary tuberculosis in some inmates.

Chest Radiograph Screening

Screening inmates with a chest radiograph is a quick and effective way to identify and immediately isolate potentially infectious persons. Radiograph screening for tuberculosis has been shown to reduce the time from intake into the correctional facility to isolation significantly, thereby reducing the risk of exposure to tuberculosis to other inmates and staff.[20] Chest radiograph screening is appropriate in settings where the incidence or prevalence of TB is high. A posterior-anterior view is the standard radiograph used initially for screening. Chest radiograph interpretations should be available within 72 hours for asymptomatic inmates. Sputum smears and culture examinations should be performed for inmates whose chest radiographs are suggestive of active TB, or who are symptomatic, regardless of their skin test results.

Inmates who are infected with HIV, and those who are at risk for HIV infection but whose status is unknown, may be anergic and consequently may have negative tuberculin skin test results even though they have latent TB infection. Therefore, these inmates should have a chest radiograph as part of their initial screening, regardless of their skin test results.

In jails, with short average lengths of stay and large numbers of individuals coming in, the principal aim of

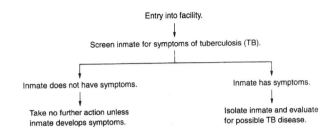

Figure 10-3. Protocol for screening inmates for TB in short-term correctional facilities that provide service to low-risk populations. (From CDC: Prevention and control of tuberculosis in correctional facilities: Recommendations of the advisory council for the elimination of tuberculosis. *MMWR* 45:13, 1996)

screening is to identify infectious persons and reduce exposure to other inmates and staff. On-site radiographic screening should be considered for large jails serving populations at high risk for TB, especially those jails with a high prevalence of HIV infection and drug injection. Radiographic screening has been successfully performed using photofluorographic imaging.[21] This technology has been superseded by digital radiography, which provides enhanced imaging and improved storage and readability.

During on-site radiographic screening, a chest radiograph is performed as part of intake screening, and radiographs are read within 24 hours by a radiologist. Those who have radiographs suspicious for tuberculosis are isolated promptly and evaluated further. In one study, compared to tuberculin skin testing as a screening mechanism, screening by radiography doubled the case finding rate of TB and reduced the time to isolation.[20] In addition, when the main purpose of screening is to identify active TB, radiographic screening at intake requires fewer follow-up visits (only those inmates with suspicious radiographs or TB symptoms) than tuberculin skin testing at intake (all of those inmates with positive tuberculin skin test results, as high as 25% of inmates in some studies).

In some prisons, selective radiographic screening at intake, in conjunction with symptom screening and tuberculin skin testing, may be useful to reduce TB transmission, depending on the prevalence of HIV infection, the prevalence of TB disease, and the quality of screening in the other facilities prior to transfer to the prison. Another successful method of reducing the risk of TB transmission used in some prisons is placing inmates in a separate intake facility until medical screening is complete.

In facilities where symptom screening with tuberculin skin testing (without radiographic screening) is used, those inmates who have positive tuberculin skin test results and no TB symptoms should have a chest radiograph with 72 hours of the skin test reading. Inmates with TB symptoms should be evaluated immediately, regardless of skin test results.

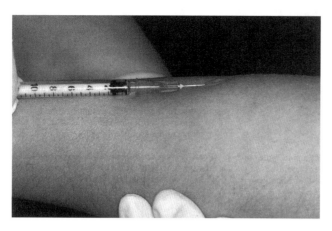

Figure 10-4. Giving Mantoux tuberculin skin test. (From CDC: Self-study modules on tuberculosis. Diagnosis of tuberculosis infection and diseases. Atlanta, GA: CDC, 1995, p 9.)

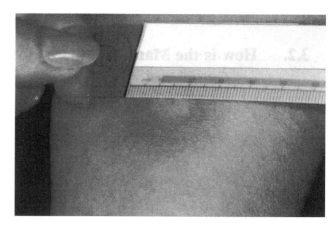

Figure 10-6. The erythema is being measured. This is **INCORRECT**. (From CDC: Self-study modules on tuberculosis. Diagnosis of tuberculosis infection and diseases. Atlanta, GA: CDC, 1995, p 9.)

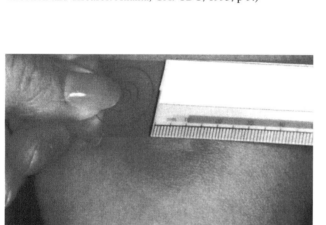

Figure 10-5. Only the induction is being measured. This is **CORRECT**. (From CDC: Self-study modules on tuberculosis. Diagnosis of tuberculosis infection and diseases. Atlanta, GA: CDC, 1995, p 9.)

Box 10-1. How to Perform the Mantoux Tuberculin Skin Test

- Perform the Mantoux test by giving an intradermal injection of 0.1 ml of 5 tuberculin units (TU) of purified protein derivative (PPD) tuberculin into either the volar or dorsal surface of the forearm.
- Inject the tuberculin with a disposable tuberculin syringe, just beneath the surface of the skin with the needle bevel facing upward. This should produce a discrete, pale elevation of the skin (a wheal) 6 mm to 10 mm in diameter.
- To prevent needlestick injuries, do not recap needles, bend or break them, remove them from disposable syringes, or otherwise manipulate them by hand.
- After dispoable needles and syringes have been used, place them in puncture-resistant containers for disposal. Follow institutional guidelines regarding universal precautions for infection control (e.g., the use of gloves).

Tuberculin Skin Test Screening

The preferred method of screening for TB infection is the Mantoux tuberculin skin test (Figure 10-4 and Box 10-1). Multipuncture tests should not be used. An experienced health care worker should read the reaction 48 to 72 hours after the injection. The area of induration should be measured and recorded in millimeters. Erythema should not be measured (Figures 10-5, 10-6). Persons with a positive tuberculin reaction and no symptoms suggestive of tuberculosis should be evaluated with a chest radiograph within 72 hours of the skin test reading. Persons with TB symptoms should be evaluated immediately, regardless of the skin test results.

The tuberculin skin test is not a good method of screening for TB disease. First, on average, 10% to 25% of patients with active TB disease have a negative reaction to tuberculin.[21, 22] Second, tuberculin skin test screening requires a follow-up visit for reading and interpretation and an additional visit for evaluation with a chest radiograph if the test is read as positive, significantly delaying diagnosis and increasing the risk of transmission to other inmates and staff. In a large urban jail with multiple inmate housing sites, follow up of tuberculin skin tests took many weeks (personal communication, M. Puisis, Cook County Jail). In one New York City jail, there was evidence of ongoing transmission of *M. tuberculosis* in the jail, despite an ongoing tuberculin skin test screening program. Despite these limitations, tuberculin skin testing may be the only practical approach to screen for TB disease in small-to-medium facilities.[15] Despite these limitations, tuberculin skin testing may be the only practical approach to screen for TB disease in small-to-medium facilities.

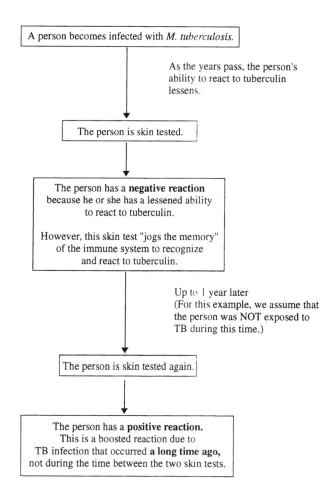

Figure 10-7. The Booster phenomenon. (From CDC: Self-study modules on tuberculosis. Diagnosis of tuberculosis infection and diseases. Atlanta, GA: CDC, 1995, p 27.)

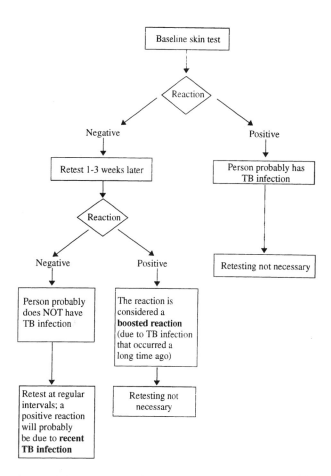

Figure 10-8. Two-step testing. (From CDC: Self-study modules on tuberculosis. Diagnosis of tuberculosis infection and diseases. Atlanta, GA: CDC, 1995, p 29.)

Two-step testing should be used for the baseline testing of persons who will receive repeated tuberculin skin tests as part of an institutional skin testing program (e.g., in prisons) (Figures 10-7, 10-8). In some persons who were infected many years ago, delayed-type hypersensitivity to tuberculin may have waned. When they are skin tested many years after infection, they may have a negative reaction, even though they are infected. However, this skin test may stimulate their ability to react to subsequent tests, resulting in the so-called booster reaction. When the next test is done, it may be misinterpreted as a new infection (recent conversion) rather than a boosted reaction.

Two-step testing can be used to minimize this problem. In two-step testing, persons who have a negative result to their baseline tuberculin skin test are retested 1 to 3 weeks later. If the second test result is negative, they are considered not infected. If the second test result is positive, they are classified as having previous TB infection. The use of two-step testing can reduce the number of positive reactions misclassified as recent skin test conversions and, therefore, reduce unnecessary evaluations of misclassified

new conversions in a facility. Tuberculin skin test screening should be performed for inmates in all prisons. Two-step testing on baseline should be strongly considered. Inmates with a positive tuberculin skin test reaction should receive a chest radiograph and thorough medical evaluation, and should be evaluated for preventive therapy if active TB is ruled out.

In jails, tuberculin skin test screening for purposes of initiating preventive therapy is often not feasible because of the high rate of turnover and short lengths of stay. Not all jail inmates have short lengths of stay, but it is often difficult to identify which inmates will be in the jail long term. In the New York City jail, half of the inmates are released within 2 weeks of admission, while the remainder have an average length of stay of 6 months (personal communication, R. Cohen).

Even if all inmates can be skin tested at intake, a large proportion will be unavailable in 48 to 72 hours for reading, and, of those who do have their skin test read, many will be released before the radiographic and medical evaluation is complete. Few can be started on preventive ther-

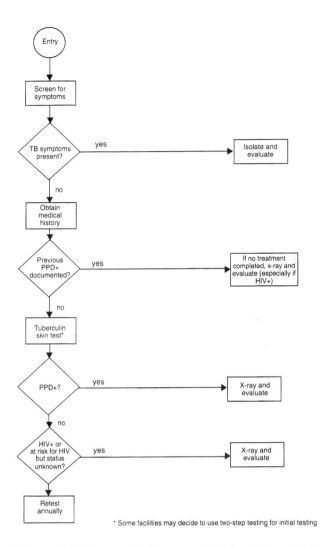

Figure 10-9. Inmates in long-term facilities. (From CDC: Controlling TB in Correctional Facilities. Atlanta, GA: CDC, 1995, Appendix 2.)

apy, and very few of those will complete preventive therapy. As few as 5% of inmates who initiated preventive therapy in a large urban jail completed therapy (M. Puisis, Cook County Jail audit, Chicago). Therefore, since the primary purpose of tuberculin skin test screening is to identify persons who require preventive therapy and to ensure that they complete preventive therapy, tuberculin skin test screening is not indicated in most jail settings. Initial screening in jails where the risk of TB is high should focus on screening for TB to reduce transmission (i.e., symptom screening with radiographic screening). For facilities in high-risk settings in which radiographic screening cannot be performed, symptom screening with physical examination, tuberculin skin testing, and matching with local health department tuberculosis registries may be an effective alternative.[23]

INITIAL SCREENING IN PRISONS

All new prison inmates should be screened for TB symptoms as soon as possible (Figure 10-9). Any inmate with TB symptoms should be placed in a TB isolation room and evaluated promptly. In addition, those who do not report TB symptoms should be questioned about whether they have been diagnosed with TB infection or disease in the past and whether they completed appropriate therapy. Those with a history of inadequate treatment should be evaluated further.

Tuberculin skin test screening should be performed on all inmates who do not have a documented history of a positive tuberculin skin test result. Two-step skin testing for baseline testing for inmates entering the facility should be considered to reduce the misclassification of boosted reactions as recent infections. Inmates who have a positive tuberculin skin test result at baseline testing should have a thorough medical evaluation, including a chest radiograph. If active tuberculosis is ruled out, the inmate should be evaluated for preventive therapy. Prisons offer an excellent public health opportunity for identifying persons at high risk for TB who can be screened for TB infection and placed on preventive therapy if indicated. By using adherence-promoting techniques, such as directly observed preventive therapy, completion of preventive therapy in infected inmates can be ensured, and future cases of TB can be prevented effectively.

Inmates who have a negative tuberculin skin test result at baseline testing should have a repeat skin test annually. Any inmate who is infected with HIV, or at risk for HIV infection but has unknown HIV status, should have a chest radiograph as part of their initial evaluation, regardless of their skin test results.

INITIAL SCREENING IN JAILS

Symptom screening should be done as soon as possible for all new inmates in jails. Any inmate with TB symptoms should be placed in a TB isolation room and evaluated promptly. Facilities without an on-site TB isolation room should have a written plan to refer patients with suspected or confirmed TB to a collaborating facility that is equipped to evaluate and treat TB patients.

The use of other screening activities depends on the risk of TB in the facility. In jails serving populations at high risk for TB, chest radiographs should be considered. In facilities where this is not possible, inmates who will remain in custody for 14 days or longer should be tuberculin skin tested within 14 days of entry (Figure 10-10). Ideally, inmates are skin tested upon entry into the facility. Inmates who have a positive tuberculin skin test result at baseline testing should have a thorough medical evaluation, including a chest radiograph. If active tuberculosis is ruled out, the inmate should be evaluated for preventive therapy. Preventive therapy should not be initiated unless there is a reasonable chance of completion. Any inmate who is infected with HIV, or at risk for HIV infection but has unknown HIV status, should

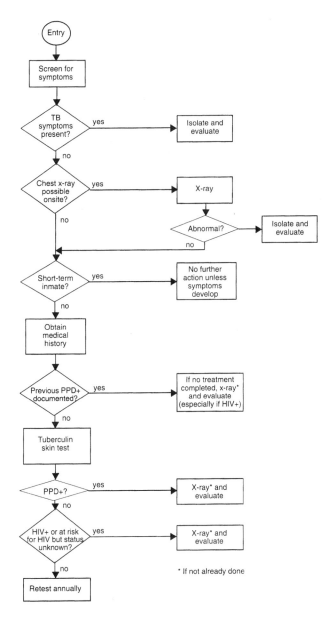

Figure 10-10. Inmates in short-term facilities serving high-risk populations. (From CDC: Controlling TB in Correctional Facilities. Atlanta, GA: CDC, 1995, Appendix 2.)

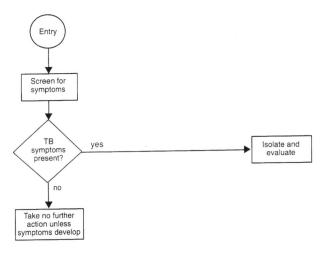

Figure 10-11. Inmates in short-term facilities serving low-risk populations. (From CDC: Controlling TB in Correctional Facilities. Atlanta, GA: CDC, 1995, Appendix 2.)

PREVENTIVE THERAPY

In prisons, screening for tuberculosis almost always includes a program of preventive therapy for inmates with positive tuberculin skin test results and normal chest radiographs. Inmates in prisons often remain incarcerated long enough to complete a course of preventive therapy, and completion of preventive therapy can be successful, especially when using adherence-promoting techniques, such as directly observed preventive therapy.

This is not true for jail inmates. Attempts to provide preventive therapy in a large urban jail have yielded completion rates as low as 5%. Most jail inmates do not remain incarcerated for the duration of a prescribed course of preventive therapy. After release, ensuring completion of preventive therapy becomes a local health department responsibility. Follow-up of infected inmates after release is generally difficult. Many patients are homeless, and others do not want their address known, or give a false address. Verification of address prior to discharge from jail may improve success. Preventive treatment programs in jails, therefore, require a cooperative arrangement with the local health department.

The cost effectiveness of preventive therapy programs in jails should be evaluated in coordination with the local health department. It is important to use available funding for tuberculosis programs in the most effective manner, based on public health priorities. Completion of therapy for persons who have active tuberculosis is the highest priority, followed by identifying contacts of infectious tuberculosis, and ensuring that infected contacts complete an appropriate course of preventive therapy. Screening persons at high risk for tuberculosis infection and ensuring that infected persons complete an appropriate course of preventive therapy is the final priority. Screening activities

have a chest radiograph as part of their initial evaluation, regardless of their skin test results.

For some large jails serving populations at high risk for TB infection and disease, on-site radiographic screening of all inmates at intake should be considered to reduce TB transmission.

In jails serving populations at low risk for tuberculosis, more extensive screening (beyond symptom screening) may not be indicated, especially if the facility and community served have low TB rates, no drug-resistant TB, and low prevalence of HIV infection (Figure 10-11).

should never take priority over completion of therapy or contact investigation activities. Screening for TB infection in jails should not be undertaken unless resources are available in the local health department to ensure appropriate follow-up and completion of preventive therapy for infected inmates after release.

LINKAGE TO LOCAL HEALTH DEPARTMENTS

Tuberculosis is a reportable disease. In all correctional facilities, officials should work closely with the state and local health departments in their jurisdictions. Correctional facilities should establish formal agreements with the health departments to delineate responsibilities and specify procedures for screening and treatment of inmates, follow-up of symptomatic inmates, follow-up of inmates who have abnormal chest radiographs, contact investigation for reported TB cases, and follow-up of inmates released before completing treatment for TB disease or preventive therapy. Correctional facilities should collaborate with health department staff to provide TB education and training to correctional facility employees.

The health department should ensure access to expert medical consultation and adequate laboratory services for the correctional facility. A specific health department person should be designated to work with the correctional facility and provide assistance. For some larger jails, health department staff have been assigned to work on site, or access to health department TB registry data has been provided to help identify new inmates who have already been identified by the health department as having or suspected of having tuberculosis. Strong linkages between correctional facilities and health departments are crucial to ensure timely identification, reporting, and appropriate treatment and completion of treatment for all cases of tuberculosis, and reducing transmission of tuberculosis in the facility and community.

REFERENCES

1. Tuberculosis Control Program, annual report. 1994.
2. Trenton, NJ: New Jersey Department of Health, 1995.
3. CDC: Probable transmission of multidrug-resistant tuberculosis in a correctional facility — California. *MMWR* 42:48-51, 1993.
4. Braun MM, Truman BI, Maguire B, et al: Increasing incidence of tuberculosis in a prison inmate population: Association with HIV infection. *JAMA* 261:393-397, 1989.
5. CDC: Reported tuberculosis in the United States, 1993.
6. CDC: U.S. Department of Health and Human Services, Public Health Service, 1994.
7. CDC: Reported tuberculosis in the United States, 1994.
8. CDC: U.S. Department of Health and Human Services, Public Health Service, Atlanta, 1995.
9. CDC: Reported tuberculosis in the United States, 1995.
10. CDC: U.S. Department of Health and Human Services, Public Health Service, Atlanta, 1996.
11. Salive ME, Vlahov D, Brewer TF: Coinfection with TB and HIV-1 in male prison inmates. *Public Health Rep* 105:307-310, 1990.
12. Spencer SS, Morton AR: Tuberculosis surveillance in a state prison system. *Am J Public Health* 79:507-509, 1989.
13. CDC: Tuberculosis prevention in drug-treatment centers and correctional facilities — selected U.S. sites, 1990-1991. *MMWR* 42:210-213 1993.
14. Alcabes P, Vossenas P, Cohen R, et al. Compliance with isoniazid prophylaxis in jail. *Am Rev Respir Dis* 140:1194-1197, 1989.
15. Bellin EY, Fletcher DD, Safyer SM: Association of tuberculosis infection with increased time in or admission to the New York City jail system. *JAMA* 269:2228-2231, 1993.
16. Stead WW: Undetected tuberculosis in prison: Source of infection for community at large. *JAMA* 240:2544-2547, 1978.
17. Snider DE Jr, Hutton MD: Tuberculosis in correctional institutions (editorial). *JAMA* 1989;261:436-437.
18. CDC: Prevention and control of tuberculosis in correctional facilities. *MMWR* 45(RR-8):1-27, 1996.
19. CDC: Controlling TB in Correctional Facilities, 1995.
20. Puisis M, Feinglass J, Lidow E, et al: Radiographic screening for tuberculosis in a large urban county jail. *Public Health Rep* 111:330-334, 1996.
21. Holder M, Dubin MR, Diamond PH: Frequency of negative intermediate-strength tuberculin sensitivity in patients with active tuberculosis. *N Engl J Med* 285:1506-1509, 1971.
22. Nash DR, Douglass JE: Anergy in active pulmonary tuberculosis: A comparison between positive and negative reactors and an evaluation of 5 TU and 250 TU skin test doses. *Chest* 77:32-37, 1980.
23. Layton M, Frieden T, Henning K: Screening of inmates for tuberculosis by chest X-rays. Thirty-fourth interscience conference on antimicrobial agents and chemotherapy, Oct 1994, Orlando.

11

Tuberculosis in the Correctional Facility

Jonathan Shuter, M.D.
Eran Y. Bellin, M.D.

Jail and prison medical services assume many different roles in the management of tuberculosis. They screen inmates for evidence of infection and order isolation for patients with suspected contagious tuberculosis; they provide treatment for active cases and offer prophylaxis to individuals who are infected but not diseased; they monitor patients for adverse reactions and manage such reactions when they occur; they protect uninfected inmates from acquiring infection and perform contact investigations when individuals are inadvertently exposed; they provide the educational and counseling services that are critical to maintaining high rates of therapy completion; they act as liaisons to providers in the community to assure therapeutic continuity for patients cycling in and out of the correctional system; and they register new cases with local public health agencies, locate cases who have been lost to follow-up in the community, and prompt the investigation of community contacts of infected detainees. The medical providers in correctional facilities are also potential disease carriers, transmitters, and victims.

Inmates may view the correctional medical service as an ally (e.g., healer or educator), or as an adversary (e.g., the inflictor of treatment-related toxicities or the enforcer of lengthy isolation). The jail or prison may act either as an ally to the public health agencies seeking to control tuberculosis or as an amplifier of disease. The correctional facility provides a unique opportunity for the diagnosis and treatment of tuberculosis in individuals whose lives are too disorganized in the outside community to maintain a relationship with a health care provider. It is an environment in which individuals may make informed health decisions at a time when mentation is not clouded by illicit drugs or by survival concerns for food and shelter. It is also a setting in which adequate nutrition and rest are provided, and inmates may recover from the weakened physiologic states associated with drug addiction and self-imposed, drug-related starvation. On the other hand, it is an environment in which most individuals have been placed against their will, which may foster an attitude of mistrust of all facility employees, including the medical providers. Moreover, it is a setting

109

characterized by congregate housing and often poor ventilation, in which endemic and epidemic tuberculosis transmission may occur,[1, 2] and may spread "through the bars" to involve the outside community.[2]

Correctional medical services occupy a crucial position within the network of organizations and individuals participating in tuberculosis control in the United States. This chapter will review the epidemiology of tuberculosis in the correctional setting and will then discuss practical issues pertaining to the diagnosis and management of tuberculosis within jails and prisons.

EPIDEMIOLOGY

The association between residence in correctional facilities and tuberculosis has long been recognized. A report on the state of the New York City almshouse in 1837, an era when correctional facilities were administered by the Department of Charities and Corrections, commented that, "The situation in one room was such as would have created contagion as the warm season came on, the air seeming to carry poison with every breath ... the lack of proper ventilation deprived the wretched inmates of even the free gift of fresh air."[3] A study of 512 New York City inmates in the early 1900s found that 15 (2.9%) had active tuberculosis and commented that, "The finding of cases of this kind in congested barrack rooms accentuates the necessity for a careful examination of all inmates."[3] The author suggested that, as a routine, sputum "should be submitted to microscopic examination if there is cough with expectoration and the physical examination of the chest leads to suspicion that tuberculosis may be present."[3] The public health law of New York State in 1902, in discussing the housing requirements of juvenile delinquents, specified that, "The beds in every dormitory in such institution shall be separated by a passageway of not less than two feet in width, and so arranged that under each the air shall freely circulate and there shall be adequate ventilation ... In every dormitory six hundred cubic feet of air space shall be provided and allowed for each bed or occupant, and no more beds or occupants shall be permitted than are thus provided for, unless free and adequate means of ventilation exist approved by the local board of health ... The physician of the institution shall immediately notify in writing the local board of health and the board of managers or directors of the institution of any violation of any provision of this section."[4] It is clear that the rudimentary elements of screening, environmental control, and involvement of public health agencies have existed, at least in New York City, for the past century.

Even as United States tuberculosis rates steadily declined between the 1950s and the early 1980s as a consequence of antimycobacterial pharmacotherapy and decreased urban squalor, high rates of tuberculosis in correctional facilities were still recognized.[2, 5] With the resurgence of tuberculosis in the mid-1980s coincident with the growth of the HIV epidemic came a recognition that jails and prisons were serving as hotbeds of tuberculosis transmission, which led to a number of studies that have better defined the epidemiology of tuberculosis in correctional institutions.

A large-scale survey of tuberculosis cases in 29 states between 1984 and 1985[6] found that the incidence rate of active tuberculosis in correctional facilities was 3.9 times greater (95% confidence intervals, 3.35–4.49) than the rate in the surrounding communities. This disparity was observed in high-, medium-, and low-incidence states. In the New York State correctional system, the incidence rate of tuberculosis increased sevenfold between 1976 and 1986.[7] In 1994, 4.6% of the incident cases of tuberculosis nationally were diagnosed in the correctional setting.[8] In New York City, the national epicenter of tuberculosis, 3.5% of individuals given diagnoses of tuberculosis were incarcerated at the time of or within the 12 months before diagnosis.[9] During the past decade, outbreaks of tuberculosis, including multidrug-resistant tuberculosis (MDR-TB), have been reported in correctional facilities across the country.[10–13]

Tuberculosis in the incarcerated population is not unique to the United States. The medical literature is replete with reports of tuberculosis in correctional settings including those of Spain,[14] Italy,[15] Ireland,[16] the Russian Federation,[17] and Madagascar.[18]

PATHOPHYSIOLOGY

Tuberculosis is caused by *Mycobacterium tuberculosis*, a slow-growing organism with a waxy cell wall that protects it from the lethal effects of human phagocytic cells. Because the only known reservoir for *M. tuberculosis* in nature is the human being, the infectious cycle begins when a patient with active tuberculosis excretes the organism into the environment, typically in a respiratory droplet transmitted into the air by coughing or sneezing. Respiratory droplets are too large to be inhaled into the lower airways where *M. tuberculosis* establishes its initial foothold, and may either settle onto surfaces and become noninfectious or develop into droplet nuclei after the evaporation of liquid from their surfaces. Droplet nuclei, which are 1–5 μm in size, may remain airborne for prolonged periods and can penetrate into the alveoli when inhaled. During the initial phase of infection, the organisms multiply within the alveolar macrophages. These macrophages, along with monocytes that are attracted from the bloodstream, are transported to regional lymph nodes via the pulmonary lymphatic system, and from the lymph nodes, an asymptomatic hematogenous dissemination occurs. Within 1 to 2 months, a protective cellular immune response develops (corresponding to the conversion to tuberculin reactivity) and halts the progression of disease throughout the body. Most individuals never advance beyond this stage, which is commonly termed *tuberculosis infection*. Five to 10% of individuals and higher numbers of immunocompromised individuals progress to *active tuberculosis disease* through the process of *reactivation,* in which one or more small foci of dormant organisms overwhelm the protective immune response and cause local and systemic disease. The highest risk of such an occurrence is within the first 2 years after the initial infection, and the most common site of disease is the lungs, particularly in the apical regions, although tuberculosis may develop virtually anywhere in the body. Certain individuals, especially children and immunocompromised individuals, may experience progressive primary tuberculosis when the initial immune response is insufficient to contain the primary focus of infection. Additionally, certain groups of patients are at greater risk for having reactivation tuberculosis because of weakened local or systemic immune responses. These groups include individuals infected with HIV and patients receiving steroids, as well as patients with diabetes, silicosis, injection drug addiction, and alcoholism. The cycle of infection and transmission is completed when the diseased individual excretes infected respiratory droplets into the environment to be inhaled by the next susceptible host.[19]

The pathophysiology of tuberculosis is of more than merely academic interest. The development of rational screening, prophylaxis, treatment, and infection control practices is predicated on a detailed understanding of these concepts.

SCREENING FOR TUBERCULOSIS

As an airborne disease, the extent of tuberculosis transmission is dependent on the infectiousness of the index case patient, the number of susceptible individuals who share air space with the case patient, the ventilation in the exposure environment, and the duration of exposure.[20] Jails and prisons are ideal environments for the transmission of tuberculosis because of the congregate housing, the prevalence of overcrowding and suboptimal ventilation, and the frequency of risk factors for tuberculous disease in the incarcerated population.[21, 22] It is, therefore, of the utmost importance to identify inmates who are likely to have contagious tuberculosis before they are housed (i.e., at the time of admission into the system). Screening programs in the correctional setting also provide the opportunity to identify large numbers of patients with tuberculosis infection who are at high risk for active disease development and who may benefit from a course of preventive therapy.

The minimum requirements for a tuberculosis screening program in a correctional facility include the following[22, 23]:

1. *History and physical examination.* All detainees should have medical histories taken and physical examinations at the time of admission to the facility that focus on symptoms and signs suggestive of tuberculosis. Of particular interest is a history of active tuberculosis prior tuberculosis infection, adequacy of prior tuberculosis prophylaxis or treatment, exposure to a friend or relative

with tuberculosis, a history of HIV disease, a history of a persistent cough (especially if continuing for more than 2 weeks), night sweats, or weight loss. The physical examination should pay particular attention to lung findings and lymph nodes.

2. *Tuberculin skin test.* All inmates without a known prior history of tuberculosis or tuberculin reactivity should receive a 5-TU tuberculin skin test at the time of admission. Inmates who are tuberculin reactors according to standard definitions should be questioned in detail about prior tuberculin testing in order to determine, if possible, the time of conversion. Individuals who were born outside the United States should be questioned about the receipt and timing of bacille Calmette-Guérin (BCG) vaccination, although a positive history should not alter the practitioner's response to tuberculin reactivity in a high-risk population, particularly if the BCG was received more than 5 years before the tuberculin screening.[22, 23] Institutions should evaluate the feasibility, merits, and costs of two-step testing according to their own local epidemiologic conditions. Two-step testing on admission may be helpful in distinguishing a remote exposure (as manifested by the "booster phenomenon") from a new conversion, particularly in an inmate population with a relatively long average duration of incarceration.[24, 25]

3. *Chest radiograph.* All inmates with symptoms or signs suggestive of tuberculosis, histories of active tuberculosis, past or present tuberculin reactivity, or with backgrounds likely to limit the sensitivity of tuberculin testing (e.g., patients with known HIV infection or patients with risk behaviors, such as injection drug use, that are associated with high rates of HIV infection) should have a chest radiograph done at the time of admission. An analysis of the yield of this strategy for each target group should contribute to the institution's protocol modification process in such a way that the process is best suited to the institution's particular population. One large study found rapid universal admission radiographs to be an economical and efficient mode of tuberculosis screening in a short-term stay facility,[26] whereas a study of universal radiographic screening in another such facility in New York City discovered few additional cases beyond those which would have been detected by a physical examination, taking a history, tuberculin testing, and cross-matching with the tuberculosis registry of the local health department.[27] The extent of radiologic screening in a given institution should be dictated by a number of factors, including local tuberculosis epidemiologic characteristics, inmate length of stay, and the ability of the health care establishment within the facility to conduct careful histories, physical examinations, and cross-matches with regional tuberculosis registries. Although the utility of radiographic examination as a screening test for tuberculosis is not questioned, no formal

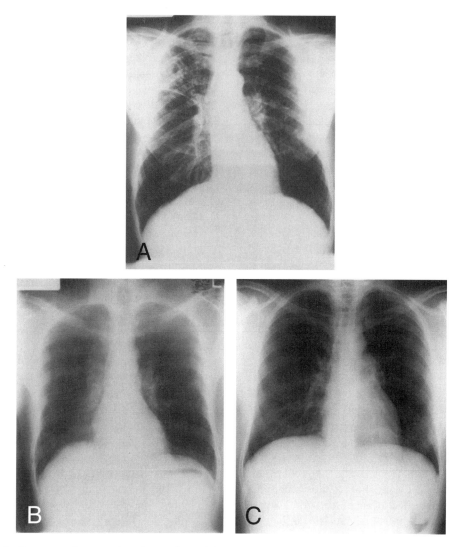

Figure 11-1. Representative screening chest radiographic presentations of patients with proven active pulmonary tuberculosis. **A**, man, 52, found to have tuberculin-positive test results for the first time on admission. He admitted to having a productive cough for 1 month, and his past medical history was significant for a partial gastrectromy. The chest radiograph shows extensive inflammatory changes and a cavitary lesion in the right upper lobe. Sputum examinations were positive for numerous acid-fast bacilli, and cultures grew *M. tuberculosis*. **B**, man, 28, with HIV infection complaining of night sweats and weight loss of 3 weeks' duration. Tuberculin test was negative as was the anergy panel. The absolute CD4+ lymphocyte count was 333/mm³. The chest radiograph shows paratracheal and hilar adenopathy. One of his initial three sputum specimens was suspicious for acid-fast bacilli. Several sputum cultures grew *M. tuberculosis*. **C**, man, 29, with AIDS and a history of tuberculin positivity 2 years before incarceration. The patient reported completing 1 year of isoniazid preventive therapy. He was housed in the general population (admission chest radiograph was normal), then persistent fevers and night sweats developed. The repeat chest radiograph (shown) is normal. Three sputum examinations were negative for acid-fast bacilli. Cultures of these sputum specimens ultimately grew *M. tuberculosis*.   (From Pedro-Botet J, Gutierrez J, Miralles R, et al: Pulmonary tuberculosis in HIV-infected patients with normal chest radiographs. *AIDS* 6:91–93, 1992, with permission.)

recommendations exist to stratify the risk level of various radiographic findings. The chest radiographs of patients with proven pulmonary tuberculosis, particularly those patients who are co-infected with HIV, may demonstrate a wide range of findings including complete normalcy[28] (Figure 11-1). Within our facility, all chest radiographic abnormalities involving the pulmonary parenchyma, pleural space, pericardium, lymphatic system, or vertebral bodies are treated seriously. When isolation beds are scarce, it seems prudent to assign highest priority to inmates with cavitary or apical disease, parenchymal infiltrates, and hilar or mediastinal adenopathy. It is our impression that the finding of an isolated granuloma, minimal parenchymal fibrosis, or pleural thickening, particularly in asymptomatic patients, is infrequently associated with a diagnosis of active tuberculosis. Of course, all chest radiographic abnormalities require a thoughtful plan of follow-up for medical considerations other than tuberculosis, and each institution should devise a protocol of response to radiologic abnormalities that meets the demands of its local inmate population.

4. ***Search for inmate membership in local health department tuberculosis registry.*** A cooperative effort with the local health department is of great importance for effective tuberculosis screening in the correctional setting. Inmates may provide faulty information on admission for a variety of reasons, ranging from forgetfulness and confusion to deliberate misrepresentation. In New York City, the department of health performs crossmatches with the city's tuberculosis registry and searches for matches on known aliases, birth dates, maternal maiden names, and other personal information to optimize their yield. Clearly, a readily accessible record of prior tuberculosis history, susceptibility patterns, treatment, and compliance can be invaluable in determining the disposition of a given patient with suspected tuberculosis.

5. ***Special circumstances.*** Short-term facilities located in communities without any active tuberculosis that house a population of inmates drawn from areas without tuberculosis and within which no cases of active tuberculosis have occurred within the previous 1 year are termed *minimal risk facilities.* Although symptomatic evaluation of all inmates should continue in these institutions, a formal program of tuberculin and radiographic screening for tuberculosis may not be necessary.[23] Screening strategies in institutions in which the vast majority of inmates leave before the 48–72 hours elapse that are necessary to interpret a tuberculin skin test may also require modification in response to these limitations.[23]

In correctional systems in which tuberculosis screening programs are in place, inmates should not only be screened on admission, but also, like employees in these facilities, be retested annually.[23] A computer database that keeps track of incarceration and release dates is indispensable for this application. During periods of increased tuberculosis transmission, more frequent testing of inmates may be indicated.

Finally, unusual housing situations may necessitate a higher level of tuberculosis screening. For example, on Rikers Island, patients may not be transferred to a dormitory reserved for patients with advanced HIV disease unless review of symptoms and a recent chest radiograph have reasonably excluded the diagnosis of active tuberculosis. The destructive potential of a single case of undiagnosed tuberculosis introduced into a group of patients with this degree of immunosuppression[29] justifies the higher level of tuberculosis screening that is required for entry.

RESPIRATORY ISOLATION AND ENVIRONMENTAL CONTROL

Any inmate with suspected active tuberculosis should be placed in an appropriate respiratory isolation facility. The principles of respiratory isolation and environmental control of tuberculosis have been reviewed comprehensively in a recent article.[20] Adequate respiratory isolation includes a negative pressure environment in the patient rooms, and at least six air changes per hour vented to the outside safely away from any intake ducts. Negative pressure anterooms are a desirable feature, and the adjunctive use of high-efficiency particulate air (HEPA) filtration or microbicidal ultraviolet radiation, or both, may be advisable in certain settings. Patients who are likely to have infectious tuberculosis must be either isolated in a suitable location within the correctional facility or transferred to an outside facility with appropriate accommodations. For the time interval preceding and during transport, the inmates should be encouraged to wear surgical face masks (to trap the large respiratory droplets), and any individuals who share air space with them should wear approved particulate respirator masks (to filter out the smaller droplet nuclei). A variety of fairly inexpensive, disposable particulate respirators carrying the designation "N-95" are now on the market, and they meet the specifications of the Centers for Disease Control, the Occupational Safety and Health Administration, and the National Institute for Occupational Safety and Health for this purpose.[30] When potentially infectious inmates must be taken out of isolation for any reason, similar precautions should be taken. Particulate respirator masks need not be worn outdoors. Cough-inducing procedures, such as sputum induction or aerosolized pentamidine administration, are particularly efficient at transmitting infectious particles into the environment, and should be performed only in an isolation booth equipped with HEPA filtration and approved for these purposes.[31] Practitioners must be mindful of the psychological stress of prolonged isolation and should ensure the availability of other stimuli, such as television and reading material. Mental health support services should be available to all isolated patients.

There is no precise guideline to determine when a specific patient may safely emerge from respiratory isolation. Most experts agree that patients with smear positive tuberculosis who have received therapy for 2 weeks, have had resolution of their coughing and fevers, and whose disease has reverted to smear negative on three consecutive daily sputum examinations, pose little infectious risk to others.[23] For cases of presumptive tuberculosis with negative sputum smears, it is our practice to allow release into the general population after 10–14 days of therapy, provided that there has been symptomatic improvement and there is no serious suspicion of MDR-TB. Because of the potentially devastating consequences of MDR-TB transmission and the greater likelihood of treatment failure, it is our practice to keep patients with MDR-TB in respiratory isolation until three consecutive daily sputum cultures are negative. Courtroom visits should be restricted in the same manner as is access to the general population. Given the severe stress induced by prolonged isolation, it is not unreasonable to relax some of the restrictions during outdoor recreation, where tuberculosis transmission is unlikely.

In our facility, we have found it helpful to use a color-coded scheme of respiratory isolation levels so that health care workers and correctional employees can easily discern the level of risk and the extent of allowable inmate activities at a glance. The four levels of isolation that are applied to patients in our respiratory isolation facility are summarized as follows:

1. Red (Highest)—Patients documented to have smear positive tuberculosis or patients with highly suspicious radiographs (e.g., upper lobe infiltrate or cavity) and cough, awaiting sputum smear results. These patients remain in respiratory isolation continuously until their color code is downgraded. Court visits and recreation are prohibited.

2. Orange (High)—Patients admitted to respiratory isolation without criteria for "Red" color coding, who are awaiting sputum smear results. Activity restrictions are identical to those of patients in red-coded isolation.

3. Yellow (Intermediate)—Patients with sputum smears that are negative, but with chest radiographs suggestive of active tuberculosis. Culture results and/or consultation for invasive diagnostic procedure pending. These patients may go to outdoor recreation, but they may not go to court.

4. Green (Low)—Patients with three negative sputum smears and chest radiographs not suggestive of active tuberculosis. Also applies to patients with active tuberculosis receiving treatment for at least 1 week who have had clinical and mycobacteriologic responses to therapy (smears either negative or decreasing in intensity of positivity). Patients may go to outdoor recreation and may go to court if their last three sputum smears are negative.

This outline provides a simple and practical framework for the stratification of respiratory isolation in a jail or prison. Of course, not all patients fit neatly into a single category, so isolation decisions must ultimately be made on a case-by-case basis. Additionally, there is some compromise of patient confidentiality inherent in these classification systems, as there is in the simple act of transferring an inmate to respiratory isolation. Although these compromises are necessary to protect the health of the inmates and correctional employees, isolation strategies should be devised with the intent of minimizing public access to personal medical information.

DIAGNOSIS

Although the process of diagnosing tuberculosis begins with a careful history, physical examination, tuberculin test, and chest radiograph, the definitive diagnosis ultimately rests on mycobacteriology laboratory testing. A patient who is designated as possibly having tuberculosis via the existing screening protocols should undergo further testing while housed in a respiratory isolation area. All patients with suspected tuberculosis, whether pulmonary or extrapulmonary, should submit three daily sputum specimens for acid-fast staining and mycobacterial culture. Standard recommendations call for three early morning spontaneously expectorated specimens in patients who have productive coughs. Patients without productive coughs should undergo sputum induction with nebulized saline, according to published protocols.[32, 33] All sputum-producing maneuvers have the potential for aerosolizing large numbers of infectious organisms and should, therefore, be performed in a respiratory isolation booth. The rationale for sputum examination in patients with extrapulmonary tuberculosis is the recognition of the lung as the initial focus of infection in virtually all cases and the frequency of positive sputum cultures, even in the absence of chest radiographic abnormalities.[34] Once collected, sputum specimens should be delivered to the laboratory with the shortest possible delay; specimens should be refrigerated if transport is not immediately available. On receipt, the laboratory should perform one of the accepted acid-fast staining techniques (Kinyoun, Ziehl-Neelsen, or fluorochrome) and inoculate the sample into the appropriate culture media. Although a description of the relative merits of the various culture media is beyond the scope of this chapter, the liquid media offer the advantage of more rapid diagnosis, whereas the solid media allow inspection of colonial morphologic characteristics and boast a lengthier record of reliable performance.[33] Genetically based rapid identification techniques are now available to provide sensitive and specific identification information on culture-positive specimens in liquid or solid media.[33] These techniques are also available for the rapid identification of *M. tuberculosis* complex organisms in smear-positive specimens, before culture, although the level of performance of these tests in the "real world" of the clinical laboratory remains to be seen.[35] All patients with culture-proven tuberculosis should have testing of at least one positive culture specimen for susceptibility to the first-line antimycobacterial drugs (isoniazid, rifampin, pyrazinamide, ethambutol, and streptomycin).[36] Isolates that are resistant to isoniazid, rifampin, or more than one other first-line agent should undergo susceptibility testing to a full panel of second-line agents. The interested reader is referred to several recent excellent reviews of existing mycobacteriology laboratory practices.[33, 37, 38]

Although the definitive diagnosis of tuberculosis rests on a positive culture result, other clinical scenarios may reasonably lead to the presumptive diagnosis of tuberculosis. For example, a patient with a new positive tuberculin reaction, an apical infiltrate, signs of fever and weight loss, and resolution of radiologic and clinical abnormalities after initiation of antituberculous therapy, would meet the classification criteria for culture-negative active tuberculosis according to most practitioners. Similarly, the observation of caseating granulomas and acid-fast bacilli on a biopsy of bone from a destructive vertebral lesion or from the pleural surface of a patient with a pleural effusion would provide convincing evidence of vertebral or pleural tuberculosis.

When tuberculosis is suspected on the basis of radiologic abnormalities, but a sputum examination does not yield a positive smear result, further steps should be taken to establish the diagnosis and to maximize the likelihood of organism recovery for the purpose of susceptibility testing. Alternative imaging procedures, such as gallium scanning[39] and chest CT,[40] may be helpful in the evaluation of a chest radiographic abnormality, although they do not substitute for mycobacteriology laboratory information. High rates of single drug and multidrug-resistance should discourage the hasty institution of empirical antimycobacterial therapy in stable patients with negative smears, even when radiologic and clinical symptoms are highly suggestive of active tuberculosis. Invasive diagnostic procedures, such as transthoracic needle aspiration or bronchoscopy, are appropriate in such cases to review histopathologic features and to maximize the likelihood of organism recovery. Empirical therapy is indicated for patients with suspected tuberculosis who refuse further evaluation or for whom further evaluation would entail intolerable delays or risks.

Because most jails and prisons do not have an on-site mycobacteriology laboratory, appropriate arrangements must be made for timely specimen deliveries to an outside laboratory and for prompt reporting of all positive and negative results. Positive smear or culture results should be treated as laboratory "panic" values and reported to the responsible practitioner immediately. All requisitions and results should be kept in a central logbook and computer database, and the review of this database should be an ongoing responsibility of the institution's infection control practitioner.

TREATMENT

The introduction of effective pharmacotherapy in the 1950s revolutionized the management of tuberculosis. More is known about tuberculosis than perhaps any other infectious disease regarding the choice and duration of medication regimens. The single resounding message taught by the resurgence of tuberculosis in the past decade has been the folly of leaving actively infected patients to their own devices, even when an adequate supply of free medication is assured. In New York City in 1988, the epicenter of the tuberculosis epidemic in the United States, only 11% of patients with newly diagnosed active tuberculosis in a large city hospital completed a course of therapy.[41] Many of the factors that are associated with medication noncompliance, such as homelessness, drug use, and psychiatric illness, are rampant in the incarcerated population. Considering this,

the present discussion will limit the traditional in-depth pharmacologic review and expand on some of the more neglected, but important, topics of education, treatment observation, and community follow-up.

1. *Education.* It is intuitively obvious that many patients will fail to comply with a complex multidrug regimen if they don't understand their disease process and the necessity for a lengthy course of treatment. Prisoners, by definition, have lost control over many aspects of their lives, including freedom of movement, freedom of communication with the outside community, and freedom of choice and timing of activities. They may perceive their health care experience with tuberculosis as yet another in a series of unpleasant intrusions on their autonomy, and much of the medication noncompliance that we have observed in our facility has revolved around the issue of control or lack thereof. Although many aspects of inmates' lives are outside of their control, they do retain the right to refuse medications, and the issue of control over medication acceptance is at the heart of much of the noncompliance. Certainly the likelihood of medication refusal is increased if the patients do not understand their diagnoses and the rationale for lengthy and complex treatment regimens. It is crucial that the medical, nursing, and, when necessary, mental health staff work together to clearly explain the medical situation and encourage ongoing compliance. All information should be understandable and culturally appropriate for the patients. Patients who are not fluent in English should receive information and counseling through translators fluent in the inmates' native languages. On Rikers Island, an educational video has been prepared in English, Spanish, Creole, and Mandarin Chinese for viewing by all new admissions to the respiratory isolation facility.

2. *Treatment observation.* The United States Public Health Service recommends that all treatment for active tuberculosis in correctional facilities be administered under direct observation.[22, 23] The success of directly observed therapy programs in stemming the tide of the tuberculosis epidemic in the United States has been well documented.[42, 43] Each facility, depending on the number of patients with tuberculosis therein, should have a health care provider or providers assigned specifically to the task of administering and overseeing directly observed tuberculosis therapy for the inmates. The observer must watch the patient swallow every pill and should listen to the patient speak, and inspect the oropharynx thoroughly after the pills are given to minimize the likelihood of surreptitious noncompliance. Even patients who swallow all pills may be noncompliant by inducing vomiting after departing from the clinical care site. Such methods of medication avoidance may be more common in inmates who receive both opiate medications and rifampin, representing an attempt to escape the increased

Table 11-1. Pharmacologic properties of medications used to treat tuberculosis*

Medication	Usual adult dosage	MIC for fully susceptible tuberculosis (μg/ml)	Expected peak serum level (μg/ml)	Elimination half-life (hr)	Dosage adjustment necessary for renal insufficiency	Dosage adjustment necessary for hepatic insufficiency	Principal toxicities
Isoniazid	300 mg PO daily	≤ 0.1	3–5	1.5–4	No	Yes	Hepatitis, peripheral neuropathy
Rifampin	600 mg PO daily	≤ 0.5	8–24	2–5	No	Yes	GI distress, hepatitis, rash, flu-like syndrome, discoloration of body fluids
Pyrazinamide	15–30 mg/kg PO daily	≤ 100	20–60	9	Yes	Yes	Hepatitis, hyperuricemia, gout
Ethambutol	15–25 mg/kg PO daily	≤ 1.0	2–6	3–5	Yes	No	Optic neuritis
Streptomycin	15 mg/kg IM daily	≤ 2.0	35–45	2–3	Yes	No	Otic and renal damage
Ofloxacin**	800 mg PO daily	≤ 1.0	8–12	4–8	Yes	No	GI distress, tremulousness
Ciprofloxacin**	750 mg PO bid	≤ 1.0	4–6	3–5	Yes	No	GI distress, tremulousness
Cycloserine	250 mg PO tid or qid	≤ 4.0	20–35	10	Yes	No	Mood changes, forgetfulness, psychosis, seizures
Ethionamide	250 mg PO tid or qid	≤ 1.0	1–5	2	No	Unknown	GI distress, metallic taste, taste, hepatitis, arthralgia, thyroid dysfunction
Para-aminosalicylic acid	3 g PO qid	Unknown	20–60	1	Unknown	Unknown	GI distress, rash, thyroid dysfunction
Capreomycin	15 mg/kg IM daily	≤ 2.0	35–45	2–4	Yes	No	Otic and renal damage
Kanamycin	15 mg/kg IM daily	≤ 2.0	35–45	2–4	Yes	No	Otic and renal damage
Clofazimine**	100–300 mg PO daily	≤ 0.06	0.5–2.0	192	No	No	GI distress, skin discoloration

Note. Abbreviations used: *PO,* orally; *IM,* intramuscularly; *BID,* twice daily; *TID,* three times daily; *QID,* four times daily; *GI,* gastrointestinal; *MIC,* mean inhibitory concentration.

*Data extracted from references [38, 44-46]. Information contained in this table, particularly dosages and toxicities, are not intended to be comprehensive lists applying to every clinical situation. The PDR or medication package insert should be consulted for further specifics.

**Not approved by the FDA for tuberculosis treatment.

metabolism of opiates that rifampin induces. Methadone recipients who require rifampin therapy should receive higher doses of the narcotic as clinically indicated. In cases in which noncompliance is suspected but not proved, an inspection of urine for the orange-red discoloration that absorbed rifampin produces, as well as serum levels of the various medications, may prove helpful.

3. ***Medication regimens.*** The pharmacologic properties of the medications commonly used in the treatment of tuberculosis are summarized in Table 11-1,[38, 44–46] and standard recommendations for the pharmacotherapy of

tuberculosis disease are summarized in Table 11-2.[47–51] The reader is referred to several excellent reviews for further details.[47, 48, 52] A number of clinical situations that necessitate a departure from "standard" treatment follow:

a. *Pregnancy.* The pregnant inmate with active tuberculosis should receive a regimen of isoniazid, rifampin, and ethambutol at the usual dosages. Pyrazinamide is not recommended because of inadequate data on teratogenicity. Streptomycin use in pregnancy is associated with unacceptably high rates of fetal malformation.[47] There is insufficient data on the safety of

Table 11-2. Treatment recommendations for active tuberculosis

Disease classification	Drug regimen*	Duration of therapy†
Initial therapy (while awaiting culture and susceptibility results)	Isoniazid, rifampin, pyrazinamide, and ethambutol or streptomycin‡	Until susceptibility information is available
Susceptible to all first-line agents	Isoniazid, rifampin and pyrazinamide for 2 months followed by isoniazid, rifampin (may be given two to three times per week after initial course of daily therapy	6–12 months
	or Isoniazid, rifampin, pyrazinamide, and ethambutol or streptomycin (three times weekly throughout)	6–12 months
	or Isoniazid, rifampin	9–12 months
Resistant to isoniazid only	Rifampin, pyrazinamide, ethambutol or streptomycin ± quinolone§	6–12 months
Resistant to isoniazid and pyrazinamide	Rifampin, ethambutol, and a quinolone§	12 months
Resistant to rifampin only	Isoniazid, pyrazinamide, ethambutol ± quinolone§	18 months
Resistant to isoniazid and rifampin (i.e., MDR-TB)‖	Three oral agents to which the isolate is susceptible and one injectable agent (injectable agent continued for at least 6 months and oral agents throughout)‖	At least 18–24 months, and for at least 12 months after sputum cultures revert to negative‖

Note: This table is intended to provide a reasonable outline of treatment options for average-sized adults with uncomplicated active tuberculosis and normal renal and hepatic function. Standard dosages for daily therapy may be found in Table 11-1. More detailed recommendations may be found in references 47 and 48.

*Twice or three times per week treatment options are available for isolates that are susceptible to both isoniazid and rifampin. Dosing schedules for these regimens may be found in references 47 and 48. All other regimens must be administered daily.

†The longer durations of therapy listed are particularly applicable to patients with HIV infection, in whom short-course therapy may be associated with high rates of failure and relapse. Four months of four-drug therapy may be adequate in the treatment of uncomplicated smear-negative, culture-negative tuberculosis.

‡Patients who are at very low risk for drug resistance, in communities where the prevalence of primary isoniazid resistance is less than 4%, may not require a fourth drug.

§The quinolone agents are not approved by the Food and Drug Administration for the treatment of tuberculosis.

‖Patients with multidrug-resistant tuberculosis (MDR-TB) should be managed by providers with expertise in the treatment of this disease. Further details regarding the treatment of MDR-TB may be found in references 49–51.

second-line medications, although fluoroquinolone agents are generally discouraged and para-aminosalicylic acid appears to be safe.[53] Pregnant inmates who require a regimen other than isoniazid, rifampin, and ethambutol should be managed under the concerted care of an infectious diseases specialist and an obstetrician/perinatologist. Furthermore, pregnant inmates who are undergoing tuberculosis treatment should be monitored closely for hepatotoxicity that may occur at an increased frequency in this population.[54]

b. *Multidrug-resistant tuberculosis.* The therapy of MDR-TB (i.e., tuberculosis resistant to at least isoniazid and rifampin) must be tailored to conform to the resistance pattern of the isolate and the range of toxicities experienced by the patient. The reader is referred to several recent excellent reviews of this subject.[49–51] It is our practice to use three oral agents to which the isolate demonstrates in vitro susceptibility together with one injectable agent for the first 6 months of treatment. The oral agents should be

continued for at least 18–24 months. All cases of MDR-TB should be managed under the supervision of a clinician with expertise in treating this disease process.

c. *Infection with HIV.* Rates of HIV infection among prisoners throughout the country, particularly among women, are substantially higher than those in the surrounding communities.[55] Although the American Thoracic Society endorses the use of short-course (i.e., 6 months) chemotherapy for uncomplicated tuberculosis in individuals infected with HIV,[47] a number of authorities have expressed concern over high relapse rates associated with this strategy.[36, 56, 57] Two large, well-designed studies[57, 58] have now demonstrated alarmingly high rates of relapse after short-course treatment of patients infected with HIV. Our practice is to treat all patients infected with HIV who have active tuberculosis for at least 1 year, and to institute lifelong secondary prophylaxis after therapy is complete[59] (see below).

d. *Ongoing therapy with HIV-1 protease inhibitor.* Patients with HIV infection who are given diagnoses of tuberculosis at a time when they are receiving therapy with one of the available protease inhibitors (including saquinavir, ritonavir, and indinavir at the time of this writing) present a difficult therapeutic problem. All of the available protease inhibitors are metabolized by the hepatic cytochrome P-450 system, a process that is accelerated by the concomitant usage of rifampin; thus, lowered serum levels of the protease inhibitors results. Suboptimal serum levels of these agents are associated with the development of viral resistance and may result in the loss of some or all of the protease inhibitors as effective modes of antiretroviral therapy. In response to this troubling drug interaction, the United States Public Health Service suggests three alternatives[60]:

   i. Prescribe conventional therapy for tuberculosis, including rifampin, and interrupt protease inhibitor therapy for the duration of this treatment.

   ii. Use rifampin only during the first 2 months of therapy, thereafter switching to an isoniazid–ethambutol-based regimen, and restart protease inhibitor treatment after the 2-month interruption.

   iii. Substitute low-dose rifabutin (150 mg daily) for rifampin and continue protease inhibitor therapy (only permissible for indinavir, not saquinavir or ritonavir). This recommendation insists on continuation of daily four-drug tuberculosis therapy for a minimum of 9 months. At least one large multinational study to date has demonstrated the therapeutic equivalence of rifabutin and rifampin in the treatment of active tuberculosis.[61]

   It is our preference to use this latter choice whenever possible to avoid the interruption of protease inhibitor therapy.

e. *Extrapulmonary tuberculosis.* In adults, the pharmacotherapy of extrapulmonary tuberculosis does not differ from that of pulmonary tuberculosis.[47] In certain cases of tuberculous meningitis and pericarditis, the adjunctive use of corticosteroids may be advisable.[47]

4. **Surgical therapy.** The optimal management of a patient with tuberculosis will occasionally require the involvement of the surgical services. Surgical resection of involved lung tissue is playing an increasingly important role in the therapy of MDR-TB, particularly when the process is limited to a single segment or lobe.[62] Surgical therapy for the constrictive sequelae of tuberculous pericarditis and pleuritis, as well as for vertebral deformities associated with Pott's disease, may also play a critical role in the long-term quality of life of affected patients.[47] In any of these situations, a surgical consultant with experience in the management of these specific processes should be sought.

5. **Record keeping.** Because of the frequency of transfers between correctional facilities and the high rate of recidivism among inmates who are released to the community, the care and the records of any given patient with tuberculosis may be divided among numerous sites. Rational therapeutic decisions can be reached only when the assorted components of these fragmented medical histories are collected and organized by the current care provider. Often, the local department of health can provide useful information through its function as a central repository of information from many or all of these diverse sites. Frequently, a diligent search for old radiographic and mycobacteriologic information yield data that are invaluable in case management, and such investigative work is to be strongly encouraged. In our facility, we use an additional tool in the care of all but the most straightforward cases of tuberculosis. Figure 11-2 is a copy of the "Drug-O-Gram," which we complete as part of the patient's record. Most cases of tuberculosis can be summarized in graphic form through the use of such a flow sheet. The prominent role that physician error plays in the development of acquired drug resistance[63] should encourage the practice of maintaining a careful record reflecting smear, culture, and susceptibility results, start and stop dates of medications, and compliance. We find that incorporation of these data into one readable sheet in the patient's record minimizes the likelihood of improper therapeutic choices.

6. **Monitoring for toxicity.** Although the list of potential adverse reactions to the antituberculous medications is lengthy (see Table 11-1), antituberculous therapy, in general, has an exceptionally favorable safety profile when medications are used according to standard regimens and the patients are monitored for toxicity. A good toxicity monitoring strategy starts with an insistence on the thorough familiarity of all involved health care providers with the common adverse effects of the antimycobacterial agents. The evaluation of all physical complaints and laboratory abnormalities in recipients of these medications must include drug toxicity in the differential diagnosis. Directly observed therapy, in addition to all of its other benefits, allows the opportunity for a health care worker to see the patient at least twice weekly and to assess for drug toxicities. Although this clinical vigilance is really the mainstay of toxicity monitoring, in the correctional setting, we require baseline, then monthly, measurements of liver function (including transaminase, alkaline phosphatase, and total bilirubin levels), as well as monthly visual acuity and color vision testing for recipients of ethambutol. Performance of the testing and recording of results are the responsibility of the practitioner who supervises directly observed therapy in the facility, and these activities should be conducted together with the routine evaluation of response to therapy (i.e., review of symptoms and follow-up of spu-

Montefiore Rikers Island Health Services, CDU Tuberculosis DRUG-O-GRAM

NAME:		AKA:			
BOOK&CASE:		NYSID:		DOB:	
		HOSPITAL:		MR#:	
PPD status and date:	Anergy status:			TB Registry No.:	

Tuberculosis Diagnosed by: Culture, Clinical, Previously diagnosed untreated   Date(S) of diagnosis:

DATE									
SMEAR									
CULTURE									

WRITE SUSCEPTIBILITIES AND DOSES USED FOR RX (EG., INH Ⓢ 300MG)

MEDS/DATES									
INH									
RIFAMPIN									
ETHAMBUTOL									
PZA									
STREPTOMYCIN									
CYCLOSERINE									
OFLOXACIN									
ETHIONAMIDE									
PAS									
CAPREOMYCIN									
CIPROFLOXACIN									
KANAMYCIN									
AMIKACIN									
RIFABUTIN									
CLARITHROMYCIN									
CLOFAZIMINE									

Adverse Events/Comments:

Figure 11-2. Montefiore-Rikers Island Health Services Drug-O-Gram. Abbreviations: *AKA,* also known as; *NYSID,* New York State Identification Number; *DOB,* date of birth; *MR,* medical record number; *TB,* tuberculosis; *PPD,* Seibert purified protein derivative of tuberculin; *RX,* treatment; *INH,* isoniazid; *PZA,* pyrazinamide; *PAS,* para-aminosalicylate.

tum examinations and radiographic findings). Although American Thoracic Society recommendations do not insist on follow-up of routine laboratory and visual function testing for asymptomatic, healthy adults with normal baseline examinations,[47] we believe that it is a prudent measure in the incarcerated population, given the high rates of alcoholism, malnutrition, chronic viral hepatitis, and HIV infection (both recognized and unrecognized) that prevail. Patients with these conditions are likely to have more of an increased risk of adverse events than that of the general population.[22] For similar reasons, we routinely prescribe pyridoxine for all recipients of isoniazid in an effort to prevent the neurotoxicity associated with this agent. Other precautionary measures that are routinely taken in our institution are baseline thyroid function testing in recipients of ethionamide and para-aminosalicylic acid (both occasionally associated with thyroid toxicity) and serum drug level determinations in recipients of cycloserine.

When toxic reactions to antimycobacterial medications develop, they must be managed in a careful, thoughtful manner. An open discussion with the patient is often helpful, as a serious adverse event is likely to threaten the trust that the inmate has in the medical system and jeopardize future compliance. An asymptomatic, mild rise in transaminase levels (less than three times the upper limit of normal or the patient's baseline) in a recipient of isoniazid is a common occurrence that does not necessarily require drug discontinuation, although careful laboratory follow-up is indicated.[64] Similarly, a mild, asymptomatic, isolated rise in the serum bilirubin level is a common occurrence in recipients of rifampin and does not, by itself, mandate drug discontinuation.[64] Patients with symptomatic hepatic dysfunction or patients with greater rises in the levels measured by their liver function tests (particularly the transaminase levels) should discontinue isoniazid, rifampin, and pyrazinamide. Our strategy in such cases is to institute a "liver sparing regimen" consisting of ethambutol, streptomycin, and a quinolone, unless the isolate is known to be resistant to one or more of these agents. This regimen provides good short-term coverage for the tuberculous disease while the laboratory abnormalities return to pretreatment levels, and may be used as a curative regimen if continued for 18 months.[65] Once the liver function abnormalities return to or approach pretreatment levels, a cautious reintroduction of the putative offending agents may be attempted. Most patients can successfully complete a course of traditional therapy using this approach, but patients who experience significant hepatotoxicity on a second challenge should receive long-term management omitting the most likely culprits. It is worthwhile to try to incorporate rifampin into the final regimen in these patients because of its unrivaled curative efficacy and the rarity of hepatotoxicity specifically attributable to this agent.[64] In cases of ethambutol-induced ocular toxicity, as evidenced by deteriorating visual acuity or color vision, it is prudent to permanently discontinue this weak agent and substitute an alternative medication. All patients who experience significant toxicity from antituberculous therapy should be treated by a practitioner with experience in managing these problems.

7. *Therapeutic failure.* With the exception of patients with MDR-TB, virtually all individuals with tuberculosis are curable using the recommended regimens. When treatment fails (i.e., cultures do not revert to negative within 3 months or cultures that had reverted to negative again become positive), several explanations should be considered. First is the possibility of noncompliance. Any portion of the treatment program not administered under direct observation (e.g., before incarceration) must automatically be considered highly suspect. Surreptitious noncompliance is a real consideration that must be confronted when therapy is not successful, and scrupulous observation of medication ingestion with continuous monitoring for 1 hour after ingestion (to eliminate the possibility of self-induced vomiting) should be instituted. Serum drug levels may be helpful when noncompliance is being considered. Another possibility that should be entertained is the development of acquired drug resistance,[66] and susceptibility testing should be repeated on the most recent positive cultures. Patients with HIV infection and patients with disorders of the small intestine may be at increased risk for therapeutic failure because of a high rate of medication malabsorption, the presence of which may be confirmed by serum drug level monitoring after witnessed ingestion.[67] Patients who malabsorb medications selectively may have their regimens adjusted to include medications that are better absorbed from the gastrointestinal tract, they may have an injectable medication incorporated into their regimens, or perhaps the administered dosages of poorly absorbed medications can be titrated upward while serum levels are followed. Other possibilities that must occasionally be considered are exogenous reinfection with a resistant strain of tuberculosis,[68] erroneous classification of the original isolate as drug susceptible consequent to a laboratory error (including mislabeling, microbiological cross-contamination of specimens, or other errors), and occasional failures that result from the imperfect efficacy of any treatment regimen. Patients whose therapy has failed should receive consultation from a specialist with expertise in the care of difficult tuberculosis cases.

8. *Secondary prophylaxis for patients infected with HIV and tuberculosis.* A number of studies have reported alarmingly high relapse rates of tuberculosis in patients with HIV infection who have completed standard therapeutic regimens.[57, 58, 69, 70] The United States Public Health Service believes that these failures are largely attributable to the absence of rifampin from the regimens in some studies and from dubious compliance; therefore, it considers ongoing preventive therapy (i.e., "secondary prophylaxis") to be unnecessary.[71] We believe that the congregate housing and high prevalence of diagnosed and undiagnosed immunosuppressive states in correctional facilities greatly magnify the potential damage caused by relapsed cases; hence, we encourage the use of lifelong secondary prophylaxis (using the same regimens as for primary prophylaxis, which are outlined below) in all patients infected with HIV completing a course of therapy for tuberculosis in our facility.[59] This recommendation is in accordance with statements made by the British Thoracic Society[72] and by investigators in France.[73]

9. *Coordination for follow-up into the community.* The arrangement of reliable community follow-up for incarcerated patients is of particular importance for jail facilities in which lengths of stay tend to be short and dates of release are often not predictable. At a minimum, at the time that the patient is given a diagnosis, he should be reported to the local department of health, provide his address and that of a close relative or friend, and receive a printed listing of tuberculosis treatment centers in the community where he can be accepted in short order after release. To optimize successful link-up to the community, the New York City Department of Health uses a voucher system, which is a component of the discharge planning for most patients in our facility. It is helpful to have designated employees responsible for this particular aspect of patient care. Using this approach, Rikers Island and the New York City Department of Health have achieved a 92% rate of successful link-up after discharge with community-based organizations for patients with active tuberculosis.

INFECTION CONTROL

In addition to excellent direct clinical care, tuberculosis control requires the services of an infection control staff. The responsibilities of this staff should include the tracking of abnormal chest radiographs and mycobacteriology laboratory information, as well as the supervision of tuberculosis contact investigations. The strategy for contact investigations within the correctional facility should parallel the "expanding circle" strategy used in the community.[22] In a jail or prison in which congregate housing and community meals are the rule and hundreds or thousands of inmates may "share air" with a given patient with tuberculosis, it is reasonable to focus the initial investigation on a group of close contacts, such as inmates in the housing area in which the index patient slept. Depending on the results of the investigation, the circle of contacts may need to be expanded to a sector of the building and, ultimately, to the entire building. All of the identified contacts who are not already known to have tuberculin-positive status should have a repeat tuberculin skin test. Patients with tuberculin-positive status discovered during the contact investigation should have histories taken and undergo physical examinations and chest radiographs to exclude active tuberculosis. If active tuberculosis is not suspected after these tests, the patient should be offered prophylactic therapy. Those patients who have tuberculin-negative status should also be examined for symptoms and signs of active tuberculosis and undergo chest radiography for suggestive symptoms or signs. Patients with tuberculin-negative status who are not suspected of having active tuberculosis should, at a minimum, have a repeat tuberculin test done 10 weeks thereafter. Asymptomatic, immunocompetent individuals whose status remains tuberculin negative may be considered uninfected. Individuals whose tuberculin tests are positive for the first time should be examined for active tuberculosis and offered prophylactic therapy if there is no evidence of active disease.[22] A high prevalence of HIV limits the sensitivity of tuberculin skin test screening and may call for a more aggressive approach to contact investigations. In our facility, in which HIV infection rates approximate 15% of the inmate population and many of the HIV infections are unrecognized, all contacts without prior histories of tuberculin positivity undergo chest radiographs and are offered prophylactic therapy. Immunocompetent patients who do not convert to tuberculin positivity 10 weeks after exposure and have no other evidence of active tuberculosis may stop the prophylactic therapy. Contacts of contagious patients who are outside of the facility (e.g., family and friends) and community contacts of other sorts, such as courtroom personnel, should be traced and investigated by the local health department.[22]

A question that arises frequently is which index patients require the initiation of contact investigations. The decision is simple for patients at the extreme ends of the spectrum of tuberculosis contagiousness. A patient with smear-positive results with cavitary tuberculosis clearly requires an aggressive and thorough investigation of contacts, whereas a patient with smear-negative, culture-negative results with presumptive tuberculosis, or extrapulmonary tuberculosis, generally does not. Any patient with smear-positive results is, by definition, excreting the pathogen in high concentrations and should prompt an investigation,[22] but it is a common error to omit the procedure for individuals with smear-negative, culture-positive results. Although it is clear that individuals with smear-negative, culture-positive results are, on the average, much less infectious than individuals with smear-positive results, they are able to transmit disease,[74] and their contacts should be investigated.

Although the health care of medical providers and correctional workers is often the responsibility of different agencies than those responsible for the inmates, the air that all these individuals breathe does not make such distinctions. A comprehensive approach to tuberculosis management in the correctional setting must include not only the systematic and periodic screening of employees as a routine, but also additional testing in the event of contact investigations. Interagency cooperation in these endeavors is critical. High rates of tuberculin conversions among employees may indicate a failure of the existing screening systems or environmental controls. They may prompt a more aggressive examination of inmates in specific locations. Conversely, low rates of tuberculin conversions are a reassuring sign that tuberculosis control strategies are accomplishing their intended goals of decreasing tuberculosis transmission within the facility. It is helpful to assign the responsibility for collecting tuberculin conversion data for employees and inmates to a specific individual within the organization, so that important trends can be detected and tracked in a systematic fashion.

PREVENTIVE THERAPY

Isoniazid prophylactic therapy is an inaccurate term because patients receiving so-called primary prophylaxis have generally already been infected with the organism. However, the term is firmly entrenched in the medical literature and will be used interchangeably with the preferable "isoniazid preventive therapy" here. Isoniazid preventive therapy is indicated for individuals with the following characteristics[47]:

1. All those who have recently (within the past 2 years) had tuberculin skin test conversions.
2. All individuals younger than 35 years of age with positive tuberculin tests.
3. All patients with known HIV infections or with HIV risk behaviors and suspected HIV infection, with present or past histories of tuberculin positivity.
4. Close contacts of patients with active, infectious tuberculosis (these patients may not need to complete a full course of therapy; see previous section on Infection Control).
5. All patients with past or present tuberculin reactivity with any of the following medical conditions:
    a. Diabetes mellitus.
    b. Steroid therapy or other immunosuppressive therapy.
    c. Hematologic malignancy or a lymphoma.
    d. Injection drug use.
    e. End-stage renal disease.
    f. Medical conditions associated with substantial weight loss or malnutrition.
    g. History of gastrectomy.

These recommendations are not generally applicable if the patient has previously completed a course of preventive therapy. Standard therapeutic recommendations are listed in Table 11-3, as are references related to that information.[75–80] Patients should be monitored for symptoms and signs of medication toxicity at least monthly.

Table 11-3. Treatment recommendations for tuberculosis prevention

Clinical characteristics*	Medication regimen	Duration of therapy
Tuberculin positive, meeting criteria for preventive therapy (see Preventive Therapy section in text), immunocompetent, normal chest radiograph	Isoniazid 300 mg PO daily[†]	6–12 months
Tuberculin positive, abnormal chest radiograph consistent with inactive ("old") tuberculosis	Isoniazid 300 mg PO daily[†]	12 months
Tuberculin positive, HIV infected	Isoniazid 300 mg PO daily[†]	At least 12 months[‡]
Tuberculin negative, anergic, HIV infected, residing in an area with tuberculosis infection prevalence greater than 2%	Isoniazid 300 mg PO daily[†]	At least 12 months[‡]
Tuberculin positive, with infecting strain presumed to be resistant to isoniazid only	Rifampin 600 mg PO daily[§]	6–12 months[§]
Preventive therapy candidate or recipient who cannot tolerate isoniazid	Rifampin 600 mg PO daily[§]	6–12 months[§]
Tuberculin positive with infecting strain presumed to be multidrug-resistant	Unknown[‖]	Unknown[‖]

Note: This table is intended to provide an overview of standard preventive regimens for average-sized adults with normal renal and hepatic function. More detailed recommendations may be found in references 75 and 76.

*The infecting strain is assumed to be isoniazid susceptible unless otherwise stated. All candidates for preventive therapy should be free of clinical, radiologic, or laboratory evidence of active disease.

†An alternative treatment regimen using a dosage of 15 mg/kg (900 mg maximum) PO twice weekly is considered acceptable,[75, 76] although its efficacy has not been verified in clinical trials.

‡Although the American Thoracic Society[47] and the United States Public Health Service[22] recommend 12 months of total therapy, other experts recommend "at least" 12 months[77, 78] or even lifelong preventive[79] therapy in patients with HIV-related immunosuppression.

§Clinical experience with rifampin as preventive therapy is inadequate to make a definitive recommendation regarding dosage or duration. The use of rifampin as preventive therapy for patients exposed to isoniazid-resistant tuberculosis is widely endorsed.[47, 77]

‖The optimal management of a patient who is exposed to multidrug-resistant tuberculosis is not known. Provisional recommendations may be found in reference 80.

Abbreviation: *PO,* orally.

The use of isoniazid preventive therapy has been endorsed as one of the major strategies to control tuberculosis in the United States. Numerous large, well-designed studies have demonstrated the efficacy of isoniazid prophylaxis in preventing the development of active tuberculosis in those with tuberculin-positive skin tests with normal chest radiographs, those with tuberculin-positive skin tests with radiographs showing inactive disease, and patients with a past diagnosis of active tuberculosis who have received incomplete therapy but who are without evidence of active current disease.[81, 82] Isoniazid prophylaxis is effective in individuals with HIV infection,[83] and a cost–benefit analysis favors its use in individuals infected with HIV who have tuberculin-negative status, are anergic, and who reside in areas where the prevalence of *M. tuberculosis* infection exceeds 2% to 3%.[84] The United States Public Health Service recommends that all isoniazid prophylaxis be given under direct observation in the correctional setting.[22, 23] In contrast to the marked success of jails and prisons in instituting directly observed therapy programs for active tuberculosis, such that greater than 90% of facilities in the United States in 1994–1995 gave all courses of active tuberculosis treatment under direct observation, comparable successes have not been achieved in the area of

directly observed preventive therapy.[85] Much lower numbers of correctional institutions comply with the recommendation for directly observed preventive therapy, most likely as a consequence of the large number of inmates that would have to be serviced. Rates of reported tuberculin reactivity among inmates range from 14% to 25%.[22] The ratio of patients receiving isoniazid prophylaxis to those receiving therapy for active tuberculosis in our facility approximates 10:1. Many correctional health services do not have the resources available to maintain a program of direct observation for the large number of eligible inmates. Moreover, a careful analysis of directly observed preventive therapy with community follow-up in the Seattle jail system,[86] as well as similar pilot programs in New York City, have yielded very disappointing completion rates. In a study of isoniazid preventive therapy on Rikers Island in 1989, the best predictors of compliance were a higher level of knowledge of the disease process and an ease of access to medication within the facility.[87] Initiatives aimed at optimizing rates of completed prophylactic therapy in the future should investigate the use of more innovative approaches to inmate education and medication distribution, development of reliable tracking systems, and inducements for ongoing compliance.

DATA MANAGEMENT

The widespread availability of computer technology in the current era provides a very powerful tool for assisting in the many aspects of tuberculosis management. The ease of use and versatility of modern data management programs have rendered the traditional written logs of mycobacteriology laboratory results obsolete. At a minimum, every correctional facility that has tuberculosis cases should maintain a computer database that contains records of sputum samples sent, smear results received, culture results, and documentation of appropriate, timely notification of the responsible health care providers. More extensive computer networks may connect databases containing laboratory, radiologic, pharmacy, clinical, and department of health information. Such systems are not only useful from the standpoint of providing a more complete set of data on each individual patient, but also have tremendous utility in tracking patients in the aggregate and thus providing insight into epidemiologic trends within the institution. On Rikers Island, for example, our computer network produces (1) daily lists of abnormal chest radiograph results so that the infection control department can independently verify that appropriate actions have been taken within the facility, (2) monthly reports tracking the usage of antituberculous medications throughout the institution, and (3) periodic analyses of the laboratory database, which permits an evaluation of trends in the rates of culture-proven tuberculosis. The collection, centralization, and distribution of such data allow for an almost endless list of quality assurance projects and for clinical research suitable for broader review by the public health community. The development and maintenance of sophisticated computer systems require an investment of resources to both purchase the equipment and fund personnel with the necessary expertise in epidemiology, biostatistics, and data management to make these extraordinarily powerful tools perform to their maximum.

ETHICAL AND LEGAL ISSUES

The fascinating topic of the ethics and legalities of tuberculosis management in correctional facilities is far too broad for a thorough review in a chapter of this length. Current views and controversies are rooted in the histories of penal systems, epidemic diseases, prisoner experimentation, and forced quarantine. The often ignoble record of mankind in dealing with these major issues has resulted, in the United States, in a system that strives to respect the autonomy of the inmate while considering the responsibility of the government to protect the health and welfare of the populace. In the abstract, the ethical obligations of correctional health services with regard to tuberculosis are very clear. It is ethical to locate and attempt to cure all patients with active tuberculosis and also to protect uninfected inmates and correctional workers from infection with the pathogen. It is unethical to refuse to treat this curable yet lethal illness, and it is unethical to refrain from taking those measures that can prevent tuberculosis transmission to uninfected individuals. In practice, however, these unassailable principles become entangled in a web of complex realities. What about patients with active tuberculosis who refuse to take their medications? What about patients who are "coerced" into taking medications because it is their only route out of respiratory isolation, then life-threatening toxicities develop from the medications? What about patients with active tuberculosis who become suicidal when faced with the stress of isolation? What about patients who enjoy isolation and refuse to provide the follow-up sputum examinations or chest radiographs that will permit their release? Dilemmas such as these are familiar to care providers in jails and prisons in which tuberculosis is common. There is no neat formula that yields the correct solutions to these questions. Rather, difficult issues must be dealt with on a case-by-case basis, and care providers must be guided by the underlying principles that in the midst of an epidemic of airborne illness, uninfected individuals must be protected, to the extent that it is reasonably possible, from contracting disease and that contagious patients must receive humane and caring therapy, the goal of which is to effect a definitive cure. Most affected inmates are compliant and cooperative when these principles are explained in a calm and respectful manner. Inmates who do not cope well with the tuberculosis management program of a facility should be involved with mental health practitioners, and multidisciplinary case conferences including nursing, medical, and mental health staff may be particularly helpful. Involvement of clergy and medical ethicists may also be necessary in problematic cases. To the extent that tuberculosis screening, isolation, treatment, and potential exposure to infection may infringe on individual rights, many of these ethical issues have been discussed and adjudicated in the courtroom setting.

The most prominent legal decisions pertaining to tuberculosis revolve around an inmate's right to be protected from exposure to the disease, the right to community-standard medical treatment, and the right to refuse tuberculosis control measures. It is beyond the scope of this chapter to cite individual court cases, but the interested reader is referred to several recent detailed reviews.[21, 85, 88, 89] The United States courts have come out squarely behind prisoners' claims to the right of protection from tuberculosis acquisition by way of adequate tuberculosis screening and control–treatment programs within the facility. For pretrial detainees, who generally comprise the majority of jail inmates, the lack of adequate programs has been judged to constitute punishment without due process of the law. For sentenced inmates, the lack of such programs has been deemed a violation of the Eighth Amendmen, prohibiting cruel and unusual punishment because it represents "deliberate indifference to serious medical needs."[21] In contrast to the unequivocal legal requirement for tuberculosis screening and control within jails and prisons, the ability of the health care provider to force an inmate to accept tuberculosis treatment is much more limited. For the sake of the public health, the courts have given the legal authority to detain patients with contagious tuberculosis in suitable respiratory isolation facilities against their will, provided that "less restrictive" measures have been unsuccessful. In New York, the epicenter of the tuberculosis epidemic early in the 1990s, the commissioner of health was granted legal authority to forcibly detain noncompliant, contagious patients until a cure was achieved (prior regulations only allowed forcible detention until the patient was rendered noncontagious). The transfer of inmates with suspected tuberculosis, even against his will, to a respiratory isolation facility is a necessary component of the legally mandated tuberculosis control program and is justifiable in that there is generally no "less restrictive" measure available in correctional facilities to avoid the imminent threat of tuberculosis transmission. Although, in certain instances, the courts have infringed on the personal autonomy of mentally capable inmates by forcing them to receive medical interventions such as vaccination,[21] in the case of tuberculosis, legal decisions support the rights of individuals to refuse treatment. The courts have, however, judged mandatory tuberculosis screening program to be permissible and have allowed for disciplinary measures against inmates who refuse screening.[21, 79] As with all informed consent and refusal processes, the right of inmates to render decisions is dependent on their mental capacity to understand both the disease process and the potential consequences of their choices.

CONCLUSION

The important role of the correctional facility in the epidemiology of tuberculosis has been recognized for many decades, and interest in this aspect of correctional health care has been reignited by the recent tuberculosis resurgence. Practitioners who manage patients with tuberculosis in the community appreciate the extraordinary effort and diligence required to achieve every single cure. Those individuals who provide care to prisoners are faced with a multitude of even greater challenges, but at the same time they have a unique opportunity to detect, prevent, and cure the disease in a population of individuals who frequently have no other interaction with the medical system. The efforts of correctional health care providers in confronting these challenges have had a profound impact on the most recent tuberculosis epidemic in the United States, and their continued successes will be vital to tuberculosis control, both in and out of correctional facilities, in the years to come.

REFERENCES

1. Bellin EY, Fletcher DD, Safyer SM: Association of tuberculosis infection with increased time in or admission to the New York City jail system. *JAMA* 269:2228–2231, 1993.
2. Stead WW: Undetected tuberculosis in prison. *JAMA* 240:2544–2547, 1978.
3. History of the care of dependents—New York City, in Wright HC, McAneny G, Cromwell G (eds): *Report of the Committee on Inquiry into the Departments of Health, Charities, and Bellevue and Allied Hospitals.* New York, J.J. Little & Ives, 1913, pp 427–448.
4. Boyce LL (ed): *The Health Officers' Manual and Public Health Law of the State of New York.* Albany, NY, Matthew Bender, 1902, pp 159–160.
5. Abeles H, Feibes H, Mandel E, et al: The large city prison—a reservoir of tuberculosis. *Am Rev Respir Dis* 101:706–709, 1970.
6. Hutton MD, Cauthen GM, Bloch AB: Results of a 29-state survey of tuberculosis in nursing homes and correctional facilities. *Public Health Rep* 108:305–314, 1993.
7. Braun MM, Truman BI, Maguire B, et al: Increasing incidence of tuberculosis in a prison inmate population: Association with HIV infection. *JAMA* 261:393–397, 1989.
8. Centers for Disease Control: Tuberculosis morbidity—United States, 1994. *MMWR* 44:387–395, 1995.
9. New York City Department of Health: Health of the city: Focus on tuberculosis. 33, 1995.
10. Valway SE, Richards SB, Kovacovich J, et al: Outbreak of multi–drug-resistant tuberculosis in a New York State prison, 1991. *Am J Epidemiol* 140:113–122, 1994.
11. Bergmire-Sweat D, Barnett B, Taylor J, et al: Tuberculosis outbreak in a Texas prison. Presented at the 35th Interscience Conference on Antimicrobial Agents and Chemotherapy, San Francisco, September 17–20, 1995, K122.
12. Centers for Disease Control: Tuberculosis transmission in a state correctional institution—California, 1990–1991. *MMWR* 41:927–929, 1992.
13. Centers for Disease Control: Probable transmission of multidrug-resistant tuberculosis in a correctional facility—California. *MMWR* 42:48–51, 1993.
14. Sanchez VM, Alvarez-Guisasola F, Cayla JA, et al: Predictive factors of *Mycobacterium tuberculosis* infection and pulmonary tuberculosis in prisoners. *Int J Epidemiol* 24:630–636, 1995.
15. Monno L, Angarano G, Carbonara S, et al: Current problems in treating tuberculosis in Italian HIV-infected patients. *Tubercle Lung Dis* 74:280–287, 1993.
16. Mundy LM, Lynch MM, Crowley BD, et al: Concomitant HIV and mycobacterial infection in Ireland, 1987–92. *Int J STD AIDS* 5:436–441, 1994.
17. Drobniewski F, Tayler E, Ignatenko N, et al: Tuberculosis in Siberia: 1. An epidemiological and microbiological assessment. *Tubercle Lung Dis* 77:199–206, 1996.
18. Auregan G, Rakotomanana F, Ratsitorahina M, et al: Tuberculosis in the prison milieu at Antananarivo from 1990 to 1993. *Arch Institut Pasteur de Madagascar* 62:18–23. 1995.
19. Garay SM: Pulmonary tuberculosis, in Rom WN, Garay SM (eds): *Tuberculosis,* ed 1. New York, Little, Brown and Company, 1996, pp 373–412.
20. Segal-Maurer S, Kalkut GE: Environmental control of tuberculosis: Continuing controversy. *Clin Infect Dis* 19:299–308, 1994.
21. Greifinger RB, Heywood NJ, Glaser JB: Tuberculosis in prison: Balancing justice and public health. *J Law Med Ethics* 21:332–341, 1993.
22. Centers for Disease Control: Prevention and control of tuberculosis in correctional facilities. *MMWR* 45(RR-8):1–27, 1996.
23. *Controlling TB in Correctional Facilities.* Rockville, Md, U.S. Department of Health and Human Services, 1995, pp 1–58.
24. Spencer SS, Morton AR: Tuberculosis surveillance in a state prison system. *Am J Public Health* 79:507–509, 1989.
25. Johnsen C: Evaluation of two-step tuberculin testing in a Massachusetts correctional facility. *Am J Infect Control* 23:209–212, 1995.
26. Puisis M, Feinglass J, Lidow E, et al: Radiographic screening for

tuberculosis in a large urban county jail. *Public Health Rep* 111:330–334, 1996.

27. Layton M, Frieden T, Henning K: Screening of inmates for tuberculosis by chest X-rays. Presented at the 34th Interscience Conference on Antimicrobial Agents and Chemotherapy, Orlando, Fla, October 4–7, 1994, J113.

28. Pedro-Botet J, Gutierrez J, Miralles R, et al: Pulmonary tuberculosis in HIV-infected patients with normal chest radiographs. *AIDS* 6:91–93, 1992.

29. Daley CL, Small PM, Schecter GF, et al: An outbreak of tuberculosis with accelerated progression among persons infected with the human immunodeficiency virus. *N Engl J Med* 326:231–235, 1992.

30. Jarvis WR, Bolyard EA, Bozzi CJ, et al: Respirators, recommendations, and regulations: The controversy surrounding protection of health care workers from tuberculosis. *Ann Intern Med* 122:142–146, 1995.

31. Centers for Disease Control: Guidelines for preventing the transmission of *Mycobacterium tuberculosis* in health-care facilities, 1994. *MMWR* 43(RR-13):1–132, 1994.

32. Pitchenik AE, Ganjei P, Torres A, et al: Sputum examination for the diagnosis of *Pneumocystis carinii* pneumonia in the acquired immunodeficiency syndrome. *Am Rev Respir Dis* 133:226–229, 1986.

33. Shinnick TM, Good RC: Diagnostic mycobacteriology laboratory practices. *Clin Infect Dis* 21:291–299, 1995.

34. Alvarez S, McCabe WR: Extrapulmonary tuberculosis revisited: A review of experience at Boston City and other hospitals. *Medicine* 63:25–55, 1984.

35. Dalovisio JR, Montenegro-James S, Kemmerly SA, et al: Comparison of the amplified *Mycobacterium tuberculosis* (MTB) direct test, Amplicor MTB PCR, and IS6110-PCR for detection of MTB in respiratory specimens. *Clin Infect Dis* 23:1099–1106, 1996.

36. Centers for Disease Control: Initial therapy for tuberculosis in the era of multidrug resistance. *MMWR* 42:1–8, 1993.

37. Witebsky FG, Conville PS: The laboratory diagnosis of mycobacterial diseases. *Infect Dis Clin N Amer* 7:359–376, 1993.

38. Heifets LB: Drug susceptibility testing. *Clin Lab Med* 16:641–656, 1996.

39. Santin M, Podzamczer D, Ricart I, et al: Utility of the gallium-67 citrate scan for the early diagnosis of tuberculosis in patients infected with the human immunodeficiency virus. *Clin Infect Dis* 20:652–656, 1995.

40. Pastores SM, Naidich DP, Aranda CP, et al: Intrathoracic adenopathy associated with pulmonary tuberculosis in patients with human immunodeficiency virus infection. *Chest* 103:1433–1437, 1993.

41. Brudney K, Dobkin J: Resurgent tuberculosis in New York City. *Am Rev Respir Dis* 144:745–749, 1991.

42. Frieden TR, Fujiwara PI, Washko RM, et al: Tuberculosis in New York City—Turning the tide. *N Engl J Med* 333:229–233, 1995.

43. Weis SE, Slocum PC, Blais FX, et al: The effect of directly observed therapy on the rates of drug resistance and relapse in tuberculosis. *N Engl J Med* 330:1179–1184, 1994.

44. Peloquin CA: Therapeutic drug monitoring of the antimycobacterial drugs. *Clin Lab Med* 16:717–729, 1996.

45. Holdiness MR: Clinical pharmacokinetics of the antituberculosis drugs. *Clin Pharmacokinet* 9:511–544, 1984.

46. Sanford JP, Gilbert DN, Sande MA: *Guide to Antimicrobial Therapy,* ed 26. Dallas, Antimicrobial Therapy, 1996.

47. American Thoracic Society: Treatment of tuberculosis and tuberculosis infection in adults and children. *Am J Respir Crit Care Med* 149:1359–1374, 1994.

48. *Treating Tuberculosis: A Clinical Guide.* Rockville, Md, U.S. Department of Health and Human Services, 1994.

49. Iseman MD: Treatment of multidrug-resistant tuberculosis. *N Engl J Med* 329:784–791, 1993.

50. Cohn DL: Treatment of multidrug-resistant tuberculosis. *J Hosp Infect* 30:322–328, 1995.

51. Yew WW, Chau CH: Drug-resistant tuberculosis in the 1990s. *Eur Respir J* 8:1184–1192, 1995.

52. Brausch LM, Bass JB: The treatment of tuberculosis. *Med Clin N Amer* 77:1277–1288, 1993.

53. Good JT, Iseman MD, Davidson PT, et al: Tuberculosis in association with pregnancy. *Am J Obstet Gynecol* 140:492–498, 1981.

54. Franks AL, Binkin NJ, Snider DE, et al: Isoniazid hepatitis among pregnant and postpartum Hispanic patients. *Public Health Rep* 104:151–155, 1989.

55. *1994 Update: HIV/AIDS and STDs in Correctional Facilities.* Washington, D.C., U.S. Department of Justice, 1995.

56. Barnes PF, Bloch AB, Davidson PT, et al: Tuberculosis in patients with human immunodeficiency virus infection. *N Engl J Med* 324:1644–1650, 1991.

57. Pulido F, Pena JM, Rubio R, et al: Relapse of tuberculosis after treatment in human immunodeficiency virus-infected patients. *Arch Intern Med* 157:227–232, 1997.

58. Perriens JH, St. Louis ME, Mukadi YB, et al: Pulmonary tuberculosis in HIV-infected patients in Zaire. *N Engl J Med* 332:779–784, 1995.

59. Shuter J, Bellin E: Secondary prophylaxis for tuberculosis in patients infected with human immunodeficiency virus. *Clin Infect Dis* 22:398–399, 1996.

60. Centers for Disease Control: Clinical update: Impact of HIV protease inhibitors on the treatment of HIV-infected tuberculosis patients with rifampin. *MMWR* 45:921–925, 1996.

61. Gonzalez-Montaner LJ, Natal S, Yongchaiyud P, et al: Rifabutin for the treatment of newly-diagnosed pulmonary tuberculosis: A multinational, randomized, comparative study versus rifampicin. *Tubercle Lung Dis* 75:341–347, 1994.

62. Pomerantz M, Brown J: The surgical management of tuberculosis. *Semin Thorac Cardiovasc Surg* 7:108–111, 1995.

63. Mahmoudi A, Iseman MD: Pitfalls in the care of patients with tuberculosis. JAMA 270:65–68, 1993.

64. Dossing M, Wilcke JTR, Askgaard DS, et al: Liver injury during antituberculosis treatment: An 11-year study. *Tubercle Lung Dis* 77:335–340, 1996.

65. Salomon N, Goldstein S, Perlman DC, et al: Utility of an ofloxacin-containing regimen in the management of hepatotoxicity in HIV-infected persons with tuberculosis. Presented at the IX International Conference on AIDS. Berlin, June 6–11, 1993, PO-B07-1242.

66. Bradford WZ, Martin JN, Reingold AL, et al: The changing epidemiology of acquired drug-resistant tuberculosis in San Francisco, USA. *Lancet* 348:928–931, 1996.

67. Peloquin C, Nitta A, Burman W, et al: Incidence of low tuberculosis drug concentrations in AIDS patients. Presented at the 34th Interscience Conference on Antimicrobial Agents and Chemotherapy, Orlando, Fla, October 4–7, 1994, M9.

68. Small PM, Shafer RW, Hopewell PC, et al: Exogenous reinfection with multidrug-resistant *Mycobacterium tuberculosis* in patients with advanced HIV infection. *N Engl J Med* 328:1137–1144, 1993.

69. Hawken M, Nunn P, Gathua S, et al: Increased recurrence of tuberculosis in HIV-1-infected patients in Kenya. *Lancet* 342:332–337, 1993.

70. Beaulieu P, Molina JM, Rouveau M, et al: Role de l'infection par le virus de l'immunodeficience humaine chez 67 patients atteints de tuberculose. *Ann Med Interne (Paris)* 144:323–328, 1993.

71. Castro KG, Blinkhorn RJ, Ellner JJ, et al: Reply to 'Secondary prophylaxis for tuberculosis in patients infected with human immunodeficiency virus.' *Clin Infect Dis* 22:399–400, 1996.

72. British Thoracic Society: Education and debate: Guidelines on the management of tuberculosis and HIV infection in the United Kingdom. *BMJ* 304:1231–1233, 1992.

73. Rogeaux O, Bricaire F, Gentilini M: Tuberculose et infection par le virus de l'immunodeficience humaine (VIH). *Rev Med Interne* 14:715–722, 1993.

74. Hertzberg G: *The Infectiousness of Human Tuberculosis: An*

Epidemiological Investigation. Copenhagen, Munksgaard, 1957, pp 57–89.

75. Centers for Disease Control: The use of preventive therapy for tuberculosis infection in the United States. *MMWR* 39(RR-8):9–12, 1990.

76. New York City Department of Health: Preventive treatment for tuberculosis. *City Health Information* 14:1-4, 1995.

77. *Handbook of Antimicrobial Therapy.* New York, Medical Letter, 1996, pp 63–65.

78. Pape JW, Jean SS, Ho JL, et al: Effect of isoniazid prophylaxis on incidence of active tuberculosis and progression of HIV infection. *Lancet* 342:268–272, 1993.

79. DiPerri G, Micciolo R, Vento S, et al: Risk of reactivation of tuberculosis in the course of human immunodeficiency virus infection. *Eur J Med* 2:264–268, 1993.

80. Centers for Disease Control: Management of persons exposed to multidrug-resistant tuberculosis. *MMWR* 41(RR-11):61–70, 1992.

81. Ferebee SH: Controlled chemoprophylaxis trials in tuberculosis: A general review. *Adv Tuberc Res* 17:28–106, 1970.

82. Falk A, Fuchs GF: Prophylaxis with isoniazid in inactive tuberculosis. *Chest* 73:44–48, 1978.

83. Selwyn PA, Sckell BM, Alcabes P, et al: High risk of active tuberculosis in HIV-infected drug users with cutaneous anergy. *JAMA* 268:504–509, 1992.

84. Rose DN, Schechter CB, Sacks HS: Preventive medicine for HIV-infected patients. *J Gen Intern Med* 7:589–594, 1992.

85. National Institute of Justice: *Tuberculosis in Correctional Facilities 1994–95.* Washington, D.C., U.S. Department of Justice, July 1996, pp 1–12.

86. Nolan CM, Roll L, Goldberg SV, et al: Directly observed isoniazid preventive therapy for released jail inmates. *Am J Respir Crit Care Med* 155:583–586, 1997.

87. Alcabes P, Vossenas P, Cohen R, et al: Compliance with isoniazid prophylaxis in jail. *Am Rev Respir Dis* 140:1194–1197, 1989.

88. Bayer R, Dupuis LJ: Ethical and legal issues in tuberculosis control, in Rom WN, Garay SM (eds): *Tuberculosis,* ed 1. New York, Little, Brown and Company, 1996, pp 965–972.

89. Safyer SM, Richmond L, Bellin E, et al: Tuberculosis in correctional facilities: The tuberculosis control program of the Montefiore Medical Center Rikers Island Health Services. *J Law Med Ethics* 21:342–351, 1993.

12

Overview of Sexually Transmitted Diseases

Michael Puisis, D.O.

William C. Levine, M.D.

Kristen J. Mertz, M.D.

An estimated 12 million new cases of sexually transmitted diseases (STDs) occur each year in the United States.[1] More chlamydial and gonococcal infections are reported than any other notifiable disease in the country.[2] Health consequences of STDs include mild acute illnesses and serious long-term sequelae, including cancer, infertility, ectopic pregnancy, and chronic pelvic pain. In addition, many STDs have been shown to facilitate transmission of HIV.[3, 4] Women are more adversely affected than men because of an increased biologic susceptibility to infection, higher likelihood of asymptomatic infection leading to delay in detection and treatment, and the serious nature of medical sequelae. Women may also transmit infections to their newborns, sometimes resulting in central nervous system damage and death to the newborn.

The burden of disease for chlamydia and gonorrhea in the U.S. is highest for women aged 15 to 19 years.[5, 6] The majority of adolescents in juvenile detention facilities are in this age group, and many have unprotected sex and are,

therefore, at high risk of chlamydial and gonococcal infection. Rates of syphilis, however, are higher in men and women older than 20 years[6]; therefore, adult facilities are more likely than juvenile facilities to admit persons at risk for syphilis. Because many detainees have been arrested for drug use or prostitution, both of which have been associated with syphilis, high rates of syphilis are not unexpected.

The Institute of Medicine recently called for expanded STD services for disadvantaged populations.[1] The Institute recommended that detention facilities provide comprehensive STD-related services, including counseling and education, screening, diagnosis and treatment, partner notification and treatment, as well as methods for reducing unprotected sex and drug use. Correctional settings have the opportunity to provide such services because they serve large populations of high-risk individuals.

Standards for medical care in correctional facilities include laboratory or diagnostic tests to detect communicable diseases, including STDs, as part of the health assessment within 14 days of admission in jails[7] and within 7 days in prisons and juvenile facilities.[8, 9] Not all facilities, however, routinely screen for STDs. In many facilities, the majority of inmates are released before getting a complete medical evaluation and, therefore, are not tested for STDs.

Most facilities performing STD tests use results to treat infections but not to assess the burden of disease. Thus, the true prevalence of STDs in correctional facilities has not been well-described. Several ad hoc studies have shown a high prevalence of various bacterial STDs in people entering correctional facilities, but these represent only a few cities. Almost no information exists on the extent of viral STDs.

In general, syphilis is more prevalent in women than men, and more prevalent in persons admitted to jails than juvenile facilities. The highest prevalence has been reported from New York City, where 26% of women tested upon admission had indications for syphilis treatment.[10] Lower rates of 2% to 10% have been reported for men entering jails.[11, 12] Studies in juvenile facilities show syphilis prevalence of less than 1% in boys[13, 14] and 0% to 2.5%[14, 15] in girls.

Gonococcal and chlamydial infection appear to be common in adolescents admitted to juvenile facilities. Reported prevalence of chlamydia ranges from 14% to 20% in female adolescent detainees[15, 16] and 7% to 12% in male adolescent detainees.[13, 17, 18] Prevalence of gonorrhea has been reported as high as 18% in girls[14, 15] and from 1% to 5% in boys entering juvenile facilities.[13, 14, 17, 18] For adult women entering jails, a study in New York City reported a prevalence of 27% for chlamydia and 8% for gonorrhea.[19] No information is available for men. For inmates admitted to state prisons, reported morbidity is considerably lower: of 101 women entering state prisons in Pennsylvania, two (2%) had positive test results for gonorrhea and five (5%) had positive tests results for chlamydia,[20] and of 2,598 men admitted to the state correctional system in Maryland, 28 (1%) had positive test results for gonorrhea.[21]

Very little information exists about the relationship between arrest code and disease. In Fulton County, Georgia, a study showed a very high prevalence of gonorrhea in women (20%) and men (15%) arrested for sexual offenses.[22] In Connecticut, women arrested for drug possession and prostitution had a high prevalence of syphilis, 7% and 14%, respectively.[23] In both of these settings, however, the prevalence in women arrested for other crimes was not reported. In Los Angeles, there was no significant association between booking charge and syphilis infection in men.[11]

The incidence of STDs acquired within correctional facilities is unknown. Cases of gonorrhea contracted during detention have been reported,[24] but most information about cases contracted while in facilities has not been published. Although sexual activity is illegal in correctional facilities

in the United States, it does occur, and transmission of STDs is possible.

REASONS TO SCREEN FOR STDS IN CORRECTIONAL FACILITIES

Considering the high prevalence of STDs in persons admitted to correctional facilities, testing and treatment is important for protecting the inmates, their babies, their sexual partners, and the rest of the community. Detection and treatment of infection can prevent long-term sequelae, which are harmful for the patient and costly to society. Given the asymptomatic nature of many infections, especially in women, many persons will not seek care for STDs. In addition, many incarcerated persons do not have a regular source of medical care in the community; the correctional facility may be the only point at which they can be tested and treated.

Many inmates who are infected at the time of admission may transmit disease to others in the community upon release if not treated. Identification and treatment of cases in detention facilities should prevent future transmission of STDs. Identifying inmates with STDs should also help to identify cases in the community if infected inmates are interviewed about their recent sex partners and these partners are evaluated.

Women infected with syphilis, chlamydia, or gonorrhea can transmit infection to their newborns. Women entering correctional facilities often have a high rate of pregnancy. Prompt detection and treatment is important in protecting infants from adverse consequences.

Persons entering correctional facilities are also at high risk for HIV. Presence of other STDs can facilitate transmission of HIV, and STD control has been shown to be effective in reducing HIV transmission.[25] Effective control programs in correctional facilities, including screening and improved clinical management, may reduce transmission of HIV in this population.

THE CORRECTIONAL ENVIRONMENT AND STD SCREENING

The correctional environment presents many obstacles to screening for STDs. Obviously, the primary purpose of correctional facilities is incarceration, and the first obstacle to screening is the viewpoint that screening for STDs is unnecessary. The responsibility of the correctional authority to screen for certain communicable diseases, such as tuberculosis, is more easily understood than the necessity of screening for STDs. Some local laws require screening for STDs, especially syphilis, as part of intake screening. In local jurisdictions where the law does not require screening, correctional officials may be reluctant to participate in such a program. In areas of high incidence and prevalence of STDs, however, correctional officials have the responsibility and opportunity to contribute to reducing the spread of STDs.

Screening for STDs is different in jails and prisons. In prisons, the rate of admission is generally low compared to that in jails. The rate of discharge from jails is approximately 20 times the rate of discharge from prisons. Prison intake areas are often housing units where inmates reside for days to weeks until all intake screening is accomplished. This permits most medical evaluations to be concluded, and allows sufficient time to provide treatment and contact tracing for those inmates with STDs.

The situation is different in jails where large numbers of inmates are admitted. Several hundred inmates may be admitted each day to large urban jails. Because of the large number of daily intakes and the short length of stay, there is usually not a single designated housing area for new inmates. The abbreviated nature of the jail intake process makes complete assessment and treatment more difficult. It is often necessary to recall patients for treatment after initial intake screening. This creates a burden for correctional staff, who must escort patients for appointments, and causes scheduling conflicts with attorneys and court appointments. Health care staff and public health personnel have to be creative in adapting to the environment; success in screening for STDs depends on not disrupting the correctional intake process.

Although each local jail may have its own particular method for processing inmates through its intake area, there are some general similarities. Inmates are asked about demographic information, prior arrests, etc. Fingerprints, photographs, identification cards, and housing assignments are all made in a predefined sequence. Successful STD screening requires integration into the intake process; however, it is often difficult for medical staff to adjust to these assembly line arrangements. For example, drawing blood for syphilis or performing urethral or cervical swabs for chlamydia or gonorrhea should be steps in the intake process, similar to fingerprinting, albeit with appropriate privacy safeguards. Unless public health or medical staff have had input into the design of the intake facility, there may not be adequate physical space to provide privacy for examinations. Although phlebotomy for syphilis serologic testing may be performed in an open arrangement, urethral or cervical swab examinations must be performed in a private setting. Acquiring space with the requisite privacy often requires careful negotiation with correctional officials.

Screening for STDs involves multiple activities, including a screening test, interpretation of test results, follow-up of positive test results with an interview, treatment, contact tracing, and post-treatment testing. In many jails, only the screening test is performed in the intake area.

UNIVERSAL SCREENING VS. SELECTIVE SCREENING

When correctional staff and monetary resources are adequate, universal screening for STDs is recommended in areas of high prevalence. Universal screening (that is,

screening of all incoming inmates) is the norm in many state prison systems. It is important, however, to assess results in terms of the prevalence of infection. In 1993 and 1994 in South Dakota, the 84 women screened for syphilis had a prevalence of 0.0%, whereas in Connecticut the 3,412 women screened had a syphilis prevalence of 17%.

In jails, universal screening is made more complicated by the chaotic nature of the intake process, which usually occurs in a half day. Nevertheless, universal screening programs in jails have been successful. Universal screening at Cook County Jail in 1993 and 1994 for 61,079 men and 8,416 women yielded syphilis rates of 2.7% for men and 10.4% for women. This program identifies as many as 16% of contagious syphilis cases in the City of Chicago (Dr. Puisis, unpublished data from Cook County Jail). Other cities conducting universal syphilis screening in jails have also reported that a large percentage of syphilis cases are identified in jails. The public health value of such programs is enormous and cannot be underestimated in the overall public health effort against STDs.

Universal screening for gonorrhea and chlamydia is seldom done in either prisons or jails. The reasons for this are not entirely established. However, when universal screening is performed in high prevalence areas, large numbers of individuals may be successfully diagnosed and treated. At Cook County Jail in Chicago, only women are universally screened for chlamydia. In 1995, 10,949 women were screened, 468 (4.5%) had positive test results, and 325 were treated before discharge from the facility. At the same facility, gonorrhea rates in a universal screening program were no less significant. In 1995, 70,692 men and 10,494 women were screened; 1,055 (1.5%) men had positive test results and 455 (4.3%) women had positive test results. Almost 70% of these individuals were treated prior to discharge from the facility (unpublished data, Dr. Puisis, Cook County Jail). In situations where universal screening may not be possible or necessary, or where resources are not available, selective screening is an option. Inmates determine to be at high risk* for STDs can be identified and tested during the intake screening process. Women are often targeted for syphilis screening because of the potential for congenital syphilis and because of higher rates of infection in female inmates.

LINKS TO LOCAL HEALTH DEPARTMENTS

In many successful STD treatment programs, particularly in jails, a crucial element is a cooperative alliance with the local health department. In most jurisdictions, medical providers, including correctional facilities, must report STD cases to the local board of health. When large numbers of inmates are screened for syphilis, it is advantageous for the board of health to provide linkage to on-line syphilis

---

*Through an epidemiologic analysis of demographic and risk characteristics.

registries. In larger facilities, it may also be cost effective for board of health personnel to be stationed on-site to provide early contact tracing interviews, HIV counseling, testing services for patients with STDs, and assistance with data collection. Medical staff at the local board of health or the Centers for Disease Control and Prevention (CDC) can also assist with treatment issues. The CDC publishes guidelines on the treatment of STDs.[26]

THE USE OF DIAGNOSTIC TESTS FOR STD SCREENING

In screening for STDs in correctional facilities, particularly in jails, it is preferable to obtain test results rapidly. On-site rapid tests may be less sensitive or specific than tests performed at an outside laboratory. However, the sooner a test result is available, the greater the chance that a patient in a detention facility can be treated before discharge.

Rapid testing is possible for syphilis, using the RPR card test. One of the most established examples of immediate testing and treatment is the "STAT RPR" program for women inmates in the New York City jail. In this program, syphilis tests are performed in the intake area and immediate access to a computerized local syphilis registry permits evaluation of prior treatment. Using established protocols, treatment decisions are made before the conclusion of medical intake screening. On-site testing increased syphilis treatment rates for women admitted to the New York City jail from 7% to 84%.[10] Of eight infants born to women treated at the jail while pregnant, seven did not need treatment for congenital syphilis because of adequate treatment of the mother.[10]

The leukocyte esterase test (LET) is a rapid dipstick test that can be performed on the first 15 to 20 mL of urine and can detect the presence of white blood cells and, thus, indicate presence of gonorrhea or chlamydia in men. These tests have been best evaluated in adolescent males, in whom sensitivity for gonococcal or chlamydial urethritis ranges from 50% to 100%, and specificity, from 80% to 100%. In many settings, men with positive LET results are treated presumptively, but specific tests for gonorrhea or chlamydia are then performed to confirm the diagnosis for purposes of reporting results to the health department, and for facilitating notification of sex partners.

Recently, rapid methods for chlamydia testing on endocervical and urethral specimens have become available; however, the sensitivity and specificity of these tests are still under evaluation. Highly sensitive and specific tests on urine now make it possible to screen women for gonorrhea and chlamydia without performing a pelvic examination and can, therefore, facilitate screening and treatment in those settings where complete examinations on female patients cannot be performed. However, these are not rapid tests, and their cost is relatively high. Until the cost of these tests declines, screening of women with these tests in jail settings may be limited.

GENERAL CONSIDERATIONS IN TREATMENT OF STDs IN CORRECTIONAL FACILITIES

When designing protocols for treatment of STDs in correctional settings, consideration should be given to STD prevalence in the population, the usual length of stay of most patients, and the possibility for completing a multi-day regimen after the initial visit. In most settings, immediate, directly observed, presumptive therapy should be provided. Medications should be available on-site, unless all patients are routinely brought to another site (e.g., a public STD clinic) for treatment. However, presumptive therapy should not preclude use of diagnostic tests, which are important for ensuring proper therapy, for reporting infections to the health department, and for management of sex partners.

MANAGEMENT OF COMMON STD SYNDROMES
Genital Ulcer Disease

In the U.S., the most common causes of genital ulcers in men and women are genital herpes simplex virus (HSV) infection, primary syphilis, and chancroid. Although the presence of vesicles is typical of genital HSV infection, even the most experienced clinicians may not be able to distinguish ulcers due to other causes. Thus, it is particularly important in most correctional facilities, where rapid and accurate diagnostic testing of ulcer specimens is unavailable, to treat patients presumptively for syphilis, and, in communities where chancroid incidence is notable, for this disease as well. In general, presumptive treatment for syphilis (and possibly chancroid) should be provided even when on-site, stat RPR test results are available, regardless of test results. The RPR test result is negative in 20% to 30% of cases of early syphilis, and patients with chancroid may have a reactive syphilis serologic test from latent or previously treated disease. All patients with genital ulcers should be offered testing for HIV infection. If the ulcer has not healed within 7 days of treatment, the patient should be re-evaluated and, if necessary, referred to a specialized facility. Patients with herpes simplex virus infection should be treated in the case of a severe, first episode, or if necessary, with chronic suppressive therapy. Patients infected with HIV may be particularly prone to severe, recurrent genital HSV infection.

Urethral Discharge

Men presenting with signs or symptoms of urethral discharge (or who have a positive LET result) should be presumed to have gonococcal or non-gonococcal urethritis; the most common cause of non-gonococcal urethritis is *Chlamydia trachomatis*, with smaller proportions due to *Ureaplasma urealyticum* and *Trichomonas vaginalis*. Although gonococcal urethritis is more often purulent than non-gonococcal urethritis, this distinction is not highly reliable. Ideally, patients with urethral discharge should have diagnostic tests for *Neisseria gonorrhoeae* (gram stain, culture, or non-culture test) and *C. trachomatis* infection. In settings where testing is not provided, and patients cannot be referred for optimal management, patients with evidence of urethral discharge should be treated presumptively with regimens that are recommended for both uncomplicated gonococcal and chlamydial infections.

Vaginal Discharge

All women with symptoms of vaginal discharge (discharge, foul odor, pruritus, dysuria) should undergo a pelvic examination by an experienced clinician, either on-site or by referral. Common infectious causes of vaginal discharge are bacterial vaginosis, vulvovaginal candidiasis, and trichomoniasis. Severe gonococcal, chlamydial, or herpetic infection may also cause discharge symptoms. Although the common causes of vaginal discharge have typical presentations that may serve to differentiate them, in most cases reliable diagnosis requires microscopic examination of secretions collected from the posterior fornix, swabbed onto two microscope slides. Clue cells (typical of bacterial vaginosis) and motile trichomonads may be found after adding one or two drops of 0.9% saline to one slide, and yeast or pseudohyphae by adding 10% potassium-hydroxide solution to the second slide. Patients with vaginal discharge should also be examined for the presence of cervical inflammation, and tested for gonorrhea and chlamydia, especially if they have an STD risk factor. Bacterial vaginosis can be treated using oral metronidazole, vaginal metronidazole, or clindamycin preparations; vulvovaginal candidiasis with many topical antifungal regimens, and by oral fluconazole; and trichomoniasis with oral metronidazole.

Pelvic Inflammatory Disease

Female patients who present with a complaint of lower abdominal pain should be suspected of having pelvic inflammatory disease (PID) if they have lower abdominal tenderness, adnexal tenderness, and cervical motion tenderness, if other causes have been excluded. Severity of tubal inflammation, scarring, and other sequelae (e.g., infertility, ectopic pregnancy, chronic pelvic pain) correlates poorly with severity of acute symptoms. All patients with suspected PID should be tested for chlamydia and gonorrhea, and therapy instituted immediately with an appropriate PID regimen; adequate therapy requires treatment of gonorrhea, chlamydia, and anaerobic bacteria. Many patients with suspected PID require further diagnostic tests and should be hospitalized, particularly when the diagnosis is uncertain, signs and symptoms are severe, or the patient cannot tolerate oral therapy.

Proctitis, Proctocolitis, and Enteritis

Acute proctitis can result from sexually transmitted pathogens through unprotected anal intercourse. The most common cause is herpes simplex virus; however, proctitis and proctocolitis may also be caused by gonorrhea or chlamydia; when ulcers are present, syphilis and chancroid should also be considered. Patients with herpetic disease may benefit from antiviral therapy for HSV infection; when purulent discharge is present or leukocytes are seen on a gram-stained smear, patients may be treated presumptively for gonococcal and chlamydial infection, pending results of further laboratory tests.

Sexually transmitted enteritis or proctocolitis may result from infection with *Entamoeba histolytica*, or *Shigella sp.* Opportunistic causes of enteritis (cytomegalovirus, mycobacterium avium intracellulare, salmonella, cryptosporidia, microsporidia, isospora) should be considered in HIV-infected patients who are immunocompromised.

Patients with sexually transmitted enteric infections (and, thus, with evidence of unprotected anal intercourse) may be at particularly high risk for HIV infection; they should be counseled and offered testing for syphilis and HIV.

MANAGEMENT OF PATIENTS WITH POSITIVE SCREENING TEST RESULTS (Table 12-1)
Syphilis

Treatment for syphilis should be based on stage of the disease. Those with primary, secondary, or latent syphilis of < 1-year duration are treated with 2.4 million units of benzathine penicillin G IM and for those with latent syphilis of longer or of unknown duration, patients should be treated with 2.4 million units of benzathine penicillin G IM each week for 3 weeks (a total of 7.2 mU). Patients who are allergic to penicillin may be treated with doxycycline 100 mg orally twice daily for 2 weeks, if duration of infection is < 1 year, however, as with any multidose regimen, ensuring adequate therapy is more difficult.

In correctional settings where patients are routinely screened for syphilis, it is necessary to decide if treatment should be based on reactive serologies alone (with or without information on titer and confirmatory testing), or if treatment should await result of an interpretation of the titer based on a complete search and examination of the patient's history of syphilis and past serologic test results. Factors that should be considered in making these decisions include prevalence of untreated syphilis in the population screened, availability of on-site diagnostic testing with or without quantitative results, availability of records on patients' previous syphilis treatment, the length of patient stay, and the probability that a patient with a reactive test result can be located once transferred or released.

In settings where prevalence of untreated disease is high, rapid syphilis serologic tests are available, most patients have not previously been treated for syphilis, and follow-up is uncertain, it may be reasonable to treat patients on the basis of a reactive serologic test result alone. Once the serologic test result is reported to the health department, and final and titer results are obtained, the health department can decide if the patient requires further therapy, and if partners should be notified and treated.

Table 12-1. Recommended therapy for common causes of bacterial sexually transmitted diseases

Disease	Recommended regimens	Alternative regimens
Early syphilis (1, 2, latent < 1y)	Benzathine penicillin G, 2.4mU	Doxycycline 100 mg PO bid x 14 d*
Latent syphilis ≤1yr or of unknown duration	Benzathine penicillin G, 2.4 mU x3 wk	
Chancroid	Azithromycin 1 g PO in a single dose, *or* Ceftriaxone 250 mg IM in a single dose, *or* Ciprofloxacin 500 mg PO bid x3 d*, *or* Erythromycin base 500 mg PO qid x7 d	
Gonorrhea† (uncomplicated anogenital)	Ceftriaxone 125 mg IM, *or* Cefixime 400 mg PO, *or* Ciprofloxacin 500 mg PO,* *or* Ofloxacin 400 mg PO*	Spectinomycin 2 g IM
Chlamydia	Doxycycline 100 mg PO bid x7 d* Azithromycin 1 g PO once	Erythromycin base 500 mg PO qid x7 d Erythromycin ethylsuccinate 800 mg PO qid or Ofloxacin 300 mg orally bid x7 d*

*Should not be used during pregnancy.

†In the absence of a negative chlamydia test result, all patients with gonorrhea should also be treated for chlamydia.

Adapted from CDC: 1998 Guidelines for Treatment of Sexually Transmitted Diseases. *MMWR* 47 (RR-1):1-116,1998.

If rapid tests and titer results are both available, treatment may be based on a titer cut-off (e.g., ≥ 1:4) to reduce the possibility of treating patients who have already received treatment (or who may have false positive test results). However, all women of childbearing age, particularly pregnant women, should be carefully observed until their infection and treatment status have been clarified. In settings where on-site tests are not available, the ability to identify and treat patients who are thought to require treatment and follow-up should be carefully assessed before embarking on a program that may have extremely low yield in terms of treatment of infected patients.

All patients with syphilis should be tested for HIV, both because syphilis is epidemiologically associated with HIV infection, and because patients with latent syphilis who have HIV infection should be evaluated for neurosyphilis. For patients co-infected with HIV who have any of the signs of neurosyphilis, therapy should not be delayed while awaiting lumbar puncture; institution of therapy will not affect diagnostic lumbar puncture results if it is performed soon after therapy is initiated.

Pregnant patients with syphilis should be treated according to the stage of their disease, and titers observed closely through the conclusion of pregnancy. Patients allergic to penicillin will require hospitalization and desensitization, since alternative therapies (e.g., erythromycin) are inadequate for preventing congenital infection of the fetus. Infants born to women with syphilis during pregnancy will require careful evaluation and follow-up, depending on the adequacy of treatment of the mother during pregnancy. Corrections officials should be certain to make optimal therapy for mother and infant available.

All correctional facilities performing syphilis serologic testing should work closely with health department staff, as they have responsibility for ensuring adequate therapy of patients and for counseling and treating sex partners.

Gonorrhea and Chlamydia

Multiple, highly efficacious options for single-dose therapy for uncomplicated gonococcal infection are available. Because of the high prevalence of resistance to penicillin, no use should be made of penicillin or amoxicillin for treatment of gonococcal infections. Other oral and injectable therapies are inexpensive and widely available. The recommended fluoroquinolones are ciprofloxacin 500 mg orally in a single dose, and ofloxacin 400 mg orally in a single dose. A regimen of an oral third-generation cephalosporin, cefixime 400 mg orally in a single dose, is also recommended, and can be used during pregnancy. Ceftriaxone is another recommended third-generation cephalosporin (125 mg IM in a single dose), but less convenient because it requires an injection. In jails, single-dose oral therapy is often preferred for reasons of ensuring compliance and to reduce risk from needlestick exposure.

Chlamydial infections can also be readily and effectively treated. Doxycycline (100 mg orally twice daily for 7 days) is inexpensive and highly efficacious. In those situations where compliance with a multiple-day regimen is considered unlikely, azithromycin 1 g orally in a single dose is preferable, although more expensive. Pregnant women with chlamydial infection should be treated with amoxicillin or erythromycin regimens; azithromycin is a less preferable alternative, because effects on the fetus have not been adequately evaluated. Because of lower efficacy of chlamydia therapy in pregnant women, test of cure should be performed.

Patients who have positive test results for gonorrhea should be treated for both gonorrhea and chlamydia, unless a chlamydia test is also performed and results are negative. When gonorrhea testing is not performed, the decision of whether or not to co-treat patients with chlamydia for gonorrhea should be based on knowledge of prevalence of gonorrhea and co-infection at that facility.

OTHER MANAGEMENT CONSIDERATIONS

All patients diagnosed with an STD should be counseled about the symptoms and risks of STDs, their potential sequelae, and where to seek STD treatment. They should also be provided information on the proper and consistent use of condoms. Infected patients should be encouraged to notify sex partners; when this cannot be performed, the health department can provide confidential partner notification.

REFERENCES

1. Butler WT (ed): Institute of Medicine. *The Hidden Epidemic: Confronting Sexually Transmitted Diseases.* Washington D.C., National Academy Press, 1997.
2. CDC: Ten leading nationally notifiable infectious diseases–United States, 1995. *MMWR* 45:883-884, 1996.
3. Wasserheit JN: Epidemiological synergy: Interrelationships between human immunodeficiency virus infection and other sexually transmitted diseases. *Sex Transm Dis* 19:61-77, 1992.
4. Mastro TD, de Vincenzi I: Probabilities of sexual HIV-1 transmission. *AIDS* 10(suppl A):S75-S82, 1996.
5. CDC: *Chlamydia trachomatis* genital infections–United States, 1995. *MMWR* 46:193-198, 1997.
6. Division of STD Prevention. Sexually Transmitted Disease Surveillance, 1995. U.S. Department of Health and Human Services, Public Health Service. Atlanta, *Centers for Disease Control and Prevention,* September 1996.
7. National Commission on Correctional Health Care: Standards for health services in jails. Chicago, *NCCHC,* 1996.
8. National Commission on Correctional Health Care: Standards for health services in prisons. Chicago, *NCCHC,* 1992.
9. National Commission on Correctional Health Care: Standards for health services in juvenile detention and confinement facilities. Chicago, *NCCHC,* 1995.
10. Blank S, McDonnell DD, Rubin SR, et al: New approaches to syphilis control: Finding opportunities for syphilis treatment and congenital syphilis prevention in a women's correctional setting. *Sex Transm Dis* 24:218-226, 1997.
11. Cohen D, Scribner R, Clark J, Cory D: The potential role of custody facilities in controlling sexually transmitted diseases. *Am J Public Health* 82:552-556, 1992.
12. Weisfuse IB, Greenberg BL, Back SD, et al: HIV-1 infection among New York City inmates. *AIDS* 5:1133-1138, 1991.
13. Oh MK, Cloud GA, Wallace LS, et al: Sexual behavior and sexually transmitted diseases among male adolescents in detention. *Sex Transm Dis* 21:127-132, 1994.
14. Alexander-Rodriguez T, Vermund SH: Gonorrhea and syphilis in incarcerated urban adolescents: Prevalence and physical signs. *Pediatrics* 80:561-564, 1987.
15. Bell TA, Farrow JA, Stamm WE, et al: Sexually transmitted diseases in females in a juvenile detention center. *Sex Transm Dis* 12:140-144, 1985.
16. Morris RE, Legault J, Baker C: Prevalence of isolated urethral asymptomatic *Chlamydia trachomatis* infection in the absence of cervical infection in incarcerated adolescent girls. *Sex Transm Dis* 20:198-200, 1993.
17. O'Brien SF, Bell TA, Farrow JA: Use of a leukocyte esterase dipstick to detect *Chlamydia trachomatis* and *Neisseria gonorrhoeae* urethritis in asymptomatic adolescent male detainees. *Am J Public Health* 78:1583-1584, 1988.
18. Brady M, Baker C, Neinstein LS: Asymptomatic *Chlamydia trachomatis* infections in teenage males.
19. Holmes MD, Safyer SM, Bickell NA, et al: Chlamydial cervical infection in jailed women. *Am J Public Health* 83:551-555, 1993.
20. Martin JW, Much DH: Sexually transmitted diseases in prison women. *Pa Med* 91:40,42; 1988.
21. Ellerbeck EF, Vlahov D, Libonati JP, et al: Gonorrhea prevalence in the Maryland state prisons. *Sex Transm Dis* 16:165-167, 1989.
22. Conrad GL, Kleris GS, Rush B, Darrow WW: Sexually transmitted diseases among prostitutes and other sexual offenders. *Sex Transm Dis* 8:241-244, 1981.
23. Farley TA, Hadler JL, Gunn RA: The syphilis epidemic in Connecticut: Relationship to drug use and prostitution. *Sex Transm Dis* 17:163-168, 1990.
24. Alcabes P, Braslow C: A cluster of cases of penicillinase-producing *Neisseria gonorrhoeae* in an adolescent detention center. *N Y State J Med* 88:495-496, 1988.
25. Grosskurth H, Mosha F, Todd J, et al: Impact of improved treatment of sexually transmitted diseases on HIV infection in rural Tanzania: Randomized control trial. *Lancet* 346:530-536, 1995.
26. CDC: 1998 Guidelines for Treatment of Sexually Transmitted Diseases. *MMWR* 47(RR1):1–116, 1998.

13

Epidemiology of HIV Infection in the Correctional Setting

David Vlahov, Ph.D.

Human immunodeficiency virus, which is the cause of AIDS, and other bloodborne pathogens are a major public health problem in prisons and jails. By the end of 1994, at least 4,588 inmates in U.S. prisons and jails died of AIDS, and during 1994, at least 5,279 inmates with AIDS were incarcerated.[1] Acquired immunodeficiency syndrome is now the leading cause of death in some prison systems.[2–4] The occurrence of AIDS in prisons and jails has stimulated the development of multiple serosurveys to identify the magnitude and scope of the HIV infection. These surveys have provided specimens with which the magnitude and scope of other bloodborne pathogens can be estimated as well.

PREVALENCE, TEMPORAL TRENDS, AND RISK FACTORS FOR HIV-1 INFECTION IN CORRECTIONAL FACILITIES

A large number of HIV-1 seroprevalence surveys have been conducted in the United States, as reported elsewhere.[1, 5, 6] In the United States, rates range from less than 1% to more than 20%[1] and vary considerably by geographic region. Rates have tended to be lowest among entrants to prisons in the midwestern region, for example, rates are less than 1% in Idaho, South Dakota, Nebraska, Wisconsin, Oklahoma, Missouri, Iowa, and Colorado. Rates among male entrants tend to be higher on the Atlantic seaboard (5% for Connecticut, 5% for Massachusetts, 3% for Rhode Island, 9% for New Jersey, 16% for New York City, 8% for Maryland, and 6% for Florida). Intermediate rates have been observed in Texas (3.5%), California (2.6%), and Illinois (4%).[1] By way of comparison, HIV prevalence rates in European prisons range from 0.3% in London, England to 34% in Catalonia, Spain.[7,8] The geographic variation in the prevalence of HIV infection in prisons and jails closely mirrors the geographic variation in both AIDS cases and HIV seroprevalence among injection drug users in the respective communities.

The prevalence of HIV-1 infection in the correctional setting tends to exceed the prevalence in the general population. For example, the 1% prevalence of HIV antibody among entrants to a military maximum security prison[9] contrasts with the 0.15% prevalence among civilian applicants to U.S. military service during a similar calendar time.[10] Although these two groups are not strictly comparable because the samples were drawn at separate times in the research subjects' respective military careers, these data are consistent with data from prison surveys and from blood donor testing that show that rates in correctional facilities are 10–100-fold higher than in general population surveys.[1,11]

In terms of the temporal trends of HIV-1 infection in correctional facilities, early reports suggested that rates were stable over time. In the Maryland State prisons, data obtained over the 3-year period from 1985 to 1987 showed stable prevalence rates among men entering prison at around 7%, which persisted in multivariate analyses.[12] Additional data for 1988 were obtained and showed the persistence of stability for HIV-1 prevalence rates among male entrants to Maryland State prisons.[13] In another survey in Maryland in 1991,[14] HIV prevalence was 7.9% in men and 15.3% in women, which was statistically similar to data obtained from the same correctional system in 1985. Similarly, stable seroprevalence rates were observed over a year's time in two other correctional systems.[15, 16] More recently, Hammett and co-workers[6] presented seroprevalence estimates from 42 state prison systems that responded to his survey instrument, which was a repeat of earlier surveys[1]; HIV rates were remarkably similar over time (Table 13-1). Such data are reassuring to correctional and public health officials and are important for planning and budgeting purposes. However, ongoing surveillance is prudent, as rates can change suddenly over time.

Risk factors for HIV-1 infection in the correctional setting have been studied extensively. The major risk factor is injection drug use before incarceration. Within the New York State prison system, which conducted risk factor investigations on diagnosed cases of AIDS, nearly 95% of inmates with AIDS reported a history of injection drug use, in comparison with 3% who claimed to be exclusively homosexual.[4] Among 1,488 male entrants to the Maryland Division of Correction between April and June 1987, 7% had HIV-1 seropositive status; 85% of the individuals with seropositive status were identified as injection drug users by history or observation of needle tracks, and injection drug users were nearly eight times more likely to be infected with HIV-1, compared with non–drug users entering prison.[12] A similar finding was reported in a seroprevalence survey of New York City inmates.[17]

Correlates of HIV-1 seropositivity among inmates (besides geographic region and injection drug use, which are closely related) include female sex, racial/ethnic minority status, and age older than 25 years.[18] In a study of ten correctional systems within the continental United States, HIV rates were twofold higher in women than in men, which was the result found in 9 of 10 systems studied.[18]

Table 13-1. HIV prevalence among entrants to prisons and jails

State/jurisdiction	Prevalence, 1989 report (%)	Prevalence, 1995 report (%)
Colorado	0.8	0.5
Idaho	0.0	0.3
Missouri	0.4	0.5
Nebraska	0.2	0.4
New York Cit	17.4	16.0
Oklahoma	0.4	0.6
Wisconsin	0.3	0.4

Modified from Hammett TM, Widom R, Epstein J, et al: *1994 Update: HIV/AIDS and STDs in Correctional Facilities*. Washington, D.C., U.S. Department of Justice, Office of Justice Programs, National Institute of Justice/U.S. Department of Health and Human Services, Public Health Service, CDC, December 1995; and Hammett TM: *Update 1989: AIDS in Correctional Facilities*. Washington D.C., U.S. Department of Justice, Office of Justice Programs, National Institute of Justice, 1990, with permission.

These results were confirmed by Hammett and co-workers' 1994 update.[1] Racial/ethnic minorities and individuals older than age 25 years also tend to have a twofold higher risk of being infected.[12–14, 18] These findings are independent of injection drug use. Other factors associated with higher HIV rates include urban residence[12] and residence in a community with a higher population density.[18] A comparison of jails and prisons located in the same state identified a similar HIV-1 prevalence by sex, which suggests no important difference between jails vs. prisons after accounting for geographic region and sex.[18]

TRANSMISSION OF HIV-1 IN THE CORRECTIONAL SETTING

Given that homosexual activity and injection drug use are acknowledged to occur inside prison[19, 20] and, as already noted, that there is an influx of individuals infected with HIV into prison, the potential for HIV transmission in prison is considerable. Although data are sparse on injection drug use while in prison within the United States,[19] studies in the United Kingdom have reported that 25% to 30% of injection drug users injected when last in custody, and, of those, 43% to 75% shared syringes.[21–23]

In terms of sexual activity in prison, rates of self-reported homosexual activity tend to be low (3.0% in Iowa and 3.6% in New Mexico)[24, 25]; however, another report noted that 10% of inmates in a New York City jail acquired gonorrhea during a 3-month period in 1986.[26] The question, then, is not whether HIV can be transmitted within correctional facilities, but how often. Also, because the median duration of sentences for prison is 2–3 years and, therefore, a large proportion of inmates return to the community, the issue is important for the general community. Put another way, to

Table 13-2. Prevalence and incidence of HIV-1 infection among prison inmates, United States

Prison System	Intake prevalence (%)	Incidence per 1,000 prison-years
Military Maximum Security	1.0	0
Nevada	2.4	1.7
Illinois	3.6	3.3
Maryland	7.0	4.2

Modified from Kelly PW, Redfield RR, Ward DL, et al: Prevalence and incidence of HTLV-III infection in prison. *JAMA* 256:2198–2199, 1986; Horsburgh CR, Jarvis JQ, McArthur T, et al: Seroconversion to human immunodeficiency virus in prison inmates. *Am J Public Health* 80:209–210, 1990; Castro K, Shansky R, Scardino V, et al: HIV transmission in correctional facilities. Presented at the International Conference on AIDS. Florence, Italy, June 16–21, 1994, Abstract M.C. 3067, p 314; Brewer TF, Vlahov D, Taylor E, et al: Transmission of HIV-1 within a statewide prison system. *AIDS* 2:363–367, 1988, with permission.

what extent do correctional facilities serve as amplifiers of reservoirs of HIV infection back into the community?

One approach to estimating the risk of intraprison HIV transmission has been to note, within community-based studies, that injection drug users with histories of incarceration have higher HIV rates than injection drug users without histories of incarceration.[27] Although suggesting that infections were acquired in prison, these results could also mean that injection drug users with more risky behavioral patterns are also more likely to be arrested and incarcerated. Alternatively, it is possible that the risk for acquiring HIV infection is low in prison but that, on release, these same individuals have a binge of risky activity that produces the resulting higher rate of HIV infection among those with histories of incarceration. In fact, studies show that levels of injection drug use tend to decline while in prison,[20, 28] and that 55% of those injecting opiates restart injecting within 6 months of discharge from prison.[29] These data suggest that it is important to educate inmates about risk reduction before their release. Thus, data from community-based studies on the higher HIV prevalence among injection drug users who have histories of incarceration are more complicated than they first appear.

That HIV-1 may be transmitted during incarceration was suggested by a study conducted by the Maryland Division of Corrections.[30] This project involved approaching 338 inmates who had been incarcerated for at least 7 years before 1985. Of the 137 volunteers tested, the 2 who had seropositive status had each been incarcerated for 9 years, and the estimated rate of infection was 2.1 per 1,000 prison-years. Although no baseline specimens were available, the extended duration of incarceration suggests that infection was probably acquired in prison. Because the response rate was low and restricted to long-term inmates, bias cannot be excluded.

Subsequently, at a military maximum security prison reporting an HIV-1 seroprevalence of 1% at baseline, serologic follow-up was performed on 567 inmates for whom negative baseline specimens were available; no seroconversions were identified.[9] In the Nevada State prisons, which report a baseline prevalence of 2.4%, the intraprison transmission rate for the entire statewide system was calculated as 1.7 per 1,000 prison-years.[31] In Illinois prisons, which report a baseline prevalence of 3.6%, the intraprison transmission rate was estimated at 3.3 per 1,000 person-years.[32]

In Maryland prisons, which report a baseline prevalence of 7.0%, the intraprison transmission rate for the entire statewide system was calculated as 4.2 per 1,000 prison-years.[33] Although the study samples in each report included only those inmates who were still incarcerated at the time of follow-up, the data suggest that the risk of intraprison transmission is low. This documentation of infrequent transmission and the observation of an apparent direct relationship between HIV-1 seroprevalence at intake and risk of transmission (Table 13-2) suggest that, for most correctional facilities in the United States, intraprison transmission is likely to be low. However, although the rates are low (relative to risks among drug users in the community), the absolute numbers of individuals infected is not trivial when considering the size of the denominator. Therefore, risk reduction in correctional settings needs attention.

To summarize, although available data on the geographic variation and temporal stability in seroprevalence in combination with data suggesting infrequent intraprison transmission appear reassuring, HIV-1 infection remains a major prison health problem. Large numbers of individuals, either at risk for infection or already infected, continue to enter correctional facilities. Prudent policies are needed so that this population can continue to be monitored, treated, and provided with interventions to efficiently prevent and control HIV-1 infection in the correctional setting.

RESPONSE TO HIV-1 IN THE CORRECTIONAL SETTING

Approaches for responding to HIV-1 infection in the correctional setting have included education of inmates about risk; screening for antibody to HIV-1 infection and segregating inmates with seropositive status; and, to a lesser extent, treatment for drug abuse. The options and constraints on each of these approaches are discussed.

Education of Inmates About Risk

In the third annual National Institute of Justice survey of U.S. correctional facilities in 1989, virtually all jurisdictions reported offering or developing some AIDS training or educational material for staff (97%) and inmates (96%).[6] Since that time, the proportion of federal and state systems that provide instructor-led HIV education for inmates has declined to 75%.[1] Although this appears discouraging, a few observation are in order. Despite the near universal application of education about risk to incoming inmates in 1989, data on the pre-existing level of knowledge about HIV and AIDS among incoming inmates was sparse. Celentano and co-workers[34] administered the AIDS Awareness Questionnaire, developed by the National Center for Health Statistics (NCHS), and administered periodically to a random sample of the U.S. population to a sample of 210 consecutive male entrants to the Maryland State prison system. These investigators reported that, within this sample, the knowledge level about HIV and AIDS, the established routes of transmission, and the prevention of transmission was high before receiving in-service education. These results were similar to a random sample of U.S. males interviewed during the same calendar time period; more than 95% correctly responded that HIV was transmitted by sexual intercourse and sharing needles. However, knowledge about causal contact transmission was lower; 57% incorrectly reported that HIV is transmitted by sharing eating utensils with someone who has AIDS. Celentano and co-workers concluded that knowledge about established routes of transmission and prevention of HIV-1 probably has been adequately disseminated before incarceration, but that clarification of unlikely sources of transmission would seem prudent.

In another study, Zimmerman and co-workers,[35] using the same NCHS AIDS Awareness Questionnaire as reported by Celentano and co-workers, conducted a survey of knowledge and perceptions about HIV-1 among 108 inmates from a prison in Pennsylvania who voluntarily participated. They found similar results with respect to knowledge but noted a strong inverse association between knowledge, about likely routes of transmission and perception of risk while in prison. This inverse association suggests that faulty knowledge about unlikely routes of transmission (i.e., through casual contact) might lead to a high perception of risk for acquiring infection while in prison. Although the extent to which the perception of risk is associated with fear and concern was not measured, studies that have identified intraprison transmission as infrequent[31–33] suggest that the risk perceptions reported by these inmates may be unnecessarily high. These findings combined with the data from Celentano and co-workers[34] suggest that education programs in the correctional setting should focus on clarifying unlikely routes of transmission. Zimmerman and co-workers[35] further noted that, among the inmates surveyed, the most trusted sources of AIDS information were television, newspapers, and programs provided by the Division of Corrections, but that the least-trusted sources were correctional officers and other inmates; these findings suggest strategies for focusing educational interventions.

In addition to clarification of concerns that arise during incarceration, education about HIV and AIDS in the correctional setting has been discussed as having a second objective. Prisons house a high concentration of injection drug users; various surveys have reported pre-incarceration drug use among 27% to 41% of prison inmates.[20–25] Also, samples taken of incoming inmates to a regional system involve large numbers of injection drug users from a wide geographic area (e.g., approximately 5,000 injection drug users in the Maryland Division of Corrections entered through a single facility in 1996, and similar numbers are released each year). This access to large numbers of injection drug users, many of whom have no history of treatment for drug abuse,[27] suggests an opportunity to efficiently reach an otherwise difficult-to-access population. However a survey of 1,580 active drug users in Baltimore, Maryland, recruited through extensive community outreach techniques, indicated that information about AIDS had been adequately disseminated[36]; therefore, education programs confined to fundamental concepts about HIV transmission and prevention would likely be redundant. Although the correctional setting provides a unique opportunity to efficiently reach large numbers of injection drug users, the most cost-effective approach to facilitate desired behavioral change requires further work.

In summary, cost-effective planning of AIDS education programs on entry into prison should recognize that fundamental concepts of HIV-1 transmission and prevention are likely to have already been disseminated to individuals entering prison. A revised focus for such programs should include clarification of unlikely sources of transmission with the objective of minimizing unnecessary fears and concerns. As previously noted, inmates being released from prison re-enter communities in which the potential for acquisition and transmission of HIV infection are high, especially if these individuals restart injection drug use. Risk reduction education targeted to inmates before release from correctional facilities is important. Such programs need to encourage continued abstinence, but also recognize that a proportion of those released will return to high-risk activities. Some correctional administrators might have reservations about risk reduction education for illegal behaviors before release, because this presents another layer of planning to identify and transport individuals to sessions in a system in which security and other resources are limited.

However, the goal is reasonable in terms of community health.

Another issue is the extent to which correctional facilities should provide condoms, bleach to disinfect needles between uses, and other public health measures. Mississippi and Vermont State prisons make condoms available, as do jails in San Francisco, New York City, Philadelphia, and Washington, D.C.. Bleach is made available in jails in Houston and San Francisco.[1] Needle exchange programs remain controversial in the United States; however, a program for prisoners in Switzerland has been implemented.[37]

Serologic Screening of Inmates

As a discrete public health policy, screening of inmates for antibody to HIV-1 and segregation of those with seropositive status has been much discussed. In a survey of U.S. correctional systems in 1987 and 1988, Hammett[6] summarized the position of proponents and opponents. Briefly, proponents argued that screening and segregation would permit identification of infected individuals and segregation would permit closer monitoring of infected individuals to reduce risk of transmission, and to initiate treatment for complications of HIV-1 infection. Opponents argued that intraprison transmission was so low that mass screening was not cost effective.

In addition, opponents argued in 1987 and 1988 that treatment of HIV-1 for asymptomatic individuals was not available. With the multitude of logistical problems surrounding mass screening and segregation in the correctional setting, it was argued that basic issues, such as confidentiality of test results and the potential for positive test results to lead to the victimization of inmates, had yet to be adequately addressed.

More recently, recommendations and guidelines for the early treatment of HIV-1 infection have been published[38,39] and updated to reflect continuing advances.[40] These guidelines call for the identification of HIV-1 infection and the monitoring of immune and viral load parameters, so that chemotherapy can be started in asymptomatic individuals with the goal of delaying onset of HIV-1–related disease.

With the advent of multiple chemotherapeutic protocols for individuals with asymptomatic HIV-1 infection, the issues surrounding serologic screening of inmates has shifted dramatically. The merits of mass screening are no longer being debated; rather, the issue now is about how to identify inmates with HIV-1 seropositive status in an efficient and cost-effective manner while protecting the confidentiality of this population. Although estimates of the cost of implementing recommendations to perform serologic screening with appropriate confirmatory testing, estimates of the cost of measuring immune and viral parameters on a semiannual basis for individuals infected with HIV-1, and estimates of the cost of administering chemotherapy are beyond the scope of this discussion, crude calculations suggest that many prison systems might need to consider supplemental budgets in terms of hundreds of thousands of dollars per year.

Two factors can potentially offset the costs of implementation of the recent recommendations for treating HIV-1 infection. First, careful attention to ethical and confidentiality considerations suggests that voluntary rather than mandatory serologic screening is the preferred approach. The proportion of inmates who might volunteer for screening is difficult to predict, but may be less than the complete population because of inmate concerns about the ability to maintain the confidentiality of test results in the correctional setting. Notwithstanding this, before publication of the recommendations for treatment of asymptomatic individuals infected with HIV-1, data from Wisconsin prisons indicated that 71% of inmates volunteered for confidential HIV-1 testing.[15]

In a prison with a higher prevalence of HIV infection, rates for voluntary testing were 40% in the first year of the program, but confidentiality issues were not cited as concerns; many who refused already knew their HIV status.[14] These studies were performed before the availability of protease inhibitors and combination therapies. With the advent of these new therapies, testing or disclosure rates might be higher. Some systems now advocate mandatory testing so that effective therapy is provided, but such an approach must be coupled with mandated, high-quality HIV clinical care.[11]

A second factor that may potentially offset costs for implementation of a comprehensive HIV-1 screening and treatment program is the ability to identify and target subgroups most likely to benefit from intervention. Although several studies have been published that identify injection drug users, minorities, women, and those older than 25 years as being at high risk for having HIV-1 infection on entry into prison,[12,18] more research is needed to refine risk categories and to examine how generalizable they are. In addition, correctional and public health officials need to discuss these data in terms of weighing the policy implications for targeting interventions from total correctional populations to subgroups that might benefit from early treatment of HIV-1 infection.

Treatment for Drug Abuse

Another HIV-1–related intervention to promote in the correctional setting is treatment for drug abuse. Injection drug users, a major risk group for HIV-1 infection, are found in large numbers in the correctional setting, and a substantial proportion report no history of treatment for drug abuse.[41] Facilitating abstinence through treatment is important so that acquisition of HIV-1 infection is prevented. Treatment may also be important for drug users infected with HIV-1, because adherence to combination antiretroviral therapies is likely to be higher in stabilized patients. Interventions, including education, counseling, treatment for HIV-1 infection, and treatment for drug abuse, conducted in the correctional setting, could have benefits for individual inmates and the surrounding community.

POLICY IMPLICATIONS

Rational policy about HIV-1 and AIDS in the correctional setting needs to balance information from multiple sources of existing data and a variety of concerns. On the one hand, general population and ecological trends suggest that the problem of AIDS in the correctional population is likely to loom even larger over time. The frequency of HIV-1 infection among entrants into the correctional setting is higher than the frequency of HIV-1 in the surrounding community. Acquired immunodeficiency syndrome is becoming more widespread in the general population, and the recent explosive growth in our nation's prison population shows signs of continuing. In addition, the prison population itself continues to change in composition. These trends suggest that there will be an increase in incarcerated infected inmates, which will lead to more AIDS and AIDS-related deaths in prisons and an increased reservoir from which intraprison transmission can occur. Clearly, overcrowding of institutions will have consequences for the problem and how it is handled; for example, segregation of infected individuals becomes more problematic as space becomes a scarcer commodity. Regulating and controlling high-risk behaviors in this situation become more difficult, particularly with the presence of "state-raised" convicts and others with long-term sentences who have "nothing to lose." In light of these considerations, some systems have responded by increasing efforts to promote abstinence from drug use through treatment of drug abuse. Some systems, such as California, New York, and Vermont, have responded to the potential for sexual transmission by providing condoms to inmates. Other policy options, such as distribution of clean needles or bleach to disinfect contaminated needles, have been considered. However, given the homosexual activity and illegality of drug use in U.S. prisons and jails, these interventions have negative political consequences. The potential for these activities to condone but not promote continuation of high-risk activities raises ethical dilemmas. In summary, the population and ecological trends indicate the need to address the correctional systems' ultimate responsibility for surveillance, monitoring, and care and treatment of infected inmates, as well as its responsibility to prevent new infection.

On the other hand, and in contrast to the general population and ecological data, prison-specific data appear to offer some reassurances about the problem of HIV-1 and AIDS in the correctional setting. Data on HIV-1 rates from correctional systems throughout the United States indicate that, for most systems, the proportion of inmates infected with HIV-1 is less than 2%. Moreover, despite the increasing size and changing composition of the incarcerated population, available data suggest that the rate of HIV-1 infection among entrants to prison has remained relatively stable over time. More importantly, four studies of intraprison transmission involving three correctional systems (two of which were statewide), in combination with data showing a similar intake and exit rate of infection in the Federal Bureau of Prisons,[1] provide the best information to date to indicate that intraprison transmission appears to be related directly to the rate of infection among inmates entering the respective system. Although the data are limited, combined they provide some reassurance about some of the current perceptions of HIV-1 and AIDS in many, if not most, correctional systems. However, reassurance does not preclude action; instead these data provide a basis for policy refinement.

To date, the epidemiologic data that identify groups at risk and geographic variation in prevalence and incidence of HIV-1 and AIDS, in combination with legal, ethical, and economic constraints, provide a basis for a rational approach to policy development. For example, epidemiologic findings might be used to efficiently target the use of combination antiretroviral therapies. The data suggest that correctional systems with higher -than-average seroprevalence rates would contain large numbers of candidates for such therapeutic intervention and should receive high priority for the use of limited resources. Similarly, such correctional systems might consider the importance and growth of providing prevention measures, such as drug abuse treatment, condoms, and safer sex education, to reduce the risk of intraprison transmission. In addition, prerelease counseling is an important activity for individuals returning to the community. Alternatively, some might consider using demographic information identified in prior epidemiologic studies as preliminary screening criteria for identifying individuals potentially in need of counseling, testing, and treatment services. Using epidemiologic data to identify institutions or individuals at high risk can assist in the daunting task of balancing the need to assume increased responsibility for the care and safety of inmates with the political, ethical, and economic consequences of meeting that responsibility.

REFERENCES

1. Hammett TM, Widom R, Epstein J, et al: *1994 Update: HIV/AIDS and STDs in Correctional Facilities.* Washington, D.C., U.S. Department of Justice, Office of Justice Programs, National Institute of Justice/U.S. Department of Health and Human Services, Public Health Service, CDC, December 1995.
2. Salive ME, Smith GS, Brewer TF: Death in prison: Changing mortality patterns among male prisoners in Maryland. *Am J Public Health* 80:1479–1480, 1990.
3. Paris JE: Mortality review: Learning from inmate death to improve health care in corrections. Presented at the 1995 Conference on Correctional Health Care. National Commission on Correctional Health Care, Washington, D.C., October 1995.
4. New York State Commission of Corrections: *Acquired Immunodeficiency Syndrome: A Demographic Profile of New York State: Mortalities 1982–1985.* Albany, NY, New York State Commission of Corrections, 1986.
5. Centers for Disease Control: Human immunodeficiency virus infection in the United States. A review of current knowledge. *MMWR* 36(Suppl 6): 1987.
6. Hammett TM: *Update 1989: AIDS in Correctional Facilities.* Washington D.C., U.S. Department of Justice, Office of Justice Programs, National Institute of Justice, 1990.
7. Public Health Laboratory Service: *Unlinked anonymous HIV seroprevalence monitoring program in England and Wales.* London, Department of Health, 1995.
8. Martin V, Bayas JM, Laliga A, et al: Seroepidemiology of HIV-1 infection in a Catalonian penitentiary. *AIDS* 4:1023–1026, 1990.
9. Kelly PW, Redfield RR, Ward DL, et al: Prevalence and incidence of HTLV-III infection in prison. *JAMA* 256:2198–2199, 1986.
10. Burke DS, Brundage JF, Herbold JR, et al: Human immunodeficiency virus infection among civilian applicants to United States Military

Service, October 1985 to March 1986. *N Engl J Med* 317:131–136, 1987.

11. De Groot AS, Hammett TM, Scheib RG: Barriers to care to HIV-infected inmates: A public health concern. *AIDS Readers* 3:78–87, 1996.

12. Vlahov D, Brewer F, Munoz A, et al: Temporal trends of human immunodeficiency virus, type 1 (HIV-1) infection among inmates entering a statewide prison system 1985–1987. *J Acquir Immune Defic Syndr* 2:283–290, 1989.

13. Vlahov D, Munoz A, Hall D, et al: Seasonal and annual variation of antibody to the human immunodeficiency virus, type 1 (HIV-1) among male inmates entering Maryland prisons: Update. *AIDS* 4:345–350, 1990.

14. Behrendt C, Kendig N, Dambita C, et al: Voluntary testing for human immunodeficiency virus (HIV) in a prison population with a high prevalence of HIV. *Am J Epidemiol* 139:918–26, 1994.

15. Hoxie NG, Vergemount JM, Frisby HF, et al: HIV seroprevalence and the acceptance of voluntary HIV testing among newly incarcerated male prison inmates in Wisconsin. *Am J Public Health* 80:1129–1131, 1990.

16. Prenderqost TJ, Maxwell R, Greenwood JR, et al: Incidence and prevalence of HIV infection during 44 months of testing prostitutes/IVDUs in the women's jail, Orange County, California (Abstract). Presented at the Fifth International Conference on AIDS, Montreal, June 4–9, 1989, p 82.

17. Weisfuse IB, Greenberg BL, Back SD, et al: HIV-1 infection among New York City inmates. *AIDS* 5:1133–1138, 1991.

18. Vlahov D, Brewer TF, Castro KG, et al: Prevalence of antibody of HIV among entrants to U.S. correctional facilities. *JAMA* 265:1129–1132, 1991.

19. Nacci PL, Kane TR: *Sex and Sexual Aggression in Prisons: Progress Reports*. Washington D.C., U.S. Department of Justice, 1982.

20. Decker MD, Vaugh WK, Brodie JS, et al: Seroprevalence of hepatitis B in Tennessee prisoners. *J Infect Dis* 150:450–459, 1984.

21. Stimson GV, Alldritt L, Dolan KA, et al: *Injecting Equipment Exchange Schemes: A Final Report of Research*. London, Goldsmith's College, 1988.

22. Turnbull PJ, Dolan KA, Stimson GV: *Prisons, HIV and AIDS: Risks and Experiences in Custodial Care*. Horsham, England, Avert, 1997.

23. Kenndy DH, Nair G, Elliott L, et al: Drug misuse and sharing of needles in Scottish prisons. *BMJ* 302:1507, 1991.

24. Glass GE, Hausler WJ, Loeffelholz PL, et al: Seroprevalence of HIV antibody among individuals entering the Iowa prison system. *Am J Public Health* 78:447–449, 1988.

25. Hull HF, Lyons LH, Mann JM, et al: Incidence of hepatitis B in the penitentiary of New Mexico. *Am J Public Health* 75:1213–1214, 1985.

26. van Hoeven KH, Rooney WC, Joseph SC: Evidence of gonococcal transmission within a correctional system. *Am J Public Health* 80:1505–1506, 1990.

27. Vlahov D, Anthony JC, Munoz A, et al: The ALIVE Study: A longitudinal study of HIV infection in intravenous drug users: Description of methods. *J Drug Issues* 21:725–750, 1991.

28. Shewan D, Gemmell A, Davis JB: Behavioral changes amongst drug injections in Scottish prisons. *Soc Sci Med* 39:1585–1586, 1994.

29. Nurco DN, Bonito AJ, Lerner M, et al: Studying addicts over time: Methodology and preliminary findings. *Am J Drug Alcohol Abuse* 2:183–196, 1975.

30. Vlahov D, Polk BF: Intravenous drug use and human immunodeficiency virus (HIV) infection in prison. *AIDS Public Policy J* 3:42–46, 1988.

31. Horsburgh CR, Jarvis JQ, McArthur T, et al: Seroconversion to human immunodeficiency virus in prison inmates. *Am J Public Health* 80:209–210, 1990.

32. Castro K, Shansky R, Scardino V, et al: HIV transmission in correctional facilities. Presented at the International Conference on AIDS. Florence, Italy, June 16–21, 1994, Abstract M.C. 3067, p 314.

33. Brewer TF, Vlahov D, Taylor E, et al: Transmission of HIV-1 within a statewide prison system. *AIDS* 2:363–367, 1988.

34. Celentano D, Brewer TF, Sonnega J, et al: Maryland inmates' knowledge of HIV-1 transmission and prevention. *J Prison Jail Health* 9:45–50, 1990.

35. Zimmerman C, Martin R, Vlahov D: AIDS knowledge and risk perceptions among Pennsylvania prisoners. *J Crim Justice* 19:239–256, 1991.

36. Celentano DD, Vlahov D, Menon AS, et al: HIV knowledge and attitudes among intravenous drug users: Comparisons to the U.S. population and by drug use behaviors. *J Drug Issues* 21:647–661, 1991.

37. Anonymous: Preventing HIV transmission in prison: A tale of medical disobedience and Swiss pragmatism. *Lancet* 346:1507–1508, 1995.

38. Public Health Service. Task Force on Anti-Pneumocystic Prophylaxis: Guidelines for prophylaxis against *Pneumocystis carinii* pneumonia for persons infected with human immunodeficiency virus. *MMWR* 38(Suppl 5):1–9, 1989.

39. Volberding PA, Lagakos SW, Koch MA, et al: Zidovudine in asymptomatic human immunodeficiency virus infection: A controlled trial in persons with fewer than 500 CD4-positive cells per cubic millimeter. *N Engl J Med* 322:941–949, 1990.

40. Carpenter CCJ, Fischl MA, Hammer SM, et al: Concensus statement: Antiretroviral therapy for HIV human infection in 1996; recommendations of an international panel. *JAMA* 296:146–154, 1996.

41. Barton WI: Drug histories and criminality: Survey of inmates of state correctional facilities. January 1974. *Int J Addict* 15:233–258, 1980.

14

Overview of HIV Care

Frederick L. Altice, M.D.

As newer treatment options become available for people living with HIV/AIDS, providing clinical care is becoming both formidable and dynamic. Obstacles to delivery of care are a particular challenge to clinicians working within prisons. These obstacles include gaining access to HIV specialists, maintaining confidentiality, having current medications available for adequate treatment of HIV, developing trust with inmates, cooperating with correctional staff, and coordinating discharge planning to ensure continuity of care. Despite impediments to providing care to inmates living with HIV/AIDS, many committed correctional health care professionals are providing beneficial care on a daily basis. With incorporation of community standards of care within correctional facilities, inmates can receive state-of-the-art treatment in a supervised setting. Optimal medical management within an organized and structured environment makes prisons a unique and underused setting for the identification and treatment of this progressive and, otherwise, fatal illness.

Over the past decade, and, in particular, the past few years, enormous clinical progress has been made in the diagnosis and treatment of HIV disease and in the prophylaxis and treatment of opportunistic infections. People with HIV/AIDS are now living longer with a higher quality of life. While management of HIV/AIDS in many correctional systems continues to improve, it has been slow to keep up with the community standard of care. Human immunodeficiency viral disease is now most effectively managed by experienced HIV clinicians due to the complexity of the disease and its many complications. This experience is gained through the inpatient and outpatient· treatment of many HIV-infected patients over time and requires access to routine, continuing medical education to keep abreast of rapid changes in HIV therapy. For instance, guidelines for the management of HIV disease changed dramatically from 1996 to 1997 so that monotherapy was no longer considered an option, and the combining of nucleoside analogues, previously thought to be optimal therapy, is now considered as less than optimal. The greatest benefit to the patient comes through experienced clinicians who are knowledgeable of newer sophisticated testing and monitoring for HIV treatment, the wide use of an array of highly active anti-retroviral agents, and the complexity of monitoring drug interactions and toxicity of therapy. Many current HIV practitioners think that HIV care should become a subspecialty.[1-9] This position has evolved as a consequence of demonstrating that morbidity, mortality, and expensive health resource utilization is reduced when patients with HIV infection receive care from an experienced HIV practitioner.[10-15] Unfortunately, correctional health care providers often lack the extensive expertise thought necessary by those proponents, and the response to train or hire experienced clinicians has fallen behind the community standard in many geographic regions.

In most geographic regions, provision of HIV services by experienced clinicians has now become the community standard of care. This standard of care should be conferred to prisoners and is supported by language in the Eighth Amendment to the United States Constitution, and through guidelines issued by the American Public Health

Association[16] and the World Health Organization.[17, 18] These community standards of care consist of comprehensiveness, continuity, competence, compassion, and cost-effectiveness. Unfortunately, the ability to achieve these standards is strongly influenced by the availability of resources, adequate clinical settings, and local expertise. Despite the special logistical and organizational obstacles encountered by these systems, it is incumbent on correctional health services to provide this level of care.

The transformation of AIDS as a relatively short-term fatal illness to management of HIV disease as a chronic disease has evolved through four recent advances. These advances include 1) improved understanding of HIV pathogenesis; 2) technologic improvements in the quantification of HIV-1 RNA levels; 3) use of combination therapy of antiretroviral agents against HIV, including the newer and more potent protease inhibitors; and 4) improved strategies for the prevention and treatment of opportunistic infections. A thorough understanding of these advances is necessary for comprehensive and competent care. However, even in the presence of adequate expertise in the management of HIV disease, correctional health care systems have unique obstacles that the community does not encounter. They must provide continuity of care to new entrants from the outside community as well as to prisoners who transfer within and between correctional facilities, as well as between systems (e.g., between local jails and state prisons or between state and federal prisons). Additionally, organizational procedures between correctional and health service staff must be in place to ensure this continuity. Movement of prisoners makes consistency of care difficult and it is unlikely that trust can be established without consistency. Furthermore, the institutional environment is designed to punish or, at a minimum, provide a site for penitence; thus, compassion as defined in health care does not necessarily translate as such in the routine treatment of prisoners. Considerable cooperation between the health services and correctional administrators, as well as with the on-line staff, is essential for overcoming the potential obstacles that may impede achievement of standard HIV care, from acceptable HIV testing practices to acceptance and adherence to antiretroviral agent therapy.[19]

Nevertheless, the provision of comprehensiveness, continuity, competence, compassion, and cost-effectiveness in the management of HIV in the prison setting offers a beneficial and underused opportunity for the introduction and the delivery of optimal health care to individuals within the correctional system. The majority of prisoners with HIV infection have histories of illicit drug use and a former reliance on acute and episodic care, often within emergency department settings.[20–22] Correctional health services may serve as entry points for the provision of primary HIV services and ultimately link individuals to community primary care settings after release.

This chapter examines the recent advances in HIV management, evaluation of the disease, and the special issues relating to detection and treatment that are unique to the correctional setting. A detailed understanding of the recent developments in the management of HIV disease is essential for practitioners and patients. This understanding will facilitate rational decision-making about new therapies and monitoring tools that will achieve the greatest and most durable clinical benefit.

RECENT ADVANCES IN THE MANAGEMENT OF HIV DISEASE
HIV Pathogenesis

It was previously thought that HIV remains virologically quiescent during the clinically latent period from HIV seroconversion to clinical AIDS. However, new data indicate that both HIV replication and CD_4 lymphocyte turnover are active throughout the natural history of HIV disease. It is this active replication of HIV that causes progressive immune damage to the infected individual. Recent studies of HIV pathogenesis indicate that newly infected persons harbor a homogeneous population of HIV that possess few mutational variants that might predispose to clinical antiretroviral resistance and therapeutic failure. Over time, mutational changes increase.

The relatively short replication cycle for HIV gives rise to 200 to 300 replicative cycles per year and 3,000 to 5,000 cycles over 10 years. This results in a total production of 10 to 12 trillion virions, and each replication is prone to increased mutational changes.[23] At the same time that HIV is active, the host's immune system is increasingly active as well. There are estimated to be 2 trillion CD_4 T-lymphocytes that turn over daily. The reserve of CD_4 lymphocytes persists, despite almost total depletion in serum associated with advanced HIV.[24–26] Despite the quantitative decline in CD_4 cells over time, there are qualitative changes that may have profound implications for treatment. That is, even a patient with a CD_4 lymphocyte count less than 10 cells/m^3 is turning over trillions of CD_4 lymphocytes; however, the T-cell repertoire by this stage of infection is limited. Unfortunately, depletion exceeds production and T-cell counts fall over time. Clinical AIDS can be expected to develop in untreated adults in approximately 10 to 12 years; for some, it will develop as early as 3 to 5 years. In only about 2% of individuals infected with HIV is HIV replication at extremely low levels and a stable CD_4 count maintained for more than 12 years. Even among this small group, many of these individuals demonstrate laboratory evidence of immune system damage.[27]

In addition to studies of HIV-1 RNA in plasma, lymphoid tissue also demonstrates marked activity and provides direct evidence of high rates of HIV-1 replication that is paralleled by detection of viral particles in plasma.[28–30] Even moderate plasma detection of HIV may underestimate the activity of HIV replication in lymphoreticular tissue.[31]

Table 14-1: Rate of disease progression by CD_4 count and corrected viral load determinations[†]

	Plasma viral load (copies/ml)*			Percent developing AIDS**		
	MACS	bDNA	RT-PCR	3 years	6 years	9 years
CD_4<350	501-3000	1001-6000	3001-14,000	0	18.8	30.6
	3001-10,000	6001-20,000	14,001-41,000	8.0	42.2	65.6
	10,001-30,000	20,001-60,000	41,001-110,000	40.1	72.9	86.2
	>30,000	>60,000	>110,000	72.9	92.7	95.6
$CD_4$351-500	501-3000	1001-6000	3001-14,000	4.4	22.1	46.9
	3001-10,000	6001-20,000	14,001-41,000	5.9	39.8	60.7
	10,0001-30,000	20,001-60,000	41,001-110,000	15.1	57.2	78.6
	>30,000	>60,000	>110,000	47.9	77.7	94.4
CD_4>500	<500	<1000	<3000	1.0	5.0	10.7
	501-3000	1001-6000	3001-14,000	2.3	14.9	33.2
	3001-10,000	6001-20,000	14,001-41,000	7.2	25.9	50.3
	10,001-30,000	20,001-60,000	41,001-110,000	14.6	47.7	70.6
	>30,000	>60,000	>110,000	32.6	66.8	76.3

*bDNA and RT-PCR values are adjusted from the original Multicenter AIDS Cohort Study (MACS) data.
**AIDS defined according to the 1987 CDC definition.
[†]Modified from the Guidelines for the Use of Antiretroviral in HIV-Infected Adults and Adolescents. National Institute of Health, Washington, D.C., 1997.

Correlation exists between HIV-1 RNA levels in plasma and in the lymphoreticular system. It appears that this correlation is less in other important body compartments, such as the cerebrospinal fluid and in genital (semen, vaginal fluid) secretions. Thus, extrapolation of plasma HIV-1 RNA levels may not correlate with the degree of infectivity through sexual contact.

HIV-1 RNA Determinations

Recent technologic advances now allow clinicians to reliably and rapidly quantitate levels of HIV-1 RNA in plasma. This laboratory tool has not only led to our improved understanding of HIV pathogenesis, but also to our understanding of antiretroviral efficacy. HIV-1 RNA determination, also known as "viral load", is a surrogate for the magnitude of HIV replication. Viral load can be quantified by either target amplification (RT–PCR), nucleic acid sequence–based amplification (NASBA), or signal amplification (bDNA) methods. Two kits for viral load determinations (bDNA and RT–PCR) are now commercially available. Values for the bDNA method are about 50% of RT–PCR values; and currently available kits detect HIV-1 RNA to levels of either 200 to 400 copies/m3 (RT–PCR) or 500 copies/m^3 (bDNA). Newer technologic advances now allow HIV-1 RNA levels to be detected to as low as 20 copies/m^3 using an ultra-sensitive method. While all three methods are similarly accurate, measurement of the same sample using two different methods may result in a two-fold difference.[32–34] Such variation suggests consistent use of one method and adherence to strict collection and processing guidelines to ensure accuracy when these are used to guide therapeutic decisions. Quantitative values can vary by threefold (~0.5 log) in either direction on repeated measurements on the same or different days.[35,36] This finding justifies a repeated measurement between 2 and 4 weeks after the initial measurement. Differences of more than threefold reflect biologically and clinically relevant changes. Intercurrent illness or immunization may transiently increase activated CD_4 cells, and, thus, lead to increased HIV replication.[37] When possible, measurement of viral load during these window periods should be avoided. Unlike CD_4 lymphocytes, HIV-1 RNA levels do not reflect diurnal variations; therefore, levels may be checked at any time of the day.

The magnitude of HIV-1 RNA is also one of the ways in which disease progression can be predicted. In studies of the natural history of HIV in controlled clinical trials, HIV-1 RNA levels have been demonstrated to be the strongest predictor of clinical outcome (development of an AIDS-defining condition or survival) over 1 to 10 years of observation.[38–49] The risk for disease progression is variable over a continuum of HIV-1 RNA levels and is depicted in Table 14-1. Target amplification (RT–PCR) and bDNA values, for the purpose of consistency, have been corrected from the original Multicenter AIDS Cohort Study (MACS) data to be consistent with HIV-1 RNA values currently obtained in clinical practice.[50] Plasma samples in MACS were collected in heparin and stored for up to 10 years and are lower than those obtained from freshly frozen plasma samples.

CD_4 lymphocyte counts, also known as T helper cells, measure the extent of immune system damage that has

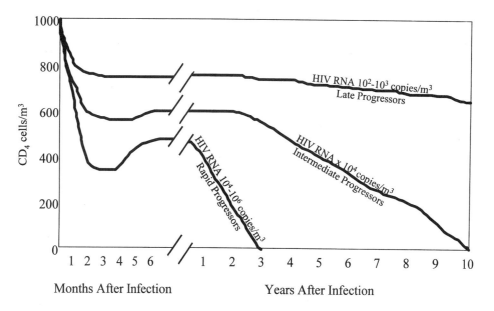

Figure 14-1. Progression of HIV disease based on set point of HIV RNA levels.

already occurred in an HIV-infected patient.[51–55] The CD_4 count also predicts risk for the development of a specific opportunistic infection or other sequelae of HIV infection.[56, 57] The CD_4 count, in conjunction with viral load determinations, enhances the accuracy for predicting disease progression and death.[58] Thus, for two individuals with the same HIV-1 RNA and differing CD_4 counts, a medical complication from HIV will likely develop more rapidly in the patient with the lower CD_4 count.

It has been found that AIDS develops in some individuals within 5 years of initial infection (~20%), and that fewer than 5% of individuals will remain asymptomatic for as long as 10 years. Thus, all those infected with HIV must be considered at risk for development of progressive disease. Therefore, antiretroviral therapy for persons infected with HIV should be based on risk of disease progression indicated by plasma HIV-1 RNA levels and the degree of immunodeficiency indicated by CD_4 lymphocyte counts.

Figure 14-1 depicts the natural history for individuals after HIV seroconversion. At the time of HIV seroconversion, there is a robust burst of viral replication, followed by the immune response of the host. Individuals respond differently. Some will have an immune system that will control HIV replication to HIV-1 RNA levels below 10^4 copies/m³ (late progressors), while others may have less containment of HIV with levels greater than 10^4 copies/m³ (rapid progressors). Even for patients with viral loads in the best prognostic category of risk for progression (e.g., HIV-1 RNA levels < 5,000 copies), the 5- or the 10-year risk is not zero. Unfortunately, there are no reliable means to prospectively identify which individuals among this group are likely to have premature progression to AIDS. This raises treatment dilemmas, particularly for this group. Denial

of treatment for these individuals may put them at risk for disease progression; therefore, implementation of therapy at any detectable HIV-1 RNA level has been suggested by many. Of course, when initiating therapy to this group, the patient must be made aware that this is long-term therapy (possibly 20 years or more) and must be willing to take medications indefinitely.

HIV-1 RNA copy number ("viral load") predicts clinical outcome not only for the natural history of HIV disease but also for response to antiretroviral therapy. Baseline viral load and response to viral load with treatment have been demonstrated to be the most reliable predictors for clinical outcome in controlled clinical trials. Reduction in viral load improves the short-term clinical outcome.[36, 59–61] When viral load is reduced by treatment with antiretroviral agents, the greater the reduction in viral load and the longer the duration, the more effective the response. Thus, routine viral load testing is indicated for initiation and monitoring of antiretroviral therapy. This has become the standard of care for HIV and is essential for providing comprehensive, competent, and cost-effective care.

HIV-1 RNA levels decrease rapidly within 2 weeks of initiation of highly active antiretroviral therapy (Figure 14-2).[62] This period, Phase I, is constant between individuals. Phase II lasts from 8 to 28 days after Phase I and accounts for approximately 1% of HIV-infected cells. Most of these infected cells are macrophages that have a longer half-life than newly or latently infected CD4 lymphocytes.

Thus, patients starting antiretroviral therapy should confirm viral load response between 2 and 4 weeks after initiation. Greater than 70% reduction (~ log 0.5) in viral load is considered significant; however, with potent antiretroviral agents, the expected response should be greater than 1.0

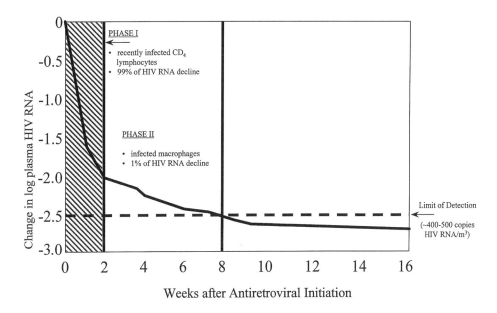

Figure 14-2. HV-1 RNA decline after initiation of potent antiretroviral therapy.

log (i.e., tenfold), and ideally 2.0 to 4.0 logs, depending on the potency of the antiretroviral combination. Peak HIV-1 RNA reductions are seen at approximately 8 to 12 weeks after initiation of therapy. If viral load becomes non-detectable, it may be further assessed using an ultrasensitive methodology (detection limit 50 copies) and may be monitored every 12 to 16 weeks. Viral load, however, should be rechecked earlier if there is a change in the patient's clinical condition or if there is a change in antiretroviral therapy. Frequent monitoring allows for early change in therapy to avoid high-level resistance. Of note, CD_4 T-lymphocytes may also increase in response to therapy; however, changes are likely to be delayed compared to changes in HIV-1 RNA levels. Peak CD_4 T-lymphocyte increases are noted after 12 weeks of therapy, thereby suggesting routine monitoring every 12 to 16 weeks.

Use of Combination Therapy

Multiple clinical trials have demonstrated clinical superiority, using combination therapy compared to monotherapy,[36, 63–68] and use of combinations including a protease inhibitor have demonstrated more profound clinical efficacy.[69–72] The rationale supporting combination therapy is based on the recent improvement in our understanding of viral pathogenesis and encompasses five essential elements: 1) to minimally provide additive — and ideally synergistic — antiretroviral activity; 2) to avoid the emergence of resistance; 3) to minimize toxicity; 4) to provide antiretroviral drug activity in different cellular dividing and body compartments; and 5) to prolong survival. Details regarding the use of antiretroviral therapy are available in chapter 15.

THE INITIAL EVALUATION

Considerable time must be allocated to the initial evaluation of the patient infected with HIV. Information regarding a patient's HIV serostatus or potential risk behaviors must be elicited in a confidential setting and in a non-judgmental fashion. For example, asking an inmate if he or she has "ever been tested for HIV or the virus that causes AIDS" is preferable to asking, "Do you have HIV/AIDS?" Additionally, stigma from being HIV-infected, or from participating in a behavior that places an individual at risk for HIV infection (unprotected sex, injection drug use, engaging in commercial sex work, and a history of a sexually transmitted disease), may limit the usefulness of the personal history if the interviewer appears judgmental.

Any inmate who self-reports being HIV-infected or who has an illness suggesting HIV/AIDS should be evaluated. First, for symptomatic patients, all acute conditions should be assessed and treated. If an inmate describes use of antiretroviral therapy immediately prior to incarceration, every attempt should be made to continue therapy without interruption. In many cases, this requires a phone call to the community clinician (with a signed patient consent) to ensure continuity of care. Patients with a remote history of antiretroviral use should be evaluated to assess clinical stage of disease (CD_4 count) and prognosis (viral load) without restarting antiretroviral agents immediately and in accordance with Figure 14-3. If the inmate has unconfirmed HIV serostatus, and reports not taking antiretroviral therapy, he or she should be referred for counseling and testing before completing the laboratory assessment. After HIV serostatus has been confirmed, the inmate infected with HIV should undergo routine laboratory evaluation (Table 14-2).

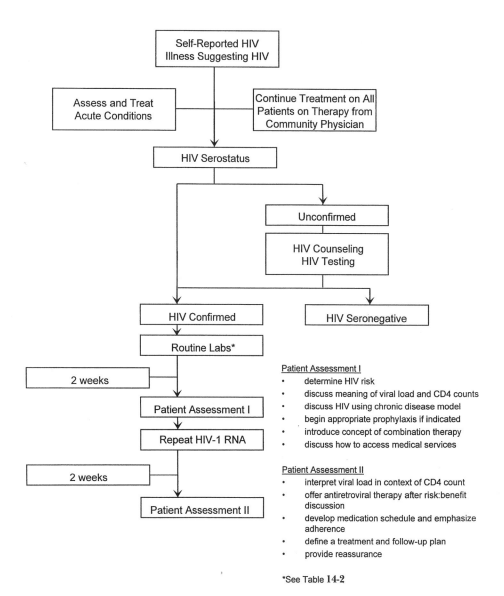

Figure 14–3. Algorithm for the assessment of patients with or suspected to be HIV infected.

Patients who receive post-test counseling and learn of their own HIV seropositivity are anxious and unsure about the meaning of being HIV-infected. This anxiety often carries over in the first meeting with the clinician. Therefore, the initial encounter between clinician and patient should explore such issues and be used to develop trust. Inmates should be assured that anything discussed between the clinician and the patient will remain confidential and in no way will be shared with the non-medical staff at the correctional facility. The first visit, then, between clinician and inmate should:

• Clarify the meaning of the reactive HIV test;
• Provide an overview of the natural history of HIV disease;
• Offer an explanation of the recent hopeful advances available for treatment that can alter the course of the disease;
• Offer reassurance that HIV, while not curable, is treatable — as with hypertension or diabetes;

• Lay the groundwork and plans for the essential follow-up visits.

In addition, the clinician should take a careful and comprehensive personal health history, conduct a physical examination, and take the necessary samples for laboratory evaluation. Some correctional systems perform the laboratory evaluation prior to the visit between clinician and inmate to expedite the evaluation process. An algorithm for patient assessment is presented in Figure 14-3. For patients who arrive at the correctional facility and who claim to be receiving antiretroviral medication, every effort should be made to confirm medication and dosage so that there is no interruption in therapy.

Some issues may be carried over to the second visit if insufficient time is available or if the process overwhelms the inmate. Updated, standardized, and comprehensive problem lists, as well as laboratory and clinical flow

Table 14-2 Laboratory testing and clinical management

Test	Indication for baseline test	Frequency of repeat test
HIV serology	All patients should have documentation of positive serology	Baseline only
CBC/diff, chemistry	All patients	As indicated by antiretroviral or other therapy
CD_4 profile	All patients	Approximately every 3–4 months
HIV-1 RNA (viral load)	All patients Two baselines separated by 2–4 weeks	Approximately every 3–4 months, and as indicated to monitor response to therapy
RPR or VDRL	All patients	Yearly
PPD	All patients without history of reactive PPD, TB treatment, or prophylaxis	Yearly or if exposed
Toxoplasma IgG	All patients when $CD_4+ < 250$	Seronegatives, when $CD_4+ < 100\text{-}200$ and unable to take TMP/SMX
Varicella IgG	Patients who cannot give history of chicken pox or shingles	Baseline only
HbsAG	All patients	Baseline only
HbsAb and anti-HBc	All patients	Consider for vaccine follow-up if both tests negative
anti-HCV	IV drug users and patients with abnormal LFTs	As clinically indicated
G-6PD	Blacks and Mediterranean descent	Only in patients whose $CD_4+ < 200$ and intolerant to TMP/SMX
Pap smear	All women	Yearly
Chest radiograph	Baseline, especially in IV drug users or patients at high risk for TB	Yearly, and as clinically indicated
Pneumovax	All patients without history of vaccination	Repeat every 5 years
dT (tetanus booster)	Patients without tetanus booster in last 10 years	Repeat every 5 years
Flu vaccine	Optional: consider in all patients during flu season	Yearly (consider holding while initially monitoring HIV-1 RNA)
Hepatitis B vaccine	Patients with negative HbsAb and anti-HBc who remain at risk for HBV	One three injection series only in patients whose sentence is > 6 months
Ophthalmological referral	All patients with $CD_4 < 50$	Determined by ophthalmologist, or if symptoms arise

sheets, are useful for the long-term treatment of patients with chronic diseases, especially those with HIV/AIDS. Tables 14–2 through 14–6 identify the issues to be addressed as part of the initial evaluation. These include the medical history, drug use history, sexual history, physical examination, and laboratory testing and clinical management. These will be discussed in more detail in the following sections.

Medical History

Either prior to or during the first assessment, information related to prior HIV testing should be obtained. This includes the dates for both negative and positive serologic testing results, as well as any CD_4 and viral load determinations (Box 14-1). To further assess the clinical degree of immunosuppression, illnesses related to or associated with HIV or HIV-related risk behavior should be assessed. Conditions associated with HIV include thrush; shingles; bacterial pneumonia; or constitutional symptoms such as fever, weight loss, or chronic diarrhea. Diagnoses related to AIDS itself include opportunistic infections, malignancies, and neurologic conditions outlined in the 1993 CDC categories for HIV. Injection drug use (IDU) is the major risk behavior associated with HIV infection among inmates. Co-morbid conditions associated with IDU include viral hepatitis B and C, endocarditis, cellulitis, skin abscesses, and drug overdose. Most inmates infected with HIV are also at high risk for tuberculosis; therefore any information regarding previous exposure, reactive PPD, or previous treatment may avoid future unnecessary testing or treat-

---

Box 14-1. Medical History

HIV testing date and place of first positive test
- date of patient's last negative test
- CD$_4$ nadir and most recent CD$_4$ count
- viral load maximum and most recent viral load result

HIV-related illnesses
- shingles (herpes zoster)
- history of pneumonia
- history of thrush
- opportunistic infections
- constitutional symptoms (fevers, weight loss, chronic diarrhea)
- extensive antiretroviral history, including types of therapy, duration, and side effects
- thrush

Other related illnesses
- skin rashes
- endocarditis
- hepatitis B and C
- skin abscesses or cellulitis
- abnormal Pap smear results

STD history and treatment: gonorrhea, chlamydia, syphilis, herpes simplex, condyloma accuminata, pelvic inflammatory disease, trichomonas

Tuberculosis history
- TB exposure
- history of positive PPD
- history of active TB
- duration and type of treatment

Health service utilization
- all previous medical and psychiatric hospitalizations
- emergency room use and diagnosis
- psychiatric history, including diagnoses, hospitalization, and treatment

Obstetric and gynecologic history
- last menstrual period (currently pregnant?)
- nature of menses
- any pregnancies after learning HIV diagnosis
- abnormal Pap smears (dates and types of treatment)

Vaccination history
- history of childhood chicken pox
- measles mumps rubella (MMR)
- last tetanus booster
- hepatitis B
- pneumovax

Box 14-2. Drug Use History

List age at first use, duration, frequency, route of use (inhaled, sniffed, injected), and date of last use for each of the following:
- tobacco
- alcohol
- marijuana
- heroin
- cocaine
- crack
- metamphetamine
- psychedelics (LSD, psilocibin)
- previous drug treatment, including outpatient, residential, or methadone maintenance treatment
- any complications of drug use (overdoses, blackouts, withdrawal seizures, delirium tremens, etc.)
- syringe-or paraphernalia-sharing

---

those who meet the vaccination requirement, it should be provided and recorded on the patient's problem list. For women, a detailed obstetric and gynecologic history should include information regarding current symptoms and past diagnoses and treatment.

Drug Use History

Inmates infected with HIV have usually used injectable or non-injectable illicit drugs. The route, duration, and frequency of drug use for each substance should be elicited (Box 14-2). Patients actively using heroin, alcohol, or benzodiazepines at the time of incarceration should be provided a medically supervised detoxification or drug maintenance. A careful drug use history may assist the HIV specialist in linking goals for HIV treatment with those learned in drug treatment programs.

Risk for HIV through the shared use of injecting equipment or paraphernalia should be elicited to adequately counsel and reduce future risk for acquiring other blood-borne infections. Information regarding prior drug treatment may be useful to counsel patients about future drug treatment options.

Sexual History

Eliciting a sexual history is challenging to even the most experienced clinician. A non-judgmental approach may include asking "How many sexual partners, including men and women, have you had in the past 5 years? Of those, how many were men and how many were women?" After the total number of partners has been established, distinguish between a primary (regular) partner and non-primary partners (casual). Risk of HIV for women inmates may differ from that of men because there is an increased proportion of women who exchange sex for money, rent, protection, or drugs. Assessing condom use for primary and non-primary partners may provide a segue to provide risk reduction

ment. Prisoners have increased age-matched morbidity for sexually transmitted diseases. Current symptoms and past treatment information are essential to avoid potential medical complications.

In addition, a detailed recent health service use history of medical and psychiatric care should be obtained to assist in acquiring hospital records. Also, a vaccination history is useful for determining risk for co-morbid conditions. For

---

Box 14-3. Sexual History

List dates and treatment for each of the following STDs:
- Gonorrhea (GC, clap, drip)
- Chlamydia (non-specific urethritis or cervicitis)
- Syphilis
- Herpes (list frequency of recurrence)
- Condyloma accuminata
- Trichomonas

Ask about sexual contact with known people with HIV/AIDS and   other high-risk individuals (sex workers or drug injectors)

Obtain non-judgmental assessment of gender of sexual contacts

Distinguish between primary (regular) and non-primary (casual) sexual partners
- Number of partners
- Condom use
- Type of contraception used

Box 14-4. Physical Examination

Overall appearance, including vital signs and weight assessment

Fundoscopic evaluation, including retinal lesions

Oropharynx
- thrush
- oral hairy leukoplakia
- Kaposi's sarcoma
- herpes simplex virus
- gingivitis
- aphthous ulcers

Complete skin examination
- rashes
- track marks
- Kaposi's sarcoma
- folliculitis
- cellulitis
- abscess
- molluscum contagiosum

Lymph nodes
- note size
- location
- mobility

Cardiovascular examination (including murmurs)

Pulmonary examination

Abdominal examination, including liver and spleen

Detailed genital and rectal examination, including internal pelvic

Neurologic assessment
- orientation
- cranial nerves
- gait
- sensory
- cerebella
- motor
- memory
- mini mental status examination

---

counseling, and may identify others who may benefit from partner notification programs. Further issues to address in the sexual history are included in Box 14-3.

Physical Examination

The physical examination is crucial in the evaluation of the inmate infected with HIV (Box 14-4). After completing the review of systems and historical information, the physical examination may provide clues about the stage of HIV disease or identify co-morbid conditions. Overall, many inmates infected with HIV may initially appear as malnourished, particularly if the pre-incarceration history identified intense illicit drug use and inadequate nutritional support. However, HIV wasting syndrome should not be diagnosed in such a setting until after adequate alimentation has been provided. A fever, however, may be the harbinger of a more serious problem and deserves a thorough assessment and observation. In patients suspected of having advanced HIV disease or visual impairment, a dilated fundoscopic examination should be performed to exclude retinitis.

The skin and mucous membranes easily provide accessible clues to secondary conditions. Thrush, oral hairy-leukoplakia (OHL), and Kaposi's sarcoma suggest more advanced HIV disease, whereas stomatitis secondary to herpes simplex virus (HSV) or *candida* species require immediate symptomatic treatment, although thrush is rarely life-threatening.

The dermatologic examination may identify many useful clues. The presence of track marks confirms injection drug use, and multiple infectious and non-infectious rashes may be detected and associated with HIV infection. Atypical dermatologic presentations or unusual responses to therapy of common dermatologic conditions may present

interesting challenges and diagnostic dilemmas in the inmate infected with HIV.

Lymphadenopathy is common at all stages of HIV disease; however, it has no prognostic significance. The HIV-related adenopathy is usually diffuse, rubbery, and mobile. However, if the adenopathy is localized or atypical, a biopsy should be performed to exclude an infectious process or a malignancy. The skin examination should also assess for complications of drug injection; cellulitis or abscesses should be sought and treated. Prior endocarditis may have left a residual cardiac murmur, and the lungs should be examined for findings associated with pneumonia. A careful examination of the liver and spleen for complications from either viral or alcoholic hepatitis and infiltrative processes should be completed.

All inmates should be evaluated for sexually transmitted diseases during examination of the genitalia. Women should also undergo a Pap smear, and, if results are abnor-

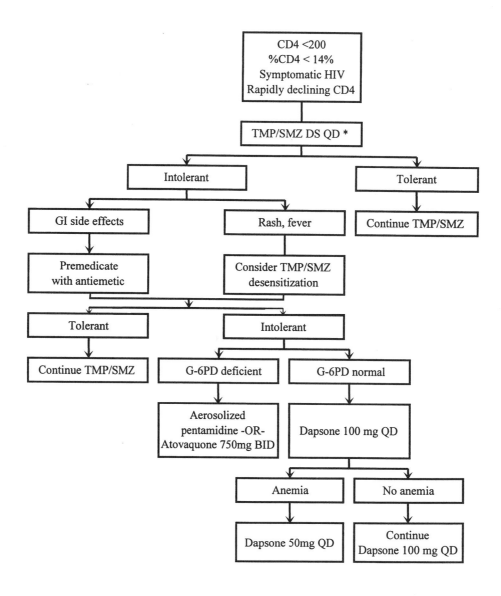

Figure 14-4. Algorithm for PCP prophylaxis.

mal, should be evaluated as described later in the section titled Human Papilloma Virus and Abnormal Pap Smear.

A careful neurologic examination may detect early encephalopathy, peripheral neuropathy, or other neurologic sequelae of HIV infection or one of its opportunistic infections. A brief mini-mental status examination should be part of each evaluation, as should an assessment for psychiatric disorders.

Laboratory Examination

The initial laboratory evaluation of the inmate with documented HIV infection minimally requires a complete blood cell count (CBC), chemistry profile including liver function tests (LFTs), CD4 lymphocyte subsets, quantitative HIV-1 RNA, VDRL, and screening serology for chronic hepatitis (HBV and HCV). Patients with HIV, particularly those with advanced disease, may demonstrate anemia, leukopenia, thrombocytopenia, and elevated levels on LFTs. Other baseline serologies may be obtained only when the patient is determined to be at risk for the disease (e.g., toxoplasma antibody when the CD4 count is < 200 cells/m^3). Other laboratory testing is detailed in Table 14-2.

All patients infected with HIV should be screened for tuberculosis through PPD and chest radiographic evaluation. This screening should be performed annually, unless the patient has been known to be exposed to tuberculosis within the facility.

Vaccination against pneumococcal pneumonia and tetanus should be performed every 5 years, and influenza vaccination should be offered seasonally. Viral load determination should not be obtained within 6 weeks of vaccination because of a transient increase in viral replication that has been observed.

PROPHYLAXIS AND TREATMENT OF OPPORTUNISTIC INFECTIONS

Opportunistic infections continue to produce excess morbidity and mortality among people infected with HIV, particularly among those who are severely immunosuppressed (i.e., CD_4 lymphocyte count < 200 cells/ m^3).[73-76] While *Pneumocystis carinii* pneumonia (PCP) continues to be the most frequent and incident opportunistic infection, PCP, along with toxoplasmosis, fungal infections, and *Mycobacterium-avium* complex (MAC) have decreased in incidence.[77] This decreased incidence appears to be influenced by two factors: the use of appropriate prophylactic regimens against these opportunistic infections, and the introduction of highly active antiretroviral therapy.

Before the introduction of highly active antiretroviral therapy (HAART), widespread use of prophylactic therapy and prompt diagnosis and treatment of opportunistic infections helped to increase survival time of people living with HIV/AIDS. Prophylaxis strategies for PCP and MAC have been systematically implemented in most community settings. Prophylaxis for other opportunistic infections is not universal and may be decided upon based on individual risk.

Initiation of potent antiretroviral therapy is often associated with some degree of recovery of immune function. In this situation, patients with advanced HIV disease and subclinical opportunistic infections, such as MAC or CMV, may develop a new immunologic response to the pathogen within 90 days of initiation of HAART and, thus, new symptoms may develop in association with the heightened immunologic and/or inflammatory response. This should not be interpreted as a failure of antiretroviral therapy, and these newly presenting opportunistic infections should be treated appropriately while maintaining the patient on the antiretroviral regimen. Unfortunately, response to potent antiretroviral therapy fails to adequately reconstitute the immune system. There is a sequential loss of specific types of immune responses,[78–80] so that patients with lower CD_4 counts prior to institution of potent antiretroviral therapy may have a less robust immune response to therapy, despite impressive increases in CD_4 counts. When CD_4 lymphocytes do increase in response to therapy, these cells may have a limited repertoire and are comprised primarily of memory cells rather than naive cells. This lack of ability to respond immunologically may predispose the host to opportunistic infections, despite the appearance of higher CD_4 T-lymphocyte counts. Additionally, antigen-specific loss of CD_4 T-lymphocytes has been reported in patients started on potent antiretroviral therapy whose CD_4 count has risen to greater than 200 lymphocytes/m^3 from a CD_4 nadir of less than 20 cells/m^3, yet CMV retinitis developed. Recent data are conflicting in this regard, suggesting an ability to immunologically respond to recall antigens (e.g., CMV) after introduction of potent antiretroviral agents. Therefore, prophylaxis regimens should be instituted based on CD_4 nadir, and not based on CD_4 count after response to potent antiretroviral therapy until further data are available.

Prevention and Treatment Recommendations

The following include a partial list of the most common disease-specific prevention and treatment recommendations that are co-supported by the United States Public Health Service and Infectious Diseases Society of America.[81] Standard and alternative treatments for these opportunistic infections are detailed, with some modification, in Table 14-7.[82]

Pneumocystis carinii **pneumonia.** *Pneumocystis carinii* pneumonia remains the most common opportunistic infection. However, the widespread use of prophylaxis has decreased this from 67% to 35% of incident AIDS cases in recent years. This pneumonia occurs in individuals whose CD_4 lymphocyte count is < 200 cells/m^3, CD_4 percentage < 14%, symptomatic HIV (thrush, sweats, diarrhea), or a rapidly declining CD_4 count. An algorithm for instituting PCP prophylaxis is provided in Figure 14-4. The mainstay for PCP prophylaxis is TMP/SMX; however, other agents demonstrated to be effective include dapsone and aerosolized pentamidine. In patients unable to tolerate TMP/SMX or dapsone, use of a systemic agent with low toxicity (e.g., atovaquone) should be considered with aerosolized pentamidine. Other agents, such as atovaquone and fansidar, may also be considered.

The major benefits of TMP/SMX include its effectiveness at preventing PCP, ease of administration, effectiveness in preventing toxoplasma encephalitis and bacterial infections, and its cost effectiveness. While TMP/SMX has been demonstrated to be the most effective agent to prevent PCP, its use has been limited by the high rate of adverse events such as gastrointestinal intolerance or dermatologic side effects. For patients who are TMP/SMX intolerant, either secondary to gastrointestinal or dermatologic side effects, both an 8-hour and a 21-day dose escalation protocol has been demonstrated to be effective to improve tolerance.[83] In other situations, reduction in dose to administration three times per week is another alternative.

For patients who are decidedly intolerant to TMP/SMX, the first alternative choice for PCP prophylaxis is dapsone. For patients in whom a rash from TMP/SMX develops, a rash to dapsone will develop in approximately 13% to 25%.

Before administration of dapsone, glucose-6-phosphate dehydrogenase (G-6PD) deficiency should be excluded, particularly among blacks and individuals of Mediterranean descent. When anemia to dapsone develops, a decrease in dose should be considered as the first alternative. However, if the anemia is refractory, use of aerosolized pentamidine, atovaquone, or the combination of the two, may be considered. Recently, atovaquone has been demonstrated to be as effective as dapsone and aerosolized pentamidine for PCP prophylaxis and may be considered as an alternative therapy.[84] However, dapsone is less expensive than atovaquone or aerosolized pentamidine and is preferable, unless the patient is dapsone-intolerant. The efficacy of the combination of aerosolized pentamidine and atovaquone compared to either agent as monotherapy has not been studied. Atovaquone may be preferred over aerosolized pentamidine because it is a systemic agent that prevents systemic pneumocystosis, is less expensive, and does not require a specialized delivery system. Conversely, atovaquone must be administered twice daily in a liquid formulation. Fansidar efficacy, compared to the other prophylactic agents, has not been established; however, like dapsone, G-6PD deficiency must be excluded.

First-line therapy for presumptive or proven PCP is appropriately dosed TMP/SMX (Table 14-3). This medication may be given orally or intravenously. Patients who demonstrate hypoxia with a $Po_2 < 70$ mmHg, an A-a gradient > 30 mmHg, or who demonstrate oxygen desaturation with minimal exertion, should receive adjuvant corticosteroid therapy. When adjuvant corticosteroids are administered, dermatologic side effects are less likely to occur to TMP/SMX; therefore, a prior non-life-threatening rash from TMP/SMX is not a contraindication for its use in treating PCP. For patients who meet the criteria for corticosteroids and are unable to tolerate TMP/SMX, second-line therapy includes intravenous pentamidine or trimetrexate. In some cases, the combination of trimethoprim with dapsone or Fansidar with clindamycin may be used for less severe PCP. Patients intolerant to the above regimens who have mild-to-moderate PCP may also receive atovaquone for therapy.

Toxoplasma encephalitis. Toxoplasma encephalitis (TE) is the most common opportunistic infection involving the central nervous system, and typically occurs when the CD_4 T-lymphocyte count is < 100 cells/mm^3. When administered for PCP prophylaxis, TMP/SMX,[85] and macrolides for the prophylaxis of MAC,[86] also provide protection against toxoplasmosis. Patients intolerant to TMP/SMX with a positive anti-toxoplasma serologic result should receive daily dapsone and once-weekly pyrimethamine for prophylaxis. Adjuvant folinic acid should be administered with pyrimethamine to avoid leukopenia.

Patients with diagnosed or suspected TE, based on computed tomography, magnetic resonance imaging, and a positive serologic result for toxoplasmosis, should be treated with a combination of pyrimethamine and sulfadiazine. Imaging should be repeated after 10 to 14 days of therapy. If no clinical response is detected, a brain biopsy should be considered, especially if the toxoplasma serologic result is negative. If the patient is intolerant to sulfa-containing medications or has an adverse reaction to this combination, pyrimethamine with oral or intravenous clindamycin may be used. Patients typically receive an induction course of anti-toxoplasmosis therapy for 6 to 8 weeks after diagnosis, and are maintained on reduced doses for life thereafter. During the induction phase, patients on combinations including sulfadiazine may require administration of a granulocyte–colony stimulating hormone (G-CSF) if neutropenia develops. Complications of combinations with clindamycin include rash, diarrhea, and Clostridium difficile colitis.

***Mycobacterium avium* complex.** The organisms responsible for disseminated MAC are common in environmental sources, such as food and water. The incidence of MAC steadily increased with the improved implementation of successful PCP prophylaxis; however, it has recently declined among some groups as a consequence of appropriate prophylaxis. When untreated, MAC is associated with increased morbidity and mortality and is most likely to occur in patients with advanced HIV disease ($CD_4 < 75$ cells/m^3). Development of MAC disease is correlated with patients who have MAC colonization of the respiratory or gastrointestinal tract; however, in one prospective series of patients, colonization was present in only 38% of patients in whom disseminated MAC developed. Thus, demonstration of MAC colonization is not an indication for institution of prophylaxis.

Three agents have been demonstrated to be efficacious in preventing disseminated MAC: clarithromycin, azithromycin, and rifabutin. The efficacies of preventing MAC infection in prospective studies using each of these medications were 69%, 59%, and 51%, respectively. Unlike rifabutin, clarithromycin and azithromycin also prevent episodes of bacterial infections and PCP. Studies combining rifabutin with either azithromycin[86] or clarithromycin[87] were conducted comparing each agent alone. The combination of agents substantially decreased the failure rate compared to monotherapy; however, combination therapy had nearly twice as many dose-limiting side effects. The increased cost and side effects associated with combination therapy limit its usefulness in clinical practice.

While clarithromycin has not been compared head-to-head with azithromycin, factors to consider in deciding between these two first-line agents is overall efficacy, adverse reactions, drug interactions, emergence of resistance, cost, and convenience. While clarithromycin was demonstrated to be more efficacious in preventing disseminated MAC (69% vs. 59%), azithromycin is more convenient, has time-limited adverse reactions, has fewer drug interactions with the protease inhibitors, is less likely to

Table 14-3. Drugs for prophylaxis and treatment of HIV-associated infections

Condition	Standard treatment		Alternative treatment	
	Drug	**Dosage**	**Drug**	**Dosage**
P. carinii Pneumonia Treatment	TMP-SMX	15 mg/kg/d* PO or IV in 3 or 4 doses × 21 days	Pentamidine Trimetrexate +Folinic acid Dapsone +Trimethoprim	3-4 mg/kg IV daily × 21 days 45 mg/m² IV daily × 21 days 20 mg/m² PO of IV q6h × 21 days 100 mg PO daily × 21 days 5 mg/kg PO tid × 21 days
	±Prednisone**	40 mg PO bid, days 1-5 20 mg PO bid, days 6-10 20 mg PO daily, days 11-21	Atovaquone susp. Primaquine +Clindamycin	750 mg PO tid × 21 days 15 mg base PO daily × 21 days 600 mg IV qid × 21 days or 300-450 mg PO qid × 21 days
Prophylaxis	TMP-SMX	1 DS tab PO daily	TMP-SMX Dapsone ±Pyrimethamine† Dapsone +Pyrimethamine‡‡ Aerosolized Pentamidine atovaquone	1 DS tab PO TIW 50-100 mg PO daily or 50 mg PO weekly 200 mg 75 mg Q week 300 mg inhaled monthly via Respirgard II nebulizer 750 mg PO bid (suspension)
Toxoplasmosis	Pyrimethamine‡‡ +Sulfadiazine	50-100 mg PO daily‡‡ 1.0-1.5 g PO q6h	Pyrimethamine‡‡ +Clindamycin	50-100 mg PO daily*** 400-600 mg PO or 600-1200 mg IV qid
Chronic Suppression	Pyrimethamine‡‡ +Sulfadiazine	25-50 mg PO daily 500mg-1.0g PO 6qhï	Pyrimethamine‡‡ +Clindamycin	50 mg PO daily 300 mg PO qid
Candidiasis Oral	Nystatin solution or tablets or Clotrimazole troches	500,000-1,000,000 U PO 3-5x per day 10 mg PO 5× per day	Fluconazole Itraconazole Ketoconazole	100-200 mg PO daily 200 mg PO daily 200 mg PO daily
Esophagal	Fluconazole	100-200 mg PO daily × 1-3 weeks	Itraconazole Ketoconazole Amphotericin B	200 mg PO daily 200-4 mg PO daily × 2-3 wks 0.3 mg/kg IV daily × 7 days
Coccidioidomycosis Chronic Suppressive Therapy	Amphotericin B Amphotericin B	0.5-1 mg/kg IV daily 1 mg/kg weekly	Fluconazole Itraconazole Fluconazole	400-800 mg PO daily 400 mg PO daily 200 mg PO bid
Cryptococcosis Chronic Suppression	Amphotericin B Fluconazole	0.3-1 mg/kg IV daily 200 mg PO daily‡‡	Fluconazole Amphotericin B	400-800 mg PO daily 0.5-1 mg/kg IV weekly
Histoplasmosis Chronic Suppressive Therapy	Amphotericin B Itraconazole	0.5-0.6 mg/kg IV daily 200 mg PO bid	Itraconazole Amphotericin B	200 mg PO bid 0.5-0.8 mg/kg IV weekly
Cytomegalovirus Retinitis, Colitis, Esophagitis	Ganciclovir	5 mg/kg IV q12h × 14-21day	Foscarnet	60 mg/kg IV weekly or 90 mg/kg IV q12h c 14-21 days
Chronic Suppression	Ganciclovir	5 mg/kg IV daily or 6 mg/kg IV 5×/wk or 1 gram PO tid	Foscarnet Cidofir	90-120 mg/kg IV daily 5 mg/kg weekly
Herpes Simplex, Primary or Recurrent Secondary Prophylaxis	Acyclovir Acyclovir	200-800 mg PO 5x/d 400 mg PO bid	Foscarnet Foscarnet	40 mg/kg IV q8h × 21 days 40 mg/kg IV daily
Varicella Zoster Primary or Disseminated	Acyclovir	10 mg/kg IV q8h x7-14 days	Foscarnet	40 mg/kg IV q8h
Dermatomal Zoster	Acyclovir	800 mg PO 5×/d x 7-10 days	Famciclovir Foscarnet	500 mg PO q8h × 7 days 40 mg/kg IV q8h

Table 14-3. Cont'd

Condition	Standard treatment		Alternative treatment	
	Drug	**Dosage**	**Drug**	**Dosage**
Syphilis			For all stages:	
Primary, secondary, or early latent	Benzathine PCN	2.4 mil U IM	Amoxicillin	2.0 g PO tid × 14 days
	or Doxycycline	100 mg PO bid × 14 days	+Probenecid	500 mg PO tid × 14 days
	or Erythromycin	500 mg PO qid × 14 days	or Doxycycline	200 mg PO bid × 21 days
Late latent	Benzathine PCN	2.4 mil U IM weekly × 3	or Ceftriaxone	1.0 g IM daily × 5-14 days
	or Doxycycline	100 mg PO bid × 28 days	or Benzathine PCN	2.4 mil U IM wkly × 3 doses
			+Doxycycline	200 mg PO bid × 21 days
Neurosyphillis	Aqueous PCN G	12-24 mil U/d IV × 10-14 d	Ceftriaxone	2 gm IV Qd × 14 d
	or Procaine PCN	12-24 mil U IM daily × 10 days		
	+Probenecid	500 mg PO bid × 10 days		
Disseminated MAC	Clarithromycin	500 mg PO bid		
	or Azithromycin	500 mg PO daily		
	+one or more of the following:			
	Ethambutol	15-25 mg/kg PO daily		
	Clofazimine	100-200 mg PO daily		
	Ciproflaxacin	750 mg PO bid		
	Rifabutin	300-450 mg PO daily		
	Amikacin	1 mg/kg IV q8h		
Prophylaxis	Azithromycin	1200 mg PO weekly	Rifabutin	300 mg PO daily
	or Clarithromycin	500 mg PO daily		

*Based on trimethoprim component.

**In moderate or severe PCP with room air PO_2 < 70 mmHg or Aa gradient > 35 mm Hg.

***After a 200 mg loading dose. Length of treatment determined by clinical response to therapy, usually 8 weeks.

†Plus folinic acid 10-20 mg with each dose of pyrimethamine.

‡‡400 mg/day for first four weeks.

have resistance isolates if prevention fails, and is less expensive.

For patients in prisons and jails who meet the criteria for MAC prophylaxis, the major considerations include ease of administration, cost for medication and dispensation, efficacy in preventing index disease, lack of pharmacokinetic interactions, and lack of development of resistance for infections that break through prophylaxis. In correctional settings, azithromycin is first-line prophylactic therapy because of its weekly administration, lack of drug interactions, lack of adverse side effects, and relative lack of resistant breakthrough isolates. Clarithromycin would be considered as an acceptable alternative, although it requires more frequent dosing, and 58% of breakthrough isolates are resistant to macrolide therapy, the mainstay of treatment. Rifabutin should be reserved for patients at high risk for MAC (i.e., colonized with MAC) and are not taking medications with known drug interactions with rifabutin.

Treatment of MAC, similar to the treatment of tuberculosis, should include a combination of several medications. First-line therapy should include a macrolide (clarithromycin or azithromycin), along with ethambutol and possibly one or more of the following second-line agents: rifabutin, ciprofloxain, and amikacin (intravenous only). Clarithromycin clears MAC bacteremia more rapidly than does azithromycin; therefore, it may be preferable as initial therapy for disseminated MAC. Third-line agents include clofazimine and rifampin. Rifabutin dose, when used with protease inhibitors, should be decreased to avoid toxicity and rifampin should be avoided with protease inhibitors.

Candida and yeast infections. Data from prospective controlled clinical trials indicate that fluconazole can reduce the risk of mucosal candidiasis[88–90] and cryptococcosis[91, 92] in patients with advanced HIV disease. The low mortality of candida infections, low prevalence of cryptococcal disease, potential for development of azole-resistant candida organisms, potential drug interactions, and the expense of prophylaxis, do not warrant routine primary prophylaxis.[93] Many experts treating patients with recurrent or severe oropharyngeal or vulvovaginal candidiasis, however, recommend secondary prophylaxis. Depending on factors such as number of episodes, severity, quality of life, cost, toxicities, and potential drug interactions, intermittent vs. prophylactic therapy may be considered. For patients receiving sec-

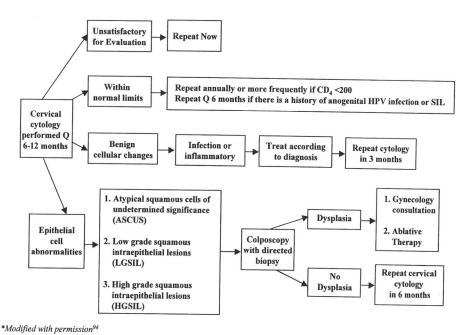

Figure 14-5. Approach to cervical cytologic evaluation for HIV-infected women.*

ondary prophylaxis, fluconazole is the preferred agent; however, itraconazole or ketoconazole may be considered.

Mucocutaneous candida infections should be treated initially with topical agents, such as clotrimazole or nystatin. For more difficult to treat infections, systemic therapy with fluconazole is recommended. For patients with symptoms suggesting esophagitis, systemic fluconazole is indicated.

Cryptococcal disease should be treated initially with intravenous amphotericin B, with or without flucytosine, followed by lifelong chronic suppression with either fluconazole or itraconazole. Most clinicians use 400 mg per day of fluconazole for 6 to 8 weeks after amphotericin induction, followed by 200 mg per day thereafter.

Cytomegalovirus. Disease from CMV has risen steadily over recent years as patients live longer. Cytomegalovirus has protean manifestations, but typically demonstrates end-organ involvement in the retina, gastrointestinal tract, and central nervous system in patients who are severely immunocompromised ($CD_4 < 50$ cells/mm^3). Oral gancyclovir (GCV) is the only agent with demonstrated efficacy in preventing CMV in patients with advanced HIV disease. Bone marrow suppression, limited efficacy, no demonstrated survival benefit, a complex regimen including twelve pills daily, and cost are important considerations when deciding about prophylaxis. Most experts do not routinely recommend CMV prophylaxis.

The most important method for preventing severe CMV disease is recognition of early manifestations of disease. Education of the "at-risk" patient to monitor for "floaters" in the eye and changes in visual field or acuity is advised.

Semi-annual fundoscopic screening in the absence of symptoms may also detect early disease before significant visual acuity is lost.

For patients with end-organ involvement due to CMV, three agents are currently available: gancyclovir, foscarnet, and cidofovir. All patients undergo a 2- to 3-week induction with therapy and must receive lifelong chronic suppressive therapy. Suppression therapy may include: 1) oral or parenteral gancyclovir; 2) parenteral foscarnet; 3) a combination of parenteral gancyclovir and foscarnet; 4) parenteral cidofovir; or 5) a gancyclovir containing intraocular implant for patients with unilateral retinitis. The intraocular implant, however, does not provide protection to the contralateral eye or other organ systems. For patients with induced neutropenia, G-CSF administration may be required.

Increased risk for cervical human papilloma virus (HPV) infection and HPV-associated dysplasia is well established among patients with HIV; however, consensus for appropriate screening protocols has not yet been established. The Centers for Disease Control and Prevention recommends two baseline Papanicolaou (Pap) smears separated by 6 months at baseline, with annual surveillance cytologic examination if both pap smear results are normal. Many experienced HIV clinicians, however, believe pap smears should be performed more frequently, because the development and progression of cervical dysplasia may be more rapid in women infected with HIV.[94, 95]

Human papilloma virus and abnormal Pap smear results. The increase in development and progression of cervical dysplasia is believed to occur because women infected with HIV have decreased tumor surveillance capacity because of their altered immunoregulatory mechanisms. Therefore, management of pre-malignant lesions should be more interventional than that in non-immuno-compromised patients. An approach to cervical cytologic evaluation for women infected with HIV is delineated in Figure 14-5. Interim Guidelines for the Management of Abnormal Cervical Cytology[96] are summarized below, based on Pap smear findings:

- Atypical Squamous Cells of Undetermined Significance (ASCUS): Treatment options vary depending on whether neoplasia is favored. If neither neoplasia nor reactive process is favored, a repeat Pap smear in 4 to 6 months without colposcopy is acceptable. If a second report of ASCUS is found within 2 years of the initial report, colposcopy with biopsy is indicated.
  Reactive Process favored: treat probable infectious etiology and repeat Pap smear in 3 months.
  Neoplasia favored: manage as if low-grade squamous intraepithelial lesion (LGSIL).
- Low-Grade Squamous Intraepithelial Lesion: patients may undergo a repeat Pap smear in 4 to 6 months or be considered immediately for colposcopy. Only patients who have had no previous abnormalities and who are very reliable for follow-up should be treated conservatively.
- High-Grade Squamous Intraepithelial Lesion (HGSIL) or Squamous Cell Carcinoma should undergo colposcopy and directed biopsy.

In the prison or jail setting, a more interventional approach is favored because 1) inmates do not necessarily remain in the correctional environment for prolonged periods; 2) if inmates are released to the community, they may not be living in stable circumstances; and 3) it is unlikely that the individual will have her gynecologic issues addressed in the community while facing issues such as securing stable housing, meeting basic needs, providing for children, and addressing issues related to treatment of her HIV/AIDS. Thus, for patients with LGSIL in the correctional setting, it is prudent to proceed directly to colposcopy with directed biopsy.[97]

If cervical dysplasia is confirmed histologically on a biopsy specimen, ablative therapy or excision should be performed for patients with HGSIL. The approach to the patient with LGSIL histologically is less clear. If the inmate has a prolonged prison sentence and her CD_4 T-lymphocyte count is < 200 cells/mm³, the gynecologist and patient may choose a conservative approach with careful monitoring. Otherwise, for patients who are pre-trial, serving shorter sentences, or who are more immunocompromised, ablative therapy or excision are encouraged for reasons stated previously in the management of abnormal pap smears.

SPECIAL ISSUES

Several potential obstacles exist within the correctional environment that may impede the provision of comprehen-

sive HIV-related health care. Careful planning and education can overcome these obstacles. First, confidentiality should never be compromised. Second, it is essential for the health services division to frequently communicate generically with the correctional authorities about health-related issues. Third, an understanding of the ramifications of interrupting or creating obstacles to receiving health care should be communicated to correctional staff, from the level of the warden to the correctional officers on the front line. Fourth, correctional administrators should participate in the development of programs that will break down unique correctional system barriers that stand in the way of providing the community standard of care. Issues involving medication dispensation, provision of HIV-related education and conduct of support groups, implementation of clinical trials, and establishing strategies for dealing with end-of-life issues, are examples of situations that require cooperation between correctional and health services staffs.

Medication Dispensation

Dispensing of antiretroviral agents pose particular problems for prisons and jails. These medications are expensive, lifelong, and may require a complex schedule. Most medications are dispensed either on the medication line or as bulk dispensation at either weekly, semimonthly, or monthly aliquots. Most systems provide only one option to inmates, and this may impede either acceptance or adherence to antiretroviral therapy. For instance, it is impractical to provide ritonavir, a medication that requires refrigeration, to prisoners at sites where bulk medication is the only method of medication dispensation. Conversely, patients receiving medications such as saquinavir or nelfinavir in bulk semimonthly aliquots must carry 126 capsules of this medication alone. The mere size of the packet of medication may identify this inmate as HIV-infected to his peers or to correctional staff, and potentially breach the prisoner's confidentiality.

For prisons that provide only directly observed therapy (DOT) for medication dispensation, several potential problems may arise. First, at prisons with a large number of prisoners with HIV, the magnitude of providing a minimal of triple combination therapy on medication line can be problematic, particularly with insufficient medical staff to dispense medications and provide the many other required duties. Second, the hours of operation for medication line may affect efficacy of antiretroviral therapies. For instance, medication line may be conducted only once or twice per day, which is inadequate for medications that must be taken more often. If medication line is provided three times per day, it may or may not coincide with meals: it is well-known that type of food and fasting states may alter drug bioavailability. Medications such as ddI and indinavir must be taken on an empty stomach and may not be taken concomitantly. Conversely, ritonavir absorption is enhanced by fatty meals, as is saquinavir by an acidic pH (e.g., grapefruit juice). Gastrointestinal side effects are minimized for several antiviral agents when dispensed with food. Therefore, prisons and jails must be creative and flexible to provide adequate life-prolonging antiretroviral therapy. Thus, it is essential for health services staff to develop flexible programs with correctional staff to minimize obstacles that would limit access to medication, which, if interrupted, may lead to irreversible resistance and antiretroviral failure.

One particular challenge is ensuring the continuity of antiretroviral therapy. Four situations merit special concern: (1) newly admitted inmates; (2) inmates transferred between facilities; (3) pre-trial detainees who have court appearances; and (4) renewal plan practices for medication by the pharmacy. Each of these situations may lead to interruption of therapy which may place the patient at risk for development of resistance. Availability of extra on-site medication may obviate delays in ordering medication from the pharmacy, and special arrangements allowing inmates to carry medication to court are essential in comprehensive HIV programs.

Several models for the delivery of medications exist within correctional settings nationwide. However, the use and misuse of expensive antiretroviral therapy and the decreased morbidity associated with adherence to medication underscores the development of novel approaches to antiretroviral dispensation. Three potential approaches can be used for the dispensation of antiretroviral agents in prisons and jails. Each approach will be discussed with regard to cost effectiveness and use of staff and resources. While each correctional system may have reasons to strive for a combination of approaches, in some settings this may not be feasible. The three approaches include bulk dispensation, DOT, and day "strip" packs.

Bulk dispensation. Bulk dispensation, or "on person medication," has been the mainstay of medication dispensation for inmates receiving "non-controlled" medication and is most consistent with the community standard of care. In community settings, individuals negotiate with their provider to take their medication, and it is the patient's responsibility for self-administering the medication.

This method of dispensation does not require large resources from either the nursing or the pharmacy staff. Unlike DOT, it does not require extensive nursing staff resources to distribute medication, nor does it require pharmacy staff to package individual pills for dispensation. While this is cost-efficient from a personnel perspective, it may be costly when patients do not consume their medication because their medication cannot be recycled once dispensed. Reasons why patients may not use the entire packet of medication include:
- Patient choice;
- Confiscation by correctional staff;
- Loss by inmate in movement from one facility to another.;
- Discontinuation by clinician because of adverse side effects.

Also, bulk dispensation makes monitoring adherence difficult because patients receive 1 to 4 weeks of medication, and a considerable amount of time may lapse before it is recognized by staff that an inmate is taking his medication incompletely. Additionally, bulk dispensation, in some settings, may be less likely to be found acceptable to inmates because they do not want to be seen carrying large medication packets that cannot be easily concealed. For example, a person taking ZDV, ddI, and nelfinavir would have large 2-week packets with 14, 28, and 126 pills, respectively.

Additionally, for patients taking ritonavir, inmates cannot carry this medication unless they have adequate access to a refrigerator for storage in their housing unit. Conversely, some inmates would not want to take their medication at the medication window three times per day, because they may be perceived by inmates or correctional staff as being "ill" (and, by association, HIV-infected), thus, bulk dispensation is the preferred option for many. Additionally, inmates who work third shift, work double shifts, or who attend school or other programs may not be able to easily interrupt their daily routines to attend the medication line at the usual limited hours of operation, and would prefer to be responsible for their own medication dispensation.

Directly observed therapy. Directly observed therapy (DOT) has been used effectively for the distribution of "controlled substances," psychiatric medications, or delivery of antituberculosis medications within correctional facilities. These medications rarely need multiple daily dosing and are not dispensed as a complex regimen involving fasting or post-prandial states. The major benefit of DOT is that adherence to therapy can be monitored most effectively. Using this method, any inmate who missed one or two doses of medication could be contacted by the appropriate medical staff to determine the reason for missed dosages. This staff person could either work with correctional or medical staff to resolve logistical constraints or counsel the inmates about the importance of adherence to therapy if the missed dose was self-imposed. Directly observed therapy would require that a medication line have long and flexible hours of operation. For instance, if a patient were prescribed ritonavir and ddI, the inmate would have to attend medication line in the morning 1 hour before mealtime to take the ddI and return again just after mealtime to take the ritonavir. If the inmate had gastrointestinal side effects from the ritonavir, this would require an additional visit to medication line 30 minutes before taking the ritonavir to receive a dose of an antiemetic. Thus, an inmate could potentially require three visits to the medication line just to complete the morning dosages of medication. In facilities where there are large proportions of inmates with HIV receiving antiretroviral agents, the duration of medication line would be prohibitive because nursing staff would have to individually prepare each inmate's medication at the time of arrival to the window. This procedure would be long and tedious, and is likely to be viewed by correctional officers as disruptive (inmates stand in line for prolonged periods outside of their usual housing units).

Some sites avoid this dilemma by sending medical staff to each housing unit to dispense medication. Such a system is unlikely to be flexible enough to deliver medications both before and after meals. Adherence may also be compromised using DOT when institutional constraints intervene, such as "lock down" status or for other security reasons. Additionally, the inconvenience to inmates may be a deterrent to either acceptance or adherence to antiretroviral agents. Directly observed therapy is the most expensive approach from a nursing staff perspective. However, it would maximize therapeutic benefit and decrease the potential for development of resistance because of the ability to monitor adherence. This would only be beneficial for those individuals accepting DOT. It would also provide a mechanism for ongoing education and counseling about antiretroviral therapy to inmates with HIV disease, as well as serve as a conduit for inmates to seek medical attention if adverse medical issues arise.

Daypack dispensation. The daypack, or "strip pack," is a hybrid of bulk dispensation and DOT. Using this procedure, the inmate would receive individual medication packets. Each pack would have the proper number of pills and time of administration directly labeled on the packet so the inmate can take his medication at the approximate prescribed time. The inmate could also be asked to take one timed dose with direct observation at retrieval of the daypack. The conceptual basis for using this procedure is that it allows for the individual to be responsible for taking the medication, yet allows the medical staff to have daily contact with the inmate to monitor adherence with therapy and to determine if complications or side effects have developed. It also decreases the likelihood that inmates with a complicated work or education schedule will have to miss taking medication because of timing or institutional constraints that impede movement within the facility.

For instance, an inmate who works third shift is unlikely to be awake for the morning medication line. He can begin his daypack with a midday or evening medication dispensation and be responsible for taking medications on his 24-hour schedule. Attendance at medication line once per day also indicates motivation on the part of the inmate to take the medication. This approach is significantly less intensive to the nursing staff than DOT and allows for daily monitoring of adherence and side effects. It also is cost-effective in recouping losses from unused pills. Any confiscated, lost, or otherwise unused medication may be reused since it is individually packed. Additionally, if an inmate's medication regimen were altered by their clinician, unused medication could also be recouped. This approach, however, may require a sophisticated and automated pharmacy that can package the medications efficiently using robotics.

For institutions with a large proportion of inmates with HIV, investment in automated pharmacy services may significantly outweigh the cost of expensive nursing staff to prepare and distribute medication as DOT. Alternatively, semi-manual systems are available for preparation of day-packs; however, these tend to be personnel-intensive. Either of these options should be strongly considered when balancing the need to minimize time that an inmate spends at medication line and the need for monitoring adherence.

Facilities able to offer multiple options of medication dispensation are likely to have the best adherence to antiretroviral therapy. For instance, programs that reward individuals for outstanding adherence by "graduating" from DOT to bulk dispensation are likely to be viewed as motivational. Alternatively, providing options allows the inmate to "participate" in the decision-making process, and thus "invests" the inmate more in his or her healthcare.

Education and Support Groups

One of the major obstacles to inmates receiving care is the lack of availability of educational material relating to treatment of their HIV disease. While many sources of HIV treatment exist, and are either free or available at a nominal fee for people living with HIV/AIDS, inmates often will not subscribe to them because possession of the information may disclose their HIV serostatus. Also, the material may be deemed contraband by correctional officials and, therefore, be confiscated. While individuals may order available information, successful ways to make information available to inmates have been implemented and include:

- Placement of medical information and periodicals in prison libraries;
- Distribution through HIV educational sessions and support groups;
- Distribution or availability of medical information at patient medical visits;
- Peer educational programs for inmates with HIV infection.

Through a health education program aimed at all prisoners, and made mandatory by the facility, treatment of HIV/AIDS can become less onerous and perhaps less stigmatizing. Given the number of inmates who meet the high-risk category for HIV/AIDS, an education program with a supportive component, and with an attitude such as "everyone here should be reading this material," will help to change the climate regarding discussion of the disease and, thereby, improve acceptance of treatment.

Additional work with correctional administrators and officers is essential to improving the educational environment for the entire prison so that flexible patterns of care can be provided that ensure inmate accessibility to education, medical care, and treatment. Such work should involve correctional officers in the development of such programs. Correctional officers, except in rare circumstances, should not conduct support and education groups for individuals who are infected with HIV, because this may limit enrollment to those who are most empowered.

Clinical Trials

Much confusion and misinformation permeates the medical, research, criminal justice, and legal communities regarding the inclusion of prisoners in research. This is particularly true regarding prisoners with HIV/AIDS. Few correctional systems have provisions or written procedures allowing the use of prisoners in clinical trials and, even fewer do so for HIV/AIDS.[98]

For prisoners who come from high HIV-prevalence areas, clinical trials are considered within the context of the community standard of care. Notwithstanding the historical reasons for excluding prisoners from clinical trials, federal guidelines exist that govern clinical trials for prisoners.[99] Additionally, several programs are already in existence that have successfully integrated clinical trials for HIV into routine clinical care.

Federal regulations restrict research on prisoners to four narrowly defined categories: 1) research on the possible causes, effects, processes of incarceration, and criminal behavior; 2) research on prisons as institutional structures or of prisoners as incarcerated persons; 3) research on conditions, particularly affecting prisoners as a class; and 4) therapeutic research. The justification for involvement of prisoners in clinical trials for HIV is included in language in categories 3 and 4. For most correctional systems, HIV disproportionately affects prisoners more than the surrounding community, and newer HIV therapeutics have marked potential of life-prolonging outcome. Additionally, the United States Department of Health and Human Services thinks that research subjects should not be deprived of health benefits, even experimental ones, simply because the subject is a prisoner.[100] Any clinical research involving prisoners must have approval by an Institutional Review Board (IRB) using guidelines developed by the National Commission for the Protection of Human Subjects in Biomedical and Behavioral Research.[101] These review boards are similar to those within universities that oversee research protocols involving human subjects. The IRB must include a prisoner advocate. Such research must not involve the use of a placebo and cannot be deemed coercive by promising privileges or other inducements. Already in existence are several linkages between academic institutions and correctional systems that have successfully integrated clinical trials into routine care, using IRBs within the academic institution.

Successful implementation of clinical trials for the treatment of HIV disease have been initiated in Maryland (in association with Johns Hopkins University), Texas (in association with the University of Texas in Galveston), New York (in association with Albany Medical Center Hospital and with St. Claire's Hospital and Health Center), and in a few other sites. Other states have made exceptions for the compassionate use of medications for the treatment of HIV or sone of its complications. The benefits to the prisoners is that it allows them access to the community standard of care, allows access to potentially life-saving or life-prolonging therapies, and improves clinical supervision of care. Such programs cannot offer incentives that would otherwise seem coercive. Benefits to the correctional system are that it provides "outside" clinical expertise, it offsets the costs of antiretroviral agents or other medications, and enhances the clinical supervision of patient care. Multiple barriers exist to implementation of such programs; however, once the institutional constraints are overcome, successful models can help pave the way for future collaborations. Existing collaborations may serve as models to other systems intending to introduce clinical trials in the future.

Indeed, the correctional health services and administrative staff must overcome administrative obstacles such as fee provision, geographic localization, access to follow-up visits, packaging and dispensation of experimental medications, and protection of confidentiality. Although complicated, these clinical care and logistical issues can be overcome through careful planning. To develop adequate introduction of clinical trials and research within the prison setting, state legislation and correctional policies must be reviewed and changed as indicated. Once legal constraints have been lifted, an appropriate collaboration and IRB must be established. Use of the affiliated academic medical center has been the most successful model. Lastly, logistical issues must be addressed proactively. These include:

- Minimization of breaches of confidentiality of inmate;
- Transportation to research site;
- Access to medical records and documentation;
- Limiting inter-institutional transfers to assure continued access to clinical trials personnel;
- Communication between DOC and research site on inmate transfer;
- Special arrangements for dispensation and provision for carrying "research" medications;
- Continuity of care within DOC, the correctional system, and to the outside community upon release.

As more academic medical institutions enter into managed care agreements with correctional systems, so will the increase in access to clinical trials. In other such settings, correctional systems will need to actively seek other such collaborations to improve the health care provision and ongoing education to staff.

End-of-Life Issues

Prisons and jails have traditionally not been equipped to deal with end-of-life issues. The recent aging of the prison population and the magnitude of HIV within correctional systems have prompted many correctional systems to explore these issues. This remains true, despite the recent decreased census of hospitalized AIDS patients and AIDS patients in hospices thought to be secondary to potent antiretroviral therapy. Important issues to be addressed by correctional health services include living wills and advance directives for inmates with terminal conditions, expertise regarding hospice nursing, medical parole or compassionate release, and family and psychological support addressing grief and loss needs for prisoners.

Caring for terminal patients and the process of dying within the correctional setting impacts the prisoner, other prisoners with similar conditions, friends and family who may be removed physically from the patient, and the health care workers and correctional staff. The impact of premature loss of life may be particularly disturbing to all parties involved. Separation of the inmate from family and friends from within and outside of the correctional system may be devastating. Death in this setting is contrary to the natural order of the dying process, as is the premature loss of life imposed by the complication of AIDS. A proactive approach to resolve these issues may obviate potential problems that may develop otherwise.

Advance directives should be addressed with all inmates with HIV who have very advanced HIV infection (e.g., CD_4 count < 50 cells/mm^3), particularly for those serving long sentences. Advance directives are, therefore, more of an issue for prison, rather than jail settings. Development of guidelines should include dialogue between the medical and legal staff. When possible, clinical staff from outside the correctional medical staff should be involved to avoid conflict of interest.

Hospice nursing and medical care expertise can be gained through arrangements between correctional settings and local or national hospice organizations. Some correctional settings may choose to reserve hospice beds in community settings to allow dying inmates to receive the expert hospice care near family and friends. Other correctional settings have developed an infrastructure to provide this care within the correctional setting. Successful correctional models have required dialogue between correctional and medical administrators to provide peer support from other inmates, allow family and friends visitation within medical units, and to implement grief and loss groups to both inmates and professional staff. Allowances of visitation rights by family and friends poses special challenges, particularly when they are on probation, parole, or are recent ex-offenders.

Another option exercised by various correctional systems includes medical parole or compassionate release stipulations provided by legislation or correctional policy. While considerable variation exists between states in both the language of the policy and in its implementation, it seems to be governed by two stipulations: 1) the inmate must not have not committed a capital offense or committed a felony using a weapon; and 2) the inmate must be deemed incapable of committing an additional crime. Interpretation of the second stipulation appears to limit the effectiveness of this policy. Medical practitioners are incapable of guaranteeing that criminal activity is impossible. Additionally, the correctional system broadly interprets this stipulation to mean that an inmate has stable living circumstances upon release. Interpretation of "stable" remains subjective and limits access to this often underused option.

Successful programs, such as the one in Maryland, seem to have effectively moved patients to the community to receive terminal care by family or hospice, and decreased the costly care necessary for patients with AIDS in their terminal 6 months of life. The Maryland program also had few problems associated with recidivist criminal behavior. Other states have been unsuccessful in implementing such programs, either because of lack of provision for medical parole/compassionate release or for its interpretation. Hopefully, with increased attention to this under-evaluated problem, correctional systems will re-examine the need for addressing end-of-life issues that are appropriate for their individual needs.

CONCLUSIONS

Despite the myriad of obstacles and complexity of care necessary for inmates infected with HIV, correctional systems can provide comprehensive programs for the treatment of HIV/AIDS. Such programs require adequate access to recent technologic advances and newer antiretroviral agents, as well as expertise in the management of HIV. National guidelines both for the treatment of HIV itself and for the treatment and prophylaxis of opportunistic infections can be effectively translated to the correctional environment. In particular, the method of antiretroviral dispensation, provision of education and support groups, access to clinical trials for the treatment of HIV, and addressing end-of-life issues are of utmost concern for correctional systems. Considerable experience has been gained to effectively link inmates infected with HIV to medical services upon release; however, this has not been universally translated to all correctional systems. Continuity of care remains one of the special challenges to correctional systems. As such, correctional systems can expand the HIV paradigm of clinical care to provide a unique model of care that would enhance the management of other chronic diseases. Implementation of such comprehensive programs can lead to a societal cost-effective program and decrease the morbidity and mortality to inmates within correctional systems, as well as to the community upon their release, if continuity of care models exists.

REFERENCES

1. Volberding PA: Improving the outcomes of care for patients with human immunodeficiency virus infection (editorial). *New Engl J Med* 334:729-731, 1996.
2. Smith S, Robinson J, Hollyer J, et al: Combining specialist and pri-

mary health care teams for HIV positive patients: Retrospective and prospective studies. *Br Med J* 312:416-420, 1996.

3. Henry K: Management of HIV infection. A 1995-96 overview for the clinician. *Minn Med* 78:17-24, 1995.

4. Paauw DS, Wenrich MD, Curtis JR, et al: Ability of primary care physicians to recognize physical findings associated with HIV infection. *JAMA* 274:1308-1382, 1995.

5. Turner BJ, McKee L, Fanning T, et al: AIDS specialist versus generalist ambulatory care for advanced HIV infection and impact on hospital use. *Med Care* 32:902-916, 1994.

6. Fulcher D, Clezy K: Managing HIV. Antiretroviral therapy. *Med J Aust* 164:607, 1996.

7. Shahmanesh M: Who Owns Aids (letter)? *Br J Hosp Med* 57:228, 1997.

8. Holmes WC: Quality in HIV/AIDS care. Specialty-related or experience-related (editorial)? *J Gen Intern Med* 12:195-197, 1997.

9. Markson LE, Turner BJ, Cocroft J, et al: Clinic services for persons with AIDS. Experience in a high-prevalence state. *J Gen Intern Med* 12:141-149, 1997.

10. Kithata MM, Koepsell TD, Deyo RA, et al: Physicians' experience with the acquired immunodeficiency syndrome as a factor in patients' survival. *New Engl J Med* 334:701-706, 1996.

11. Bennett CL, Garfinkle JB, Greenfield S, et al: The relation between hospital experience and in-hospital mortality for patients with AIDS-related PCP. *JAMA* 261:2975-2979, 1989.

12. Bennett CL, Adams J, Gertler P, et al: Relation between hospital experience and in-hospital mortality for patients with AIDS-related Pneumocystis carinii pneumonia: Experience from 3,126 cases in New York City in 1987. *J AIDS* 5:856-864, 1992.

13. Turner BJ, Ball JK: Variations in inpatient mortality for AIDS in a national sample of hospitals. *J AIDS* 5:978-987, 1992.

14. Stone VE, Seage GR III, Hertz T, et al: The relation between hospital experience and mortality for patients with AIDS. *JAMA* 268:2655-2661, 1992.

15. Markson LE, Cosler LE, Turner BJ: Implications of generalists' slow adoption of zidovudine in clinical practice. *Arch Intern Med* 154:1497-1504, 1994.

16. Cohen RL, Altice FL, Greenspan J,et al: Standards for HIV-AIDS care in prisons & Jails. Update to the APHA Publication: Standards for Health Care Services in Correctional Institutions, 2nd ed. Washington D.C., American Public Health Association, 1996.

17. World Health Organization: Health in prisons: Health promotion in the prison setting: Summary report on a WHO meeting, London, 15-17 October. Copenhagen WHO Regional Office for Europe, 1996.

18. World Health Organization: WHO guidelines on HIV infection and AIDS in prisons. Geneva World Heath Organization, 1993.

19. Altice FL, Mostashari F, Thompson AS, et al: Perceptions, acceptance, and adherence to antiretrovirals among prisoners. The 4th Conference on Retroviruses and Opportunistic Infections, Washington D.C., January 1997.

20. Cherubin C: The medical sequelae of narcotic addiction. *Ann Intern Med* 67:23-33, 1967.

21. Sapira JD: The narcotic addict as a medical patient. *Am J Med* 45:555-558, 1968.

22. Louria DB, Hensle T, Rose J: The major medical complications of narcotic addiction. *Ann Intern Med* 67:1-32, 1967.

23. Ho DD, Neumann AU, Perelson AS, et al: Rapid turnover of plasma virions and CD_4 lymphocytes in HIV-1 infection. *Nature* 373:123-126, 1995.

24. Pantaleo G, Graziosi C, Demarest J, et al: HIV infection is active and progressive in lymphoid tissue during the clinically latent stage of disease. *Nature* 362:355-358, 1993.

25. Wei X, Ghosh SK, Taylor ME, et al: Viral dynamics in human immunodeficiency virus type 1. *Nature* 373:117-122, 1995.

26. Perelson AS, Neumann AU, Markowitz M, et al: HIV-1 dynamics in vivo: Virion clearance rate, infected cell life-span, and viral generation time. *Science* 217:1582-1586, 1996.

27. Haynes BF, Panteleo G, Fauci AS: Toward an understanding of the correlates of protective immunity to HIV infection. *Science* 335:1091-1098, 1996.

28. Haase AT, Henry K, Zupancic M, et al: Quantitative image analysis of HIV-1 infection in lymphoid tissue. *Science* 274:985- 989, 1996.

29. Cohen OJ, Pantaleo G, Schwartzentruber DJ, et al: Pathogenic insights from studies of lymphoid tissue from HIV-infected individuals (review). *J AIDS* 10(Suppl 1):6-14, 1995.

30. Tamalet C, Lafeuillade A, Yahi N: Comparison of viral burden and phenotype of HIV-1 isolates from lymph nodes and blood. *AIDS* 8:1083-1088, 1994.

31. Cohen OJ, Pantaleo G, Lamb GK, et al: Studies on lymphoid tissue from HIV-infected individuals: Implications for the design of therapeutic strategies. *Springer Semin Immunopathol* 18:305-322, 1997.

32. Yen-Lieberman B, Brambilla D, Jackson B, et al: Evaluation of a quality assurance program for quantitation of human immunodeficiency virus type 1 RNA in plasma by the AIDS clinical trials group virology laboratories. *J Clin Microbiol* 24:2695-2701, 1996.

33. Schuurman R, Descamps D, Jan Weverling G, et al: Multicenter comparison of three commercial methods for quantification of human immunodeficiency virus type 1 in plasma. *J Clin Microbiol* 34: 3016-3022, 1996.

34. Revets H, Marissens D, de Wit S, et al: Comparative evaluation of NASBA HIV-1 RNA QT, AMPLICOR-HIV monitor, and QUANTIPLEX HIV RNA assay, three methods for quantification of human immunodeficiency virus type 1 in plasma. *J Clin Microbiol* 34: 1058-1064, 1996.

35. Raboud JM, Montaner JSG, Conway B, et al: Variation in plasma RNA levels, CD_4 cell counts, and p24 antigen levels in clinically stable men with human immunodeficiency virus infection. *J Infect Dis* 174:1191-1199, 1996.

36. Deeks SG, Coleman RL, White R, et al: Variance of plasma HIV-1 RNA levels measured by branch DNA (bDNA) within and between days. *J Infec Dis,* 176(2):514-517, 1997.

37. Stanley SK, Ostrowski MA, Justement JS, et al: Effect of immunization with a common recall antigen on viral expression in patients infected with human immunodeficiency virus type 1. *New Engl J Med* 334:1222-1230, 1996.

38. Mellors JW, Kingsley LA, Rinaldo CR, et al: Quantitation of HIV-1 RNA in plasma predicts outcome after seroconversion. *Ann Intern Med* 112:573-579, 1995.

39. O'Brien TR, Blattner WA, Waters D, et al: Serum HIV-1 RNA levels and time to development of AIDS in the multicenter hemophilia cohort study. *JAMA* 276:105-110, 1996.

40. Jurriaans S, van Gemen B, Weverling GJ, et al: The natural history of HIV-1 infection: Virus load and virus phenotype independent determinants of clinical course? *Virology* 204:223-233, 1994.

41. Saksela K, Stevens CE, Rubenstein P, et al: HIV-1 messenger RNA in peripheral blood mononuclear cells with an early marker of risk for progression to AIDS. *Ann Intern Med* 123:641-648, 1995.

42. O'Brien WA, Hartigan PM, Martin D, et al: Changes in plasma HIV-1 RNA and CD_4 lymphocyte counts and the risk of progression to AIDS. *N Engl J Med* 334:426-431, 1996.

43. O'Brien TR, Rosenberg PS, Goedert JJ: Longitudinal HIV-1 RNA levels in a cohort of homosexual men. Submitted.

44. Katzenstein DA, Hammer SM, Hughes MD, et al: The relation of virologic and immunologic markers to clinical outcomes after nucleoside therapy in HIV-infected adults with 200 to 500 CD_4 cells per cubic millimeter. *New Engl J Med* 335:1091-1098, 1996.

45. Dickover RE, Dillon M, Gillette SG, et al: Rapid increase in load of human immunodeficiency virus correlate with early disease progression and loss of CD_4 cells in vertically infected infants. *J Infect Dis* 170:1279-1284, 1994.

46. McIntosh K, Shevitz A, Zaknun D, et al: Age-and time-related

changes in extracellular viral load in children vertically infected by human immunodeficiency virus. *Pediatr Infect Dis J* 15:1087-1091, 1996.

47. Mofenson LM, Korelitz J, Meyer WA, et al: The relationship between serum human immunodeficiency virus type 1 (HIV-1) RNA level, CD_4 lymphocyte percent, and long-term mortality risk in HIV-1–infected children. *J Infect Dis* 175:1029-1038, 1997.

48. Dickover RE, Dillon M, Leung K-M, et al: Early prognostic indicators in primary perinatal HIV-1 infection: Importance of viral RNA and the timing of transmission on long-term outcome. *JAMA,* in press.

49. Shearer WT, Quinn TC, LaRussa P, et al: Viral load and disease progression in infants infected with human immunodeficiency virus type 1. *New Engl J Med* 336:1337, 1997.

50. Mellors JW, Rinaldo CR Jr, Gupta P, et al: Prognosis in HIV-1 infection predicted by the quantity of virus in plasma. *Science* 272:1167-1170, 1996.

51. Enger C, Graham N, Peng Y, et al: Survival from early, intermediate, and late stages of HIV infection. *JAMA* 275:1329-1334, 1996.

52. Stein DS, Korvick JA, Vermund SH: CD_4 lymphocyte cell enumeration for prediction of clinical course of human immunodeficiency virus disease: A review. *J Infect Dis* 165:352-363, 1992.

53. Mellors, JW, Munoz A, Giorgi J, et al: Plasma viral load and CD4 lymphocytes as prognostic markers of HIV-1 infection. *Ann Intern Med,* in press.

54. USPHS/IDSA Prevention of Opportunistic Infections Working Group: USPHS/IDSA guidelines for the prevention of opportunistic infections in persons infected with human immunodeficiency virus: A summary. In press.

55. El-Sadr W, Oleske JM, Agins BD, et al: Evaluation and management of early HIV infection. Rockville, MD, U.S. Department of Health and Human Services, Public Health Service, Agency for Health Care Policy and Research, January 1994, DHHS publication no. (AHCPR)94-0572.

56. Finkelstein DM, Williams PL, Molenberghs G, et al: Patterns of opportunistic infections in patients with HIV infection. *J AIDS* 12:38-45, 1996.

57. Mellors JW, Munoz A, Giorgi JV, et al: Plasma viral load and CD_4 lymphocytes as prognostic markers of HIV-1 infection. *Ann Intern Med* 126:946-954, 1997.

58. Sandberg J, Slikker W: Developmental pharmacology and toxicology of anti-HIV therapeutic agents: Dideoxynucleosides. *FASEB J* 9:1157-1163, 1995.

59. Philips AN, Eron JJ, Bartlet JA, et al: HIV-1 RNA levels and the development of clinical disease. *AIDS* 10:859-865, 1996.

60. Coombs RW, Welles SL, Hooper C, et al: Association of plasma human immunodeficiency virus type-1 RNA level with risk of clinical progression in patients with advanced infection. *J Infect Dis* 174:704-712, 1996.

61. Welles SL, Jackson JB, Yen-Lieberman B, et al: Prognostic value of plasma human immunodeficiency virus (HIV-1) RNA levels in patients with advanced HIV-1 disease and with little or no prior zidovudine therapy. *J Infect Dis* 174:696-703, 1996.

62. Perelson AS, Essunger P, Cao Y, et al: Decay characteristics of HIV-1–infected compartments during combination therapy. *Nature* 387:188-191, 1997.

63. Caliendo AM, Hirsch MS: Combination therapy for infection due to human immunodeficiency virus type 1. *Clin Infect Dis* 18:516- 524, 1994.

64. Yarchoan R, Lietzau JA, Nguyen BY, et al. A randomized pilot study of alternating or simultaneous zidovudine and didanosine therapy in patients with symptomatic human immunodeficiency virus infection. *J Infect Dis* 1994; 169:9-17.

65. Collier AC, Coombs RW, Fischl MA, et al: Combination therapy with zidovudine and didanosine compared with zidovudine alone in HIV-1 infection. *Ann Intern Med* 119:786-793, 1993.

66. Katlama C, Ingrand D, Loveday C, et al: Safety and efficacy of lamivudine-zidovudine combination therapy in antiretroviral-naive patients: A randomized controlled comparison with zidovudine monotherapy. *JAMA* 276:118-125, 1996.

67. Fischl MA, Stanley K, Collier AC, et al: Combination and monotherapy with zidovudine and zalcitabine I patients with advanced HIV disease. *Ann Intern Med* 122:24-32, 1995.

68. Meng TC, Fischl MA, Boota Am, et al: Combination therapy with zidovudine and dideoxycytidine in patients with advanced human immunodeficiency virus infection: A phase I/II study. *Ann Intern Med* 116:13-20, 1992.

69. Cameron DW, Heath-Chiozzi M, Kravcik S, et al: Prolongation of life and prevention of AIDS complications in advanced HIV immunodeficiency with ritonavir: Update. XI international Conference on AIDS, Vancouver, July 1996 (Abstract MoB411).

70. Steigbigel R, Berry P, Teppler H, et al: Extended follow-up of patients in a study of indinavir at 800 mg q8h (2.4 g/D), 100 mg q8h (3.0 g/D) and 800 mg q6h (3.2 g/D). XI international Conference on AIDS, Vancouver, July 1996 (Abstract MoB412).

71. Collier AC, Coombs RW, Schoenfeld DA, et al: Treatment of human immunodeficiency virus infection with saquinavir, zidovudine, and zalcitabine. *N Engl J Med* 334:1011-1017, 1996.

72. Gulick R, Mellors J, Havlir D, et al: Potent and sustained antiretroviral activity of indinavir, zidovudine, and lamivudine. XI international Conference on AIDS, Vancouver, July 1996 (Abstract ThB931).

73. Kaplan JE, Maur H, Holmes KK, et al: USPHS/IDSA guidelines for the prevention of opportunistic infections in persons infected with human immunodeficiency virus: Introduction. *Clin Infect Dis* 21(suppl 1):S1-S11, 1995.

74. Selik RM, Chu SY, Ward JW: Trends in infectious diseases and cancers among persons dying of HIV infection in the United States from 1987 to 1992. *Ann Intern Med* 123:933-936, 1995.

75. Moore RD, Chaisson RE: Natural history of opportunistic disease in an HIV-infected urban clinical cohort. *Ann Intern Med* 124:633-642, 1996.

76. Jones JL, Hanson DL, Ward JW, Kaplan JE: Incidence trends in AIDS-related opportunistic illnesses in injecting drug users and men who have sex with men (Abstract We.C.3418) vol 2. XI International Conference on AIDS. Vancouver, July 7-12, 1996.

77. Moore RD, Chaisson RE: Natural history of opportunistic disease in an HIV-infected urban clinical cohort. *Ann Intern Med* 124:633-642, 1996.

78. Shearer G, Clerici M: Early T-helper cells defects in HIV infection. *AIDS* 5:245-253, 1991.

79. Schnittmam S, Lane HC, Greenhouse J, et al: Preferential infection of CD4 memory T cells by human immunodeficiency virus type 1: Evidence for a role in selective T cell functional defects observed in infected individuals. *Proc Natl Acad Sci USA* 87:6058-6062, 1990.

80. Connors M, Kovacks JA, Krevath S, et al: HIV infection induces changes in CD4 T cell phenotype and depletions within the CD4 T-cell repertoire that are not immediately restored by antiviral or immune-based therapies. *Nature Med* 3:533-540, 1997.

81. Kaplan JE, Maur H, Holmes KK, et al: USPHS/IDSA guidelines for the prevention of opportunistic infections in persons infected with human immunodeficiency virus: Introduction. *Clin Infect Dis* 1995;21(suppl 1):1-11, 1995.

82. Abramowicz M, ed: Drugs for AIDS and associated infections. *Med Letter Drugs Ther* 959:90-91, 1995.

83. Simonds RJ, Hughes WT, Feinberg J, Navin TR: Preventing Pneumocystitis carinii pneumonia in persons infected with human immunodeficiency virus (review). *Clin Infect Dis* 21(suppl 1): 44-48, 1995.

84. El-Sadr W, Murphy R, Luskin-Hawk R, et al: Atovaquone (ATV) versus dapsone(DAP) in the prevention of P. carinii pneumonia (PCP) in patients intolerant to trimethoprim and/or sulfamethoxazole

(TMP/SMX) CPCRA 034/ACTG 277. Presented at the 35th Annual Meeting of the Infectious Diseases Society of America, September 13-16, 1997, San Francisco, CA (Abstract 769).

85. Leoung G, Stanford J, Giordano M, et al: A randomized, double-blind trial of TMP/SMX dose escalation vs. direct rechallenge in HIV+ persons at risk for PCP and with prior treatment-limiting rash or fever (Abstract LB-10). 37th ICAAC, Toronto, 1997.

86. Havlir DV, Dube MP, Sattler FR, et al: Prophylaxis against disseminated Mycobacterium avium complex with weekly azithromycin, daily rifabutin, or both. *New Engl J Med* 335:392- 398, 1996.

87. Benson CA, Cohn DL, Williams P, et al: A phase III prospective, randomized, double-blind study of the safety and efficacy of clarithromycin vs. rifabutin vs. CLA+RBT for prevention of Mycobacterium avium complex disease in HIV+ patients with CD4 counts < 100 cells/mL (Abstract 205). Presented at the 3rd Conference on Retroviruses and Opportunistic Infections, Washington, D.C., 1996.

88. Manfredi R, Mastroianni A, Coronado OC, et al: Fluconazole as prophylaxis against fungal infection in patients with advanced HIV infection. *Arch Intern Med* 157:64-69, 1997.

89. Powderly WG, Finkelstein D, Feinber J, et al: A randomized trial comparing fluconazole with clotrimazole troches for the prevention of fungal infections in patients with advanced human immunodeficiency virus infection. NIAID AIDS Clinical Trials Group. *New Engl J Med* 332:700-705, 1995.

90. Schuman P, Capps L, Peng G, et al: Weekly fluconazole for the prevention of mucosal candidiasis in women with HIV infection. A randomized, double-blind, placebo-controlled trial. Terry Beirn Community Programs for Clinical Research on AIDS. *Arch Intern Med* 126:689-965, 1997.

91. Singh N, Barnish MJ, Berman S, et al: Low-dose fluconazole as primary prophylaxis for cryptococcal infection in AIDS patients with CD4 cell counts of < or = 100/mm³: Demonstration of efficacy in a positive, multicenter trial. *Clin Infect Dis* 23:1282-1286, 1996.

92. Quagliarello VJ, Viscoli C, Horwitz RI: Primary prevention of cryptococcal meningitis by fluconazole in HIV-infected patients. *Lancet* 345:548-552, 1995.

93. Reef SE, Mayer KH: Opportunistic candidal infections in patients infected with human immunodeficiency virus: Prevention issues and priorities. *Clin Infect Dis* 21(Suppl 1):99-102, 1995.

94. Williams AB: Gynecologic care of women with human immunodeficiency virus infection. *Clin Excellence Nurse Practitioners* 1: 115-123, 1997.

95. Maiman M, Fruchter R, Serur E, et al: Recurrent cervical intraepithelial neoplasia in human immunodeficiency virus-seropositive women. *Obstet Gynecol* 82:170- 174, 1993.

96. Kurman RJ, Henson DE, Herbst AL, et al: Interim guidelines for management of abnormal cervical cytology. The 1992 NCI Workshop. *JAMA* 271:1866-1869, 1994.

97. El-Sadr W, Oleske JM, Agins BD, et al: Evaluation and management of early HIV infection. Clinical practice guideline No. 7. Agency for Health Care Policy and Research, Public Health Service, US Department of Health and Human Service, Rockville, MD, 1994.

98. Potler C, Sharp VL, Remick S: Prisoners' access to HIV experimental trials: Legal, ethical, and practical considerations (review). *J AIDS* 7:1086-1094, 1994.

99. Code of the Federal Register, 46.306. Washington D.C., Department of Health and Human Services, 1996.

100. Code of the Federal Register, 53.654. Washington D.C., Department of Health and Human Services, 1978.

101. Code of the Federal Register, 46.103 (e) and 46.109 (a). Washington D.C., Department of Health and Human Services, 1989.

15

Use of Antiretroviral Agents in the Treatment of HIV

Frederick L. Altice, M.D.

The treatment of patients infected with the human immunodeficiency virus (HIV) is becoming increasingly more complex as newer medications and technologies are approved. Over the past 2 years, the rapid rate of development of technology and antiretroviral agents has provided new options for optimal management of HIV itself. The recent advances include: 1) a better understanding of viral replication kinetics leading to our improved understanding of HIV pathogenesis; 2) the development of quantitative viral load assays and the demonstration of their ability to predict disease progression and response to therapy; 3) the development and availability of new and more potent antiretroviral agents; and 4) clinical data documenting the superiority of combination therapy, particularly combinations that include a protease inhibitor.

Optimal suppression of HIV replication is best accomplished through the use of a combination of anti-HIV agents. Several studies have demonstrated the superiority of

combination therapy over monotherapy. Studies in the United States (ACTG 175)[1, 2] and in Europe (DELTA)[3] both demonstrated that zidovudine (ZDV) monotherapy is suboptimal and that clinical outcomes were improved when ZDV was combined with didanosine (ddI) or zalcitabine (ddC). These trials also demonstrated that instituting combination therapy at $CD_4 < 500$ cells/mm^3 resulted in a clinical and survival benefit.

Other trials comparing ZDV with the combination of ZDV plus lamivudine (3TC) resulted in clinical and survival benefits as well.[4] Recently, ACTG 320 demonstrated a 50% reduction in mortality in patients whose CD_4 was < 200, using a triple combination which included the protease inhibitor, indinavir, with ZDV and 3TC, compared to ZDV plus 3TC alone. Other studies using combinations that include a protease inhibitor have been demonstrated to have both an increase in magnitude in reduction of viral load as well as in duration, compared to combinations that do not include one.[5, 6] Similar studies involving combinations using a non-nucleoside reverse transcriptase inhibitor (NNRTI) have shown sustained reductions in viral load, however less efficacious than combinations using a protease inhibitor.[7] Thus, the current data provide clinical justification for starting patients on potent protease inhibitor combinations at both late and early stages of disease.

For antiretroviral-naïve patients, the most potent combination of nucleoside analogues include the use of a thymidine analogue (ZDV or d4T) combined with a purine analogue (ddl, ddC, 3TC, or abacavir). Combinations of d4T with ddC should be avoided because of concern for neurotoxicity and combinations of d4T with ZDV should be avoided because of competition for phosphorylation, thus leading to clinical deterioration. Appropriate nucleoside analogue combinations may produce an average peak viral load reduction of 1.2 to 1.7 logs; however, this may not be sustained in combinations using 3TC because of the rapid rate of development of resistance. This means that, for patients whose viral load is > 30,000 copies/mm^3, it is unlikely that one can achieve a sustained non-detectable viral load level (HIV-1 RNA < 400 copies/mm^3) using any of these combinations. Therefore, to achieve maximal viral suppression, one should combine a protease inhibitor, or at a minimum, an NNRTI, with double nucleoside analogue combinations.

Selected combinations should be administered with a predefined target regarding degree of suppression. Each agent used should permit further therapeutic options if possible, and should not be cross-resistant with the other antiretroviral agents in the combination. For example, patients administered a regimen containing ZDV and 3TC who do not achieve sustained "non-detectable" viral load may not respond to other nucleoside analogues that may be cross-resistant with either agent (e.g., both 3TC and ddl have important mutations at 184V that confer resistance to HIV and prior ZDV therapy may limit future options using d4T). Where mutations are identical, cross-resistance may occur.

The recent data suggesting incomplete suppression of viral replication and the emergence of resistant isolates of HIV to administered antiretroviral agents indicate that combinations should be maximally effective and combined in ways that are at least additive in antiviral activity and, at best, synergistic. Combination antiretroviral therapy that maximally suppresses viral replication delays the emergence of resistance, is more potent in reducing viral load, may attack the virus at multiple points in its replication cycle, and has been demonstrated to delay the progression to AIDS or death and prevent progressive immune deficiency. Factors to be considered in selecting combinations of antiretroviral agents include:
- Prior antiretroviral exposure
- Baseline HIV-RNA level
- Co-morbid medical conditions (e.g., anemia, pancreatitis, peripheral neuropathy)
- Potential drug interactions
- Ease of administration (meals, number of times per day, number of pills, taste, etc.)
- Agents to which HIV is less likely to become resistant.

A major obstacle to suppression of HIV replication is its inherent ability for developing drug resistance. Rational use of combination therapies can prevent or delay the development of drug resistance and provide the patient with optimal clinical benefit. It is particularly beneficial if treatment begins before viral load exceeds the expected ability of a drug combination to completely suppress replication. In these situations (e.g., HIV-1 RNA > 100,000 copies/mL), it may be prudent to initiate patients with four potent antiretrovirals.

Potential risks of combination therapy include increased toxicity, reduction in the quality of life, increased problems with adherence, and increased cost. Careful consideration and discussion between the clinician and patient is necessary to avoid the potential complications of combination therapy, especially given that monotherapy and dual nucleoside analogues combinations are no longer considered to be viable options.

OVERVIEW FOR TREATMENT OF HIV

Based on the understanding of the pathogenesis of HIV, the use of viral load testing and the new highly active antiretroviral agents, the International AIDS Society/USA (IAS/USA)[8] and the NIH consensus panel[9] have issued guidelines for initiating antiretroviral therapy for individuals with HIV seroconversion and for those with established HIV infection. A brief overview of the existing antiretroviral agents approved by the Food and Drug Administration (FDA) will be presented along with the guidelines for initiation and treatment of HIV.

There are three classes of antiretroviral agents that are available for the treatment of HIV disease. These include the nucleoside analogue reverse transcriptase inhibitors (RTIs), the non-nucleoside analogue reverse transcriptase inhibitors (NNRTIs), and the protease inhibitors (PIs). Tables 15-1 through 15-3 provide summary information about each of the agents within each class of antiretroviral agent.

Nucleoside Analogue Reverse Transcriptase Inhibitors

The RTIs were the first class of antiretroviral agents developed. Clinicians have had the most experience using RTIs initially as monotherapy, and more recently, in combination therapy (Table 15-1). The primary mechanism of action of this class is through inhibition of viral RNA-dependent DNA polymerase (reverse transcriptase). The five drugs in this class in the order of FDA approval are zidovudine (ZDV), didanosine (ddl), zalcitabine (ddC), stavudine (d4T), and epivir (3TC). For the purposes of combining these agents, it is useful to divide these agents into the

Table 15-1. Characteristics of nucleoside reverse transcriptase inhibitors

| | Thymidine analogues | | Purine analogues | | |
Generic name	Zidovudine	Stavudine	Didanosine	Zalcitabine	Lamivudine
Abbreviation	(AZT, ZDV)	(d4T)	(ddl)	(ddC)	(3TC)
Trade name	Retrovir®	Zerit®	Videx®	Hivid®	Epivir®
Dosing recommendations	200 mg tid or 300 mg bid	> 60K: 40 mg < 60K: 30 mg	Tablets > 60K: 200mg < 60K: 125mg	0.75 mg	150 mg
Doses per day	BID or TID	BID	BID*	TID	BID
Oral bioavailability	60%	86%	Tablet: 40% Powder: 30%	85%	86%
Serum $t^{1/2}$	1.1 hours	1.0 hour	1.6 hours	1.2 hours	3-6 hours
Intracellular $t^{1/2}$	3 hours	3.5 hours	12 hours	3 hours	12 hours
CNS penetration	20-60%	16-97%	20%	9-37%	20%
Route of elimination	Hepatic glucuronidation	Renal excretion	Renal excretion 50%	Renal excretion 70%	Renal excretion unchanged
Log HIV RNA ↓	0.6	0.8	0.7	< 0.5	1.2
Major toxicity	Bone marrow: —anemia —neutropenia Subjective complaints: GI intolerance, headache, insomnia, malaise	Peripheral neuropathy Nausea Diarrhea	Pancreatitis Peripheral neuropathy	Peripheral neuropathy Oroesophageal ulcers	Minimal toxicity Mild rash Headache

*ddl: there is increased support for new daily dosing.

thymidine analogues (ZDV, D4T) and the purine analogues (ddl, ddC, 3TC). The thymidine analogues, in general, are most effective in actively dividing HIV-infected CD_4 T-lymphocytes. Among this class, these drugs achieve the highest levels in the central nervous system. On the other hand, ddl concentrates in slower dividing cells, like macrophages, and is slow to develop resistance. The most limited antiretroviral activity is seen with ddC monotherapy. Mutational changes conferring resistance develops rapidly with 3TC; this occurs within 1 month of initiating therapy. However, despite this mutation, antiviral activity is not entirely lost since this mutation gives rise to a mutant virus that replicates less efficiently than the wild type variant (i.e., it is less "fit"). All RTIs are administered twice daily, except ddC, and recent data may suggest a role for daily dosing of ddl. The first combination nucleoside analogue pill, Combivir®, combines ZDV with 3TC at doses of 300 mg and 150 mg, respectively. Less frequent dosing and combination agents may have the added benefit of improving acceptance and adherence to antiretroviral therapy, because it limits the complexity and number of pills that must be taken.

Preliminary data on the soon-to-be FDA-approved purine analogue abacavir (1592U89) suggest that it is the most potent agent among RTIs.[10] It achieves a mean 1.5 log

reduction in viral load in antiretroviral naive patients is administered twice daily, penetrates the CSF similarly to ddl and 3TC, develops resistance slowly, is not cross-resistant with ZDV (however, it may be cross-resistant with other purine analogues[11]), and has few adverse side effects except a recently described hypersensitivity syndrome which occurs in about 4% of patients. Patients who experience this "serum sickness"-like reaction should not be rechallenged with abacavir. In addition, it appears to be synergistic with ZDV and nevirapine, and at least additive when combined with ddl, ddC, D4T, and 3TC.[12] Its role in combination therapy has yet to be established. It will, however, provide more potent options in the future.

Unlike the other classes of antiretroviral agents, few drug interactions between the RTIs and other common HIV medications exist. Patients receiving either high-dose cotrimoxazole (TMP/SMZ) or ganciclovir may be at increased risk for the development of neutropenia if administered with ZDV. However, this complication may be treated with granulocyte-colony stimulating factor (G-CSF). Patients taking ddl should not be administered dapsone, indinavir, or quinolones within 2 hours of taking ddl, because the ddl-containing buffer decreases absorption of these agents and, therefore, decreases their bioavailability. Both ddC and d4T should be administered cautiously with other agents known

Table 15-2. Non-nucleoside reverse transcriptase inhibitors

Generic name	Nevirapine	Delavirdine
Trade name	Viramune®	Rescriptor®
Form	200 mg tabs	100 mg tabs
Dosing recommendations	200 mg po qd x 14 days, then 200 mg po bid	400 mg po tid (four 100 mg tabs in ≥ 3 oz water to produce slurry)
Oral bioavailability	> 90%	85%
Serum t$^{1/2}$	25-30 hours	5.8 hours
Log HIV RNA ↓	1.5	1.0
Elimination	Cytochrome P$_{450}$ Metabolism; 80% excreted in urine; 10% in feces	Cytochrome P$_{450}$ metabolism; 51% excreted in urine; 44% in feces
Drug interactions	*Induces* cytochrome P$_{450}$ enzymes The following drugs have suspected interactions that require careful monitoring if co-administered with nevirapine: rifampin, rifabutin, oral contraceptives and protease inhibitors Nevirapine decreases the levels of protease inhibitors (saquinavir, ritonavir, indinavir, nelfinavir)	*Inhibits* cytochrome P$_{450}$ enzymes Contraindicated drugs: terfenadine, astemizole, alprazolam, midazolam, cisapride, rifabutin, rifampin (avoid H$_2$ blockers) Drugs that decrease delavirdine levels: phenytoin, rifabutin, rifampin, carbamazepine, phenobarbitol Delavirdine increases the levels of protease inhibitors (saquinavir, ritonavir, indinavir, nelfinavir), clarithromycin, dapsone, rifabutin, ergot alkaloids, dihydropyrides, quinidine, warfarin, Antacids and didanosine: separate administration by ≥ 1 hr
Major toxicity	Rash (25-30%); only 6% discontinued secondary to severity	Rash (20-25%)

to cause peripheral neuropathy. Cotrimoxazole, when administered in high doses, may also increase levels of 3TC and potentiate toxicity.

Non-nucleoside Analogue Reverse Transcriptase Inhibitors

Non-nucleoside reverse transcriptase inhibitors (NNRTIs) are an additional group of agents for the treatment of HIV. They must be used in combination with, and are similar to, the RTIs because they inhibit reverse transcriptase and prevent infection in newly dividing cells. Human immunodeficiency virus develops resistance in as few as 2 to 7 weeks when this drug is used as monotherapy. However, when used in combination with the RTIs, development of resistance to the RTI is decreased and there is a more pronounced and sustained antiviral effect.

Two NNRTIs have been approved for use against HIV (Table 15-2). Nevirapine, which was the first agent approved, is taken twice daily. Its major side effects are fever, muscle soreness, or a rash that appears to be a dose-related effect. Rash, usually not life-threatening, is managed by starting treatment at 200 mg per day and escalating to the higher dose (200 mg twice per day) after 2 weeks. Nevirapine appears to induce hepatic P$_{450}$ enzymes that are responsible for its own degradation. Thus, higher doses are

tolerated once the rate of degradation is increased. Unfortunately, the induction of P$_{450}$ by nevirapine may create drug interaction problems, most notably, up to 25% decreased bioavailability of many of the protease inhibitors, the dose of which must then be increased when prescribed in combination with nevirapine.

Delavirdine is well-absorbed and rash is seen in about 20% to 25% of patients receiving it. Similar to nevirapine, this side effect is usually not life-threatening and can be managed conservatively. Unfortunately, delavirdine is dispensed as 100 mg tablets and the recommended dose requires 12 pills per day. The pills must be dissolved in a water slurry and are best absorbed in an acidic stomach. Therefore, H$_2$ antagonists in general, antacids, and ddI should be avoided within 1 hour of dosing. The requirement of a water slurry preparation makes dispensation of delavirdine in the correctional setting a problem. Limited studies of drug interactions have been conducted with delavirdine and the protease inhibitors. Unlike nevirapine, delavirdine appears to increase the levels of the protease inhibitors, particularly indinavir, saquinavir, and nelfinavir. In patients receiving these combinations, careful monitoring for hepatotoxicity should be instituted. Perhaps after the pharmacokinetic interactions have been delineated, the use of delavirdine may be used favorably with the protease inhibitors to

Table 15-3. Characteristics of protease inhibitors

Generic name	Saquinavir	Ritonavir	Indinavir	Nelfinavir
Trade name	Invirase®/Fortavase®	Norvir®	Crixivan®	Viracept®
Form	200 mg caps	100 mg caps 600 mg/7.5 ml po solution*	200, 400 mg caps	250 mg tablet 500mg oral po
Dosing recommendations	600 mg q8h‡ Take with food	600 mg q12h† Take with fatty meals	800 mg q8h (Fasting)	750 mg q8h
Pills per day	9/18	12	6	9
Oral bioavailability	hard/soft gel capsule: 4%, erratic	60-80%	30%	20-80%
Serum half-life	1-2 hours	3-5 hours	1.5-2 hours	3.5-5 hours
Log HIV RNA ↓	0.5	1.5-2.0	1.5-2.0	1.5-2.0
Route of metabolism	Biliary metabolism P_{450} cytochrome 3A4	Biliary P_{450} cytochrome 3A4, 2D6, 2C9/10	Biliary metabolism P_{450} cytochrome 3A4	Biliary metabolism P_{450} cytochrome 3A4
Adverse effects	GI intolerance, nausea, and diarrhea Headache Elevated transaminase enzymes	GI intolerance, nausea, vomiting, diarrhea Paresthesias -circumoral -extremities Asthenia Taste perversion Lab: Triglycerides increase > 200%, transaminase elevation, elevated CPK and uric acid	Nephrolithiasis GI intolerance Lab: Increased indirect bilirubinemia (inconsequential) Misc: headache, asthenia, blurred vision, dizziness, rash, metallic taste, thrombocytopenia	Diarrhea

*Must be refrigerated.

†Dose escalation for ritonavir: Day 1-2: 300, mg bid; day 3-5: 400, mg bid; day 6-13: 500, mg bid; day 14: 600, mg bid.

‡Combination treatment regimen with saquinavir (400-600 mg po bid) plus ritonavir (400-600 po bid).

decrease the frequency of dosing. Cross-resistance between NNRTIs limits change from one agent to the other, and resistance has been detected for more than1 year after discontinuation of nevirapine.[13]

Protease Inhibitors

The introduction of the class of protease inhibitors has provided considerable clinical benefit to people affected by HIV/AIDS. As a class, they are the most potent antiretroviral agents. However, they differ in their potency, bioavailability, dosing, side effects, drug interactions, and drug resistance profiles (Table 15-3). The agents have demonstrated clinical efficacy at all CD_4 counts and a survival benefit when combined with RTIs at all CD_4 strata, including CD_4 counts < 50 cells/m³.

The current formulation of saquinavir has poor bioavailability, and as such, may rapidly develop resistance. A newer formulation has recently been released, but until its long-term efficacy is determined, saquinavir should not be used as a sole protease inhibitor combined with other agents. The new, soft gel formulation appears to have improved bioavailability and is more potent than its predecessor. Preliminary data on the use of saquinavir

combined with ritonavir are compelling. The favorable drug interaction between the two agents allows for decreased dosing of both and is associated with decreased toxicity, which should ameliorate the currently unpleasant side effects of ritonavir. These side effects of ritonavir may also be minimized through careful counsel before initiation, and through using antiemetics and a dose-escalation scheme.

Timing of dosing for these agents is crucial. Ritonavir, and the combination of ritonavir and saquinavir, are the only viable options for twice-daily dosing. Recent pharmacokinetic data suggest that nelfinavir may be dosed 1250 mg twice daily. Indinavir must be administered every 8 hours however, clinical trials are under investigation to determine efficacy in twice daily regimens. Furthermore, indinavir must be taken in a fasting state, not administered concomitantly with ddl, and a patient taking indinavir should be encouraged to drink large amounts of fluids to minimize the risk of nephrolithiasis. Access to adequate water and restroom facilities may limit options for some prisoners.

Resistance between protease inhibitors appears to overlap, at least partially, and for ritonavir and indinavir these

Table 15-4. Indications for initiating antiretroviral therapy in patients with chronic HIV infection

Clinical category	CD$_4$ Count and HIV-1 RNA level	Recommendation
Symptomatic (AIDS, thrush, unexplained fever)	Any Value	Therapy recommended for all
Asymptomatic	CD$_4$ count < 500 cells/mm^3 or HIV-1 RNA > 10,000[1]-20,000[2]	Therapy should be offered to all*
Asymptomatic	CD$_4$ count > 500 cells/mm^3 and HIV-1 RNA < 10,000[1]-20,000[2]	Some experts would treat, others would monitor and observe

*Strength of recommendation based on prognosis of disease progression and willingness of patient to accept therapy.
[1]Using b-DNA method.
[2]Using RT-PCR method.

agents require at least three mutations to develop irreversible resistance and cross-resistance between the two agents is nearly complete. The resistance patterns to the other protease inhibitors have not been completely elucidated; however, a single mutation has been associated with resistance to saquinavir, and high-level resistance to nelfinavir has partial cross-resistance to the other agents.

Many identified pharmacokinetic drug interactions exist between the four available protease inhibitors and with other common therapeutic agents. Ritonavir is the most potent inhibitor of cytochrome P$_{450}$; however, all agents have the potential for creating adverse events for patients on multiple therapeutic agents. Review of described drug interactions is essential for each patient on a regular basis. The pharmacist can also be extremely useful in the co-treatment of patients receiving protease inhibitors.

Ritonavir may increase the serum levels and, therefore, the potential for adverse side effects for several agents such as antihistamines, many benzodiazepines, calcium channel blockers, antidepressants, cisapride, some neuroleptics, opiates, anti-epileptics, oral hypoglycemics, coumadin, azoles, and rifamycins. Some of these agents are contraindicated with ritonavir; however, others may only need a dose adjustment or more careful observation for toxicity. The other protease inhibitors are less potent inhibitors of cytochrome P$_{450}$. As such, astemizole, cisapride, rifamycins, and terfenadine all have described interactions with saquinavir, indinavir, and nelfinavir. The protease inhibitors also have known interactions with each other, and when co-administered, each raise the serum levels of the other agent.

In addition, agents that induce cytochrome P$_{450}$ (e.g., rifampin, phenytoin, nevirapine) may decrease the efficacy of the protease inhibitors by decreasing their serum levels. When such interactions are anticipated, it may be necessary to increase the dose of the protease inhibitor. Therefore, optimal management includes a careful review of all prescribed medications at each visit, with assured supervision by a skilled HIV specialist who is aware of such interactions.

INITIATING ANTIRETROVIRAL THERAPY

Antiretroviral therapy has been demonstrated to provide optimal clinical benefit in individuals infected with HIV, especially for those with advanced HIV disease.[14–18] In addition, our newer understanding of HIV pathogenesis also suggests benefit to treatment for patients with CD$_4$ T-cells < 500 cells/mm^3, however, long-term clinical trials have not been conducted for this group. Therefore, questions remain concerning the early use of antiretroviral therapy.

A major dilemma confronting patients and practitioners is that the antiretroviral regimens currently available with the greatest potency in terms of viral suppression and CD$_4$ T-lymphocyte preservation are therapeutically complex. They are associated with a number of specific side effects and drug interactions, and they pose a substantial challenge for adherence. Thus, clinicians should base decisions on a combination of viral load determinations, CD$_4$ T-lymphocyte count, symptomatic disease, and preference of the patient. The clinical indications for treatment are outlined in Table 15-4.

Asymptomatic HIV Infection

Decisions regarding treatment of asymptomatic, chronically infected individuals must balance a number of competing factors that influence risk and benefit (Box 15-1). A patient and physician should carefully weigh these considerations before initiating therapy. To maximize the potential for adherence to the medication regimen, several discussions with the patient may be necessary before initiation of therapy is indicated.

Decision-making factors for physicians include:
- The willingness of the individual to begin therapy;
- The degree of existing immunodeficiency, as determined by the CD$_4$ T-lymphocyte count;
- The risk of disease progression, as determined by the level of plasma HIV-1 RNA;
- The potential benefits and risks of initiating therapy in asymptomatic individuals;
- The likelihood of adherence to the prescribed treatment regimen after counseling and education;

Box 15-1. Benefits and Risks of Early Antiretroviral Initiation in Asymptomatic Patients with HIV

Potential Benefits
- Control of viral replication, mutation, and reduction of viral burden;
- Delayed progression to AIDS and increased survival;
- Prevention of progressive immunodeficiency and potential maintenance of an intact immune system;
- Decreased risk of selection of a resistant strain of virus;
- Decreased risk for transmission of HIV to others;
- Decreased drug toxicity risk.

Potential Risks
- Limitation of future choices of antiretroviral agents;
- Decreased quality of life from adverse drug effects;
- Unknown long-term toxicity of antiretrovirals;
- Unknown duration of effectiveness of antiretroviral;
- Earlier development of drug resistance;
- Risk of dissemination of drug-resistant virus.

- The ability of the physician to provide intensive follow-up, both in terms of treatment and continued emotional support.

Many studies have demonstrated that clinicians and other health care providers poorly predict adherence.[19–22] The likelihood of patient adherence to a complex drug regimen should be discussed and determined by the individual patient and physician before therapy is initiated. Therefore, individual patients should not be excluded from consideration for antiretroviral therapy simply because he or she exhibits a behavior that might be interpreted to lend itself to non-adherence.

To achieve the level of adherence necessary for effective therapy, providers are encouraged to use strategies for assessing and assisting adherence that have been developed in the context of other chronic diseases (e.g., diabetes, hypertension, asthma). These strategies include:
- Motivation and creating a sense of optimism;
- Intensive patient education regarding the critical need for therapy and adherence;
- Establishment of specific goals that should be mutually agreed upon (best accomplished by a handshake contract);
- Reassurance of careful follow-up and laboratory monitoring;
- Ability to address potential complications or toxicity from medication in a timely manner;
- Development of a long-term treatment plan.

When possible, clinicians should minimize the number of medications, frequency of dosing, complexity of regimen, and the potential for side effects. For example, twice-daily therapies are preferable to thrice-daily ones. Use of one antiviral requiring food with another requiring a fast-

ing state increases complexity and, therefore, may decrease adherence. In prisons and jails, where ability to take a complicated regimen is limited by structural barriers outlined in Chapter 14, adherence to therapy is particularly challenging.

Intensive follow-up should take place to assess adherence to treatment, monitor progress or complications of therapy, and to continue patient counseling for the prevention of sexual and drug injection-related transmission. Use of trained nursing or pharmacy staff to monitor adherence and counsel inmates is a useful way to avoid development of resistance. In this manner, counseling and re-identification of purpose can be instituted before a follow-up visit with the treating physician.

Initiation of treatment. Once the asymptomatic patient with HIV and physician have decided to initiate antiretroviral therapy, treatment should be aggressive, with the goal of maximal suppression of plasma viral load to undetectable levels. Box 15-2 summarizes current recommendations for antiretroviral therapy and what regimens to use. As was noted in Table 15-4, in general, patients with $CD_4 < 500$ cells/mm^3, or HIV-1 RNA > 10,000-20,000 copies/mL of plasma should be offered therapy.

Because HIV disease is virtually always progressive, two general approaches exist for initiating therapy in the asymptomatic patient: 1) an interventional approach that would treat most patients early in the course of HIV infection; and 2) a more cautious approach in which therapy may be delayed because the balance of the risk of disease progression benefits noted in Box 15-1 favor observation, continued monitoring, for three to six months, and delayed therapy.

Interventional approach. The interventional approach is predicated on our current understanding of HIV, which suggests treatment before the development of significant immunosuppression. The goal of treatment is to achieve undetectable viremia; thus, almost all patients with > 500 CD_4 T-cells/mm^3 would be started on therapy as would patients with higher CD_4 lymphocyte counts who have detectable plasma viral load. The conservative approach for asymptomatic patients would be to delay treatment of the patient with CD_4 counts > 500 cells/mm^3 and low levels of viremia who have a low risk of rapid disease progression. With a conservative approach, careful observation and laboratory monitoring would be necessary to determine a change in risk evidenced by an increase in HIV-1 RNA or a decrease in CD_4 T-lymphocyte count. Patients with an elevated HIV-1 RNA level, irrespective of CD_4 count, should be offered therapy.

If the decision is made to initiate therapy in the antiretroviral-naïve patient, a regimen that is expected to reduce viral replication to undetectable levels should be selected. Based on the weight of experience, the preferred regimen to accomplish this is two nucleoside analogues (RTIs) and one potent protease inhibitor (Box 15-2).

Alternative regimens may be used; these include substituting an NNRTI for the protease inhibitor, or, as a third, less desirable choice, regimens consisting of 2 RTIs alone if the patient has a high viral load and is unable or unwilling to take a three-drug regimen. Substituting a NNRTI for a protease inhibitor is likely to be most effective in antiretroviral-naïve patients with lower levels of viremia (e.g., HIV-1 RNA levels < 50,000 copies/mm^3).

Although one may choose an alternate regimen, these do not suppress and sustain viremia to below detectable levels with the same success rate as do combination treatment with two RTIs and a protease inhibitor. If potent treatment is not possible, then alternate regimens may be considered. There is, however, some debate among the experts who suggest insufficient data to choose between a three-drug regimen containing a protease inhibitor and one containing NNRTI in the drug-naïve patient with a modestly elevated HIV-1 RNA level. This is being further studied. Although 3TC is a potent RTI when used in combination with another RTI, in situations in which suppression of virus replication is not complete, resistance to 3TC develops rapidly.[23, 24] Therefore, the optimal use for this agent is a part of a three or more drug combination that includes a protease inhibitor which will increase the opportunity for complete suppression of virus replication. Other agents in which a single genetic mutation can confer rapid drug resistance, such as the non-nucleoside reverse transcriptase inhibitors (NNRTIs) nevirapine and delavirdine, should also be used as part of a multi-drug combination. The use of monotherapy is contraindicated and is not recommended.

Detailed information comparing the different nucleoside RTIs, the NNRTIs, and the protease inhibitors is presented in Tables 15-1 through 15-3. Many potential drug interactions are known between the protease inhibitors and other agents. Thus, therapy may often require dose modification of various drugs. Toxicity assessment requires an ongoing process; assessment at least twice during the first month of therapy and every 1 to 3 months thereafter is a reasonable management approach. Laboratory testing may be required at least monthly, given the complexity of therapy. Adherence should be monitored initially after starting therapy, and between 2 and 4 weeks thereafter.

Advanced HIV Disease

All patients diagnosed with advanced HIV disease should receive antiretroviral therapy regardless of plasma viral levels. Advanced HIV disease includes those patients who have a CD$_4$ count less than 200, a history of opportunistic infection, an HIV-related malignancy, neurologic sequelae (or wasting, as defined in the 1993 CDC definition of AIDS), or those with symptomatic HIV (defined as the presence of thrush or unexplained fever). The recommendations for antiretroviral therapy as described for the asymptomatic are applicable for this group. However, these patients may be more susceptible to the toxicity of anti-

---

Box 15-2. Antiretroviral Therapy Recommendations for Treatment of HIV

Preferred: There is strong evidence of clinical benefit and sustained HIV-1 RNA suppression.

Two RTIs and a highly active protease inhibitor.

RTI Combination	Protease Inhibitor*
ZDV + ddI	ritonavir
D4T + ddI	
ZDV + ddC	indinavir
ZDV + 3TC†	
D4T + 3TC†	nelfinavir
	ritonavir + saquinavir

Alternative: Less likely to provide sustained viral suppression; clinical benefits undetermined.

Two RTIs (see column above) + NNRTI**
-OR-
Two RTIs (see column above) + saquinavir

Not generally recommended: Clinical benefit demonstrated but initial viral suppression not sustained in most patients.

Two RTIs (see column above)

Not recommended: Evidence against use and virologically undesirable

All monotherapies‡
D4T + ZDV
ddC + ddI
ddC + D4T
ddC + 3TC

---

*Current hard gel Saquinavir formulation not recommended; however, newer formulation with improved bioavailability is under consideration. Combination protease inhibitors using Ritonavir 400mg bid + Saquinavir 400mg bid is used in place of a singly highly active protease inhibitor by many clinicians.

**All combinations using a NNRTI were with ZDV and ddI.

†High-level resistance to 3TC develops within 2-4 weeks; therefore, it should be used optimally in 3-drug combinations expected to reduce viral load to non-detectable levels.

‡ZDV monotherapy may be considered in pregnant women who are antiretroviral-naïve with high CD4 T-lymphocyte counts, and low viral loads to prevent perinatal transmission.

---

retroviral agents, or experience adverse complications secondary to drug interactions with agents used for prophylaxis or treatment of opportunistic infections.

Delay of initiation of antiretroviral therapy may be prudent in situations where the patient presents with an opportunistic infection or other complication of HIV when therapy is being considered. The clinician must consider drug interactions, as well as co-morbidity of additional medication, at the time of treatment of an opportunistic infection. Additionally, the clinician must be aware of potential psychological distress. Emotional distress may be overwhelming to the patient and ultimately affect adherence to a complicated medical regimen. However, once the patient is stabilized, therapy should be initiated with a maximally suppressive regimen (e.g., 2 RTIs and a protease inhibitor). In patients unlikely to achieve a non-detectable viral load with therapy (e.g., HIV-1 RNA > 100,000 copies), the use of 2 RTIs and either an NNRTI and a protease inhibitor or with two protease inhibitors may be necessary to achieve adequate viral suppression. When stabilized on a maximally suppressive and tolerable regimen, therapy should not be discontinued during an acute opportunistic infection or malignancy, unless there are concerns regarding drug toxicity, intolerance, or drug interactions.

There is always a potential for drug interactions when multiple medications are used to treat patients with advanced HIV. When choosing antiretroviral agents, potential drug interactions and overlapping drug toxicities must be considered. For example, in a patient with active tuberculosis, receiving rifampin is a problem if the patient is also receiving a protease inhibitor. The protease inhibitor adversely affects the metabolism of rifampin, causing elevated levels and potential toxicity. Conversely, rifampin lowers the blood level of protease inhibitors, potentially decreasing efficacy and possibly inducing antiretroviral resistance. Rifabutin, an agent similar to rifampin, might be used at a reduced dose in certain selected patients on protease inhibitors. Other factors complicating advanced disease are wasting and anorexia, which may prevent patients from adhering to the dietary requirements for efficient absorption of certain protease inhibitors. Bone marrow suppression associated with ZDV and the neuropathic effects of ddC, D4T, and ddI may combine with the direct effects of HIV to render the drugs intolerable. Hepatotoxicity associated with certain protease inhibitors may limit the use of these drugs, especially in patients with underlying liver dysfunction. The absorption and half-life of certain drugs may be altered by antiretroviral agents, particularly the protease inhibitors and NNRTIs, the metabolism of which involves the hepatic cytochrome P_{450} enzymatic pathway. At times, this metabolism can be exploited to improve the pharmacokinetic profile of selected agents such as saquinavir (by dosing with ritonavir); however, these interactions can also result in life-threatening drug toxicity. Thus, health care providers should inform patients of the importance of discussing with them any new drugs, including over-the-counter agents and alternative medications, that they might be taking. Also, they should give careful attention to the relative risk versus benefits of specific combinations of agents. Clinicians must also pay serious attention to any complaint by patients since some adverse events and drug interactions are not well described.

CRITERIA FOR ALTERING THERAPY

Improving the length and quality of the patient's life is the goal of antiretroviral therapy. It is accomplished through suppression of viral replication to below detectable levels sufficiently early to preserve immune function. When this is not achievable with a specific therapeutic regimen, it should be modified. The plasma HIV-1 RNA level is considered the most important parameter in evaluating therapeutic response. Significant increase in levels of viremia not attributable to non-adherence, intercurrent infection, or vaccination is a clear indication of drug regimen failure, regardless of stability of CD_4 T-cell counts. Clinical features and sequential changes in CD_4 T-cell counts may complement the viral load test in evaluating a response to treatment. The most common cause of an increase in viral load is medication non-adherence. Adherence should be checked before altering therapy. If the adherence was incomplete and sustained for a prolonged time, the likelihood of development of resistant strains is increased. If the insufficient adherence is of a short duration, or if the patient has completely discontinued all medications, the regimen should not be considered a failure, and therapy may be restarted with appropriate counseling. Specific criteria that should prompt consideration for changing therapy after non-adherence has been addressed include:

- Less than a 10-fold (1.0 log) reduction in plasma HIV-1 RNA by 4 weeks following initiation of therapy;
- Failure to suppress plasma HIV-1 RNA to undetectable levels within 4 to 6 months of initiating therapy;
- Repeated detection of virus in plasma after initial suppression to undetectable levels, suggesting the development of resistance;
- Any reproducible significant increase, defined as three-fold or greater (≥ 0.5 log), from the nadir of plasma HIV-1 RNA not attributable to intercurrent infection, vaccination, or test method;
- Persistently declining CD_4 T-cell counts, as measured on at least two separate occasions;
- Clinical deterioration; that is, a new AIDS-defining diagnosis that was acquired ≥ 90 days after the time treatment was initiated. While this suggests clinical deterioration, it may or may not suggest failure of antiretroviral therapy.

In the decision to change therapy, one must also recognize that there are limited choices of agents available. Therefore, a decision to change may reduce the patient's future treatment options. As such, the physician may be somewhat more conservative when deciding to change therapy and may take into consideration alternative options such as potency of the substituted regimen, probability of tolerance, or ability to adhere to the alternative regimen. While partial suppression of the virus is considered superior to no suppression of the virus, some physicians and patients may prefer suspension of treatment to preserve future options. Sometimes treatment is suspended when it is not possible to achieve a sustained antiviral effect. When considering a change in therapy, referral to or consultation with an experienced HIV clinician is key. These patients should be given the option for inclusion in an appropriate clinical trial when indicated and available.

Antiretroviral Resistance

Viral resistance is one of the major causes of virologic rebound and subsequent therapeutic failure. This may occur either as a consequence of inadequate potency of treatment (e.g., use of nucleoside RTI combinations without a protease inhibitor) or from sustained partial adherence to therapy. Other less common factors that may secondarily lead to resistance through suboptimal drug levels include malabsorption, altered intracellular metabolism, or distribution to cellular compartments (e.g., central nervous system, lymphoreticular system). Resistance develops because pre-existing HIV-1 mutations are present at low levels in the trial population, even among antiretroviral-naïve patients. Incomplete viral suppression creates selective pressure to allow minority mutant strains to emerge and ultimately become dominant over the wild-type strain found in antiretroviral-naïve patients. Once mutations begin, there is a cascading effect that leads to a predominance of resistant viruses. The development of resistance to one agent may reduce the efficacy of another agent used at a later date. Therefore, it is essential to maximally use the most potent agents at the time of initiation of therapy.

Resistance to reverse transcriptase inhibitors. Resistance to RTIs is characterized by the gradual evolution of mutations that substitute with the wild-type virus at various codons of the reverse transcriptase enzyme. Initial base pair substitutions selected for ZDV occur at codons 215 and 219, while later substitutions occur at sites 41, 67, and 70 of the reverse transcriptase enzyme. In general, mutations are overlapping and associated with cross-resistance for ddI and ddC; the exception is a mutation at codon 69, which is highly resistant to ddC, and less so for ddI. Prior use of ZDV may render future use of d4T ineffective based on altered intracellular phosphorylation.[25]

While many mutations are associated with development of resistance, some may be beneficial. The 3TC-selected mutation at codon 184 and the ddI-, ddC-, and abacavir-selected mutation at codon 74 have both been demonstrated to reverse the effects of resistance to ZDV-selected mutants and restore some of the antiretroviral activity of ZDV. The mutation at codon 184 develops as the dominant form of the virus within 4 to 6 weeks after initiating therapy with 3TC. Codon 75 mutations have been demonstrated to confer resistance *in vitro* with exposure to D4T; however, such mutations have not been found *in vivo*. Additionally, there may be many more mutations associated with combination therapy that do not reflect resistance to a single agent. Some of these mutations are described at codons 62, 75, 77, and 116; however, they are uncommon. Less is known about mutations that occur in combinations of RTIs with other classes of antiretroviral agents.

Resistance to NNRTIs. Broad cross-resistance exists between nevirapine, delavirdine, and many of the NNRTIs being developed. Described mutations for this class are many and include substitutions at codons 100, 103, 106, 188, and 190. The mutations that occur with this class of agents develop rapidly, suggesting they should be combined maximally with other agents. The most common NNRTI mutation occurs at codon 181, which can suppress resistance to ZDV.

Resistance to protease inhibitors. The majority of mutations selected by the protease inhibitors are located throughout the protease enzyme. In general, multiple, stepwise mutations must occur before phenotypic resistance occurs. That is, there may be genotypic mutations that develop which do not have clinical significance until three or more mutations occur. While more than eleven mutations have been well described for this class, the greater the number of mutations, the greater the likelihood that broad cross-resistance to all other protease inhibitors will develop. For saquinavir and nelfinavir, a single mutation may confer high-level phenotypic resistance. Thus, if a patient adherent to therapy converts from having a non-detectable to a detectable viral load while on a combination containing a protease inhibitor, careful consideration should be given to alter therapy immediately before high-level resistance with many mutations has occurred.

Therapeutic Options When Changing Antiretroviral Therapy

Theoretical considerations should outweigh specific strategies for changing therapy, since there are limited clinical trials. Treatment should ideally involve replacement of the regimen with different drugs to which the patient is naïve, using two new nucleoside analogue agents and one new protease inhibitor or NNRTI agent. However, two new protease inhibitors and another agent might also be beneficial. This option may not be possible because of the prior use of antiretroviral agents, toxicity, or intolerance. If the patient with detectable viremia for whom an optimal change in therapy is not possible, and who remains clinically stable, it may be best to delay changing therapy in anticipation of the availability of newer and more potent agents. It is recommended that the decision to change therapy and design a new regimen should be made in consultation with, or on referral from, a clinician experienced in the treatment of patients infected with HIV.

Considerations for Changing a Failing Regimen

When one decides to change regimens, several complex factors must be considered, such as:
- Recent clinical history and physical examination;
- Plasma HIV-1 RNA levels measured on two separate occasions;
- Changes in absolute CD_4 T-lymphocyte count;
- Remaining effective treatment options;
- Possible resistance patterns that have already developed from prior therapy;
- Tolerance levels to potential side effects;
- Adherence to medications assessment;

• Preparation of the patient for the new regimen, with particular attention to side effects, drug interactions, dietary requirements, and possible need to alter medications.

Diligent assessment of adherence prior to changing antiretroviral therapy is indicated if HIV-1 RNA levels are rising; appropriate patient education is indicated to improve adherence if it has been deemed insufficient. Unfortunately, once resistance has developed for many agents, it may not be reversible solely by increasing adherence.[26]

There are two principal reasons for changing therapy: drug failure versus drug toxicity. With drug toxicity, it is appropriate to substitute one or more alternative drugs (same potency and same class) as the agent suspected to be causing the toxicity. With drug failure, where more than one drug had been used, it will be important to take a detailed history of current and past antiretroviral medications, and a record of other HIV-related medications should be obtained before selecting an alternative regimen.

Patients who should be considered for a change in therapy include:

• Those receiving single or double nucleoside therapy, with detectable plasma viral load or evidence of clinical progression;

• Those on potent combination therapy (with a protease inhibitor) whose viremia, while initially suppressed, has become detectable once again;

• Those whose viremia was never suppressed to below detectable limits, and whose potent combination therapy included a protease inhibitor.

The regimen should be changed to drugs not previously taken whenever possible. With triple combinations of drugs, at least two–and preferably three–new drugs should be used to prevent drug resistance. The addition of a single agent to a failing regimen is strongly discouraged. For instance, in a patient whose viral load was previously non-detectable on the combination of ZDV and ddC and whose viral load has risen to 50,000 copies/mm^3, the addition of a protease inhibitor would be the equivalent of using protease inhibitor monotherapy, because essentially all 50,000 copies are resistant to ZDV or ddC or even to both agents. Although not routinely recommended, in some instances where decisions are complicated, use of either phenotypic or genotypic resistance testing may assist decision-making. Unfortunately, the exact utility of these tools has not yet been established and awaits standardization.

In many instances, options are limited when clinicians decide that therapy must be altered in the setting of therapeutic failure. Patients may have received prolonged sequential monotherapy in the past or, alternatively, inadequate combination therapy in the setting of a high viral load and, therefore, have developed resistance to many of the available antiretroviral agents. Unfortunately, limited options exist for these patients who may require unique combinations of antiretroviral agents not outlined in the existing guidelines. Combinations of protease inhibitors, combining a protease inhibitor with an NNRTI, and seeking antiretroviral agents only available through compassionate use protocols has become the reality of treatment for heavily antiretroviral, pre-treated patients. Experienced HIV specialists are best suited to address such complicated issues.

SPECIAL CONSIDERATIONS FOR TREATMENT
Acute HIV Infection

At least 50%, and as many as 90%, of patients acutely infected with HIV will present with symptoms of the acute retroviral syndrome and, as such, are candidates for early therapy.[27–29] In the primary care setting, however, acute HIV infection is often not recognized because of the similarity of the symptom complex with those of the "flu" or other common illnesses. Additionally, there may be acute primary infection without symptoms. However, physicians should consider HIV infection in all patients with a compatible clinical syndrome and should confirm suspicions with appropriate laboratory work-up, including a test for HIV-1 RNA. There is evidence for a short-term effect of therapy on viral load and CD$_4$ T-cell counts, but long-term outcome data demonstrating a clinical benefit of using antiretroviral treatment have not been completed. Clinical trials have been limited by small sample sizes, short duration of follow-up, and often treatment that results in suboptimal antiviral activity. However, ongoing clinical trials are in effect and are investigating the long-term clinical benefit of more potent treatment regimens for this population. The theoretical rationale for early intervention, at the time of HIV seroconversion, is five-fold:

• To suppress the initial burst of viral replication and decrease the magnitude of virus dissemination throughout the body;

• To potentially decrease the severity of acute disease;

• To potentially alter the initial viral "set point" (Figure 14-1, previous chapter), which may ultimately affect the rate of disease progression;

• To maintain the immunologic repertoire of CD$_4$ "naïve" T-cells;

• To possibly reduce the rate of viral mutation, due to the suppression of viral replication.

Because of reported delays in diagnosis of HIV infection and subsequent advancement to the acute stage, therapy of primary HIV infection is based on theoretical considerations. Therefore, the potential benefits and risks must be weighed accordingly. With quality of life issues often the most important consideration for the patient, a candid discussion between physician and patient is essential.

The risks of initiating therapy for acute HIV infection include the following *possible* adverse effects, and are similar to those for initiating therapy in the asymptomatic patient:

• A compromised quality of life resulting from drug toxicities;

• Development of drug resistance;

- Limited future treatment options;
- Need for therapy indefinitely;
- Blunting the evolution of an appropriate immune response.

Who To Treat During Acute HIV Infection

All patients with laboratory evidence of acute HIV infection should be candidates for treatment; that is, those with detectable HIV-1 RNA in plasma using sensitive PCR or bDNA assays and a negative or indeterminate HIV antibody test. Plasma HIV-1 RNA measurement is the preferred method of diagnosis; however, a test for p24 antigen is sometimes useful, particularly when RNA testing is not readily available. A negative p24 antigen test *does not* rule out acute infection, and when acute infection is suspected, a test for HIV-1 RNA should be performed.

Therapy for patients in whom seroconversion has occurred within the previous 6 months should also be considered. If viremia in infected adults has resolved by 2 months, treatment during this phase should be based on the likelihood that virus replication in lymphoid tissue is still not maximally contained by the immune system during the first 6 months following infection. For patients who test antibody-positive, and who believe the infection is recent—but for whom the time of infection cannot be documented—treatment consideration should be made using the "Assessment of Patients With or Suspected to be HIV Infected" algorithm in Figure 14-4 of Chapter 14.

Testing for plasma HIV-1 RNA levels and CD_4 T-cell count and toxicity monitoring should be performed repeatedly before initiation of therapy, between 2 and 4 weeks, and every 3 to 4 months thereafter. Some experts think that testing for plasma HIV-1 RNA levels at 4 weeks is not helpful in evaluating the effect of therapy for acute infection, because viral loads may be decreasing from peak viremia levels, even in the absence of therapy.

Duration of Therapy for Primary HIV Infection

Once therapy is initiated, many experts would continue to treat the patient with antiretroviral agents indefinitely, because viremia has been documented to reappear or increase after discontinuation of therapy. However, some experts would treat for 1 year and then re-evaluate the patient with CD_4 T-cell determinations and quantitative HIV-1 RNA measurements. The optimal duration and composition of therapy are unknown, and ongoing clinical trials are expected to provide data relevant to these issues. The difficulties inherent in determining the optimal duration and composition of therapy initiated for acute infection should be considered when first counseling the patient regarding therapy.

Considerations for Antiretroviral Therapy in Pregnant Women With HIV

For optimal antiretroviral therapy in pregnant women with HIV, clinicians should follow the same guidelines as those for non-pregnant adults. Although ZDV therapy during the second and third trimester has demonstrated a three-fold reduction in maternal-fetal transmission, the question of initiating therapy in the pregnant woman with HIV remains controversial. In weighing the concern about the mother's health and the risk of antiretroviral therapy to the fetus, one must keep in mind the documented risk of transmission of the HIV virus to the newborn. As such, primary consideration should be given to the mother's virologic and immunologic status. In recognition of the fact that the first trimester of pregnancy is one of maximal organogenesis and risk for teratogenicity, initiation of antiretroviral therapy when possible should be delayed until after the fetus is 14 weeks of gestational age. Some clinicians recommend that those mothers who were receiving therapy at the time of conception may consider discontinuing treatment until after the 14-week period, unless risk of HIV progression in the mother is too great. While this practice is not universally agreed upon, initiation of antiretroviral therapy or temporary discontinuance should take place only after a thorough and clear discussion between the mother and the clinician.

Regarding discontinuance of therapy, no data currently address the risk or harm of transient discontinuance of antiretroviral therapy. However, one can anticipate a rebound in HIV-1 RNA levels during this period, and a rebound might increase the risk of *in utero* HIV transmission as well as potentiate progression of the disease in the mother. Thus, many other experts recommend use of a maximally suppressive regimen even during the first trimester, especially if the mother's risk of disease progression is high (e.g., high viral load) or if the mother was maximally suppressed on antiretroviral agents at the time of conception.

Treatment Regimen

Of the antiretroviral agents used for treatment of pregnant women infected with HIV, the pharmacokinetics of only ZDV and 3TC have been evaluated. Both ZDV and 3TC are well tolerated and cross the placenta. Additionally, concentrations in cord blood are similar to those in maternal blood observed at the time of delivery. However, ZDV has most effectively been shown to reduce the risk of HIV transmission from mother to child.[30, 31] Other than ZDV, there are no data on both the pharmacokinetics and safety of most other RTI antiretroviral agents used for pregnant women infected with HIV.

Based on data from ACTG 076, ZDV should be administered orally after 14 weeks' gestation and continued until the child is delivered. During the peripartum period, ZDV should be administered intravenously to the mother, and orally to both the mother and to the newborn for the first 6 weeks of life. Using this regimen, the risk of perinatal transmission is reduced by approximately 70% to 80%.

Since data are limited or unavailable, ZDV is the drug of choice for the purpose of reducing the risk of perinatal transmission of HIV/AIDS to the newborn. No data presently justify substitution. Nonetheless, choices for treatment must be based on data from pre-clinical and clinical testing of other drugs, as well as a thorough discussion of the risks and benefits between patient and clinician. Prior antiretroviral history of the mother may justify using other agents. Additionally, antiretroviral response may be diminished in patients previously treated with ZDV, thus emphasizing the need to use alternative agents. For example, a woman with a several-year history of taking the combination of ZDV plus 3TC, and who now has an elevated viral load on therapy, may benefit from switching to an alternative RTI combination, perhaps in conjunction with a protease inhibitor.

In the class of non-nucleoside reverse transcriptase inhibitors, the only one evaluated that also appears to be well tolerated is nevirapine. When administered to pregnant women infected with HIV who are in labor, a single dose crossed the placenta and the neonatal blood concentration was at a level equivalent to that of the mother. There are no studies to date on the use of other non-nucleoside reverse transcriptase inhibitors for use in pregnancy, nor are data available on multiple dosing during pregnancy.

As with all patients with HIV/AIDS, there must be careful and close monitoring of prescribed treatments, especially when decision-making is not based on extensive clinical trial information. Although HIV transmission from mother to child can occur at any level, those receiving treatment with ZDV have been shown to have a reduced risk of transmission to their child, regardless of HIV-1 RNA levels. Untreated women have higher HIV-1 RNA levels than women who receive treatment. This factor correlates with increased risk of transmission to the child. Thus, antiretroviral therapy should be offered to all pregnant women with HIV. The choice of therapy should minimally be ZDV monotherapy for antiretroviral naïve patients with high CD_4 cell counts and low viral loads. Like patients who are not pregnant, complete suppression of viral replication is indicated if the patient and clinician deem the risk/benefit ratio to be in favor of treatment.

CONCLUSIONS

The rapid development of new antiretroviral agents provides renewed hope in their ability to suppress viral replication and prolong life when prescribed appropriately. The wide array of agents within and between the three classes also presents new challenges in the treatment of HIV. Our challenges, however, are to minimize toxicity and promote adherence among our patients. Correctional systems are likely to interface with a large number of antiretroviral-naïve patients, and, therefore, have an important place in our public health system for treatment of HIV using optimal therapeutic regimens. Suboptimal use of antiretroviral agents in this population may lead to the development of resistance and limit future options. Inadequate therapy may lead to multidrug resistant strains that may be rendered non-treatable with

existing or future antiretroviral agents. Limited resources, lack of availability of potent combinations, inadequate access to viral load testing to monitor therapy, and lack of expertise in treating patients on a complicated medication regimen continue to be obstacles in some correctional settings. These obstacles, however, should be a priority for innovation and can be overcome. It is particularly cost-effective to provide maximal antiretroviral therapy to patients to offset the expensive cost of care associated with patients whose risk for disease progression is high.[32] Development of systems that link patients to care after release have been successful in many settings; however, correctional health services should develop HIV programs in collaboration with those in the community. In this manner, the integration of HIV services may assist transition of HIV care between the correctional and community setting, and lead to a continuum of care. Despite these obstacles, many systems have successfully developed programs that are comprehensive, cost-effective, and provide a continuum of care.

REFERENCES

1. Katzenstein DA, Hammer SM, Hughes MD, et al: The relation of virologic and immunologic markers to clinical outcomes after nucleoside therapy in HIV-infected adults with 200 to 500 CD_4 cells per cubic millimeter. AIDS Clinical Trials Group Study 175 Virology Study Team. *New Engl J Med* 335:1091-1099, 1996.
2. Hammer SM, Katzenstein DA, Hughes MD, et al: A trial comparing nucleoside monotherapy with combination therapy in HIV-infected adults with CD_4 counts from 200 to 500 per cubic millimeter. AIDS Clinical Trials Group Study 175 Study team. *New Engl J Med* 335:1081-1090, 1996.
3. Delta Coordinating Committee. Delta: A randomised double-blind controlled trial comparing combinations of zidovudine plus didanosine or zalcitabine with zidovudine alone in HIV-infected individuals. *Lancet* 348:283-291, 1996.
4. CAESAR Coordinating Committee: Randomized trial of addition of lamivudine or lamivudine plus lovirride to zidovudine-containing regimens for patients with HIV-1 infection: The CAESAR trial. *Lancet* 349:1413-1421, 1997.
5. Hammer SM, Squires KE, Hughes MD, et al: A controlled trial of two nucleoside analogues plus indinavir in persons with human immunodeficiency virus infection and CD_4 cell counts of 200 per cubic millimeter or less. *N Engl J Med* 337:725-733, 1997.
6. Gulick RM, Mellors JW, Havlir D, et al: Treatment with indinavir, zidovudine, and lamivudine in adults with human immunodeficiency virus infection and prior antiretroviral therapy. *N Engl J Med* 337:734-739, 1997.
7. Gerstoft J, AVANTI Study Group: AVATI 2. A randomized double-blind comparative trial to evaluate the efficacy, safety, and tolerance of combination antiretroviral regimens for the treatment of HIV-1 infection: AZT/3TC vs AZT/3TC/indinavir in antiretroviral-naïve patients (Abstract I-94). Presented at the 37th ICAAC, Toronto, 1997.
8. Carpenter C, Fischl M, Hammer S, et al: Consensus statement—Antiretroviral therapy for HIV infection in 1996. Recommendations of an international panel. *JAMA* 276:145-154, 1996.
9. National Institute of Health: Report of the NIH panel to define principles of therapy of HIV infection. Washington D.C., 1997.
10. Daluge SM, Good SS, Faletto MB, et al: 1592U89. A novel carbocyclic nucleoside analog with potent, selective anti-human immunodeficiency virus activity. *Antimicrob Agents Chemother* 41:1082-1093, 1997.
11. Tisdale M, Alnadaf T, Cousens D: Combination of mutations in human immunodeficiency virus type 1 reverse transcriptase required for resis-

tance to the carbocyclic nucleoside 1592U89. *Antimicrob Agents Chemother* 41:1094-1098, 1997.

12. Faletto MB, Miller WH, Garvey EP, et al: Unique intracellular activation of the potent anti-human immunodeficiency virus agent 1592U89. *Antimicrob Agents Chemother* 41:1099-1107, 1997.

13. Havlir DV, Eastman S, Gamst A, et al: Nevirapine-resistant human immunodeficiency virus: Kinetics of replication and estimated prevalence in untreated patients. *J Virol* 70:7894-7899, 1996.

14. Fischl M, Richman D, Grieco M, et al: The efficacy of azidothymidine in the treatment of patients with AIDS and AIDS-related complex: A double-blind, placebo controlled trial. *N Engl J Med.* 317:185-191, 1987.

15. Fischl M, Richman D, Hansen H, et al: The safety and efficacy of zidovudine in the treatment of subjects with mildly symptomatic human immunodeficiency virus type 1 infection: A double-blind, placebo controlled trial. *Ann Intern Med* 112:727-737, 1990.

16. Volberding P, Lagakis S, Koch M, et al: Zidovudine in asymptomatic human immunodeficiency virus infection: A controlled trial in persons with fewer than 500 CD_4-positive cells per cubic millimeter. *N Engl J Med* 322:941-949, 1990.

17. Volberding P, Lagakis S, Grimes J, et al: The duration of zidovudine benefit in persons with asymptomatic HIV infection: Prolonged evaluation of protocol 019 of the AIDS Clinical Trials Group. *JAMA* 272:437-442, 1994.

18. Hammer SM, Katzenstein DA, Hughes MD, et al: A trial comparing nucleoside monotherapy with combination therapy in HIV-infected adults with CD_4 cell counts from 200 to 500 per cubic millimeter. *N Engl J Med* 335:1081-1090, 1996.

19. Hayes RB, Taylor DW, Sackett DL, et al: Can simple clinical measurements detect patient noncompliance? *Hypertension* 2:757-764, 1980.

20. Stewart M: The validity of an interview to assess a patient's drug taking. *Am J Prev Med* 3:95-100, 1987.

21. Gilbert JR, Evans CE, Haynes RB, et al: Predicting compliance with a regimen of digoxin therapy in family practice. *Can Med Assoc J* 123:119-122, 1980.

22. Inui TS, Carter WB, Pecoraro RE: Screening for noncompliance among patients with hypertension: Is self-report the best available measure? *Med Care* 19:1061-1064, 1981.

23. Schuurman R, Nijhuis M, van Leeuwen R, et al: Rapid changes in human immunodeficiency virus type 1 RNA load and appearance of drug-resistant virus populations in persons treated with lamivudine (3TC). *J Infect Dis* 171:1411-1419, 1995.

24. Keulen W, Back N, van Wijk A, et al: Initial appearance of the 1841le variant in lamivudine-treated patients is caused by the mutational bias of human immunodeficiency virus type 1 reverse transcriptase. *J Virol* 71:3346-3350, 1997.

25. Sommadossi JP, Zhou XJ, Moore J, et al: Impairment of stavudine (d4T) phosphorylation in patients receiving a combination of zidovudine (ZDV) and d4T (ACTG 290). Presented at the 5th Conference on Retroviruses and Opportunistic Infections, Chicago, 1998.

26. Molla A, Korneyva M, Gao Q, et al: Ordered accumulation of mutations in HIV protease confers resistance to ritonavir. *Nature Med* 2:760-766, 1996.

27. Schacker T, Collier A, Hughes J, et al: Clinical and epidemiologic features of primary HIV infection. *Ann Intern Med* 125:257-264, 1996.

28. Kinloch-de Loes S, de Saussure P, Saurat J, et al: Symptomatic primary infection due to human immunodeficiency virus type 1: Review of 31 cases. *Clin Infect Dis* 17:59-65, 1993.

29. Tindall B, Cooper D: Primary HIV infection: Host responses and intervention strategies. *AIDS* 5:1-14, 1991.

30. Sperling RS, Shapiro DE, Coombs RW, et al: Maternal viral load, zidovudine treatment, and the risk of transmission of human immunodeficiency virus type 1 from mother to infant. Pediatric AIDS Clinical Trials Group Protocol 076 Study Group. *New Engl J Med* 335:1621-1629, 1996.

31. Bryson YJ: Perinatal HIV-1 transmission: Recent advances and therapeutic interventions. *AIDS* 10 (Suppl) 13:33-42, 1996.

32. Moore RD, Bartlett JG: Combination antiretroviral therapy in HIV infection: An economic perspective. *Pharmacoeconomics* 10(2):177109-113, 1996.

Women's Health Care

16

Preferred Care of the Pregnant Inmate

Stamatia Z. Richardson, M.D.

The management issues surrounding pregnancy and the care of infants of incarcerated women have become increasingly complex. This is primarily due to an increase in the number of women in prison by 313% from 1980 to 1990.[1] In addition, approximately 80% of these women are of child-bearing age. With overcrowding, decreasing health budgets per capita, facilities and methods that seem ancient to the "free world," the incidence of poor outcome secondary to poor care would seem an obvious and predictable consequence. Logically, the biggest risk would be to those of short-term incarceration who have little chance of intervention with good prenatal care, drug abuse treatment, good nutrition, and educational programs prior to release.

Although no studies have compared control subjects with equal socioeconomic, substance abuse, and perinatal histories with those in jail or prison less than 120 days, it is arguable that timely identification of pregnancy and early intervention prior to release—followed by case management—should have favorable outcomes. Studies done with long-term (greater than 120 days) incarceration have shown significant decreases in perinatal morbidity.[2]

Women who are now behind bars tend to have been at highest risk for perinatal morbidity and mortality when they were in the community-at-large. These are poor women, women of color, drug abusers, smokers, drinkers, and those who are more likely to have sexually transmitted diseases, including HIV and hepatitis B. They have poor social support systems and are often victims of battering, incest, and sexual abuse. Most are single moms who have custody of dependent children. Many are repeat offenders who are in and out of jail frequently, and some have significant psychiatric issues. For many, the environment of jail is so significantly better than "home" that perinatal morbidity and mortality can only be expected to decrease. Incarceration is such a major stress even to those who are frequently "in and out," that education and case management are a must for continued good pregnancy outcome once these women are released into the community.[3]

IMMEDIATE POST-ARREST CARE

The greatest risk of poor perinatal outcome occurs between the time of arrest and presentation to the medical staff at the jail. For booking jails this time delay may be a matter of hours, but for large city or county systems where inmates are first placed in a local lockup, then appear before a bond court and only then are sent to jail, this time delay may last 4 days.

Drug and alcohol withdrawal can be particularly harmful to the fetus during this time. Pregnant women who are addicted to heroin should be promptly identified so that methadone can be started. For the safety of the fetus, methadone should be maintained for the duration of pregnancy. Lack of nutritional support, adequate fluid intake,

---

┌───┐
│ **Box 16-1. Questions for the Intitial Interview** │
│ ─── │
│   │
│ 1. Have you been experiencing severe nausea, vomiting, or │
│   diarrhea?   │
│ 2. Do you have any bleeding, cramping, abdominal pain, or │
│   vaginal discharge?   │
│ 3. Have you been feeling the baby's usual movements (after │
│   22 weeks' gestation)?   │
│ 4. What illicit drugs or alcohol have you been using? How │
│   much? When was your last use?   │
│ 5. Do you have any infections, or have you been exposed to │
│   any during your pregnancy?   │
└───┘

and an absence of medical services are also problematic during this time. Intake medical staff must be acutely aware that pregnant women may arrive at their facilities without having had care for some time, and may be withdrawing from alcohol or other drugs.[4]

When bleeding, contractions, abdominal pain, or exacerbation of chronic illness occurs, the correctional officers in charge of the inmate are least prepared to deal with the problem at hand. Until processing is completed by the local municipality, an inmate (male or female, pregnant or not) has very little access to medical personnel. The local hospital is very likely to be superficial in dealing with an incarcerated pregnant woman. The potential accompanying publicity and disturbance to their private patients is thereby minimized.

Women, on the other hand, who are fully evaluated by the prenatal personnel—be they nurse practitioners, physician assistants, nurse clinicians, family practitioners, obstetricians, or even a perinatologist—are rarely abandoned, rushed, or superficially treated by local hospitals if transferred there. This is because those same correctional medical personnel that intervene hopefully have a relationship with and/or admitting privileges at these hospitals when emergencies do occur.

INTAKE SCREENING

A major task of the intake process is to identify pregnant women quickly. Beta-hCG urine testing is acceptable. Full assessment by the medical prenatal team should be performed within 24 hours. Staffing considerations may make this impractical in many facilities. Therefore, realistically, this should be accomplished within 1 week. It is important to identify those pregnant women who have had a prior complicated pregnancy. This is best accomplishesd as part of the intake medical questionnaire. Box 16-1 provides a list of questions that should be asked in this questionnaire.

Beta-hCG urine testing should identify pregnant women within 1 to 2 days. In small prisons or jails, these women would be immediately housed in areas nearby medical personnel so that medical complaints or emergencies can be identified. This may also be accomplished by special nurs-

ing rounds. In larger jails or prisons, special tiers or cell blocks for pregnant women may be used so that medical personnel can concentrate their staff on these special housing units. Correctional staff and medical staff on these units should be trained to recognize the signs and symptoms of labor and complications of pregnancy. Pregnant women should be screened for sexually transmitted diseases (STDs). This is ideally performed as part of the intake process. If STD screening is not routinely performed at intake, then it should be performed as soon as the urine test identifies a woman as pregnant. Immediate intake RPR syphilis testing with follow-up treatment ("stat RPR") has been shown in New York to reduce congenital syphilis (unpublished data, Sue Blank, M.D., New York Department of Health). In jails where pregnant women may be quickly released from jail, intake STD screening and treatment may reduce complications of pregnancy in those who would otherwise not be involved in prenatal care upon release from jail. If immediate intake STD testing is performed, but treatment is not provided, then positive test results should be forwarded to the local board of health immediately for civilian follow-up. The relationship with the local board of health should be formalized so that these referrals are appropriately addressed.

ROUTINE PRENATAL CARE

Following American College of Obstetrics and Gynecology guidelines for prenatal care should be standard practice to ensure quality of care. Monthly prenatal visits by physicians or midlevel providers (physician assistants or nurse practitioners) trained in obstetrical care should be done every month up to 28 weeks, then bi-weekly during 28 to 36 weeks, and finally weekly until delivery. If such a qualified practitioner is unavailable at the facility, all pregnant women should receive prenatal care at a nearby qualified physician's office.

At the first visit, a full history should be obtained, including chronic disease history (diabetes mellitus, hypertension, asthma, seizure disorder, thyroid disorder), substance abuse, sexually transmitted diseases such as HIV and syphilis, and history of past perinatal morbidity. A full examination follows and should include a pelvic examination with PAP screening, testing for gonorrhea and chlamydia, and a wet mount to detect bacterial vaginosis, trichomoniasis, and candidiasis. Also at the first visit, serologic testing for anemia, sickle trait, blood group, Rh factor, antibody screening, rubella immunity, hepatitis B surface antigen, and syphilis screening is performed. Urine is collected for analysis and culture to detect asymptomatic bacteriuria. Tuberculosis testing with PPD placement from the intake process should be read within 7 days. Furthermore, in large facilities where the incidence of tuberculosis is higher in the community, screening with radiographs to identify patients with tuberculosis may be indicated. In any case, every woman recieving radiographs

---

Box 16-2. Initial Aspects of the First Clinical Encounter

Full history, especially about prior pregnancies.
Full family history.
Substance-abuse history, including tobacco and alcohol.
Full physical examination with fundal height measurement, fetal heart tone assessment, and pelvic examination.
Gonorrhea and chlamydia screen.
Wet mount with saline KOH.
PPD placement.
HSV screening for suspicious lesions.
Pap smear.

Box 16-3. Laboratory Tests

At the initial visit:
  Blood group
  Antibody screening
  Rh factor
  CBC
  Sickle cell screen
  RPR
  Rubella immunity
  Hepatitis B surface antigen
  Urinalysis
  Urine culture
  HIV counseling and anitbody testing
At 13-17 weeks:
  AFP or AFP/beta-hCG/estrogen neural tube defect screening
At 26-28 weeks:
  50-g 1-h glucose tolerance test
At 35-37 weeks:
  Beta strip screen of the vagina, perineum, and rectum

---

for tuberculosis screening in the facility should have her abdomen shielded with a lead apron in case pregnancy is suspected. Case management, education/counseling about HIV risks, and voluntary testing should be offered initially. In this way, a "team" approach can be established. This calls for the "over-1-hour" encounter, but time is of the essence where incarceration is likely to be 90 days or less. Diet supplements (usually a 3200-calorie diet is sufficient to offer a 25-40 pound weight gain) should be offered at time of identification, as well as vitamin, calcium, and iron supplements.

At subsequent visits, size/date discrepancies should be assessed, ultrasound ordered, and diabetes screening (glucola test) ordered at 26-30 weeks' gestation. Alpha fetoprotein (AFP), or combination AFP/beta-hCG/estrogen, tests should be used with caution since accuracy of dates is needed to make wise decisions with the results. Needless anxiety is caused when AFP tests are too high or too low, based on poor gestational dating from unsure last menstrual periods. These women's menstrual histories are sketchy at best, and most have had no prenatal care or ultrasound in the first trimester. Alpha-fetoprotein testing should be done on those with reliable dates and size or ultrasound that correlates with the patient's dates (Boxes 16-2, 16-3).

Termination of pregnancy counseling should be offered appropriately as well.[5] The controversy of whether termination should be offered free of charge or subsidized by tax monies for poor women is a hot political issue for women—incarcerated or not. However, those pro-life or pro-choice rights that exist for women in the community should exist for those behind bars. Timely ultrasounds for determination of accurate fetal age should be offered to all women. Transportation to and from scheduled tests and medical encounters by correctional staff should be a priority for these women.

The logistics of offering all these services varies from setting to setting. Many areas have very small jails where one medic or nurse may comprise the "medical team" for any man or woman who may be arrested. Other prisons may detain 1,000 or more inmates, all women, and should

provide comprehensive services on site. The vast majority of correctional institutions fit somewhere in between. The challenge is to provide optimum care for all. Certainly dietary concerns need to be specialized, no matter the size of the institution or its subset who are pregnant. At Cook County Jail, approximately 80 pregnancy diet trays are prepared along with the 9,000 other trays for the mostly male population. There is no excuse, even with budgetary concerns and constraints, for not providing care that will decrease morbidity and mortality. For many institutions, that means frequent local visits to community health centers for community-based care, social services, and education. In larger jails and prisons, social workers, case managers, etc, for other illnesses, such as HIV disease, chronic renal failure, or paraplegia should be cross-trained to case manage and assist in continuity of care into the community, once the woman is released from jail or prison.

Substandard care within a smaller institution only invites trouble with significant perinatal morbidity and mortality. Even in larger institutions, a tertiary care center (where high-tech monitoring and hospitalization are possible) should be readily available for frequent consultation as needed for obstetric and medical complications. Without a neonatal intensive care unit on-site, inmate-patients will need to be referred to a perinatal unit for stress testing, amniocentesis, and other more invasive procedures. It is also inappropriate to monitor patients in pre-term labor or even term labor without full neonatal back-up on site. An on-site monitoring unit should be used only for the most stable patient requiring fetal monitoring, non-stress testing, and ultrasound amniotic fluid measurements in a routine manner (e.g., in gestational diabetics, multiple-fetus gestations, or in post-dates situations). Most facilities are so far from having such on-site services that the key is recognition by less-trained staff of those times when more than routine care is required, and the cooperation of correctional institution authorities.

ENVIRONMENTAL FACTORS

By far the most crucial aspect of prenatal care within correctional settings is the day-to-day environment. Is the correctional authority, the superintendant, warden, director, etc., supportive of frequent movement to local hospitals, or in some cases local clinics? Patients may be shackled to and from these sites.[6] No pregnant woman should be shackled for prolonged periods, or at all during labor, for obvious humane reasons, but also because the hypercoagulable state of pregnant women may result in clotting abnormalities, including pulmonary embolism.[7]

Often the correctional authority may not be willing to take inmates to and from abortion clinics in a confidential and non-threatening way. Correctional officials must understand that immediate transport in an emergency or in a precipitous delivery can reduce morbidity, mortality, and litigation from obstetric complications. This becomes a bigger issue in rural areas, where the nearest perinatal center may be up to 50 miles away.

Correctional environments are often anti-therapeutic. In a mileau of punishment, usual and customary prenatal activities frequently are not provided. Correctional officials and medical staff must understand the societal importance of encouraging a positive pregnancy outcome. It is recommended that adequate space and time are set aside for parenting and prenatal group classes. Private space and time are necessary for proper case management. Many institutions are more concerned about having a punitive environment than providing supportive services. It should be realized, however, that parenting, perinatal, and case management services may assist the mother in behavior or attitudinal changes that may positively affect the future relationship between the mother and child.

Whether one considers a small lock-up of 50 or less, or a large jail of 9,000, the attitude of the correctional staff and the "front-line" medical workers is often more important in providing suppport during a stressful pregnancy than what specific programs are provided. If the obstacle course to getting to the doctor, the laboratory, the x-ray technician, or the health educator is so insurmountable, it doesn't matter how well "the prenatal team" does its job. The act of living day to day with the "line" officers, medics, and nurses needs to be tolerable.[8]

As an example: Jane (a fictional character made of a composition of real ones) was arrested 4 days ago and processed and placed on the tier 2 days ago. Having been without her usual $50-per-day heroin habit, she is having vomiting, diarrhea, and abdominal cramps, and is in her 15th week of gestation. First, she needs to gain the attention of her correctional officer ... who will call the medication

nurse ... who needs to call the dispensary doctor, nurse practitioner, or physician assistant to address this patient's needs. It doesn't matter how qualified, how comforting, how understanding her final provider is. She first needs to reach that point. That means the less-than-qualified officer, medic, and nurse need some basic triage skills in obstetrics. It is also so easy to be empowered by anger and self-righteousness against the individual who has self-destructive behavior and who may be harming a fetus. Without sensitivity training, the stress of dealing with women who are at the lowest point in society can be overwhelming for staff. This stress often manifests itself in unprofessional, demeaning behavior by both correctional personnel and medical staff. It can be as difficult, yet delicate, as weeding a flower bed to strike the perfect balance of tough standards and self-motivation that these women desperately need, without imposing cynicism or hopelessness.[9]

HOUSING

Often, because jail and prison populations remain overwhelmingly male, housing arrangements for women may not be given priority. Arrangements for customary and required services, such as infirmary units, clinic examination rooms, specialized housing, counseling rooms, drug treatment, etc., may not be available for female inmates until their numbers justify separate facilities. Nevertheless, women must have access to these services. Anecdotal reports of pregnant women being housed on acute psychiatric units during pregnancy because of unavailability of appropriate housing confirm an unacceptable practice.

Medical staff must help correctional authorities to understand that certain housing considerations must be granted to pregnant women. For example, during pregnancy the bladder is compressed, resulting in a need to urinate more frequently than normal. Pregnant women, therefore, must not be locked in cells (segregation or otherwise) that do not have toilets. Gravid women near term or at risk for abruptio placenta must be housed in areas where immediate access to correctional staff is available. It makes sense to offer all pregnant women lower bunks. Overcrowding, which results in housing pregnant women on tiers where health care staff have to decide who is awarded a top bunk, results in conflict, anger, unnecessary medical work, and increased risk to the mothers and fetuses. Housing arrangements also need to provide for liberal movement. Correctional authorities need to know that lack of freedom to move, which is often a consequence of segregation housing or shackling, may result in increased risk for pulmonary embolism or deep vein thrombosis.

The recommendation to house pregnant women in a single tier has advantages and disadvantages. In larger systems with multiple pregnant women, single-site housing permits easier access to parenting and prenatal classes. Delivery of special diets is also made easier for correctional staff. Other specialized treatments (drug treatment) can also be centralized or provided in groups on the housing unit.

The disadvantage to centralized housing is that congregate housing promotes exposure to airborne infection and contagious diseases, such as tuberculosis or influenza. While the risk of exposure on a pregnancy tier may be no different than on any other tier, once an exposure occurs all the pregnant women on the unit might be exposed.

Also, issues of pregnancy termination, adoption, and foster care, whether state-mandated or not, create hostilities between those who favor abortion and those who do not. These hostilities can result in altercations between inmates, which can be disruptive of clinic care. Health care staff need to be vigilant in maintaining an appropriate professional demeanor during these situations.

It is important that the provider actually physically assess the patients' living areas on a regular basis. It is the only way to understand how some unfortunate is being bullied or harassed, or how gang activity can impact an entire area and cause significant stress. It is not uncommon that extra food is traded for cigarettes or an extra blanket. Nor is it uncommon that a patient is pressured or threatened with physical harm for sex acts. Frequently, an older woman may support a primagravida who has been frightened by a roomful of experienced pregnant women's stories of what labor and childbirth is like. The biggest ally or foe to the prenatal clinic process is the impression the health care providers make on the "strong" ones, usually the women that "lead" the whole "tier." Animosity, distrust, and unfounded accusations can undermine even the best prenatal care. Patients even in this setting do have to meet you halfway. The most difficult task is to remain patient no matter what the attitude, be very slow to be offended no matter the remark, and remain firm in the limits that are set for discontinuing an encounter (cursing, threatening behavior, or language). Even with a poor start, a clean start with a disgruntled patient should be attempted–if not later the same day–then at least within a week. Judgmental behavior and accusations flung back at an incarcerated pregnant woman only backfire as she becomes more defensive and angry. Remember that as the provider one can leave, take the next day off, or go home and cool down, while the patient has lost her freedom and has lost many controls.

DIETARY ISSUES

Prison or jail food is frequently unappetizing. Many of the social cues that enhance consumption of food are absent in the prison setting. Food may be cold or poorly heated, and mass-produced for its calorie and vitamin content rather than for its taste. To the average patient the food is barely tolerable and very repetitive. Nevertheless, at the very least, the pregnant woman's diet should have more calories with extra iron and calcium sources and should be low in nitrates that are harmful to the fetus. It is important to rec-

ognize that because of a distaste for prison food, many inmates frequently sustain themselves from items purchased from the prison "commissary" (the institution's makeshift, all-purpose store for personals, cigarettes, and junk food). Health care staff need to appreciate that the poorest women who have no means to pay for commissary items have no means to supplement their diets, since bread and peanut butter are favorite substitutes from the commissary for a meal that is particularly not palatable. Often very picky eaters, borderline hyperemesis patients, and those with multiple-fetus gestations, need expensive liquid nutritional supplements to gain the minimum weight requirements.

DRUG WITHDRAWAL

As already discussed, drug withdrawal is a major cause of morbidity in the correctional setting. Luckily, it rarely lasts longer than 5 to 7 days. Heroin withdrawal in the late second and third trimester can precipitate fetal distress, preterm labor, and meconium complications after birth. When deemed necessary, heroin-addicted women should be started on methadone to prevent these complications. Cocaine abuse can precipitate abruption of the placenta and intrauterine fetal demise. Certainly alcohol withdrawal should be assessed in a hospital, since progression to delerium tremens is an obstetric emergency. Also, fetuses with fetal-alcohol syndrome need to be identified as quickly as possible. These patients in the late third trimester need frequent antepartum, non-stress testing even after the acute withdrawal symptoms have subsided.

GESTATIONAL DIABETES AND SPECIAL PROBLEMS

Multiple-fetus gestations, gestational diabetics, Rhogam candidates, and post-dates occur fairly frequently and are provided for in the same manner as in the community (with non-stress testing and biophysical profiles). The difficulty for the gestational diabetic is getting the screening done as soon as possible for those with risk factors. It is recommended to perform screening for those at risk at the first prenatal clinic. All other women should be screened at 26 to 28 weeks' gestation. Once identified, the intense monitoring of up to four-times-a-day chemstrips (fasting and several post-prandial), and provision of a proper ADA diet (to permit weight gain, yet allow tight control of blood sugars) are very difficult in a correctional setting. Medical personnel in correctional settings frequently need inservicing on managing the treatment and education of the gestational diabetic.

Because of the intensity of services required by gestational diabetics, infirmary housing is recommended. Tight control of blood sugar must be matched with appropriate weight gain. Once the right balance of food, weight gain, and insulin is in place, the surveillance can be eased; however, this rarely happens with the erratic eating habits of prisoners. When appropriate housing for monitoring purposes and trained and qualified health care staff are unavailable, these patients should be referred to an off-site qualified physician's office. In this case, the correctional health care staff must understand and carry out the recommendation of the off-site physician.

SELECT MEDICAL CONDITIONS AND PREGNANCY

Certain medical conditions, such as asthma, tuberculosis, hypertension (not pre-eclampsia), cardiac disease, thyroid disorders, hemoglobinopathies, seizure disorder, peptic ulcer disease, and general surgical conditions, may require consultation with a tertiary care center. Pre-eclampsia, toxemia, and hepatic abnormalities with hemolysis that can occur in late pregnancy should be monitored in a hospital setting.

Obstetric conditions that may also require consultation or inpatient management include hyperemesis gravidarum, intra-uterine growth retardation, abruption, placenta previa, history of first-and second-trimester fetal loss (i.e., cerclage candidates), and patients requiring IV tocolytics. Oral tocolytics can be attempted in the jail/prison setting if frequent monitoring is possible.

Infection with HIV is an ever-increasing concern in pregnancy, and testing should be offered to all. Not by any means, however, should it be mandatory. The percentage of female AIDS cases reported to the CDC from 1987 to 1995 increased from 10% to 20%. In Illinois in 1995, 0.13% of all child-bearing women had HIV. For perspective, this equals the percentage of women who had babies with neural tube defects. That percentage is five to six times higher in black women and probably even higher in incarcerated women. Not only is the number of HIV-positive women increasing rapidly, but the results of the 1991 NIH ACTG-076 trial should compel all providers to test all pregnant women for HIV disease. The use of Zidovudine (ZDV) during the last two trimesters, during labor and delivery, and during the first 6 weeks of the newborn's life reduced HIV transmission from 25.5% (the placebo group) to 8.3%.

When women are known to be HIV positive, their prenatal care should focus not only on the fetus, but also on providing the best care to the mother in her stage of the disease. Opportunistic infection prophylaxis and multiclass antiviral agents should be used. When she is pregnant, ZDV should be added to her regimen and frequent consultation to an HIV specialty center is recommended. For the woman who is first diagnosed while pregnant, the disclosure can be devastating and counseling should be available for all the emotions she needs to deal with. Unfortunately, there is usually very little time for this woman to make a decision on whether she wants to terminate the pregnancy or if she wants to take ZDV during the pregnancy. Supportive services such as health education and case management should be offered.

PSYCHIATRIC ILLNESS AND PREGNANCY

Another class of inmate is the chronic psychiatric patient who is pregnant. Again, health education and counseling are paramount to include this gravida in the process of pregnancy, labor, and delivery. Antidepressants, antipsychotics, and other medications should be given as needed for better outcome. Very few drugs cause any significant teratogenicity and using these drugs may give profound improvement in symptoms in the gravida. The exception is the use of lithium in the first trimester, but again, in severe mania, it should be used in the latter trimesters.

LABOR, BIRTH, AND THE POSTPARTUM PERIOD

Like most pregnant women, those behind bars worry about how difficult labor and birth will be. They also worry if they will be believed and taken to the hospital in time for the delivery. They worry if it will be a dignified experience. The answer depends on inservicing of correctional officers and medical staff to triage and transfer appropriately. Correctional staff should not be allowed in the delivery room, nor should the patient be shackled. Emphasis should be on as safe and natural an experience as possible. Analgesia and anesthesia should be administered per protocol. If possible, family should be allowed to support the laboring patient, and the health care team should be the same as the antenatal team in clinic. The fear of ridicule and stigmatization by other patients and unknown providers is very real. It is not unusual for this patient to be overly sensitive and to cling to her infant after delivery. The inservicing of hospital staff who may not deal with predominantly incarcerated women may not be easy or practical. Very few women's jails and prisons have arrangements for mothers to take care of their own infants, so separation and bonding issues are terrifying. Transferring guardianship to other loved ones—mothers, sisters, husbands, boyfriends, etc.—may be confusing. Panic, profound sadness, or anger may be some of the emotions when the day of separation does arrive (usually 24 to 72 hours after the birth).

PRECIPITOUS DELIVERY

With good triage skills, staff can usually transport women to the hospital prior to delivery. Sometimes, women in labor are not transported in a timely fashion and precipitously deliver at the correctional facility. In addition, multigravida patients may also deliver precipitously at the facility. Failure to appropriately monitor women near term, or housing arrangements that do not permit women near term to be close to staff, may result in a precipitous delivery in the inmate housing units or cells. These events are unsettling to other inmates and have negative risk-management consequences.

If the inmate begins delivery in the health care unit before transportation can be arranged, it is best to create a quiet and secluded area within the health care unit. Officers and onlookers should be asked to leave so that privacy is afforded the woman in delivery. Transportation should be by ambulance, and phone consultation with the local area hospital should be made early to guide care of the mother and infant.

All health care staff in correctional facilities housing pregnant women should be trained in infant basic life support and basic delivery skills (e.g., supporting the perineum, suctioning the infant's nose and mouth, checking for a nuchal cord, etc.). Immediate transportation is crucial, especially for preterm deliveries and meconium-stained amniotic fluid.

After mother and infant are safely transported, precipitous deliveries at the facility should be reviewed so that flaws in the facilities practices can be corrected. Any early signs of labor that had been missed or ignored should be discussed among the staff. Inservicing and additional educational support may be necessary. The goal is to prevent any precipitous delivery in the correctional facility.

Pregnancy Loss

Pregnancy loss, at any time, can be devastating, but added grief and anger can exist for the incarcerated woman. Misconceptions about the cause of the loss and her role or the staff's role in the loss should be addressed with the patient. Answering any questions honestly and openly alleviates anger toward the staff and the facility, and reduces the chance of displaced guilt over her own part in the event. Reassurance and group discussion with other pregnant women also fosters more trust and support.

POSTPARTUM CARE

Postpartum care is fairly routine, with most complications such as episiotomy or wound infection, bleeding, and breast engorgement manifesting within the first week. For those who have breast-fed babies in the past, and for those who would have chosen to were they not incarcerated, it is a time of grief and loss. What is not routine is the emotional loss the woman feels. Psychiatric consultation should be liberal. These women should be returned to their original housing assignments after their immediate recovery. That is where their few support systems have been built with other inmates and staff. They want to share their experience (even if it was negative) and brag about their child. When they are housed with those who have known them, even subtle postpartum depression is noted sooner by the appropriate health care workers. They need support from health educators and case managers to feel that, since they delivered, they have not been forgotten.

Again, the actual assessment and care of the stable inmate and the emergent care when complications occur do not differ from guidelines for any pregnant woman. Moreover, the demographics are very similar to inner-city

public health clinics.[10] The major difference is to understand the loss of freedom, and the desolation and despair that affects the attitude of these patients. There is also physical loss of freedom that prevents movement to the health care team at will. Even in the prenatal clinic there is a loss of freedom, for they cannot choose a provider or switch to a different one. The sensitivity required for health care workers goes beyond being empathic. The realization should be made that full control of management belongs to the health care provider in a situation that, for most women, is a major change and an initiation to a new phase of the life cycle. That control should not be abused, care should not be coerced, and as many choices as possible should be alotted these women. Non-judgmental, non-punitive, but still directive care will usually yield a good outcome in this unnatural environment during such a profound time as labor, delivery, and childbirth in these women's lives.

Good outcomes also depend on thorough prenatal care, with emphasis on substance-abuse counseling and case management, which will help link patients to various resources when they return to the community.[11] This is crucial for those who are incarcerated less than 120 days. For those who do deliver in jail or prison, even minimal prenatal care and sobriety from drugs and alcohol usually have great effects on outcome.[12] Apart from good clinical care, environmental factors and the sensitivity of "line staff," medical and correctional, have the most significant effect on the patient's perception of pregnancy, labor, delivery, and the postpartum period as having been dignified and humane.

REFERENCES

1. Safyer SM, Richmond L: Pregnancy behind bars. *Semin Perinatol* 19(4):314-322, 1995.
2. Cordero L, Hines S, Shibley KA, et al: Duration of incarceration and perinatal outcome. *Obstet Gynecol* 78(4):641-645, 1991.
3. Fogel CI, Harris BG: Expecting in prison: Preparing for birth under conditions of stress. *J Obstet Gynecol Neonatal Nursing* 15(6):454-458, 1896.
4. Egley CC, Miller DE, Granados JL, et al: Outcome of pregnancy during imprisonment. *J Reprod Med* 37(2):131-134, 1992.
5. Philipp E: Pregnancy in prison. *Br J Clin Pract* 1985; 39(9):331-334.
6. Ogden J: Labour chains. *Nursing Times* 91(31):18, 1995.
7. Dillner L: Shackling prisoners in hospital. *Br Med J* 312(7025):200, 1996.
8. Hufft AG: Psychosocial adaption to pregnancy in prison. *J Psychosoc Nursing Mental Health Serv* 30(4):19-22, 1992.
9. Shelton BJ, Gill DG: Childbearing in prison: A behavioral analysis. J Obstet Gynecol Neonatal Nursing 18(4):301-308, 1989.
10. Fogel CI: Pregnant inmates: Risk factors and pregnancy outcomes. *J Obstet Gynecol Neonatal Nursing* 22(1):33-39, 1993.
11. Breuner CC, Farrow JA: Pregnant teens in prison. Prevalence, management, and consequences. *West J Med* 162(4):328-330, 1995.
12. Cordero L, Hines S, Shibley KA, et al: Perinatal outcomes for women in prison. *J Perinatol* 12(3):205-209, 1992.

17

Women's Health Care in the Incarcerated Setting

Lisa Keamy, M.D.

INTRODUCTION

Although the absolute numbers of women in correctional facilities remain at less than 10% of the total prison and jail population, the rate of increase of incarcerated women from 1985 to 1995 is approximately one and a half times that of males[1] (Table 17-1). Women are one of the fastest growing populations of incarcerated individuals. Although women often are provided separate facilities when they are detained or imprisoned, they are often subjected to the same programs, policies, and procedures governing their male counterparts. When this occurs, the health care policies that specify the care that the women receive may fail to address issues related to reproductive function as well as the complex psychosocial issues surrounding the incarceration of single female heads of household. Health assessments, preventive screening, and treatment for many conditions must be gender specific. In the civilian setting, lack of gender-specific research and treatment guidelines has prompted efforts such as the National Institutes of Health Women's Health Initiative, which funds studies that will eventually increase the women's health database as it pertains to not only gynecologic and psychological issues but also internal medicine issues.

Despite the growing number of women who are incarcerated, the numbers were still small in 1997. There is very little gender-specific research of various disease rates in correctional facilities. Data and audits from Cook County Jail in Chicago, Illinois have demonstrated greater rates of HIV infection, syphilis, chlamydia and gonorrhea, illegal substance abuse, and mental illness for women entering the institution, relative to either their male counterparts or women in civilian settings.[2] It is suggested that these differences may be related to a greater percentage of women engaged in commercial sex work, as well as a higher soci-

Table 17-1. Number of adults in state and federal prisons or jails, by sex and race

	Total males	White males	Black males	Total females	White females	Black females
1985	692,600	382,800	309,800	40,500	21,400	19,100
1995	1,438,100	726,500	711,600	113,100	57,800	55,300
1985–1995 % increase	108	90	130	179	170	190

Note: populations estimated rounded to the nearest 100.

Modified from National Institute of Justice: *Correctional Populations in the United States.* Washington, D.C., U.S. Department of Justice, Office of Justice Programs, Bureau of Justice Statistics, 1995, with permission.

etal threshold for the incarceration of women. Although the differences may be multifactorial in their origin, they rest heavily on the fact that, with a smaller, absolute census, a relatively greater percentage of the incoming female population, as compared with the male population, is composed of drug users and commercial sex workers. In addition to health problems directly related to these practices, another factor is a general absence of health care before incarceration. Although some women may be apathetic to health care needs secondary to drug use or a chaotic lifestyle on the street, there are many more whose access to adequate health care has been blocked by virtue of their existence within the socioeconomic underclass of our society. Women who are unable to hire adequate legal assistance or who are unable to pay their bond are probably no more able to obtain health care while not incarcerated. Additionally, the majority of women entering jails and prisons do so during their reproductive years. Many have young children and have been single heads of household. Two studies from the early 1990s suggest that two thirds of incarcerated women have one or more children younger than the age of 18 years.[3] With arrest and detention come uncertainty regarding the immediate whereabouts and well-being of one's children, accompanied by the possibility that custody may be moved outside the extended family, either temporarily or permanently. This can be a psychological stressor of enormous proportion, in addition to the "regular" stress of being behind bars. Its impact on health and health care-seeking behaviors should not be underestimated. Women entering correctional settings may also have a much higher than average prevalence of prior victimization through physical, sexual, or psychological violence.[2]

Taken together, these factors create unique care needs for both short- and long-term female detainees and prisoners. Any facility housing women should have appropriate resources for the delivery of care from midadolescence through old age. Family physicians, given their training in internal medicine, obstetrics and gynecology, pediatrics, and psychiatry, are ideally equipped to care for this population. This is especially true when a single physician is responsible for all care. Because many centers do not have

staffing by family physicians, physicians must receive additional training to provide appropriate gynecologic care. Alternately, a system may choose to spend extensive resources by bringing in specialists or by sending many patients off site for care. Midlevel providers, if used, should have skills that range from obstetrics and gynecology to internal medicine and mental health. As the specialties of obstetrics–gynecology and primary care medicine seek to broaden the scope of their training programs to include more internal medicine and gynecology, respectively, these providers may work singly in a female correctional setting. Adequate support services such as a resource library, private examination rooms equipped for the performance of gynecologic examinations, a working microscope with dark-field capabilities, a Doppler stethoscope (for prenatal care), and the on-site capability to perform urine pregnancy tests and dipstick urinalyses are useful components of any system providing care for women.

This chapter is not written primarily for family physicians or obstetrician–gynecologists; it is directed to other clinicians who may find daunting the task of caring for women who are of reproductive age in the full context of their health care needs, be they medical, gynecologic, obstetric, or psychological.

INTAKE SCREENING

In addition to an appropriate general medical and psychiatric history, a number of questions are pertinent specifically to women, and special attention should be paid to substance abuse during intake screening (Box 17-1). In a prison, women should have their own history and physical forms to accommodate these specific questions. Jails might find it easier to include a women's health addendum to their general history and physical form. The intake history, like the physical examination that follows, must take place where privacy is assured, both to protect the woman from inappropriate scrutiny and to increase the likelihood of reliable responses. Two important features of the history—the assessment for domestic violence and the sexual history—are vital in directing the course of care, and women must feel that their privacy is ensured before they will reveal intimate details of their lives.

Box 17-1. Intake History—Addendum for Females

Past medical history (gynecologic and obstetric)
1. Last menstrual period and last normal menstrual period
2. Last sexual intercourse, use of contraception, perceived risk of pregnancy
3. Age at menarche, cycle length, amount of flow (days and quantity)
4. Prior menstrual abnormality
5. Prior STD
6. Most recent Pap smear, history of previous abnormal pap smears, prior colposcopy
7. Prior gynecologic surgery, prior history of cysts or tumors
8. History of DES exposure
9. Prior pregnancies—with outcomes regarding miscarriage or abortion, full or pre-term, birth weight, complications of pregnancy or delivery
10. History of prior breast abnormalities, mammograms, biopsies

Family history
1. Breast or ovarian cancer
2. Osteoporosis

Social history
1. Assessment of family and household structure, with attention to issues related to number, location, safety of children
2. Brief assessment of history of past or ongoing domestic violence
3. Sexual history to elicit high-risk practices for STDs, especially HIV and hepatitis, including questions that assess HIV risk for prior sex partners

Abbreviations: *STD*, sexually transmitted disease; *DES*, diethylstilbestrol.

Box 17-2. Physical Examination—Addendum for Females

1. Breast examination with self breast examination instruction.
2. Pelvic examination, with attention to external genitalia, speculum and bimanual examination, with collection of cervical cultures for chlamydia and gonorrhea, evaluation of vaginal discharge if present. Pap smears should be performed as indicated (see discussion). Bimanual examination should assess tenderness of uterus or adnexae, uterine enlargement, or adnexal mass.
3. Laboratory procedures as indicated—see discussion in text.

When assessing for HIV risk, the physician needs to initiate a thorough discussion of all previous partners and their risk factors to help identify the risk from heterosexual spreading of the disease that accounts for 38% of female AIDS cases.[4] In civilian populations, the rate of heterosexual spread is rising more rapidly than that caused by injection drug use. From 1990 to 1996, heterosexual acquisition rose by 146%; acquisition secondary to injection drug use rose by 60%.[4] In civilian urban emergency departments, there is underdiagnosis of HIV infection in women relative to men. This is thought to be secondary to too low an index of suspicion for possible heterosexual spread in women with minimal risk otherwise.

The examination should consist of a general physical examination focused on areas identified during the past history interview and systems assessment, as well as additional gender-specific items (Box 17-2). Performance of laboratory examinations as part of the routine intake screening should be directed toward the rapid identifica-tion of processes, such as infection or pregnancy, so that morbidity is minimized and, in the case of early release, so that the ongoing spread of disease back into the community is minimized. To this end, all women should, in addition to gonorrhea and chlamydia cultures, have blood drawn for a syphilis serologic test. Where resources permit, women who have childbearing potential should have rubella titers performed. Admission screening at Cook County Jail revealed that almost 10% of women who were of reproductive age were not immune.[2] Pregnancy testing, Pap smear performance, and HIV serologic determinations are more complicated in their indications and in their practical and administrative ramifications, and will be addressed one by one.

Human immunodeficiency virus serologic determination, although important to obtain in any woman with risk factors who would voluntarily undergo testing, reasonably cannot be performed at intake in those settings in which evaluations happen immediately on entry to a facility. Intake testing in jails is difficult as a result of a lack of privacy, the inability of staff to perform appropriate pretest counseling in an often-rushed receiving area, and the inability to guarantee return of results and, therefore, posttest counseling, before discharge. Testing for HIV status should be reserved for women at risk who will have long enough stays to undergo adequate pretest and posttest counseling and who will be able to benefit from that knowledge while incarcerated (i.e., those that will be able to receive appropriate further workup and therapy). An extremely important subgroup is that of pregnant women, for whom identification and treatment can reduce perinatal transmission by two thirds (from 25.5% to 8.3%), as demonstrated in the AIDS Clinical Treatment Group 076.[5]

Pap smears should be performed on all women entering prison facilities. Indications within a jail setting are different, mostly because of administrative reasons. Performance of Pap smears is not useful if the result will not be available to the patient before she leaves the facility. Many laboratories have a turnaround time of 2–4 weeks for processing. In addition, women entering jails may give false names, phone numbers, or addresses. If a woman leaves before the return of an abnormal Pap smear result, an administrative burden is placed on the physician, who must attempt to locate and notify the patient. Additionally, Pap smears performed on women with active vaginal and cervical infections are frequently read as abnormal, and repetition of the test is needed after treatment. An unpublished study of 100 consecutive female admissions to Cook County Jail, Chicago, Illinois in 1989 revealed 62 abnormal Pap smears, of which more than half had clear evidence of specific, treatable infection. Pap smears should not be performed in the presence of acute inflammation or active menstruation, but should be scheduled for some later time within the first few weeks of incarceration and after any indicated treatment has been instituted. Likewise, Pap smears should be deferred in women who expect to be discharged from the correctional facility before test results could reasonably be expected to be returned, unless they are willing, in confidence, to provide a stable address or phone number in the community to which results could be given. Such an approach conserves valuable health care resources and improves the utility of screening.

Pregnancy tests are yet more complicated. It is important to identify pregnant women within a correctional setting to ensure early prenatal care for women whose pregnancies are often high risk. Early identification also ensures early access to methadone for pregnant narcotics abusers. Last, early identification prevents the use of medications, vaccines, or radiologic procedures that might be contraindicated early in pregnancy. National Commission on Correctional Health Care standards suggest that all women undergo pregnancy testing at admission. Most currently available urine pregnancy tests are easy to perform and are reliable, detecting pregnancy at 10–14 days after conception—up to a day or two before a missed menstrual period. Result limiting factors are that the woman's urine is to be adequately concentrated (specific gravity greater than 1.015) and that the time elapsed since last possible conception is at least 10–14 days. This last feature makes routine pregnancy test screening at admission problematic, as a woman entering may have recently conceived but may be within the 2-week "window," which results in a false-negative test. The intake study from Cook County Jail evaluated 100 consecutive detainees, of which 8 had positive pregnancy tests on entry; 1 of the 8 was unaware of her own pregnancy and had not yet missed a menstrual cycle. Of the remaining women with negative pregnancy tests, 65% gave histories of recent sexual intercourse (within 1 week of incarceration). Thus, at least 65% of women in that study group were at possible risk for falling within the window. Although the study failed to retest those women with negative results at intake, to estimate how many false-negative results one might expect by testing immediately, such a study is needed.

PREVENTION
Cancer Screening

Breast cancer. Breast cancer screening modalities include patient-performed breast examination, clinician-performed breast examination, and mammography. Although a highly publicized test exists to establish the presence of a genetic marker for cancer (the *BrCa* gene), the familial breast cancer for which it represents increased risk is rare; therefore, this test has no utility for widespread screening. Differences exist between various professional organizations regarding initiation of screening and the time interval between screenings. The U.S. Preventive Health Services (USPHS) Task Force, after review of studies and recommendations from other organizations, recommends mammograms and clinical breast examinations every 1–2 years for women from the age of 50–69 years. It further states that little evidence exists to support the use of mammography or clinical breast examination screening in women aged 40–49 years, although the American Cancer Society, the American College of Obstetricians and Gynecologists, and the American Medical Association recommend them both every 1–2 years during this time period.[6] The latter recommendation is followed by many practitioners in the community. There is also no consensus with respect to cessation of surveillance; although the American Geriatric Society recommends cessation at age 85 years, the USPHS again cites a lack of clear evidence of benefit in women older than the age of 70 years. The decision to stop screening should be made by both the physician and the patient individually, based on issues such as desire or willingness to undergo treatment, overall quality of life, and other coexisting illnesses. Increased surveillance in women younger than 50 years who have first-degree relatives with breast cancer, especially cancer of premenopausal onset, has no basis in studies, per the task force. Nonetheless, many practitioners would choose to begin surveillance by mammography at 35–40 years or earlier to relieve patient anxiety. In the presence of a strong multigenerational history of breast and ovarian cancer, genetic testing might be warranted, and a woman should be referred for counseling with specialists to address this extremely complex issue.

Beyond official screening recommendations, which should be adhered to in the case of long-term (more than 1 year) detainees or inmates, the decision about whether to offer mammography to women who will be incarcerated for less than the age-specific screening interval is an individual facility decision. It needs to be made on the basis of available resources measured against the level of medical care the detainee or inmate is likely to receive on the outside. Thus, an uninsured or dysfunctional woman in her 50s who has never had a prior mammogram and who is unlikely to seek one on the outside should be offered one even if her jail stay is for only 1 or 2 months.

Ovarian cancer. Ovarian cancer is diagnosed more frequently than invasive cervical cancer and carries a higher mortality rate than cervical and endometrial cancer combined. Cancer statistics for 1995 cite 26,600 cases and 14,500 deaths from this cancer.[7] Nonetheless, there are no routine screening recommendations for this malignancy because a 1994 National Institutes of Health Consensus Conference found no evidence that screening the general population using pelvic examinations, serum CA 125 levels, and ultrasound had any effect on mortality or morbidity.[8] Three large screening trials are currently in progress comparing no screening to various combinations of ultrasound, pelvic examinations, and blood tests, and their target completion dates range from 2002 to 2008. Although no longer within the realm of asymptomatic screening, any adnexal mass in a woman who is going through or has already gone through menopause must be evaluated aggressively for possible cancer. Although many practitioners believe that ovarian cancer is not seen with any symptoms until it is far advanced, complaints of pelvic pain or a new onset of abdominal distention occur as presenting symptoms in more than half of women given diagnoses of stage I disease.[9] Women with these complaints deserve a closer evaluation using pelvic examination and ultrasound. Women with first-degree relatives who have ovarian cancer have a lifetime risk of between 6.5% and 8%,[10] and their examinations should be approached with a higher-than-usual index of suspicion.

Cervical cancer. There are approximately 15,000 new cases of cervical cancer diagnosed yearly in the United States, and more than 4,000 deaths were documented for 1994.[11] Pap smears can detect premalignant changes of the cervix; since widespread use of routine screening, mortality from cervical cancer has fallen by as much as 60%.[12] Current recommendations for cervical cancer screening include Pap smears every 1–3 years for all women, beginning at age 18 years or at the age of first sexual intercourse, whichever comes first in life. After three or more consecutive normal annual smears, the test may be performed less frequently at the discretion of the provider, according to guidelines endorsed by the American Cancer Society, American College of Obstetricians and Gynecologists, the National Cancer Institute, the American Academy of Family Physicians, and the American Medical Association.[13] In those women deemed at higher risk for cervical cancer (having three or more previous sex partners, a history of human papilloma virus or sexually transmitted diseases [STDs], a previous abnormal pap smear result, HIV infection, or being a smoker), screening should continue on at least a yearly basis. In women who are at very low risk (virginal women with prior normal Pap smears, those who have had a hysterectomy for benign disease, or those with multiple normal Pap smears earlier in life and who are now older than 65–70 years old), Pap smears may be stopped entirely,[14] although pelvic examinations to assess for uterine and ovarian pathologic conditions are still in order. The vast majority of women entering jail or prison

will fall in the normal-to-high risk category and will require yearly Pap smears. Old records may be difficult to obtain, and efforts to do so should be reserved for those with histories of prior abnormal cytologic results or prior treatment for dysplasia, or both. All women entering a correctional setting should be screened for cervical cancer, with their consent. The National Commission on Correctional Health Care strongly suggests Pap screening for jail settings and mandates it for prisons.[15] Optimal screening takes place at midcycle, without a history of recent (24–48 hour) douching, foreign-body insertion, or sexual intercourse. Concurrent discharge, infection, or menstrual flow can confound results, and collection should occur after resolution of these conditions. The smear should be prepared before other specimens, such as cultures, are taken. A wooden spatula is rotated full circle around the exocervix and is spread on a slide. Immediately after, a cervical cytology brush or, if they are unavailable, a saline-moistened cotton swab is inserted just within the endocervical canal, is rotated, and is then withdrawn and rolled over the slide, and fixative liquid or spray is applied. Results return anywhere from 1 to 4 weeks later. When possible, laboratories with shorter turnaround times should be used (as long as they are accredited). Appropriate follow-up notification is mandatory, whether the woman is still incarcerated or is free.

Currently, cytologic results are classified according to the Bethesda system, which is a system of descriptive diagnoses developed to help clarify both the degree of abnormality and further management. The usefulness of performing cytologic screening extends only so far as the health care provider's ability to understand the results and provide appropriate treatment, follow-up, or referral. Figure 17-1 shows one algorithm for responding to cervial cytologic results.

Abnormal readings that require prompt colposcopy and, therefore, in most settings, referral to a gynecologist, include:

- Atypical squamous cells of uncertain significance—favor dysplasia
- Atypical squamous cells of uncertain significance—favor reactive/inflammation in a short-stay patient for whom follow-up after treatment or at 6 months cannot be guaranteed
- Carcinoma-in-situ
- Cervical intraepithelial neoplasm
- Dysplasia
- Atypical glandular or endocervical cells of uncertain significance
- High-grade squamous intraepithelial lesion
- Low-grade squamous intraepithelial lesion
- Hyperkeratosis or parakeratosis or both

Because continuity of care is difficult to predict in jail settings, prompt colposcopy is suggested when a choice exists. In more stable prison settings, providers may opt to follow the new onset of mild abnormalities, such as a low-

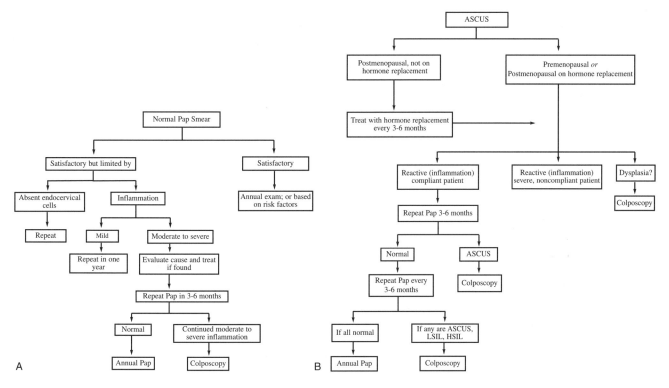

Figure 17-1. Algorithm for responding to cervical cytologic results of a Pap smear: **A,** normal; **B,** atypical squamous cells of uncertain significance (ASCUS).

grade squamous intraepithelial lesion with Pap smears every 4–6 months as long as they remain normal. An exception to this is that any woman with HIV-positive status with an abnormal Pap smear (other than one resulting from a specific infection) should be referred immediately for colposcopy.[16] It is advantageous to maintain clear communication lines with both the pathologist and a gynecologic consultant, as guidance can be provided in many cases by phone. If a woman requires treatment for an infection or close Pap smear surveillance after having had a colposcopy, these can be performed on site. In some facilities, such as those with a large number of women and a high prevalence of abnormalities, it may be most cost-effective to purchase a colposcope and to bring either a gynecologist or a family physician with colposcopy training on site to evaluate women as needed.

Sexually Transmitted Disease

A number of sexually transmitted infections are easily diagnosed and can be treated by the primary care provider. Human immunodeficiency virus related disease, hepatitis, ulcerative genital disease, gonorrhea, and chlamydia have been discussed in the chapter, "Overview of Sexually Transmitted Diseases in Correctional Facilities." The importance of offering zidovudine to pregnant women with HIV as well as the appropriate treatment of pregnant women with syphilis has already been emphasized.

Similarly, treatment for gonorrhea or chlamydia must take into account that some agents frequently used for treatment, such as ciprofloxacin or doxycycline, are contraindicated during pregnancy. Erythromycin, used as an alternative, is poorly tolerated, especially in pregnancy, because of its gastrointestinal side effects. Additionally, treatment regimens for asymptomatic carriers of gonorrhea or chlamydia on routine screening are different than regimens for women with pelvic inflammatory disease (PID). Therefore, detainees and prisoners given diagnoses of positive screening tests require bimanual pelvic examinations to confirm or rule out a suspicion for mild PID. All pregnant women with prior histories or recurrence of herpes simplex virus must inform their obstetric providers, as there is a perinatal transmission risk. Last, as many STDs are diagnosed within days of entry to jails, correctional clinicians should always consider the possibility of early pregnancy when choosing treatment.

Vaginal discharge. Vaginal discharge is a frequent presenting complaint in female populations. Although women outside the correctional setting are often encouraged to invest in over-the-counter therapies for the possibility of a candidal infection before seeking medical care, such an approach is unwise in prison or jail settings. Delayed treatment may lead to a failure to diagnose PID or a systemic infection, and there may be possible adverse effects on future fertility. In an environment in which access to care is

Table 17-2. Therapy for vulvovaginal candidiasis

Drug	Dosing regimen	Relative cost
Clotrimazole (GyneLotrimin, Mycelex)	1% vaginal cream intravaginally daily for 7 days 100-mg tablet intravaginally daily for 7 days 500-mg tablet intravaginally for 1 day	$
Fluconazole (Diflucan)	150-mg tablet orally for 1 day	$+
Miconazole (Monistat)	2% vaginal cream for 7 days 100-mg vaginal suppository for 7 days 200-mg vaginal suppository for 3 days	$$
Terconazole (Terazol)	0.4% vaginal cream for 7 days 0.8% vaginal cream for 3 days 80-mg vaginal suppository for 3 days	$$+

not always prompt, the danger of further delays in appropriate diagnosis and treatment is coupled with a population that tends, at least early in incarceration, to be at higher risk for many STDs. Therefore, all women with symptomatic episodes of vaginal discharge should be adequately evaluated. Although discharge can be uncomfortable or troublesome, it is seldom life threatening in the absence of a fever, pelvic or abdominal pain, or immune compromise, and triage decisions may be made accordingly.

Typically, symptoms of vaginal infection include any combination of discharge, vaginal odor that the woman experiences as unusual or foul, pruritus, labial erythema or swelling, and dysuria. The physician should elicit information from the patient about the other salient features of the history for this complaint; this information would include a concurrent complaint of abdominal or pelvic pain, a fever, chills, a menstrual history with the date of the woman's last menstrual period so that the possibility of pregnancy can be evaluated, a recent sexual history, including change in partners before incarceration, a history of condom use, a prior history of similar symptoms, and any drug allergies. The woman should also be asked about the possibility of a vaginal foreign body, which may be intentional, as in secreted contraband, or accidental, as in retained tampons. The evaluation of vaginal discharge is made predominantly on the basis of a microscopic examination, augmented by visualization of vaginal and labial mucosa and findings on the bimanual pelvic examination. At the time of the speculum examination, notice should be taken of mucosal erythema or lesions. The cervix may be erythematous as well, or it may demonstrate the punctate markings known as a strawberry cervix, which suggest a trichomonal infection. The discharge itself, on gross examination, may appear thick and white or cream colored, often somewhat dry in appearance as in candidiasis; it may appear yellowish-green and frothy, as in trichomoniasis; or it may appear to be a thin, homogenous, grayish-white color, as in bacterial vaginosis. However, as there is significant overlap among these conditions in terms of the gross appearance, both the whiff test

and microscopic evaluation are indispensable. The question of whether to perform tests for other sexually transmitted infections such as gonorrhea, chlamydia, syphilis, or herpes often arises and should be guided by the clinical impression as well as by a working knowledge of intake procedures within a facility. If screening results for gonorrhea, chlamydia, and syphilis from intake are not yet available or if these tests were not performed, they would certainly be performed at the time of an evaluation for vaginal discharge. Finally, the bimanual examination of a woman with uncomplicated vaginitis and an otherwise normal genital tract should be essentially nontender. If significant cervical motion tenderness exists (elicited by gentle intravaginal movement of the cervix by two examining fingers) or if there is adnexal or uterine tenderness on palpation, an upper genital tract infection must be entertained as a diagnosis. (See the section on abdominal pain and PID.)

Once a diagnosis is made, treatment can be fairly straightforward. In the case of vulvovaginal candidiasis, treatment is best achieved with an azole derivative cream, of which several exist. Although vaginal tablets are more convenient for use, creams offer the advantage of allowing application to external genitalia for relief of pruritis. In general, a 3–7-day course of therapy is preferred over shorter regimens that have a higher failure rate. Treatment options among topical agents are listed in Table 17-2 and appear in order of increasing cost. In addition, an immediate dosing regimen with 150 mg fluconazole is highly effective and is less expensive than several of the topical formulations. One runs the risk of systemic side effects, as well as a theoretical danger of eventual resistance, in the face of overuse. Nonetheless, it offers the advantage of ensured compliance in a setting and population known to be variable in their adherence to treatment regimens, and it should be strongly considered for use in clearly documented infection. Furthermore, immediate dosing therapy removes the risk of a 3–7-day supply of cream being lost, stolen, or bartered in the general population. Treatment of trichomoniasis vaginalis is with 2.0 g of metronidazole given in an immediate dose. For treatment failures, metronidazole may be given for 7 days (500 mg twice a day). If treatment again fails, metronidazole can be administered in a dose of 2.0 g every day for 3–5 days. In addition, patients should be queried about ongoing exposure to infection via intimate sexual contact between women or possibly via shared use of personal hygiene items between detainees, although this latter mode of transmission does not appear widely in gynecologic literature. Patients and, if possible, partners should be treated. While taking metronidazole, patients must avoid alcohol (including that sometimes produced within confinement) because a disulfiram-like reaction may occur. Because there is currently no alternative treatment available for women who are allergic to metronidazole or whose treatment fails repeatedly, they are best referred to a specialist. Some women experience unpleasant gastrointestinal side effects to metronidazole, including emesis. An intravaginal metronidazole gel is recommended for use in bacterial vaginosis. At 5 g intravaginally twice a day for 5 days, it is more expensive than 500 mg oral metronidazole that is administered twice a day for 7 days or 2 g immediately. Alternately, clindamycin may be used at 300 mg twice a day for 7 days or may be used intravaginally in a cream form (5 g at bedtime for 7 days). Clindamycin is attractive for women who do not tolerate metronidazole or who are pregnant, because the latter drug is contraindicated early in pregnancy. Because several studies have linked persistent bacterial vaginosis and trichomoniasis to adverse pregnancy outcomes (e.g., preterm labor or preterm rupture of membranes), either infection should be treated as soon as is feasible, and the proscription against metronidazole use early in pregnancy should be kept clearly in mind.

Condyloma. Human papilloma virus, thought etiologically responsible for cervical cancer, causes condyloma acuminata, or venereal warts, although different subtypes are responsible for the two conditions. They are seen as painless rough growths with the texture of the surface of cauliflower on the perineum and anal/genital mucosa. They are not difficult to remove, but it is difficult to prevent recurrence. Removal may be attempted on skin with 25% podophyllin in tincture of benzoin, which is applied to the warts weekly up to six times after protecting surrounding healthy tissue with water-insoluble ointment. A 0.5% podofilox solution for self-treatment is applied twice a day for 3 days with 4 days off, then repeated up to 4 times. Neither of these agents is safe for use during pregnancy. Condylomata may also be treated with bichloroacetic acid or trichloroacetic acid, again applied after protecting the surrounding skin. Cryotherapy with either a cryoprobe or liquid nitrogen may also be effective. Patients with anal and cervical lesions must be referred to a gynecologist for evaluation and treatment. Venereal warts, when mild, are predominantly a cosmetic concern, but an individual can carry the dormant virus in normal adjacent skin even after treatment. Patients should be counseled regarding the infectious

nature of condylomata, and they should be aware of the fact that transmission may occur in the absence of visible lesions. In pregnant women, condylomata should be removed, as they may otherwise grow quite large, become extremely vascular, and interfere with the birthing process. Furthermore, human papilloma virus can cause laryngeal papillomatosis in newborns, whether they are delivered vaginally or by cesarean section.[17]

Preventive measures. Although the diagnosis and treatment of a primary infection caused by an STD is important, perhaps even more crucial is the effort to educate and change the behavior of patients, who have invariably engaged in high-risk sexual behaviors to acquire the STD in the first place. Women undergoing evaluation for or treatment of an STD should have as complete sexual histories as possible taken at the time of their diagnoses. Questions regarding sexual practices, numbers and types of sex partners, and protective measures used (or not used) must all be asked in a matter-of-fact manner to elicit honest responses. The information gathered may be used to show the patient their risk for contracting other STDs, including hepatitis and HIV, as well as their risk for pregnancy. Information can be shared regarding ways to decrease risk, and recommendations can be made regarding surveillance for disease. Some facilities have educators on site that work to provide disease prevention counseling, as well as peer counseling programs for HIV and other STDs. If a woman does not leave treatment with a clear understanding of her infection, how to avoid either spreading or recontracting it, and how to protect herself from other infections, the health care system has failed to fulfill a primary responsibility to the patient and to the community to which she may return.

Domestic Violence

Handgun violence has assumed epidemic proportions among young urban men of color, and has received increasing attention from health care providers with an interest in public health. Likewise, the burgeoning problem of domestic violence arouses the concern of providers of health care to women and children across all racial and socioeconomic classifications. Statistics from the early 1990s suggest that 2–4 million American women are victims of domestic violence yearly.[18] In 1 year, husbands or boyfriends killed 30% of all women murdered.[19] A large midwestern urban jail study reported that 48% of incoming women reported a prior history of being shot, beaten, or stabbed. The 20% shooting or stabbing rate was similar to the prevalence in a study of males at the same institution. The history of prior rape in the women entering was almost 20%.[2] Of importance in correctional health care is the fact that victims can also be victimizers; an estimated one third of female state prison inmates in 1991 were convicted of violent crimes, and one third of that number served time for homicide.[20] Two thirds had victimized someone they knew; women

> **Box 17-3. Screening Questions for Domestic Violence**
>
> 1. Do you have a partner or family member who makes you afraid for your own safety or for the safety of your children? Have you ever had such a partner or family member?
> 2. Do you and your partner ever fight? What happens when you do?
> 3. When you are in your own home, do you feel safe?
> 4. Have you ever been made to have sex against your will?
> 5. Do you feel physically safe in jail/prison?
> 6. Has another individual threatened you while in jail? Who?

From U.S. Healthcare: Current Concepts in Women's Health: Domestic Violence and Primary Care, Monograph, 1994, with permission.

> **Box 17-4. Questions to Assess Lethality**
>
> 1. Does your partner abuse alcohol or drugs?
> 2. Does he have a gun or knife readily available to him? Has he ever attacked or threatened you with either?
> 3. Does he threaten other family or household members?
> 4. Is he violent outside of your home?
> 5. Has your partner ever hurt you while you were pregnant?

From U.S. Healthcare: Current Concepts in Women's Health: Domestic Violence and Primary Care, Monograph, 1994, with permission.

who had been previously abused were more likely to have victimized a relative or intimate partner.[3]

Although physical violence such as beating, hitting, pushing, or forcibly restraining, and emotional or psychological abuse such as constant criticism, intimidation, or threatening future physical violence, come to mind when discussing domestic violence, violence with weapons such as knives and guns is also prevalent. Outside prison, it is estimated that more than a million women each year may seek medical care for injuries caused by battering. Some estimates suggest that domestic violence is implicated in 20% of the cases of women who seek treatment for serious injury by reporting to a hospital, in 25% of the cases of women who attempt suicide, and in 25% of the cases of women who seek prenatal care.[21] Because women who are in relationships complicated by violence are at high risk for revictimization, and because children in homes in which violence is present are more likely to lead adult lives that include violence, the public health dimension of identifying and treating victims and perpetrators of domestic violence is obvious.

Few jails and prisons that house females have extensive programs for victims of violence. Many fail to screen incoming detainees or prisoners, fearing to open a Pandora's box of needs that cannot be met. What constitutes an appropriate approach to identification and treatment of domestic violence within a correctional setting? Although incarcerated women are at least temporarily safe from their abusers, without appropriate interventions and reasonable alternatives, many women return to the same setting they left. Although incarceration is a stressful time for almost every woman, the period away from an abuser may offer a unique window of opportunity to address the problem of violence in a relatively safe environment. Questioning women about domestic violence must be done carefully and nonjudgmentally. Privacy must be provided at intake screening to enhance the reliability of the response.

General questions appropriate for screening are listed in Box 17-3,[22] and might be adapted for use at either intake or in the context of a routine clinical visit.

Positive responses must be explored and documented in as noncritical a manner as possible. Although it is impossible to accurately predict levels of risk, some questions that may help assess lethal potential in a battering relationship (positive responses indicate higher risk) are listed in Box 17-4.[22]

Patients should be informed that domestic violence affects many different types of women; that it often becomes more severe with time; that violence is not safe or acceptable; that it may severely affect not only a woman's health but also the health of her children; and that there are ways to remove herself and her children from danger, as difficult as that may seem. It is also important, given the unique environment in which correctional health care is delivered, to be sensitive to the possibility that the patient may be in detention or prison because of retaliatory violence against her abuser or because of violence she has inflicted on her own children. Additionally, jails and prisons themselves often foment violent behavior. Within the complex social setting of jails and prisons, same-sex partnerships as well as "family" groupings often form, and the concept of "home" assumes a different meaning. When combined with the potential risk of psychological or physical violence at the hand of correctional staff, the possibility of "domestic violence"—psychological, physical, or sexual—is far from remote. Assessing such violence behind bars is fraught with difficulty and poses a challenge for the health care provider who may have little recourse with respect to changing housing assignments, addressing the behavior of correctional staff toward prisoners, or otherwise protecting women who choose to report. Furthermore, the possibility that reports may be falsely generated on the part of a woman for purposes of alleviating uncomfortable living arrangements or to cause disciplinary action against another prisoner must be carefully considered. Any information must be treated with strict confidentiality and be carefully documented. With permission from the patient, medical staff can work with security to increase the personal safety of the woman in question and to monitor the behavior of other inmates or correctional staff.

Once a pattern of violence has been documented, either on the outside or within a facility, what is appropriate ongoing care? Obviously the answer to this question will differ based on a woman's estimated length of stay, whether she is immediately safe or experiencing violence behind bars, and the level of resources that are available both within the correctional facility and in the community at large. Some facilities have mental health programs that include possibilities for individual or group therapy. Classes that focus on building self-esteem, as well as parenting classes to help teach women alternatives to violence within their own childraising practices, exist at some sites and should be encouraged at more. Although programs that address handgun and weapon violence for men exist in some correctional settings, these programs should be expanded to identify and treat domestic batterers who, by and large, are male. Every state has an organization for domestic violence victims,[23] and it may be instrumental in providing information and resources. The possibility of bringing community programs behind bars is a creative approach to providing staff to fulfill special needs. This approach has worked for some major urban jails with respect to other health care issues such as HIV prevention and prenatal care, which, like domestic violence, greatly affect the community to which inmates return. Such a model could also lend itself to domestic violence prevention. Many local communities have domestic violence hotlines as well as emergency women's shelters (some also accommodate children). At the very least, short-stay detainees should be made aware of hotline and shelter numbers and should be encouraged to seek help, either before their discharge or shortly thereafter. Longer-stay detainees may be encouraged to participate in on-site programs. Within correctional settings, it has become standard to screen for infectious diseases, psychiatric diseases, and chronic medical diseases, some of which are easily treatable, but many of which are not. Screening for domestic violence and encouraging the beginning of a journey toward treatment may be even more important to the long-term health of the women who are put behind bars and then who are eventually allowed to return to their families and the community outside.

PROBLEM-ORIENTED TOPICS
Breast Masses

For most women, the finding of a breast lump by self-examination or by physician examination is extremely anxiety provoking. Although breast cancer is curable in its early stages (about 15% to 20% of newly diagnosed cancers are localized), overall mortality has not yet fallen. The incidence has risen to about 11%, doubling since 1951.[24] The increase is thought to be caused, in part, by the increasing longevity of American women and increased screening practices, as well as by changes in diet, hormone use, earlier menarche, older age at time of first pregnancy, and, possibly, environmental factors. Fear of breast cancer cuts across many social and cultural lines and may seem disproportionate, compared with feelings about illnesses such as cardiovascular disease, which often carries a worse prognosis. Appropriate management of a breast mass brings reassurance to the woman, and assures prompt biopsy of suspicious lesions while avoiding unnecessary biopsies of benign lesions. (Many appropriate and necessary biopsies will be benign as well.)

Modalities for imaging breast masses include mammography and ultrasound. The former has been discussed with respect to screening guidelines in asymptomatic women, but may also be used effectively to characterize a palpable mass, especially in older women or in women with less dense breasts (a radiologic characteristic, not a physical characteristic). Ultrasound is the imaging modality of choice in women younger than the age of 35 years because the majority of masses in this age group are benign. Mammography tends to be more difficult to interpret in young breasts, and ultrasound can effectively assess whether a mass appears cystic, solid, or a complex of the two.

A mass identified on physical examination in a young (younger than 35 years) woman and characterized by mobility, discrete margins, and tenderness, may be aspirated after local anesthesia in the primary provider's office, and its contents should be sent for cytologic evaluation. If fluid is aspirated and the mass resolves (presumably, therefore, a cyst), the patient may be followed up for recurrence. If no fluid is obtained, the patient should be sent for an imaging study and a specialist evaluation. A solid mass with a benign appearance, consistent with fibroadenoma, may be followed with a sequential physical examination and mammogram or ultrasound. In women for whom such continuity of follow-up is unlikely, because of either expected early discharge from jail or transfer and for postmenopausal women, more aggressive management including fine-needle or excisional biopsy is warranted. A biopsy, which may sometimes be preceded by imaging studies, should be performed on any mass that appears to be fixed, irregular, or nontender, regardless of the age of the woman. Additionally, a biopsy should be performed on a palpable mass in the absence of mammographic or ultrasound abnormalities, which is a less-likely occurrence. The importance of having access to an experienced surgeon and accurate radiologic services cannot be overemphasized, as they can provide excellent guidance in the decision-making process and can minimize excessive use of open biopsies, while making an early diagnosis of malignancy.

Contraception

Many women entering correctional facilities will be using various forms of contraception at the time of their arrest. Presumably, they will not have heterosexual relations while imprisoned (a small minority of prisons allow conjugal visits, and some jail detainees leave for work release or home, monitoring programs, only to reappear in jail days or weeks later). Although most incarcerated women are not in need of contraception in a formal sense, anyone providing health care for them should be aware of issues related to the use of various contraceptive agents.

Oral contraceptive pills. On entering correctional facilities, women taking oral contraceptive pills may have missed taking their pill for several days by the time they arrive. These women need to be informed that the contraceptive efficacy for their current pill cycle is destroyed, even if they begin taking their pills again after an early discharge to home. These women may also experience withdrawal bleeding within a few days of pill interruption as a normal response, although women often perceive this bleeding as highly abnormal. Some women take oral contraceptive pills for their noncontraceptive benefits in controlling dysmenorrhea, endometriosis, dysfunctional bleeding patterns, acne, or premenstrual syndrome. A physician evaluation must occur to determine whether therapy should be continued or other therapy should be substituted. In settings in which appropriate gynecologic care is not available on site, therapy interruption may necessitate off-site referral early in incarceration. There is no indication for the long-term contraceptive use of birth control pills in prisons in the absence of conjugal visitation programs. In jails, however, the patient and the physician should make a decision based on the estimated length of stay. In correctional settings, oral contraceptive pills may be misused or may become a black market commodity. Their administration should be regulated as part of daily documented medication passage to avoid sporadic use and its consequences (irregular cycles and bleeding).

Depot medroxyprogesterone acetate (DMPA). Depot medroxyprogesterone acetate is an injectable progestational contraceptive agent given intramuscularly every 12 weeks. It may cause weight gain, headaches, and irregular bleeding patterns, as well as amenorrhea, with repeated use. It works by preventing ovulation, although ovulatory function usually returns within 5 months of the last injection. Because DMPA is a highly effective contraceptive agent, amenorrhea in a recently incarcerated woman who was within the therapeutic 12-week window at the time of entry should not be cause for concern.

Long-acting implantable contraception (Norplant). Norplant consists of six injectable silastic tubes containing norgestrel, a progestational agent. Inserted subcutaneously in the upper arm, it provides long-term contraception for up to 5 years. Side effects include bleeding irregularities, headaches, acne, and weight gain. Indications for removal include completing 5 years of use as well as a woman's desire to alleviate known side effects. Women who know they will be incarcerated beyond the contraceptive efficacy remaining should have their implants removed early in their stay. To avoid capsule rupture, a provider who is well versed in the procedure should perform the removal. Training kits for removal are available from the manufac-

turer, and practice enhances removal, which may be a time-consuming process.

Intrauterine devices. Intrauterine devices provide a safe contraceptive option for women who are at low risk for STDs, are multiparous, have no undiagnosed bleeding disorders or histories of ectopic pregnancy, and are able to check their own IUD string. Many women entering correctional facilities will not have been good candidates for this method. Women entering with recent IUD insertion may have menorrhagia or dysmenorrhea. If at any time the IUD string is not located in the vagina by the patient or the provider, it must be localized via ultrasound. If the IUD is located within the uterus, a gynecologist may retrieve the string so that it can once again rest in the vagina. If it has perforated the uterus, it must be surgically removed. The risk for infection with an IUD is higher in women with multiple sexual partners, and, in the setting of PID, IUD removal is advised at the time of treatment. Long-term prison inmates should consider removal if their sentence is longer than the efficacy period for their particular type of IUD.

Disorders of Menstruation

Few complaints elicit more consternation on the part of nongynecologically trained providers of care to women than those involving menstrual abnormality. The "normal" menstrual cycle ranges from 25 to 35 days. The cycle is divided into two phases, the first being the follicular phase, marked by menstrual flow, which occurs in response to declining hormonal levels from the previous cycle, and by the concurrent development of new ovarian follicles with subsequent stimulation by hormones (follicle stimulating hormone [FSH]) released by the pituitary. The maturing follicle produces estrogen, which stimulates the uterine lining to proliferate and thicken. The estrogen produced also stimulates the pituitary to release luteinizing hormone (LH), which, in turn, stimulates progesterone production. The production of LH peaks shortly before ovulation or before rupture of the ovarian follicle, which releases a mature oocyte. With follicular rupture, the luteal phase begins: the remnants of the follicle reorganize into the corpus luteum, and estrogen and progesterone production continues. The luteal phase lasts an average of 14 days (range, 12–17) and is a remarkably consistent time period from woman to woman. The hormones released help maintain the endometrial lining; if pregnancy and implantation occur, the corpus luteum is maintained to enable continued hormone production until the placenta develops and takes over. If pregnancy does not occur, the corpus luteum involutes, progesterone and estrogen levels fall, and the cycle continues with the entry into the follicular phase and menstruation. On average, menstrual flow occurs for the first 5–6 days of each cycle. In general, although the amount of blood lost ranges up to about 30–40 mL, the assessment is confounded by the fact that women frequently overestimate the amount of bleeding they experience. Reporting "pad counts" (i.e., the number of sanitary pads or tampons used) is likewise unreliable. Nonetheless, although the amount of blood lost is difficult to quantify absolutely, most women can accurately describe relative changes in their menstrual flow compared with their perceived baseline.

Amenorrhea. Amenorrhea is defined as an absence of menstruation and is termed *primary*, in which case a woman has not had the onset of menses whatsoever by age 16 years, or *secondary*, in which case a woman has had a history of regular, cyclic menstruation followed by cessation. The vast majority of women in jails and prisons seen with a complaint of amenorrhea will fall into the latter category. However, in facilities that also house adolescents, some cases of primary amenorrhea may be seen. The most important cause of amenorrhea is pregnancy. An undiagnosed pregnancy may result in early pregnancy loss, rupture in an ectopic pregnancy, or iatrogenic exposures to radiation or medications that are contraindicated in pregnancy. A current-generation urine pregnancy test performed on a suitably concentrated urine specimen (specific gravity greater than 1.015) and performed at least 14 days after the last possible sexual intercourse should be diagnostic. The possibility of conception behind bars must be evaluated in any woman with amenorrhea during a jail or prison stay.

Amenorrhea not associated with pregnancy may be treated differently in jails than in prisons. Women with very short lengths of stay may be safely referred to a civilian physician for follow-up after discharge. For longer-term detainees in jails and for prison inmates, a workup should be undertaken because hypoestrogenic states resulting in amenorrhea may result in long-term increased cardiovascular mortality or osteoporosis risk. Hyperandrogenic anovulation may carry an increased risk of diabetes, hypertension, and lipid abnormalities. An undiagnosed prolactinoma may result in destruction of CNS tissue contiguous to it. Likewise, either primary or secondary amenorrhea may be a manifestation of an eating disorder, albeit not a frequent diagnosis made in correctional settings.

During clinical visits, a general medical history should be augmented by a careful menstrual history, including age at onset, frequency, length of flow, and last normal period. A history of contraceptive use, a history of prior gynecologic procedures, a prior obstetric history, and a recent sexual history must be explored. A number of medications, including antipsychotics, tricyclic antidepressants, calcium channel blockers, methyldopa, and cancer chemotherapeutics, can cause amenorrhea, as can illicit drug use, especially use of cocaine and amphetamines. Likewise, recent users of oral contraceptive pills, DMPA, or Norplant may experience amenorrhea for several months after the cessation of use. In the review of systems, differences in skin texture, acne, hair distribution changes, and voice, weight, energy, or libido changes are important to elicit. In women older than 30 years, symptoms of early menopause can be elicited, such as vasomotor symptoms, mood swings, and a history of increasingly irregular menses.

The physical examination should include a blood pressure check, attention to signs of secondary sexual development, such as axillary and pubic hair, and breast development. Breasts should be checked for galactorrhea. The presence of virilization, as evidenced by a male distribution of body hair, such as terminal hair on the face, hair on the chest, upper back, or extensor surfaces of the upper arm, a male escutcheon on the abdomen, or temporal thinning, should be noted. The thyroid should be assessed. A pelvic examination must be performed to assess for clitoromegaly, an imperforate hymen, a vaginal septum, and the presence of a uterus and ovaries, as well as any pelvic mass. Any woman with an absence of secondary sex characteristics and amenorrhea beyond the age of 14 years should be referred to a gynecologist or endocrinologist for evaluation of primary hormonal failure.

Assuming that pregnancy has been suitably excluded, amenorrhea can be thought of as the result of an abnormality in the estrogen level, the androgen level, or regulation at the level of the hypothalamus. An evaluation of amenorrhea combines the assessment from a physical examination in conjunction with laboratory determinations, an observance of various responses to hormonal stimuli, and, in some cases, imaging studies or exploratory surgery. Thyroid-stimulating hormone and prolactin levels should be measured because either subclinical thyroid disease or a pituitary adenoma can cause amenorrhea. Women who are using narcotics, as well as women taking some phenothiazines, may demonstrate galactorrhea and mildly elevated prolactin levels. Retesting after cessation of drugs or medications is useful. When medications cannot be stopped, the upper limit of acceptable should be changed from 20 ng/dL to 50 ng/dL. The patient's estrogen status should then be evaluated by administering a progesterone challenge, for example, 10 mg of medroxyprogesterone acetate daily for 10 days. In the presence of an anatomically normal genital tract, normal endometrium, and an adequate level of endogenous estrogen, such a challenge results in withdrawal bleeding within 2–7 days of the last dose. The absence of withdrawal bleeding suggests either a hypoestrogenic state or damaged endometrium (fairly rare, but possible in situations in which there has been previous overvigorous instrumentation of the uterus, as in dilatation and curettage, with subsequent scarring). The two can be differentiated by administering a "priming" dose of 1.25 mg of estrogen daily for 3 weeks, with 10 mg of medroxyprogesterone acetate concurrently for the last 5 days (days 16–21). An absence of bleeding suggests that the endometrium is scarred and unresponsive. If there is a menstrual response to this regimen, a low estrogen state is implicated and the FSH level should be measured. An elevated FSH level signifies primary ovarian failure or premature menopause. A low FSH level in the presence of hypoestrogenism suggests a disorder of hypothalamic or pituitary origin and would prompt imaging of the pituitary. A normal study would lead one to consider a stress-related cause (something seen frequently but which remains a diagnosis of exclusion).

If the physical examination has pointed toward an excess of androgens (truncal obesity, hirsutism, clitoromegaly, acne, male-pattern baldness), the initial lab workup may include determinations of serum testosterone, dehydroepiandrosterone sulfate (DHEAS), and 17α-hydroxy-progesterone levels. A mild-to-moderate elevation in testosterone (80–200 ng/dL) may cause chronic anovulation. A testosterone level greater than 200 ng/dL is strongly suggestive of an androgen-secreting tumor (adrenal or ovarian). Likewise, a highly elevated DHEAS level (greater than 7,000 ng/dL) is highly suggestive of an adrenal tumor. The possibility of a tumor prompts imaging studies such as ultrasound or CT, and exploratory surgery should be performed as needed.

If, at any point in the evaluation of amenorrhea, the practitioner becomes uncertain of his results or has a suspicion that there is an adrenal, ovarian, or pituitary tumor or adrenal hyperplasia, the patient should be referred to a specialist for definitive diagnosis and treatment. If a progesterone challenge results in withdrawal bleeding, the conclusion is that there is chronically unopposed endogenous estrogen. To prevent endometrial hyperplasia, medroxyprogesterone acetate may be administered for 5–10 days monthly or bimonthly. Alternately, combined oral contraceptive pills may be used monthly. If a woman demonstrates evidence of low estrogen and is either in a premenopausal state with hypothalamic or pituitary dysfunction or has premature menopause, she is at an increased risk for osteoporosis and cardiovascular disease. She should receive combined oral contraceptive pills, which closely mirror premenopausal hormone levels. If she is experiencing menopause and is in her mid-40s or older, she should receive treatment as outlined in the section on menopause and hormone replacement.

Increased bleeding. Increased bleeding is difficult to quantify. The terminology in discussing abnormal menses that are heavier or longer than normal includes menorrhagia (bleeding for more than 7 days or 80 mL total blood loss), metrorrhagia (more frequently than every 21 days), or a combination of the two. Although the term *dysfunctional uterine bleeding* has become a popular term, it really refers to abnormal bleeding patterns that have no fixed anatomical cause and that occur in the absence of pregnancy, infection, clotting disorders, or neoplasms. The evaluation of abnormally heavy or frequent menses rests on a careful history and physical examination, in which factors of age, cancer risk, infection risk, and desire or lack of desire for maintenance of reproductive function all enter into decisions regarding laboratory and diagnostic tests and therapy options. Historical features to note include risk factors for endometrial neoplasms such as obesity, diabetes, advancing

age, a family history of endometrial cancer, or a history of anovulation (with persistent low levels of unopposed endogenous estrogens). The age of onset of bleeding irregularity is important for other reasons as well: the prevalence of uterine leiomyomas (fibroids) may be as high as 33% in older black women who are of reproductive age; the prevalence is slightly lower in whites (about 20% to 25%).[25] Adenomyosis, the presence of endometrial tissue within the muscle layers of the uterus, can also cause menorrhagia, as well as dysmenorrhea, but can only be diagnosed histologically. In young adolescents with menorrhagia, concurrent clotting disorders may exist in as many as 20%.[26] A recent sexual history is critically important; metrorrhagia or menorrhagia of fairly recent onset in women who are of reproductive age may signal a pregnancy; it could be an intrauterine pregnancy with a threatened or missed abortion, an ectopic pregnancy, or a molar pregnancy. Untreated endometritis or cervicitis may be a cause of intermenstrual bleeding or spotting, as well as heavier than usual menses. Cervical polyps are often highly vascular and may bleed intermenstrually. Additionally, although thyroid disease does not usually make its appearance solely in the form of a menstrual disorder, it can cause menorrhagia and amenorrhea.

The laboratory evaluation should begin with a pregnancy test, unless the patient is known to have gone through menopause, in which case episodes of vaginal bleeding need to be evaluated immediately for the presence of an endometrial neoplasm. The evaluation also includes a Pap smear (if one has not been performed within the last 6–12 months or visible abnormalities appear on examination), a complete blood cell count, and a determination of the level of thyroid-stimulating hormone for all patients. Cervical cultures and coagulation studies also could be performed if the history and examination are suggestive of either an infection or a clotting disorder. Endometrial sampling is a valuable, inexpensive, and easily acquired outpatient skill for the primary care provider and can reduce off-site gynecologic visits. It should be performed in any case in which the possibility of an endometrial neoplasm is raised, by virtue of positive risk factors (increasing age, obesity, diabetes) and/or by the persistence of abnormal bleeding. If an endometrial biopsy cannot be performed at the facility, the patient should be referred to a gynecologist, who can perform either a biopsy or dilatation and curettage. Transabdominal and transvaginal ultrasound can be used to diagnose leiomyomas, or the information obtained can suggest a diagnosis of adenomyosis. Transvaginal ultrasound is more expensive but less invasive than endometrial biopsy, and also demonstrates the thickness of the endometrial lining or "stripe." An endometrial stripe greater than 6 mm in a patient who has gone through menopause is indicative of endometrial hyperplasia. In women who have not yet gone through menopause, the endometrial stripe fluctuates with the menstrual cycle, but is usually less than 12–14 mm in width.

Treatment and referral decisions must be made on the basis of diagnostic findings and the correctional clinician's expertise. Underlying conditions, such as infection or thyroid disease, and pregnancies with threatened abortions can be treated in the jail or prison setting. Ectopic pregnancies obviously require immediate, urgent, or emergent referral, depending on the stability of the patient. Hydatidiform moles, as well as endometrial hyperplasia, must be referred for specialty evaluation and care. A diagnosis of a leiomyoma may be safely observed in the absence of profound and refractory anemia, intractable pain, or symptoms secondary to compression of contiguous organs. Iron supplementation may be given to replace heavy blood loss. If more definitive therapy is needed, a referral may be made for interventions that range from myomectomy to total hysterectomy. In some cases of menorrhagia, gonadotropin-releasing hormone antagonists may be given to induce atrophy, which is an expensive option. If no other treatable cause is found, bleeding can be treated with both hormonal and nonhormonal therapies. Hormone therapy includes the use of 10 mg of medroxyprogesterone acetate daily for 10 days each month. Alternately, women may be treated monthly with monophasic combined oral contraceptive pills, given that there are no pre-existing contraindications to their use. Either approach can reduce bleeding and will prevent the increased endometrial cancer risk associated with chronic or intermittent anovulation. Although there is a small risk of estrogenic stimulation of leiomyomas, it is not often significant and can be monitored with serial pelvic examinations or ultrasound. If a woman is in the midst of a period of menorrhagia, monophasic combined oral contraceptive pills are sometimes used to cause bleeding cessation. Pills are administered sequentially one pill at a time three times daily for 7 days, during which time bleeding should cease. Withdrawal bleeding occurs at termination of the pack, then oral contraceptive pills can be used in a routine manner thereafter to maintain the patient's menstrual cycle. Nonhormonal therapy can be given in the form of nonsteroidal anti-inflammatory agents, whose inhibition of prostaglandin synthesis activity may be responsible for decreased endometrial blood flow. A referral to a specialist is warranted at any point in the diagnosis and treatment if the primary provider lacks expertise or is technically unable to perform a needed examination or test, if abnormal results are obtained on biopsy, or if medical treatment fails. In many cases, however, the primary care provider will accomplish evaluation and treatment, with less delay and less cost.

Abdominal Pain

An approach to abdominal pain in female patients must take into account both gynecologic and nongynecologic origins and whether the pain is acute or chronic. Box 17-5

Box 17-5. Causes of Acute Abdominal Pain

Gastrointestinal	Ovarian torsion
Appendicitis	Pelvic inflammatory
Cholecystitis	disease
Diverticulitis	Tubo-ovarian abscess
Gastroenteritis	Infectious
Inflammatory bowel	Bacterial Peritonitis
disease	Hepatic or splenic
Irritable bowel	abscess
syndrome	Trauma
Peptic ulcer disease	Abdominal wall
Obstruction	hemorrhage
Genitourinary	Splenic rupture
Cystitis	Vascular
Polynephritis	Acute hemorrhage from
Nephrolithiasis	ruptured viscus
Gynecologic	Aneurysm rupture
Dysmenorrhea	Sickle crisis
Ectopic pregnancy	Other
Endometriosis	Diabetic ketoacidosis
Leiomyoma (Fibroids)	Narcotics withdrawal
Ovarian cyst	

---

lists some possible causes of pain, quickly reminding the clinician that, although many causes are relatively benign and self-limited, others are potentially life-threatening if unrecognized. Common to the evaluation of abdominal pain in either men or women is the taking of a history to elicit characteristics of the pain. The onset, severity, and location, whether there is radiation, whether the pain is intermittent or continuous, and qualities such as sharpness, dullness, or cramping, can all offer clues as to the diagnosis. Additional symptoms such as a fever, nausea, heartburn, vomiting, diarrhea or constipation, shortness of breath, lightheadedness, jaundice, hematuria, and dysuria, as well as the frequency, may help differentiate between gastrointestinal, genitourinary, or vascular causes. A history of prior medical illness, prior surgery, long-term medication use, illicit drug or alcohol use, or recent trauma, is also useful. In women, additional information related to the pelvic organs is obviously critical. The history should include questions regarding any relationship of the pain to the menstrual cycle, questions regarding both the last menstrual period and the last normal menstrual period, questions regarding the last episode of sexual intercourse and the method of contraception used, if any was used at all. A prior history of pregnancy or childbirth, a prior history of STDs, and the presence or absence of vaginal bleeding, discharge, or dyspareunia, help complete the history. The physical examination should include observation of the patient's ability to walk or position herself on an examination table, the taking of full vital signs, and cardiac, pulmonary, and abdominal auscultation followed by palpation and a rectal examination. In women, a pelvic examination with speculum and bimanual components is mandatory unless the pain is clearly nongynecologic. Useful laboratory tests and data such as a complete blood count with a differential test, the sedimentation rate, electrolyte levels, liver function tests, amylase and glucose levels, a urinalysis with a pregnancy test, cultures, or wet mounts have specific indications, as do studies such as abdominal or chest radiographs, ultrasounds, CT, or endoscopy. Laparoscopy or open laparotomy may be required for diagnosis. A complete discussion of abdominal pain is beyond this chapter's scope, so the focus will now turn to causes that are specific to the female genital tract.

The history guides the clinician's physical examination and further workup. Severe pain that is sudden in onset and without clear relation to menses or the menstrual cycle should arouse concern about a possible organ or structure rupture, such as an ovarian cyst, a tubo-ovarian abscess, or, that which is most catastrophic, an ectopic pregnancy rupture. Ovarian torsion may also result in severe, sudden pain. Peritoneal signs such as guarding on palpation, pain with coughing or walking, or increased pain with maneuvers such as hip extension or external rotation, help support such a diagnosis. A pelvic examination may be significant for diagnosing asymmetric pain with a palpable mass; however, there may be no mass palpable, and by the time of the rupture, symptoms may be rather generalized. A history of fevers and an elevated white blood count and sedimentation rate may favor a diagnosis of an abscess or appendicitis. Lack of a fever, but a missed menses or abnormal last menses coupled with a positive pregnancy test, or an unstable blood pressure or hematocrit, favors suspicion of ectopic pregnancy rupture, a true gynecologic emergency. At any point that the diagnosis of ectopic pregnancy seems likely, staff and transport must be mobilized to ensure rapid access to an emergency department for ultrasonography and surgical evaluation. There is little to no excuse acceptable for loss of life secondary to this treatable entity, which is still the third-ranking cause of obstetric mortality.

Pain that is less sudden in onset, gradually worsening over time to become moderate to severe, may include entities such as functional ovarian cysts, ovarian cancer, or PID. The first is caused by a maturing ovarian follicle that fails to rupture at the time of ovulation and that persists into the luteal phase and beyond. It usually resolves on its own with time, but may sometimes rupture and leave little trace behind on ultrasound besides a small amount of free pelvic fluid. Large (greater than 8 cm) cysts usually require laparoscopic surgery for resolution. Likewise, masses or cysts found on a pelvic examination or ultrasound that are solid or complex (both solid and cystic) require surgical evaluation for diagnosis. Last, any palpable mass in a woman who has gone through menopause should be explored, regardless of its ultrasonographic appearance.

Pelvic inflammatory disease occurs most frequently in adolescence and early adulthood. When rates of commer-cial sex workers entering the correctional facility are high, PID should even be suspected in middle-aged and older women. The pain is usually progressive, but may be either very mild or severe enough to mimic appendicitis, a ruptured ectopic pregnancy, or ovarian torsion. Failure to treat PID adequately may result in short-term sequelae, such as tubo-ovarian abscesses, or long-term sequelae, such as infertility or chronic pelvic pain secondary to adhesions. The diagnosis is usually made on the basis of bilateral pelvic pain on examination, with cervical motion tenderness and an absence of a palpable mass. There may be a fever, an elevated white blood cell count with left shift, or positive cervical cultures for gonorrhea or chlamydia. A speculum examination may show leukorrhea or a purulent discharge. The inflammation may be severe enough to cause peritoneal signs on examination, making it easy to confuse this diagnosis with appendicitis or a critical ectopic pregnancy.

Pelvic inflammatory disease is usually a polymicrobial infection. Treatment regimens are aimed at a broad range of anaerobic and aerobic organisms, including *Neisseria gonorrhoeae* and *Chlamydia trachomatis*, *Escherichia coli*, streptococci, and mycoplasmas. Treatment may be provided on an outpatient or inpatient basis. The Centers for Disease Control recommends inpatient treatment if the diagnosis is uncertain and an ectopic pregnancy or appendicitis cannot be ruled out, if an abscess is suspected, or if the patient is also pregnant, has HIV infection, fails to tolerate the treatment regimen, or fails to improve within 72 hours.[27] In many correctional settings, all but extremely mild cases of PID belong in a supervised infirmary setting or hospital because of the high risk that follow-up will not be timely or access rapid enough in case of clinical deterioration. Specific treatment regimens have been reviewed in the chapter on STDs. Partners of incarcerated women with PID should be traced and treated by correctional clinicians if also incarcerated. The local board of health can trace partners who are not incarcerated.

Acute pelvic pain often has a fairly indolent course. When a history is taken, the patient may be able to describe a recurrent pattern of pain that is cyclical. If the pain occurs at the time of menses and is of a cramping or dull nature localized to the lower abdomen or lower back, then dysmenorrhea, endometriosis, or adenomyosis are likely possibilities. Early pregnancy with threatened abortion must also be considered in a woman with a new onset of dysmenorrhea, especially in the population of women entering correctional facilities, because prior menses may have been irregular or unremarked by the woman herself. In the absence of pregnancy, patients may benefit from the use of nonsteroidal therapy, usually begun before the onset of menses and continued for 3–4 days, or they may benefit from oral contraceptive use to regulate their menstrual cycles. Pain that is unilateral and related to the menstrual cycle, but that occurs at about midcycle, or 12–15 days before the next expected menses, may be a result of ovulation. Mittelschmerz is unlikely in women who are known to be anovulatory, either through hormonal derangement or because of oral contraceptive pill or long-acting progesterone use.

Menopause

With the aging of prison populations, increasing numbers of incarcerated women may pass through menopause. Hormone replacement ameliorates local and systemic symptoms of menopause such as vaginal and peri-urethral atrophy and vasomotor symptoms such as hot flashes, and its use is approved by the Food and Drug Administration for this indication as well as osteoporosis prevention. There is a significant benefit in terms of prevention of osteoporosis,[28] as well as cardiovascular disease,[29] the leading cause of death in American women. This last benefit is probably of greatest magnitude; a meta-analysis of 21 studies showed a 50% reduction in the risk of coronary events.[30] There are also studies supporting a role for estrogen in the prevention of strokes in women who have passed through menopause.[31]

The risks of hormone replacement therapy are not completely known. Unopposed estrogen was previously used in women with intact uteri who had gone through menopause, but has been shown to increase the risk of endometrial cancer; this problem has largely been minimized with the concurrent use of progesterone. In fact, the endometrial cancer risk in women receiving cycled estrogen and progesterone may be lower than the risk experienced by women not receiving hormone therapy.[32, 33] The issue that continues to elude consensus is the extent to which hormone replacement therapy, specifically the estrogen component, may affect breast cancer risk. Studies funded through the Women's Health Initiative will provide data on this subject over the next 10 years.

All women should be counseled regarding hormone replacement therapy at the time of menopause, or as soon thereafter as possible. Even women with a remote menopause history should be offered therapy in the absence of contraindications, as a benefit still exists, although it does so to a lesser degree than if therapy begins immediately.[34] Regimens for hormone replacement must take into account the presence or absence of an intact uterus in the patient, the major benefits being sought, and the risks that are specific to the patient. Contraindications to estrogen use include breast cancer, invasive endometrial cancer, undiagnosed vaginal bleeding or a breast mass, previously diagnosed activated protein C resistance, current deep venous thrombosis, or a recent stroke. Whether patients with a distant history of breast cancer or with a history of noninvasive endometrial cancer can be safely offered hormone replacement is uncertain.

The forms of hormone used most frequently in the United States are conjugated equine estrogens (Premarin) and medroxyprogesterone acetate (Provera). An alternative estrogen form is estradiol-17β (Estrace). The minimum dose of estrogen shown to confer a cardioprotective and osteoporosis prevention benefit is 0.625 mg of conjugated equine estrogens daily (1.0 mg estradiol or 50–100 µg transdermal estradiol), although some women may initially require a higher dose, typically 1.25 or 2.5 mg to control vasomotor symptoms. As soon as is possible, this dose should be brought back down to the lowest dose (0.625 mg or above) that will control symptoms. Women who have had hysterectomies for benign disease may receive unopposed estrogen on a daily basis without interruption. In those women who have intact uteri, a progestational agent, usually medroxyprogesterone acetate, must be given with the estrogen. It can be given cyclically with estrogen (as in 0.625 mg of conjugated estrogens on days 1–25 each month, with 10 mg medroxyprogesterone acetate on days 16–25 each month or days 1–14 of each month) or can be used continuously with the estrogen (as in 0.625 mg of conjugated estrogens every day with 2.5 mg medroxyprogesterone acetate every day, also marketed as a single pill called Prempro). The advantage of this latter regimen is its ease of administration—one pill every day, as opposed to remembering different pills on different days in the cycle. It is also slightly less expensive. The disadvantage of this regimen is a greater amount of irregular spotting, especially for the first 6–9 months of use, which may generate a need for transvaginal ultrasound or endometrial biopsy to evaluate the possibility of endometrial hyperplasia.

Estrogens can also be administered via transdermal delivery systems; however, this mode is significantly more expensive, which may discourage its use in correctional settings. It still provides vasomotor symptom relief and osteoporosis prevention, and, although once thought to provide less cardiovascular benefit than when taken via the oral route, studies show similar benefit with long-term use.[35] Some women have difficulty with progesterone side effects such as bloating, breast tenderness, and depression. An alternative agent, norethindrone, may be used at a dose of 0.35 mg for continuous combined therapy, and at a dose of 0.70 mg for sequential therapy. For women who do not tolerate systemic hormone replacement therapy, symptoms of urogenital atrophy may be treated with vaginal estrogen creams or a newly released vaginal ring that is impregnated with estrogen. The extent to which these forms of estrogen can be systemically absorbed is small. Nonetheless, concerns regarding the possible risk for endometrial hyperplasia must still be kept in mind, and there must be appropriate evaluation of bleeding by transvaginal ultrasound or endometrial biopsy, depending on the services that are locally available.

Osteoporosis

Osteoporosis affects 15–20 million individuals in the United States, and most are women in their postmenopausal years.[36] It is defined as a loss of bone mineral density to 2.5 standard deviations below the mean for a healthy young adult. Risk factors for its development include a poor calcium intake earlier in life (with consequent decreased peak bone mass), an ongoing poor calcium intake, having passed through menopause either naturally or surgically through oophorectomy, a sedentary lifestyle, a slender frame, smoking or heavy drinking of alcohol, and heavy caffeine use. Additionally, long-term glucocorticoid use or hyperthyroidism, as well as excessive therapy with exogenous thyroid hormones or seizure medications, can result in loss of bone mineral density. Bone loss begins to a small degree before menopause, but the loss is greatly accelerated during the first 10–15 years after menopause.[37] Osteoporosis predisposes to vertebral compression fractures that cause pain, loss of height, and kyphosis; to an increased risk of femoral neck fractures with resulting immobilization and up to a 20% mortality rate in the year afterward; and to increased wrist fractures.

Attention must be focused on prevention and then treatment for this condition. The mainstay of prevention efforts revolve around educating women from adolescence onward about the need for an increased calcium intake, increased weight-bearing exercise, and avoidance of risk-increasing behaviors such as smoking and caffeine and alcohol use. Current recommendations regarding calcium intake are for females older than age 11 years to consume 1,200 mg of calcium daily, either through a normal diet or a supplement in the form of calcium carbonate (Tums or vitamin preparations) or calcium citrate. At the time of menopause, the amount should increase to 1,500 mg. Formulations that contain at least 400 IU of vitamin D are preferred. If Tums is used, vitamin D supplementation should be added separately. (Only milk is supplemented with vitamin D—dairy products such as cheese or yogurts are not). At the time of menopause, women should be counseled regarding hormone replacement therapy, as previously mentioned. Women in whom hormone replacement therapy is contraindicated, women who are undecided about whether they will take hormone replacement therapy, and women who have not yet gone through menopause whose risk is thought to be a result of long-term glucocorticoid use, should be offered bone densitometry evaluation via a dual-energy x-ray absorptometry (DEXA) scan. If results show a loss greater than 2 standard deviations below peak mass, treatment for osteoporosis should begin. Dual-energy x-ray absorptometry scanning can also help assess a woman's response to therapy. A consensus about who should have DEXA scans and how often they should be performed has not yet emerged from the various foundations and task forces that are concerned with women's health issues.

In women who cannot receive hormone replacement or who do not have a relative estrogen deficiency, calcium, vitamin D, and exercise are the mainstay of therapy. New pharmacologic therapy in the form of alendronate, a bis-phosphonate, given at a dose of 10 mg every day, has been shown to increase bone mineral density by up to 9% over 3 years of use.[28] Side effects limiting use are abdominal pain, nausea, constipation, and diarrhea. Results from studies that look at the combined use of alendronate and hormone replacement therapy are still pending.

For women incarcerated for only short periods of time, the provision of diets that provide 1,200–1,500 mg of calcium daily, and the provision of opportunities for weight-bearing exercise, are probably adequate interventions when combined with patient education regarding the reduction of modifiable risk. Women who enter an institution while receiving active therapy for osteoporosis prevention or for the treatment of a documented disease should continue receiving their medications. For those women who will be long-term residents, prevention and treatment must be instituted as soon as the risk is identified and must be continued throughout their stay. In some cases, a referral will need to be made, most likely to an endocrinologist, especially in the face of a need for second-line agents or in cases in which accelerated bone density loss occurs despite therapy.

REFERENCES

1. National Institute of Justice: *Correctional Populations in the United States.* Washington, D.C., U.S. Department of Justice, Office of Justice Programs, Bureau of Justice Statistics, 1995.
2. Herdegen J, Keamy L, Raba J: Health status of incarcerated urban females. Unpublished study, 1989.
3. Greenfield LA, Minor-Harper S: *Women in Prison.* Washington, D.C., U.S. Department of Justice, Office of Justice Programs, Bureau of Justice Statistics, NCJ-127991, 1991.
4. Data from the Centers for Disease Control, within lecture at Johns Hopkins Hospital, 1996.
5. Connor EM, Sperling RS, Gelber R, et al: Reduction of maternal–infant transmission of human immunodeficiency virus type I with zidovudine treatment. *N Engl J Med* 331:1173–1180, 1994.
6. U.S. Preventive Services Task Force: *Guide to Clinical Preventive Services,* ed 2. Baltimore, Md, Williams and Wilkins, 1996.
7. Wingo PA, Tong T, Bolden S: Cancer statistics, 1995. *CA Cancer J Clin* 45:8–30, 1995.
8. National Institutes of Health Consensus Development Conference Panel: Ovarian cancer: Screening, treatment, and followup. *NIH Consensus Statement,* no 12, April 5–7, 1994.
9. Finn CB, Luesley DM, Buxton EJ, et al: Is stage I epithelial ovarian cancer overtreated both surgically and systemically? Results of a five-year cancer registry review. *Br J Obstet Gynaecol* 99:54–58, 1992.
10. Schildkraut JM, Thompson WD: Familial ovarian cancer: A population-based case control study. *Am J Epidemiol* 128:456–466, 1988.
11. Boring CC, Squires TS, Tong T, et al: Cancer Statistics, 1994. *CA Cancer J Clin* 44:7, 1994.
12. Cramer DW: The role of cervical cytology in the declining morbidity and mortality of cervical cancer. *Cancer* 34:2018–2027, 1974.
13. American Cancer Society: *Guidelines for the Cancer Related Checkup: An Update.* Atlanta, Ga, American Cancer Society, 1993.
14. U.S. Preventive Services Task Force: *Guide to Clinical Preventive Services,* ed 2. Baltimore, Md, Williams and Wilkins, 1996, p 112.
15. *Standards for Health Services in Prisons, 1992;. Standards for Health Services in Jails, 1996.* Chicago, National Commission on Correctional Health Care.
16. Agency for Health Care Policy and Research: *Managing early HIV*

infection. Rockville, Md, U.S. Public Health Service, Publication No 94.0573:32, 1994.

17. Centers for Disease Control and Prevention: 1993 sexually transmitted diseases treatment guidelines. *MMWR* 42(RR-14):87, 1993.

18. Stark E, Flitcraft A, et al: *Wife Abuse in the Medical Setting: An Introduction for Health Personnel*, Monograph No 7. Washington, D.C., National Clearinghouse on Domestic Violence, 1981.

19. *Crime in the United States. Uniform Crime Rates for the United States, 1992*, Washington, D.C., Federal Bureau of Investigation, 1993.

20. Snell TL, Morton DC: *Women in Prison. Survey of State Prison Inmates 1991*. Washington, D.C., U.S. Department of Justice, Office of Justice Programs, Bureau of Justice Statistics, NCJ-145321, 1991.

21. AMA: *Diagnostic and Treatment Guidelines on Domestic Violence*. Chicago, American Medical Association, 1992.

22. U.S. Healthcare: *Current Concepts in Women's Health: Domestic Violence and Primary Care*, Monograph. 1994.

23. U.S. Healthcare: *Current Concepts in Women's Health: Domestic Violence and Primary Care*, Monograph. 1994, pp 61–64.

24. Ries LAG, Miller BA, Hankey BF, et al (eds): *SEER Cancer Statistics Review 1973–1991: Tables and Graphs*. Bethesda, Md, National Cancer Institute, NIH Publication No 94-2789, 1994.

25. Lemcke DP, Pattison J, Marshall LA, et al (eds): *Primary Care of Women*. Norwalk, Conn, Alleton and Lange, 1995, p 444.

26. Lemcke DP, Pattison J, Marshall LA, et al (eds): *Primary Care of Women*. Norwalk, Conn, Alleton and Lange, 1995, p 443.

27. Centers for Disease Control and Prevention: 1993 sexually transmitted diseases treatment guidelines. *MMWR* 42(RR-14):75–81, 1993.

28. Bellantoni MF: Osteoporosis prevention and treatment. *Am Fam Physician* 54:986–992, 1996.

29. Effects of estrogen or estrogen/progestin regimens on heart disease risk factors in postmenopausal women. The postmenopausal estrogen/progestin interventions (PEPI) trial. *JAMA* 273:199–208, 1995.

30. Barrett-Connor E, Bush TL: Estrogen and coronary heart disease in women. *JAMA* 265:1861–1867, 1991.

31. Finucane FF, Madans JH, Bush TL, et al: Decreased risk of stroke among postmenopausal hormone users. *Arch Intern Med* 153:73, 1993.

32. Persson I, Adami HO, Bergkvist L, et al: Risk of endometrial cancer after treatment with estrogens, alone or in conjunction with progestogens: Results of a propective study. *BMJ* 298:147, 1989.

33. Voigt LF, Weiss NS, Chu JR: Progestogen supplementation of exogenous estrogens and risk of endometrial cancer. *Lancet* 338:274, 1991.

34. Felson DT, Zhang Y, Kreger BE, et al: The effect of postmenopausal estrogen therapy on bone marrow turnover in elderly women. *N Engl J Med* 329:1141–1146, 1993.

35. Crook D, Cust MP, Ganger KF, et al: Comparison of transdermal and oral estrogen/progestin replacement therapy: Effects on serum lipids and lipoproteins. *Am J Obstet Gynecol* 166:950, 1992.

36. Speroff L, Glass H, Kase N: *Clinical Gynecologic Endocrinology and Infertility*, ed 5. Baltimore, Md, Williams and Wilkins, 1994, p 597.

37. Speroff L, Glass H, Kase N: *Clinical Gynecologic Endocrinology and Infertility*, ed 5. Baltimore, Md, Williams and Wilkins, 1994, p 598.

Mental Health

18

Psychiatric Intake Screening

Leslie Stein, Psy.D., R.N.
Carl Alaimo, Psy.D.

INTRODUCTION

The deinstitutionalization of America's seriously mentally ill population has transferred responsibility for psychiatric care from large, publicly funded hospitals to community-based providers. This phenomenon, labeled *transinstitutionalization,*[1] documents the movement of the mentally ill from state psychiatric hospitals to nursing homes and correctional facilities. Holcomb and Ahr[2] argued that the criminal justice system has replaced state hospitals as agents of social control for young, violent individuals with psychiatric disorders. Ironically, jail or prison was the most common treatment for seriously mentally ill individuals 200 years ago.[3]

PREVALENCE OF MENTAL HEALTH ILLNESS IN CORRECTIONAL SETTINGS

The increased prevalence of inmates with mental health problems has resulted in an increased burden on those who provide treatment, thus limiting access to treatment. Recent statistics illustrate the enormity of this demand. Bureau of Justice figures compiled for 1994 document that the United States has approximately 5.2 million adults under correctional supervision of one sort or another: almost 3 million on probation; 690,159 on parole; 483,717 in jail and 991,612 in prison; in 1995, America's prisons housed more than 1 million prisoners.[4] A considerable portion of this population is seriously mentally ill. Linda Teplin conducted studies finding that 6.1% of male detainees and 12.3% of female detainees admitted to the Cook County Department of Corrections (CCDOC) in Chicago, Illinois had a serious mental illness.[5]

The San Diego County Jail reported that, in 1995, 14% of the 4,572 male inmates and 25% of the 687 female inmates received psychotropic medication, and the assistant sheriff described the San Diego County Jail as "the bottom-line mental health provider in the county."[6] Cermak Health Services of Cook County, the on-site health care provider for the CCDOC, documented 6,301 admissions to its Department of Mental Health Services in 1996, which were more than those of any state psychiatric facility in the entire State of Illinois. In January, 1997, 857 inmates received ongoing mental health services at the Cook County Jail, representing close to 10% of the entire inmate population of Cook County Jail. Statistics from King County Jail in Seattle, Washington in July, 1993 reported that, on average, 160 of the jail's 2,000 inmates had a serious mental illness; Travis County statistics for the same period record that 14% of inmates in the county jail

---

Box 18-1. Elements of First-Level Mental Health Screening

1. Observation and structured inquiry immediately on arrival at facility.
2. Prevention of integration of those who are acutely or chronically mentally ill into general population housing.
3. Identification of inmates in need of more complete mental health evaluations.
4. Identification of inmates at risk for suicide.
5. Identification of past and present psychotropic medication history.
6. Identification of prior mental health history, including hospitalization.
7. Use of a standardized form as part of the receiving or screening process.
8. Provision of oral and written information to inmates about access to mental health services.
9. Screening by trained individual.

From *Psychiatric Services in Jails and Prisons.* Washington, D.C., American Psychiatric Association, Task Force Report 29, 1989, with permission.

Box 18-2. Second-Level Intake/Receiving Screening Components

1. Occurrence within 24 hours of admission into facility.
2. Completion of a standard intake mental health screening form.
3. Performance of the screening by health care staff.
4. More focused evaluation of mental health.
5. Provision of more detailed information about mental health services to inmate.

From *Psychiatric Services in Jails and Prisons.* Washington, D.C., American Psychiatric Association, Task Force Report 29, 1989, with permission.

---

in Austin, Texas had a serious mental illness; and Miami's Dade County Jail housed an average of 350 inmates per day who were mentally ill. Each of these institutions reported that they were the largest provider of mental health services in their respective counties.[7] The Los Angeles County Jail System documented that 3,300 of its 21,000 inmates received mental health services on a daily basis during this time period, making it "de facto the largest mental institution in the country."[7]

STANDARDS AND LEGAL REQUIREMENTS

The courts have mandated that mentally ill offenders be treated for their disorders (*Bowring v Godwin*,[8] *Estelle v Gamble*,[9] *Jones v Wittenberg*[10]). Some of the case law sets minimum standards for mental health treatment in jails, requiring structured programs for screening and evaluating inmates for the presence of mental disorders (*Alberti v Sheriff of Harris County, Texas*,[11] *Campbell v McGruder*,[12] *Dawson v Kendrick*,[13] *Inmates of Allegheny County Jail v Pierce*,[14] *Pugh v Locke*,[15] and *Ruiz v Estelle*[16]).

In an effort to bring attention to the critical function of correctional screening for mental illness, the American Public Health Association, the American Psychiatric Association (APA), and the National Commission on Correctional Health Care (NCCHC) have each furnished sets of guidelines or standards so that this function can be implemented.

The NCCHC standards define the minimums for mental health screening. During receiving screening, which is done immediately on arrival into the facility, structured inquiry is performed that identifies individuals in need of

immediate attention because they may be an immediate danger to themselves or others. According to the 1996 NCCHC jail standards, this screening should be performed by "health trained or Qualified Health Care Personnel." The NCCHC makes exceptions for small facilities that do not have around-the-clock staff by permitting "health trained correctional staff" to perform receiving screening. This first-level receiving screening is intended to prevent suicide and to identify inmates at risk for drug withdrawal (including alcohol), which may mimic mental illness. Observation of behavior at the time of the interview should include a focus on the state of consciousness, mental status (including suicidal ideation), appearance (e.g., tremors or sweating), and conduct. The latter physical signs may indicate acute drug withdrawal or intoxication that may mimic mental illness.[17]

The NCCHC also requires a mental health evaluation within 14 days of incarceration in prisons.[18] This is a more thorough interview meant to identify inmates with mental illness so that treatment can be initiated. For clinical appropriateness and risk management prevention, our recommendation is that the staff who provide the mental health portion of receiving screening be trained and exhibit competency in mental health interviewing. Mental health evaluations should be performed by individuals who have mental health credentials and training consistent with the type of evaluation to be performed. These evaluations must be performed under the requirements of all applicable practice acts.

The APA's 1989 task force report gives recommendations for mental health screening that involve two levels of screening activities and the possibility of a follow-up evaluation by a mental health professional. The first level identifies inmates with mental illness or symptoms of mental illness so that suicide, inappropriate housing assignment, or drug and alcohol withdrawal can be prevented at the receiving, or intake, level. Box 18-1 gives a partial listing of the core components for mental health screening and evaluation. Level 1 screening is reception screening and may be

---

Box 18-3. Components of Full Mental Health Evaluation

1. Occurrence within 24 hours of referral or immediately when clinically indicated.
2. Referral from receiving screening, other health care staff, correctional officers, or inmates themselve.
3. Use of a standardized form that is incorporated into medical record.
4. Performance of evaluation by appropriately trained mental health professional.

From *Psychiatric Services in Jails and Prisons.* Washington, D.C., American Psychiatric Association, Task Force Report 29, 1989, with permission.

Box 18-4. Initial Screening of Inmates in Prisons

1. Evaluation of dangerousness to self or others.
2. Observation of the presence of psychotic symptoms and/or extreme emotional states.
3. Requirement of a psychotropic medication history.
4. Requirement of a psychiatric history.
5. Evaluation of cognitive functioning.
6. Identification of impairment of psychosocial functioning that may interfere with integration into the prison environment.

From Steadman HJ, Cocozza JJ (eds): *Mental Illness in American Prisons.* Seattle, National Coalition for the Mentally Ill in the Criminal Justice System, 1993, with permission.

---

performed by an appropriately trained individual. The APA and NCCHC do permit screening by correctional officers. Level 2 screening is performed by mental health staff, and consists of a detailed mental health evaluation that is a component of the admission workup (Box 18-2). Professional mental health evaluations are reserved for those inmates with suspected or actual functional disabilities that may be indicative of mental illness or developmental disability (Box 18-3).[19]

In addition to formalized standards, Steadman and Cocozza[20] have provided screening guidelines specifically for prison facilities. They indicated that all inmates should have a brief initial screening for severe mental illness immediately on admission to prison. Box 18-4 lists components of that screening process.

PRIMARY PSYCHOLOGICAL SCREENING

Mental health evaluation instruments that can be used as part of the screening process include the Minnesota Multiphasic Personality Inventory, second edition, the Structured Clinical Interview, the Diagnostic Interview Schedule, the Referral Decision Scale, the Millon Personality Inventory, and the Brief Psychiatric Rating Scale, to name a few. In jails, use of these psychometric instruments may be cause problems from a practical standpoint, given the high level of noise and activity in most jail receiving areas, the requirement for administration of these instruments by highly trained and qualified mental health care professionals, and the length of time required for administration of these instruments.

The NCCHC and APA standards already cited give templates on which to base mental health screening programs. The general goal of any mental health screening program is to prevent unrecognized mental illness from causing harm to the inmate or to other inmates or staff. In addition, screening identifies inmates in need of continued mental health treatment. Screening at intake provides a crucial assessment of inmates' mental status, including behav-

ioral cues indicating suitability for placement in the general population of the correctional facility or highlighting a need for mental health services in a segregated environment. Screening should include, at a minimum, inquiry into common mental health problems; observed, severe behavioral abnormalities that may preclude general population housing; and an inquiry into suicidal ideation.

Screening should be conducted in a setting respectful of the privacy and dignity of the inmate and where sensitive and valid information may be obtained. For example, Cermak Health Services designed simple booths of wood and plexiglas in the receiving area of the jail to facilitate psychological screening. The booths provide sound reduction and enhance confidentiality but allow the examiner to remain in full view of correctional staff, ensuring the examiner's safety. Inmates should be informed about the nature, purpose, and results of the screening process. Screening is best accomplished using a semistructured interview with a standardized measure. Wherever possible, ancillary information should be incorporated (e.g., medical records, presentencing reports, previous custodial records, information from family members). This may require informed consent releases from the inmate.

There are important differences in jail vs. prison mental health screening. Prisons have considerably fewer intake assessments than jails of comparable size. In prisons, inmates generally arrive at the facility on a regular schedule, usually during the daytime on a weekday. In jails, inmates arrive at all hours of the day and night. In large jails, staff may be available 24 hours a day for the purpose of mental health screening. In small jails, it may be impractical to hire 24-hr/day health care staff to perform reception screening. For this reason, the initial receiving screening in small jails is often performed by correctional staff; existing standards of the NCCHC and APA permit officer screening when correctional officers are appropriately trained.

Those who perform the screening must have training to identify symptoms of mental disorders and to competently administer the screening instrument(s). If the individuals doing the screening identify a mental health concern or cannot obtain what would appear to be critical screening information, they should make a referral for a follow-up assessment. If a detainee expresses suicidal ideation or homicidal ideation, or appears to have a florid psychotic condition, the individual performing the screening should arrange for immediate intervention treatment.

Cook County Jail processes an average of 300 inmates each day. Each inmate receives a brief initial psychological screening at intake to determine his need for further mental health services. Mental health specialists, personnel with bachelor's and master's degree level training in psychology, perform this initial screening with supervision from a clinical psychologist. All inmates with any evidence of current mental health problems are referred to advanced degree level mental health staff (those with Doctor of Psychiatry or Doctor of Philosophy degrees, or a psychiatrist) for an in-depth interview within 24 hours of the initial assessment. Having trained mental health staff perform the initial screening helps to reduce the volume of secondary screenings by higher degree level mental health staff. All institutions must have provisions for the evaluation of psychiatric emergencies. Large jails and prisons usually maintain a psychiatric unit that is open and staffed 24 hours a day to provide treatment to inmates in severe psychological distress. In smaller correctional settings without a psychiatric unit, isolating detainees in severe psychological distress from the general population in a safe cell in full view of security personnel is essential until treatment is secured through a local mental health provider, through a consulting psychiatrist, or through another community resource. Transferring a detainee, in custody, to the nearest hospital may also provide rapid access to needed treatment. Someone responsible for on-site psychiatric care must assume responsibility for the care of the inmate on discharge from the local hospital.

PRIMARY PSYCHOLOGICAL SCREENING INSTRUMENTS

Standardized screening forms should be used for primary receiving mental health screening. Figure 18-1 illustrates one such form. This instrument is designed to address various aspects of memory, psychiatric history, drug and alcohol use, suicide history, and current risk of suicidal and/or homicidal behavior. The tool also permits an assessment of behavioral appropriateness at the time of screening. Based on the responses on the screening tool, an inmate is assessed as appropriate for general population housing or in need of a more in-depth evaluation using the secondary assessment screening procedures to determine alternate placement needs.

In the example screening form, inmates provide a minimal amount of personal information as well as specific answers to eight questions pertaining to their mental health history and current treatment needs. There should be follow-up of all inmates with positive responses to a history of mental illness, usage of psychotropic medication, or any suicidal ideation or recent history of a suicide attempt. At Cermak Health Services, mental health personnel refer all inmates who are receiving psychiatric treatment and taking psychotropic medication at the time of intake for a secondary evaluation. Many inmates express suicidal ideation at the time of intake, as the shame of arrest and fear of incarceration causes them to consider suicide as an alternative to facing prosecution. Interventions at intake targeted toward reducing fear and realistically examining legal options frequently eliminate the need for psychiatric treatment. However, inmates who insist that they will harm themselves (or others) should always receive a secondary evaluation.

At the CCDOC, mental health personnel routinely review inmates' charges with them during receiving screening. There are three reasons for this. First, at CCDOC, the booking officers inform the inmates of their charges just before mental health screening so that the inmate's level of knowledge of the charges, bond, and court date provide clues to the individual's short-term memory and concentration abilities. Inmates with difficulty in concentration and impaired short-term memory frequently require specialized housing to ensure their safety, even in the absence of a psychiatric disorder. Occasionally, inmates verbalize delusional perceptions associated with their charges, and this, too, provides useful information for dispositional planning. Second, in jail settings, mentally ill offenders frequently are charged with disorderly conduct, theft of services, simple battery, criminal damage to property, or criminal trespass; inmates who are seen with these charges deserve careful consideration during intake screening. Often these offenses suggest a long-term history of mental health problems. Third, at the CCDOC, the Department of Mental Health Services has a practice of referring all inmates charged with aggravated criminal sexual assault of a minor and those charged with murder of a first-line relative (e.g., parent, child, grandparent, sibling, spouse, partner) for a secondary evaluation. Individuals charged with these types of crimes tend to experience extreme emotional states and frequently require psychiatric intervention.

Many mentally ill offenders deny all history and symptoms of psychiatric illness. Observation of an inmate's ability to cooperate with the booking procedures of the jail or the intake prison procedures, as well as his physical appearance and presentation, provide invaluable clues to discerning the presence of a mental illness. Care must be taken, however, to differentiate between an offender who is deliberately provocative and refusing to follow intake correctional procedures and one whose uncooperative behavior is a symptom of a mental illness.

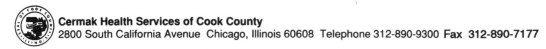

Cermak Health Services of Cook County
2800 South California Avenue Chicago, Illinois 60608 Telephone 312-890-9300 **Fax 312-890-7177**

Cermak Health Services Department Of Psychiatry
Brief Primary Psychological Screening Tool

Last Name_____ First Name_____ DOB_____ DOC#_____

Home Address_____Phone_____

Charge_____ Bond_____ Court_____

Race: W__ B__ Sp__ Other___ SS#_____ Employed: yes/no

Occupation: labor clerical food service sales other_____

1. Has the detainee ever been in Cook County Jail before? yes/no

    If yes, what division(s)?_____

2. Has the detainee ever been hospitalized for psychiatric treatment?
    yes/no

    If yes, number of hospitalizations_____ most recent (date)_____

    location_____ reason_____

3. Does the detainee currently receive outpatient psychiatric treatment?
    yes/no

    If yes, most recent visit (date)_____ location_____

4. Does the detainee take medication? yes/no

    If yes, name(s) of medication(s)_____

5. Does the detainee drink alcohol? yes/no Use drugs? yes/no

    If yes, what kind of drugs are used?_____

6. Has the detainee ever attempted suicide? yes/no

    If yes, when (date)_____ how?_____

7. Does the detainee feel suicidal now? yes/no

8. Is the detainee expressing homicidal ideation? yes/no

9. Is the detainee's behavior appropriate in the RCDC area? yes/no

    If no, please describe_____

    _____

Recommended Plan: General Population____ Secondary Assessment____

_____   _____

signature of psychiatric staff member performing   date/time
primary evaluation

_____

signature of psychiatric staff member performing
secondary evaluation

1/95
F-2981

Figure 18-1. Brief primary psychological screening tool. *Abbreviations: DOB*, date of birth; *DOC*, department of corrections; *W*, white; *B*, black; *Sp*, Spanish; *SS*, social security; *RCDC*, Receiving, Classification, and Diagnostic Center. (From Cermak Health Services of Cook County, Department of Psychiatry, 2800 South Carolina Avenue, Chicago, Illinois 60608, with permission.)

Box 18-5. Minimal Requirements for Mental Health Evaluation

---

1. Structured interview by mental health worker.
2. Hospitalization and outpatient mental health treatment history.
3. Current psychotropic medication history.
4. Evaluation for suicidal ideation and history of suicidal behavior.
5. Notation of drug usage.
6. Notation of alcohol usage.
7. History of sex offenses.
8. History of expressly violent behavior.
9. History of victimization as a result of criminal violence.
10. Special education placement history.
11. History of cerebral trauma or seizure disorder.
12. Notation of emotional response to incarceration.
13. Testing, when indicated, for mental retardation (e.g., with revised Wechsler Adult Intelligence Scale, WAIS-R).

From *Standards for Health Services in Prisons.* Chicago, National Commission on Correctional Health Care, 1996, with permission.

SECONDARY SCREENING EVALUATIONS

Secondary mental health evaluations are more detailed and thorough evaluations that occur as a result of referrals from receiving screening. Inmates referred for a secondary evaluation receive an in-depth assessment, documented on standardized forms. Figure 18-2 is an example of a secondary evaluation form (admission/evaluation form). The purpose of secondary evaluations is to further elucidate the potential for mental health problems in individuals identified as at-risk on receiving screening. Appropriate disposition can then occur to prevent harm to the inmate or others. The examiner conducting a secondary evaluation obtains a detailed history of prior psychiatric treatment, verifies current treatment modalities, conducts a thorough mental status examination, makes a provisional diagnosis, and institutes a dispositional plan, which may include admission to specialized housing. At CCDOC, in the event that an examiner decides to admit an inmate to Mental Health Services, the evaluator completes a secondary interview (Figure 18-3) with the inmate. This interview, whose scope and focus are in compliance with standards set by the NCCHC, is designed to obtain information relevant to the inmate's psychosocial history. Inmates requiring any level of treatment provided by the Department of Mental Health Services at Cermak Health Services are admitted to a mental health unit for evaluation of those needs. Follow-up care in the general population of the jail is arranged by the Department of Mental Health Services after discharge from a mental health unit. Intake personnel are not involved in arranging routine follow-up care in the general population of the jail. This level of organization and the quantity of

mental health housing is seldom available at most correctional facilities. When mental health housing is unavailable, a mechanism of tracking patients with mental health conditions in general population units should be in place. Secondary evaluations should include a mechanism to decide whether mental health housing is appropriate for any individual inmate based on availability.

MENTAL HEALTH EVALUATION

Inmates with chronic or acute mental illness need some type of follow-up treatment of their mental health condition. The purpose of the mental health evaluation after admission is to evaluate individuals in need of such treatment and to initiate the treatment process.

It should not be assumed that a chronic mental illness is less life-threatening than a medical illness. Untreated mental illness may result in suicide, in physical harm to the inmate because of psychotic thought processes, or in harm to other inmates or staff. A mental health evaluation, performed by professional mental health staff, is indicated for every inmate with a history of recent mental health treatment or for inmates exhibiting symptoms or signs of mental illness. Most prisons will perform these evaluations on all incoming inmates. This activity not only has a clinical purpose but also assists the correctional authority in classifying inmates for housing purposes. In jails, it may be impractical to perform an in-depth mental health evaluation on every inmate. The NCCHC standards are different for jails and prisons. Mental health evaluations are essential standards (required for accreditation) for prisons, but are only important (not mandatory for accreditation) for jails. Regardless of standards, it is important that, in jails, any individual with a history of mental illness or who exhibits signs of mental illness be assessed via an evaluation. Use of mental health staff for receiving screening permits triaging of inmates and selectively referring those for full evaluations.

Mental health evaluations are similar to history and interview evaluations by mental health professionals in civilian settings. Standardized questionnaires emphasize those items that may particularly affect individuals who are incarcerated, as determined by population studies. Box 18-5 lists items that should be addressed in a mental health evaluation.

Incarcerated populations present a unique challenge for determining whether inmates have psychopathologic conditions and the need for mental health services, or whether they are just exhibiting malingering behavior. When in doubt, the evaluator is advised to not only choose a conservative alternative but also to assume that the behavior is pathologic in origin. Input from other clinicians and assessment over time usually clarify the "true" psychiatric needs of inmates. The following vignettes illustrate actual use of the Brief Psychological Screening Tool with inmates at Cook County Jail.

CERMAK HEALTH SERVICES DEPARTMENT OF PSYCHIATRY

2800 SOUTH CALIFORNIA AVENUE   CHICAGO, ILLINOIS 60608-5107

ADMISSION/EVALUATION FORM

Evaluation Site: RCDC   BackDoor   Other:_____   Date:_____

Reason For
Referral:

History:

Current Symptoms:

Current Treatments:

Mental
Status
Exam:

Diagnosis: Axis I:

          Axis II:

          Axis III:

Plan:

_____   _____

(ER/Admitting Physician - If Applicable)   (Evaluator's Signature)

                                                                                F-2749

                                    Patient Name:_____

                                    CCDOC Number:_____

                                    Date of Birth:_____

                                    Location :_____

        IMPRINT PLATE

(Blue = **ER/3-North/South Medical Records**   Yellow = **Psych Intake Basket**   Pink = **Evaluator**)

Figure 18-2. Admission/evaluation form. *Abbreviations: RCDC,* Receiving, Classification, and Diagnostic Center; *ER,* emergency room; *CCDOC,* Cook County Department of Corrections. (From Cermak Health Services of Cook County, Department of Psychiatry, 2800 South Carolina Avenue, Chicago, Illinois 60608, with permission.)

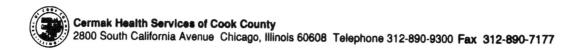

Cermak Health Services of Cook County
2800 South California Avenue Chicago, Illinois 60608 Telephone 312-890-9300 **Fax 312-890-7177**

CERMAK HEALTH SERVICES DEPARTMENT OF PSYCHIATRY
SECONDARY INTERVIEW

Name:_____ DOB:_____ SS#:_____ DOC #:_____

Orientation: Time:_____ Place:_____ Person:_____ Situation:_____

Development History: Place of Birth:_____ #of Siblings:_____ Raised by:_____

History of Abuse: Physical_____ Emotional_____ Sexual_____

Duration of Abuse:_____ Perpetrator of Abuse:_____

Family Psychiatric History:_____

Family Substance Abuse History:_____

Educational History: Highest Level Achieved_____Special Classes_____Problems_____

Reason for Termination_____

Interpersonal Relationships: Intimate Relationships_____ Marriage(s)_____ Duration_____

Friendships_____ Children_____ Age(s)_____

Current Living Situation:_____

Vocational History: Most recent type of work_____ Type/duration of longest job_____

Military Service: Yes/No Branch_____ Type/Year of Discharge_____Current means of support_____

Medical History (circle all that apply): Hypertension Asthma Diabetes Mellitus Gun Shot Wound/Location_____

Allergic To:_____

History of Head Trauma/LOC Yes/No   Duration_____ Seizures_____ Other_____

ETOH/Substance Use History: Amount   Frequency   Duration   Treatments:_____
ETOH
Marijuana
Opiates
Cocaine
PCP
Other

History of Black Outs: Yes/No   DTS Yes/NO   DUI Yes/No   #of DUI Arrests_____

Criminal History: Current Charge:_____ Past Convictions: Yes/No   Bond:_____
Sentence(s)_____ Paroled From_____ Court Date_____
Currently on parole/probation: Yes/No From:_____
Previously Housed In Division VIII: Yes/No   Date_____ Team_____

Diagnostic Impression: Axis I_____ Axis II_____ Axis III_____

Date:_____

_____
Evaluator's Signature

Time:_____

Blue Copy=Patient Chart   Yellow Copy=Psych Intake Basket   Pink Copy=Evaluator

Revised: 03/14/93
F-2873

Figure 18-3. Secondary interview form. *Abbreviations: DOB,* date of birth; *SS,* social security; *DOC,* Department of Corrections; *LOC,* loss of consciousness; *ETOH,* ethanol; *PCP,* phencyclidine; *DTS,* delirium tremers; *DUI,* driving under the influence. (From Cermak Health Services of Cook County, Department of Psychiatry, 2800 South Carolina Avenue, Chicago, Illinois 60608, with permission.)

Garage Door Transmissions

James B is a 37-year-old white man charged with criminal damage to property. Mr. B provided appropriate personal identification information but, when questioned about the nature of the charges against him, he became indignant and reported, "it's the same old thing over and over again." He admitted to a history of multiple psychiatric hospitalizations, but indicated that he had no outpatient followup, nor did he take medications. He denied drug or alcohol use and denied any past or present suicidal ideation. When questioned about homicidal ideation, he stated, "I think I may have to kill Carlos." The examiner also noted that Mr. B spoke incoherently into his hand at frequent intervals. The examiner referred Mr. B for further evaluation because of his peculiar behavior and veiled threats of homicide.

On further evaluation, Mr. B revealed that he thought his neighbor, Carlos, had implanted a device in his garage door opener that sent "special signals" directly into Mr. B's brain. These signals scanned his thoughts, broadcast his sexual fantasies to the neighborhood, and ridiculed him to his neighbors. The police had arrested Mr. B after he broke into his neighbor's garage and destroyed his neighbor's garage door opener. Mr. B expressed dismay that the signals continued after he destroyed the garage door opener but surmised that his neighbor must be an undercover police officer with ties to the jail, as the transmissions continued after Mr. B's arrest, during court arraignment, and in the receiving area in jail. Mr. B denied needing any psychiatric intervention and became agitated, loud, and verbally abusive at the suggestion that his report of the "transmissions" indicated a need for psychiatric treatment. He denied that he would act on his thoughts of killing his neighbor because "killing an undercover cop would be more trouble than he's worth."

Despite his protestations, the examiner determined that the inmate experienced auditory hallucinations, had paranoid delusions, and warranted immediate psychiatric attention with a provisional diagnosis of "schizophrenia, paranoid type." This type of patient requires psychiatric hospitalization or management in a short-term correctional psychiatric unit.

Jane Doe

Jane Doe is a 24-year-old black woman charged with criminal trespass to land. At the screening, she refused to answer any questions posed by the examiner, insisting that everyone address her as Jane Doe, and citing her "fifth amendment right" even when questioned about simple details of her life, such as her date of birth and age. She grinned and appeared to experience delight at the frustration expressed by correctional personnel and health care providers as she thwarted their information-gathering efforts. The examiner noted she had an extremely foul body odor. She also attempted to strike another female inmate without any obvious provocation, and she kicked at correctional officers who intervened. She refused to cooperate with booking procedures and required two officers to physically direct her through processing. Arrest reports indicated that she had refused to leave a downtown church and verbally threatened others worshipping at the church.

Despite her refusal to cooperate with the psychological screening at intake, the examiner made a decision to admit her to a short-term psychiatric care unit for women, with a provisional diagnosis of "psychotic disorder, not otherwise specified." The examiner believed that the inmate's lack of cooperation stemmed from an underlying mental illness. Distinguishing between volitional, uncooperative behavior and uncooperative behavior prompted by an underlying mental illness presents one of the biggest challenges to mental health providers performing screening at intake.

Spider Man

Todd G, a slightly built white man of approximately 23 years of age, was isolated from other inmates in a small bullpen in the receiving area when the examiner arrived to perform the intake screening. He rocked back and forth on his heels and shouted, "I am God!" He responded to all the examiner's questions in a bizarre, incoherent manner, frequently growling and moaning. Without warning and without external provocation, he suddenly climbed the bullpen wall and crawled onto the duct work approximately 15 feet above the receiving area. With lightning speed, he crawled along the ducts and jumped down into another bullpen. As several officers approached to apprehend him, he lashed out at the officers and fought them with full force for approximately 10 minutes. Eleven officers finally subdued him and assisted in transporting him to a short-term care psychiatric unit where he was placed in full leather restraints. The inmate's bizarre behavior, coupled with his extraordinary strength, caused the examiner to provisionally give him a diagnosis of suspected phencyclidine (PCP)-induced psychosis.

The drug screen performed on Todd G revealed the presence of PCP in his system. It was also discovered that both Todd's ankles were broken, presumably in his jump from the duct work. Despite two broken ankles, he had fought vigorously for 10 minutes against 11 officers and subsequently against the full leather restraints. To this day, correctional officers and civilian personnel affectionately refer to him as "spider man." This vignette illustrates how intake personnel must make rapid assessments, often with very little concrete information to substantiate a diagnosis. Safety needs in these situations are the examiner's priority.

Boohoo Blues

Edward W is a 42-year-old black man charged with possession of a controlled substance. At the intake screening, he appropriately provided all identifying information and indicated that he had been jailed multiple times on similar charges. Curiously, he gave a Chicago street address but a suburban telephone number. He explained that it was "easier" to contact him via his cellular telephone, which had a suburban area code. Initially, he reported no history of psychiatric treatment but admitted to a $100-per-day heroin habit. He denied any history of suicide attempts but stated that he was suicidal at the time of intake. The examiner noted that he wiped his nose repeatedly during the screening interview, complained of abdominal cramping, and left the interview once to vomit in a nearby trash can. On his return to the interview, he stated that he "forgot" to tell the examiner that he takes amitriptyline hydrochloride (Elavil) for his "nerves" and for "hearing voices." He reported that his mother "gives it" to him, and "she goes to the doctor" for him. When confronted about the inconsistencies in his story, he stated that without his medication he would kill himself. He articulated no specific suicidal plan but demanded medication to "help" his "nerves." The examiner explained the procedure for admitting someone to the short-term care unit for men, and the necessity of using full leather restraints to ensure his safety and the safety of the others in the milieu. The inmate replied, "No, I don't need that, I just need something for being sick." After gaining the assurances of the inmate that he would not harm himself, the examiner found him appropriate for housing in the general population of the jail, confident that the inmate had engaged in malingering behavior calculated to obtain drugs.

This inmate provided many clues to his malingering. The nature of his charges, his heroin habit, and his use of a cellular telephone rather than providing a residential telephone number all are indicative of an individual engaged in purposefully deceptive behavior. He displayed opioid withdrawal symptoms, and his story of receiving amitriptyline hydrochloride from his mother seemed extremely implausible. Many drug addicts attempt to gain access to the Department of Mental Health Services with the hope of receiving medication to alleviate withdrawal symptoms or to obtain a substitute drug. Occasionally, inmates will not give assurances that they will not harm themselves. Admission to the Department of Mental Health Services with suicide-preventive measures is always appropriate when inmates express an imminent plan to harm themselves.

I Can't Believe I Killed Her

Marcus M is a 26-year-old black man charged with first-degree murder. Mr. M provided appropriate identifying data and indicated that he had been jailed twice previously on drug charges. He reported no history of psychiatric treatment, but readily admitted to smoking upward of $200 per day of crack cocaine for the last 3 years. He denied any history of suicide attempts and denied suicidal or homicidal ideation at intake. On closer questioning, the examiner learned that Mr. M was charged with murdering his moth-

er. He spoke very softly, appeared disheveled, and tears welled up in his eyes several times during the intake screening. He reported feeling depressed, unable to concentrate, and unable to sleep, and had profound feelings of helplessness since his arrest. He repeatedly stated, "I can't believe I killed her" during the intake interview. Despite the absence of a significant history of treatment for a major mental disorder, the examiner referred him for further evaluation and admission to the Department of Mental Health Services with a provisional diagnosis of "adjustment disorder with depressed mood."

At Cook County Jail, as previously mentioned, the Department of Mental Health Services refers all individuals accused of murdering a first-line family member for an in-depth evaluation. The trauma of losing a close relative and, of course, the burden of responsibility for the death, often precipitate a psychological crisis. During the in-depth interview, Mr. M revealed an extensive history of physical and sexual abuse at the hands of his mother and her boyfriends. He reported that they argued about his drug use and that he "snapped," strangling her in the kitchen. He spent approximately 6 months in the Department of Mental Health Services, where his psychological condition stabilized, allowing him to be released to the general population of the jail.

You Were Driving

Javier T is a 47-year-old Hispanic man who had multiple warrants for traffic violations. He had been in a local police lockup for 3 days before his admission to the Cook County Department of Corrections. At the screening, the examiner noted that he had severe tremors of all extremities, perspired profusely, and was disoriented with regard to the time and place. He admitted to a history of social drinking and denied any drug use. He gave mostly incoherent responses to questions posed by the examiner, and stated, "How should I know where we are, you were driving." The examiner determined that the inmate underreported his alcohol consumption and suspected that the inmate's disorientation and bizarre speech content resulted from delirium tremens rather than from psychotic thought processes. His lengthy detainment in the local lockup, without access to alcohol, made him vulnerable to severe withdrawal symptoms. The examiner referred the inmate to the medical department for immediate treatment. The examiner recognized the physiological signs of alcohol withdrawal and identified the inmate's need for urgent treatment. Often, inmates seen with bizarre behavior are routed to mental health personnel for management of their symptoms. However, frequently, organic or physical conditions, such as alcohol withdrawal or severe head trauma, can have signs and symptoms similar to mental illness. The mental health examiner in the intake area must always consider organic and physical causes as a possible explanation for any bizarre presentation.

Gifts From God

Louis R is a 28-year-old white man charged with the aggravated criminal sexual assault of two minor boys, aged 7 and 8 years. At the screening, he provided appropriate identifying information and denied any history of treatment for mental health problems. However, the examiner referred the inmate for a secondary evaluation because of the nature of the charges against him. On closer inquiry, the inmate revealed that an angel from God came to him and told him he could use the two minor boys for his sexual pleasure as a gift from God. He described seeing a vision of a "ghost-like" angel and repeatedly hearing the voice of God for approximately 5 years. He stated that initially the angel told him to sacrifice the two boys, but later "God" told him to use the boys for his "sexual pleasure." The examiner initially expressed skepticism at the inmate's reported symptoms because they all related to the charges against him and possibly represented his defense strategy. On further inquiry, the inmate revealed that his family had attempted to hospitalize him many times in psychiatric facilities. He stated that they did not recognize his "divinity" or his "chosen status," and he believed that many of his family members had made a deal with the devil to destroy him. He also stated that the devil invented psychiatric medication as part of a plan to destroy him. The examiner determined that the inmate might possibly have a major mental disorder, and admitted him to the diagnostic unit for further evaluation with a provisional diagnosis of "rule out schizophrenia, paranoid type, rule out malingering."

Recognizing that responsibility for determining innocence or guilt falls outside the purview of mental health providers in correctional settings, the examiner took a conservative approach and admitted the inmate to the Department of Mental Health Services. In this case, the inmate continued to verbalize delusional ideas and continued to report auditory hallucinations, but refused to take psychotropic medication. Ultimately, the inmate had a court-ordered fitness evaluation. He was found unfit to stand trial and was remanded to the Illinois Department of Mental Health for restoration. These cases can confuse an intake examiner because many factors influence the evaluation, including the examiner's own feelings about individuals who perpetrate these types of crimes. Sometimes, the sexual abuse charges stem from custody fights, which may render them suspect. Consider the following vignette as an example.

That Is Not True

Judith P is a 32-year-old Asian woman charged with aggravated criminal sexual assault of her 3-year-old daughter. Mittimus papers from court indicated that Ms. P penetrated her daughter's vagina with her fingers and other household objects. At intake, Ms. P offered appropriate identifying information, denied any history of psychiatric treatment, and denied any suicidal ideation. She stated repeatedly that she had never harmed her daughter in any way, and reported that she and her husband were locked in a bitter fight to obtain custody of the daughter. She stated that her husband brought these charges against her in an effort to discredit her parenting skills. She produced paperwork from a local hospital stating that the daughter showed no signs of abuse and recommending that Ms. P retain custody of her daughter. Ms. P reported that her family had assisted her in retaining a private defense attorney and that she expected vindication on all charges. She denied any need for mental health services and joked that, while she felt like killing her husband, she would not want to come to jail again because of him. As Ms. P displayed no symptoms indicating that she had a major mental disorder, the examiner found her appropriate for housing in the general population of the jail. The examiner explained the procedure for obtaining mental health services in the future should Ms. P believe she had a need for them.

In a case such as this, the examiner has no direct knowledge of the detainee's innocence or guilt. Admission to the Department of Mental Health Services in a pretrial situation for treatment of pedophilia would not be appropriate, however, given the inmate's vehement denials of engaging in such behavior and the absence of any contrary evidence. Giving the inmate a diagnosis of a sexual deviancy disorder would serve only to prejudice the case against her.

CONCLUSION

Proper screening and assessment are essential for protecting the correctional institution from legal liability and for safeguarding both the legal and the medical rights of the individual detainee. All inmates should be screened on admission. The screening can be relatively brief and should focus on the broad concepts and symptoms presented. The screening and identification of those individuals with mental illness for purposes of placement and treatment assure that new arrivals who need to be are separated from the general inmate population and from other inmates who may be mentally ill, intoxicated, or violent.

REFERENCES

1. Johnson AB: *Out of Bedlam: The Truth About Deinstitutionalization.* New York, Basic Books, 1990.
2. Holcomb WR, Ahr PR: Arrest rates among young adult psychiatric patients treated in inpatient and outpatient settings. *Hosp Community Psychiatry* 39:52–57, 1988.
3. Torrey EF, Stieber J, Ezekiel J, et al: *Criminalizing the Seriously Mentally Ill: The Abuse of Jails as Mental Hospitals.* Washington, D.C.: Public Citizen's Health Research Group and National Alliance for the Mentally Ill, 1992.
4. Bureau of Justice Statistics: *Sourcebook of Criminal Justice Statistics—1995.* Washington, D.C., U.S. Department of Justice, 1996.
5. Teplin L: Psychiatric and substance abuse disorders among male urban jail detainees. *Am J Public Health* 84:290–293, 1994.
6. Torrey EF: Jails and prisons: America's new mental hospitals. *Am J Public Health* 85:1611–1613, 1995.

7. Torrey EF: Jails and prisons: America's new mental hospitals. *Am J Public Health* 85:1611–1613, 1995, p 1612.

8. *Bowring v Godwin*, 551 F2d 44 (4th Cir 1977).

9. *Estelle v Gamble*, 429 US 97 (1976).

10. *Jones v Wittenberg*, 509 F Supp 653 (ND Ohio 1980).

11. *Alberti v Sheriff of Harris County, Texas*, 406 R Supp 649 (SD Tex 1975).

12. *Campbell v McGruder*, 580 F2d 521, 549 (DC Cir 1978).

13. *Dawson v Kendrick*, 527 F Supp 1252 (SD WVa 1981).

14. *Inmates of Allegheny County Jail v Pierce*, 487 F Supp 638, 642–643 (WD Pa 1980).

15. *Pugh v Locke*, 406 R Supp 318 (MD Ala 1976).

16. *Ruiz v Estelle*, 503 F Supp 1265, 1323 (SD Tex 1980).

17. *Standards for Health Services in Jails*. Chicago, National Commission on Correctional Health Care, 1996.

18. *Standards for Health Services in Prisons*. Chicago, National Commission on Correctional Health Care, 1996.

19. *Psychiatric Services in Jails and Prisons*. Washington, D.C., American Psychiatric Association, Task Force Report 29, 1989.

20. Steadman HJ, Cocozza JJ (eds): *Mental Illness in American Prisons*. Seattle, National Coalition for the Mentally Ill in the Criminal Justice System, 1993.

ADDITIONAL SOURCES

1. Bubler NN (ed): *Standards for Services in Correctional Facilities*, ed 2. Washington, D.C., American Public Health Association, 1986.

2. Bureau of Justice Statistics: *Jail Inmates 1990*. Washington, D.C., U.S. Department of Justice, 1991.

3. Solomon P, Draine J: Issues in serving the forensic client. *Soc Work* 40:25–23, 1995.

19

Mental Health Outpatient Services in Correctional Settings

Andrea Weisman, Ph.D.

INTRODUCTION

A considerable body of literature has developed during the last 10–15 years with regard to the issue of providing mental health services to individuals under the jurisdiction of the criminal justice system. This work is fairly broad-based with representation from professional organizations, consumer-oriented mental health and legal advocacy groups, criminologists, private practitioners, and federal agencies, all of whom are concerned with the exploding incidence of incarceration of the mentally ill and with the paucity of services with which they are provided wherever they may be found—from their initial experiences in local lockups to county jails to state and federal prisons and, ultimately, through their return to their communities via probation or parole supervision.[1–10]

Taken together, this body of literature supports the propositions that mental health services should be provided in correctional settings; that good mental health care does

not interfere with security concerns in the correctional setting; and that screening, evaluation, suicide prevention, treatment, and discharge or transfer planning constitute essential services, regardless of the correctional setting within which they may be provided.

This chapter will describe some of the issues involved in attempting to develop and implement outpatient mental health services for individuals in correctional settings. Outpatients are inmates receiving mental health services while housed in the general populations of jails or prisons, as compared with inmates in special mental health housing units or areas. Delineating the parameters of the group(s) requiring mental health services, while housed in general population cell blocks, is often based on factors such as whether there is a specialized unit for their care, whether there are designated beds available for them, or to what extent there are existing personnel resources. Large urban facilities, such as the Fulton County Jail in Atlanta, Georgia, the Boulder County Jail in Colorado, the Salt Lake City County Jail in Utah, or Rikers Island in New York, are more likely to have separate housing units or infirmaries with psychiatric and nursing coverage to address the needs of the inmates with the most severe psychiatric illnesses.[11, 12]

This capacity is particularly critical in urban facilities because they have a greater concentration of inmates with serious mental illnesses housed within them. According to the report published by the National Alliance for the Mentally Ill (NAMI) and the Public Citizen's Health Research Group, *Criminalizing the Seriously Mentally Ill: The Abuse of Jails as Mental Hospitals*, which was based on a nationwide survey of 1,391 jails—or 41% of jails in 45 states, the estimated percentage of individuals with serious mental illnesses in facilities with populations greater than 1,000 was 8.7%. In small facilities with average populations less than 50, this percentage was estimated to be roughly 3.3%.[11] The greater density of untreated individuals with serious mental illnesses in urban areas accounts for their increased prevalence among incarcerated populations. Those who are homeless and mentally ill—a condition both caused by and consequent to lack of treatment—have extraordinarily high arrest and incarceration rates. In a study of more than 200 homeless individuals in Los Angeles,[13] 74% had previously been arrested and spent time in the Los Angeles County Jail. In addition, as the NAMI–Public Citizen's report documents, 29% of jails had detained individuals who were mentally ill with no known criminal charges against them.[11]

Understanding the magnitude of the issue is critical in beginning to think through the kinds of mental health services, both inpatient and outpatient, that need to be developed within correctional settings. One way to capture this magnitude is to attend to the figures Torrey[14] presents in his latest polemic decrying national mental health policy, *Out of the Shadows*:

> In 1955, there were 558,239 severely mentally ill patients in the nation's public psychiatric hospitals. In 1994, this number had been reduced by 486,620 patients, to 71,619 … however, the census of 558,239 patients in public psychiatric hospitals in 1955 was in relationship to the nation's total population at the time, which was 184 million.
>
> By 1994, the nation's population had increased to 260 million. If there had been the same proportion of patients per population in public mental hospitals in 1994 as there had been in 1955, the patients would have totaled 885,010. The true magnitude of deinstitutionalization, then, is the difference between 885,010 and 71,619. In effect, approximately 92 percent of the people who would have been living in public psychiatric hospitals in 1955 were not living there in 1994 … that [still] means that approximately 763,391 severely mentally ill people are living in the community today who would have been hospitalized 40 years ago [emphasis added].

Various facility-specific and field survey methodologies have been used in estimating the incidence of mental illness within correctional settings, producing figures ranging between 3.3% and 25%.[11, 15–19] In large part, the range is accounted for by differences in the definition of mental illness used among researchers. Reports on the low end of the range, as previously noted, estimated incidence not only in smaller facilities but also used more restrictive definitions requiring a major Axis I diagnosis, such as schizophrenia or a major affective disorder. Reports that produced estimates at the high end used more expansive definitions capturing individuals with primary Axis II diagnoses. Consider for a moment that if we used the reasonably conservative figure of 8.7% to estimate the incidence of serious mental illness represented among the 2,200 detainees at the Fulton County Jail, we would expect to find 185 inmates with serious mental illnesses on any given day. Given that the jail has a 14-bed infirmary, that means that 171 inmates with serious mental illness will have to have their needs met on an outpatient basis, that is, in the general population.

Facilities with insufficient or inadequate space for the separate housing of patients with mental illnesses will inevitably house inmates with serious mental illnesses in the general population. Procedures for screening the most severely ill patients—those considered to be a danger to self or others and whose dangerousness is evaluated to be a consequence of their mental illness—will be particularly critical. In facilities with minimal or no specialized housing, establishing necessary linkages to hospitals with inpatient psychiatric services will be of paramount concern. Inevitably, this will still mean that facility-based outpatient services will require the resources to manage a wide range of acute psychiatric conditions.

In general, a full array of services, including medication management, ongoing screening and evaluation, and crisis intervention, a variety of psychotherapeutic treatment modalities, including behavioral management strategies, and clinical case management will be core components of any outpatient mental health program.[8–10] The parameters determining the development of outpatient services for particular facilities will vary to some extent based on the accessibility to inpatient services, both on and off site. This chapter begins at the point of considering some of the clinical and administrative issues entailed in developing an outpatient mental health program, including the goals and objectives of corrections-based mental health programs, the clinical and nonclinical populations requiring interventions on an outpatient basis, and what some of the barriers are to the provision of mental health programs in correctional settings.

MENTAL HEALTH GOALS WITHIN CORRECTIONAL SETTINGS

Toughening attitudes among policy makers and lawmakers and society generally have resulted in longer sentences and harsher, more punitive attitudes and environmental realities within correctional settings. Jails and prisons are usually environments that are hostile to the provision of mental health services, and even dedicated public sector professionals are presented with fundamental challenges to their basic beliefs or principles. The devastating consequences of even limited lengths of stay in some extreme correctional environments frequently lead to a deterioration in the level of functioning of some inmates or even, some believe, in their ability to exercise moral reasoning.[20–22]

In what may be the most extreme case, the desolating consequences of protracted lengths of stay in super-maximum security facilities in which inmates are kept entirely isolated and disconnected from each other, security staff, and, generally, external stimulation has been identified as a discernible clinical syndrome, referred to, alternately, as the Secure Housing Unit (SHU) Syndrome,[22] Administrative Segregation (AD SEG) Syndrome,[23] or the condition known as restricted environmental stimulation (RES).[24] Practitioners studying the environmental effects of prolonged social isolation report observing such symptoms as confused thought processes, hallucinations, irrational anger, emotional flatness, violent fantasies, social withdrawal, oversensitivity to stimuli, and chronic depression.[25–28]

Although the most extreme symptoms may often be associated with the most extreme environmental conditions, there is by no means a uniform effect across inmates, and some amount of variability is undoubtedly attributable to the individuals themselves. For example, some experience negative psychological repercussions after stays in much less restrictive settings. There are clearly individual differences in inmates' abilities to tolerate correctional environments. For many, incarceration may exacerbate pre-existing mental illnesses. For others, being incarcerated may lead to the development of some degree of personality reorganization or disorganization, in attempts to accommodate themselves to the social realities imposed among peers and between themselves and those in authority.[21, 29]

Providing mental health services in this context can be formidable. In large measure, mental health professionals in these settings are in the position of having to undo or minimize the psychological effects of the standard operational policies and procedures implemented in the correctional setting. The American Public Health Association Standards (1986)[30] address this directly by recommending that psychiatric services work toward the improvement of institutions' mental health. The American Psychiatric Association (APA) task force report can also be read as addressing the importance of mental health professionals' concern for the correctional environment because these environments may provide "insufficient attention to basic human needs [which can] seriously compromise the delivery of ... services. Unless specific attention is paid to these

environments, they may negate or overwhelm therapeutic interventions and indeed all programming."[9]

Identifying the goals of a corrections-based outpatient mental health program raises some difficult questions. Correctional administrators want mental health services to assist them in addressing management issues and in avoiding liability by reducing dangerous and disruptive behavior. In jails, in pretrial cases, the courts are interested in mental health staff working to restore inmates' competency so that they may stand trial. Metzner[7] recalled Cohen and Dvoskin on the matter of goals of mental health programs in correctional settings, by observing these to be the "reduction of the disabling effects of serious mental illness in order to maximize inmates' ability to participate in correctional programs; decreasing the needless extremes of human suffering caused by mental illness; and helping to keep the [prison] safe for staff, inmates, volunteers and visitors."[7]

American Psychiatric Association standards discuss the goal of mental health services primarily in terms of providing access to basic services "at a level that is consistent to those that are available in the community,"[9] which is not necessarily a high standard. As previously mentioned, the NAMI–Public Citizen's report[11] noted that the incarceration rate of those who are seriously mentally ill had risen in direct relation to the paucity or inaccessibility of services provided by the departments of mental health. Indeed, underscoring the reality of worsening accessibility to services with the advent of mental health managed care, NAMI's recent efforts have lately been directed at identifying and raising awareness about the barriers to accessing mental health services faced by Medicaid recipients in the 49 states now contracting with managed health care organizations.[31]

Mental health professionals must also struggle with a host of nonclinical issues that determine the parameters of therapeutic contracts. Typically, the frequency or duration of a therapeutic contract is based on legal or security concerns that cannot be modified by clinical interests or issues. In the face of this, they must also struggle with establishing goals with clients that are life enhancing and, to the extent practicable, afford inmates a degree of privacy and control over the terms of the therapeutic contract.

- Programs that strive to address individuals' institutional adjustment and that enhance their skills in living more successfully in the community upon release seems desirable. Both these foci are encompassed in the following goals for outpatient mental health programs;
- To establish therapeutic opportunities that seek to moderate the effects of incarceration by providing support and by promoting positive social behavior among individuals;
- To reduce dangerous and disruptive behavior;
- To provide the opportunity to address the particular issues and offenses that may have caused or contributed to the individual's detainment;
- To ensure access to these services by providing them in a consistent, reliable, and structured manner;

- To establish linkages to community service-providing agents or agencies at the point of release.

In addition, among the most critical interventions in moderating the institutional culture, or Zeitgeist, is a comprehensive mental health training program for correctional staff and supervisors that focuses on the signs and symptoms of mental illness and that helps them to distinguish volitional behavior from behavior that may be beyond the control of the individual, or that is made more intractable or extreme by correctional circumstances.

WHOSE RESPONSIBILITY IS IT, ANYWAY?

The issue of who should provide mental health services to an incarcerated population has been quite controversial. The ongoing issue has been whether departments of mental health (or their subsidiary agencies), who are acquainted with the particulars regarding identification and treatment of mental illness but who are unfamiliar with the correctional setting, should provide mental health services to individuals in correctional settings or whether departments of corrections, who are unfamiliar and frequently uncomfortable with issues of mental illness, should be obligated to develop the resources necessary to provide corrections-based mental health services.

Overwhelmingly, researchers argue that correctional facilities, particularly jails that house individuals not yet convicted of crimes, should not be "considered isolated institution(s)," but rather that these facilities and their populations should be perceived as belonging to the community.

Broadly speaking, the community includes departments of mental health, private service-providing agencies or individuals, universities, the courts, the police, and others, all of whom, it is believed, have a responsibility to partner with jails in developing solutions for the care and management of detainees with mental illnesses.[32]

A variety of effective solutions for service provision have worked in different localities. At the Cook County Jail in Chicago, Illinois, a full range of in- and outpatient psychiatric services are provided by Cermak Health Services, which is part of the Cook County Bureau of Health. Professional psychiatric services are provided by the Isaac Ray Center, an organization associated with Rush–Presbyterian Medical College. In Lexington, Kentucky, Fayette County Detention Center inmates are provided assessment and referral services by the local community mental health center, the Bluegrass East Comprehensive Care Center. The Mental Health Center of Boulder, Colorado also provides mental health services to inmates at the Boulder County Jail. In Bellingham, Washington, the Whatcom County Jail's 190 inmates receive mental health services through a combination of contractual arrangements with in-house department of corrections nursing staff and community-based private practitioners who travel to the jail to provide services ranging from substance abuse counseling to rape counseling.[11]

Model programs or program components can be established in a variety of ways using state and local resources. Universities have served in critical capacities in terms of responding to the mental health needs of incarcerated individuals. In New York, HealthLink is a Hunter College program that establishes community-based aftercare linkages for individuals requiring medical or mental health services on release from the Rikers Island jail. HealthLink, which began as a 5-year privately sponsored demonstration project, is a model public–private partnership that collaboratively arranges or provides critical services.

In Seattle, the University of Washington and the department of corrections, along with other service-providing community agencies, designed a work plan to address issues and strategies for an ongoing public awareness campaign, with the premise that at least part of the problem in establishing necessary services was a need to educate the public about the mental health needs of incarcerated individuals, as well as to educate the various stakeholders about each others' problems and limitations in providing services.

In Texas, establishing a structure for more coordinated service delivery to children vastly improved the quality of services provided. Texas established, by legislation, what they referred to as community resource coordination groups (CRCGs) to create a structure and forum for integrating services delivered to children and their families by multiple public agencies. In 1994, Texas had about 110 CRCGs across the state, serving more than 800 children and their families each year. Texas' plan was to use this same principle in developing services for adult offenders.

Some states have been successful in bringing together policy makers and high-level administrators in the systems involving mental health, substance abuse, and criminal justice to jointly identify the barriers to the provision of mental health services to individuals in the justice system. In some states these efforts have resulted in the development of blueprints for multiagency collaborations to more effectively coordinate service delivery, beginning at the point of the diversion of those with the most serious mental illnesses from the justice system altogether, and including the provision of services to individuals incarcerated in jails and prisons. Technical assistance to governors' task forces consisting of key stakeholders with decision-making authority has been, and continues to be, available to all states. For example, the federally funded National GAINS Center for People with Co-Occurring Disorders in the Justice System, in Delmar, New York, serves as a resource center and provides just this sort of consultation to states.

The federal court orders in effect in some states, regarding either the mental health system or mental health service delivery in facilities operated by departments of corrections, can be used to leverage necessary services for those with mental illnesses. In Washington, D.C., the repeated failure of the Commission on Mental Health Services and the department of corrections to effectively coordinate the delivery of mental health services to inmates in the Central Detention Facility (the D.C. jail) resulted in the court mandating that these agencies terminate their arrangement and that the department of corrections develop the resources to provide necessary services.[33] In 1995, the D.C. jail was placed under receivership when the department of corrections failed to do so. The receivership established the necessary structure and resources for the development and implementation of critical mental health services. The fact that the District's Commission on Mental Health Services was also under independent federal court orders regarding general issues of mental health service provision to its class members has been used by the D.C. jail receivership to make headway in establishing a more viable partnership between the agencies. The focus of these efforts has been on both the establishment of procedures for aftercare linkages and the initiation of a dialogue regarding the diversion of misdemeanants with serious mental illnesses.

Although there are alternatives to arranging for the provision of basic mental health services in correctional settings, some principles seem clear. In systems in which multiple agencies may provide services, there need to be well-articulated memorandums of understandings and/or policies and procedures that direct the interactions between agencies and their staffs, and there needs to be one consistent reporting structure for on-site service providers. There need to be designated representatives for the specific agencies that participate in the partnership and an on-site administrator or director of the whole spectrum of services provided. There need to be regularly scheduled meetings for agency representatives and the on-site administrator, so that service provision in terms of improved outcomes for inmates can be reviewed and so that any obstacles individuals or agencies may experience in the course of fulfilling their responsibilities can be addressed.

OUTPATIENT SERVICES

Outpatient treatment programs are uniformly identified as one among an array of needed corrections-based mental health services.[1, 7, 9, 12, 33–36] Critical components of any outpatient program include:

- Intake screening on admission, especially to jails that have individuals arriving from the street with little or no accompanying information;
- More comprehensive mental health evaluations for those who evidence unstable mental status or who report current use of services or a past history of mental health treatment or a past history of self-inflicted injuries;
- Crisis intervention;
- Suicide prevention.

These, however, are topics that provide the basis for other chapters in this volume and so are not handled here.

As a general matter, aside from these necessary services, other program components are more likely to be provided as elective treatments to inmates. Although some individual therapy will surely be necessary in addressing individuals' needs in crisis situations, the most useful modality will be group interventions because it will maximize the allocation of resources.[32] Among the more common groups will be those dealing with general support, anger management, conflict resolution, stress reduction, grief and loss, and the learning of assorted occupational and leisure skills. The discussion here will focus on more specialized outpatient services, such as medication management, substance abuse services, sex offender treatment, and behavioral management, and on programmatic issues specific to specialized populations such as women and juveniles.

Provision of specific outpatient services will, in part, be predicated by a number of factors, such as whether the facility is a jail or prison, what the size and location of the specific facility is, and what the relationship is or can be between the department of corrections and the department of mental health or other private service-providing agencies, practitioners, or universities. For inmates with chronic mental illnesses, the extent of care that will fall back on corrections-based outpatient programs will be dependent on the success of these linkages in providing services before, during, and after incarceration.

Mental health programs will differ between jails and prisons in terms of not only what specific services may be offered, but also what the clinical focus of services needs to be, given the anticipated duration of therapeutic contracts. Pretrial jail inmates are more likely to be in emotional crisis, newly cut off from children, family, or friends, uncertain about their charges or future. Because jail stays are likely to be brief relative to prisons, the clinical focus of services needs to be on providing individuals with support and preparing them for longer-term work in either the community or prison.

For example, some estimates place the incidence of abuse or trauma experienced among incarcerated women at more than 90%.[37] Arguably, a mental health program with a clinical component focused on abuse and trauma will be critical for women's long-range recovery. However, attempting to elicit disclosures from women in the context of a brief jail stay would be imprudent, inasmuch as the disclosures of more fragile individuals may put them at greater risk for the occurrence or exacerbation of predictable clinical crises such as intrusive flashbacks and dissociative episodes.

A more clinically appropriate focus in a jail setting would be to help women gain greater control of those symptoms that put them at greater risk for conflict with other inmates or staff during their incarceration. Doing this involves teaching women skills and tools that keep them focused in the present, such as how to gain control of intrusive imagery and the use of relaxation techniques. In a jail setting, teaching women how *not* to deal with abuse material and how to focus, instead, on strategies to stay safe, including learning techniques for compartmentalizing experiences, seems more clinically appropriate. Issues that involve longer-term work such as disclosing, reliving, identifying the dysfunctional sequelae to the abuse, and so on, are probably more judiciously left to contexts in which lengthier therapeutic engagements are more likely.[38–41] Clinical interventions need to be designed to address the individual's needs in the particular context within which the services will be provided. The basic safety needs of patients and the likely duration of the therapeutic contract will be key in planning interventions. These same principles apply, regardless of the content of the issues being addressed.

Medication Management

Effective medication management programs will consist of (1) a tracking and monitoring system, (2) regularly scheduled clinics staffed by a psychiatrist–nurse team who together review compliance and institutional behavior and first-person reports of inmate, and (3) regularly scheduled patient educational groups related to the use of psychoactive medications.

Although most correctional facilities prefer a policy of arranging psychoactive medication administration on a watch-take basis to reduce the incidence of patients hoarding and bartering medication for other goods and services, for individuals who don't require this oversight, this becomes another area of their lives over which they exercise little control. Perhaps as a consequence, the issue of medication compliance, as Dvoskin[12] and others note, can tend to become a battleground between inmates and medical staff, which is all the more reason why effective education programs need to be implemented as part of successful medication management strategies.

Substance Abuse Services

The explosive increase in the incarceration rate is attributable in large part to mandatory sentences for drug offenses. According to the 1995 report, *Young Black Americans and the Criminal Justice System: Five Years Later*,[42] issued by the Sentencing Project, between 1983 and 1993 the number of drug offenders grew from roughly 9% to more than 25% of populations incarcerated in either jails or state and federal prisons. The figure for prior drug use among incarcerated individuals is an astronomical 83%.[43]

The rising rate of co-occurring substance abuse and mental disorders among incarcerated individuals has also received attention from both researchers concerned with tracking incidence rates and program administrators concerned with designing services.[4, 12, 44] According to the National GAINS Center figures, the co-morbidity from substance abuse or dependence and serious mental illness among a prison population is 13%. This figure is much higher, of course, if the co-occurrence of antisocial personality disorder and substance abuse disorders are assessed. The GAINS Center's estimate for the co-occurrence of sub-

stance abuse or dependence and the mental health diagnoses of schizophrenia, major affective disorders, and antisocial personality disorder among a jail population, reaches as high as 90%.[45]

Although based on a limited sample, Steadman et al.[1] reported that 60% of jails responding to their survey (N = 42) provided some in-house substance abuse services. Peters and Hills[44] however examined a larger sample of jails (N = 1,737) and found that only 28% offered substance abuse services that went beyond detoxification. Another survey of substance abuse services, reported by Metzner,[34] found that most states provide some form of intervention, from assessment on intake to individual and group counseling. As many as 30 states reported some type of intensive residential program, "often based on the therapeutic model."[46]

In jails, where the stays are briefer, the development of a program that focuses on the evaluation of the need for services and results in specific recommendations for community-based services that can be used in planning for services seems desirable. More structured residential programs that proceed in stages are more likely to be effective in prison settings.

A promising approach is offered by the GAINS Center, which promotes a model involving the cross-training of mental health and substance-abuse-treatment staff for more effective, integrated service delivery. The Center is scheduled to introduce this model in New York City's Rikers Island substance abuse program, Casa Montalvo, later in 1997.

Although there are a wide array of program types, there is a paucity of data on the effectiveness of any of these models. One promising opportunity to assess the effectiveness of an in-house jail substance abuse treatment program was recently reported by the Department of Mental Health Law and Policy (DMHL&P) at the Florida Mental Health Institute. The DMHL&P developed a program in conjunction with the Hillsborough County Sheriff's Office. It was one of three sites funded by the Bureau of Justice Administration with a commitment to evaluate performance-based outcomes in assessing program effectiveness.[47] This is an area in need of considerable further exploration.

Sex Offender Treatment

The Bureau of Justice Statistics (BJS)[48] reports that about 234,000 sex offenders are under the care, custody, or control of correctional agencies and that, of these, roughly 60% are under conditional supervision in the community. The BJS estimates that just less than 5% of the total correctional population in the United States are male offenders convicted of rape or sexual assault. The rise in the rates of rapes and sexual assaults since 1980 is staggering. The BJS compares the average annual growth of prison populations in general, which is estimated at around 7.6%, with the annual growth rate for violent sexual assaults other than rape, which is estimated to be 15%. These are crimes whose rate of growth is second only to drug trafficking.

Data from Minnesota reveal that more than 94% of inmates convicted of sex offenses were acquainted with their victims, and that only about 30% of adults convicted of felony sex offenses received state prison terms, which averaged 7.4 years. The legal course in the other 70% of the cases resulted in a relatively brief jail stay—around 6 months—with court-mandated treatment during conditional release on probation.[49]

The BJS[50] statistics indicate that the average sentence for convicted rapists released from state prisons is about 10 years, and the average time served has risen slightly to 5 years. For sexual assaults, sentence length is around 6 1/2 years, and the average time served has risen to just less than 3 years.

Although the recidivism data are equivocal on the matter of duration of treatment and length of time in the community before a repeat offense, there does seem to be modest evidence to support the claim that there is some reduction in the repeat offense rates of offenders who elect to attend and remain in treatment.[51, 52] A recent report by the National Center for Institutions and Alternatives, which runs the Augustus Institute, a community-based program for sex offenders in Alexandria, Virginia, looked at the results of 12 separate studies assessing the repeat offense rates of offenders participating in treatment. Their review found far more studies reporting positive than negative or inconclusive results; of the 12 studies, 9 found positive results, 3 found inconclusive results, and none of the studies found negative consequences to offender participation in treatment.[52]

In spite of the inconclusiveness of outcome data, given the growing prevalence of sex offenses, including sex offender services as a component of an outpatient mental health treatment program would seem judicious. Programs are typically defined and constructed in discrete, staged component parts corresponding to patient ownership of the offending behavior, the ability to identify antecedents or triggers to offending, and the ability to manage one's own risk factors and generalize to novel situations.[49]

As with other clinical issues discussed in terms of the jail setting, given the brevity of some arrestees' detainment, focusing treatment on formal assessments of those individuals who admit responsibility for the offense, who ask for treatment, or who may be ordered by the court to undergo evaluations, may be most appropriate. More comprehensive treatment services, which may be established as a residential program, can be planned for prison settings. Because of the stigma and potential for harassment from other inmates, ongoing treatment for sex offenders may best be accomplished in residential programs. In general, these programs tend to be more intensive, and the patient may average as much as 1,000 hours of treatment before completion.[51]

There appear to be a variety of structures available for implementing programs. Specialized community-based sex offender programs in the jurisdiction in which the correctional facility is located can provide valuable resources, including consultation and training to department of corrections staff. The Augustus Institute provides training and technical assistance to departments of corrections in the development of sex offender services. The Sex Offender Accountability and Responsibility (SOAR) Program located at Harnett Correctional Institution in Lillington, North Carolina is run by the department of corrections through contracts with private providers for facility-based services.[52] In Minnesota, where sex offender treatment services are independently provided by both the department of corrections and the department of human services, the recommendation was offered that the two departments work more cooperatively to both provide services and develop policy for the regulation of these services.

Alaska's Department of Corrections developed treatment programs in conjunction with private vendors in three regions throughout the state. When the programs were found to lack consistency and to have duplicated resources, they were refashioned to provide a continuum of services among the regions so that the needs of inmates were met at the different points in their treatment. The Hiland Mountain Sex Offender Treatment Program is a notable example of a multiphase, multi-institutional treatment program for offenders.[51]

Developing a broad-based continuum of services model for the provision of treatment to sex offenders is exemplified by the development of these services in Canada. In 1994, the Correctional Service of Canada Regional Psychiatric Centers decided to implement a national strategy by bringing together sex offender assessment and treatment specialists from all service regions in both the private and public sectors. The resulting committee developed standards for treatment that were subsequently reviewed by administrative and legal representatives as well as by consumers. A directive was adopted in 1996 that describes assessment, treatment, and outcomes for offenders. The standards specify that

Treatment should typically motivate the offenders to take full responsibility for their offense(s), help them identify their crime cycle (the internal and external events that lead to offending), teach them to deal with deviant sexual fantasies and urges, and help them learn to cope with barriers to meaningful consensual and age-appropriate relationships. Other treatment goals include learning to appropriately channel anger, loneliness and sadness, understand how others feel, and avoid or cope with high-risk situations.[54]

As these programs exemplify, to maximize outcomes for offenders, the developers of these programs should coordinate expertise and resources among private practitioners and departments of corrections and human services to achieve an integrated approach that offers a continuum of care from facility-based programs to community supervision. Given the complexity of these partnerships, as well as the uncertainty of treatment effectiveness, it is recommended that agencies develop interagency agreements that include standards for service provision and strategies for assessing the effectiveness of programs in terms of both the consumers and systems involved.

Behavioral Management Programs

Among the most vexing problems for mental health, medical, and correctional staff is the management of individuals who demonstrate an apparent willingness to injure themselves for reasons seemingly independent of underlying psychiatric disorders.[55–57] This acknowledges three distinguishable types of self-inflicted injuries: those that are intended to result in death, those that are intended for affective discharge, and those that are designed for secondary gain. Suicidal behavior is the subject of a chapter in this volume and will not be dealt with here. The second type is usually referred to as self-mutilation and involves intentional cutting, burning, or other self-inflicted injuries for the purpose of cathartic release or the self-inflicted injury is the goal (see Winchel and Stanley[55] and Jones[57]). The motivations for these types of self-inflicted injuries are distinct from those individuals engage into effect an institutional response. It is critical that a mental health professional evaluate individuals who injure themselves so that the reason for the injury can be determined, and so that appropriate treatment interventions can be devised.

The *Diagnostic and Statistical Manual of Mental Disorders,* ed 4,[58] defines malingering as the voluntary production of psychological symptoms for reasons having to do with individuals' circumstances and not with their internally residing pathologic conditions. The motivations for the manufacture of behaviors suggestive of mental illness are varied but are usually related to individuals' understanding of the role mental illness potentially plays in housing assignments, off-site placements to psychiatric hospital settings, and the mitigation of legal outcomes, among other desirable ends. The context creates the circumstances for self-injury to gain a currency, and this makes the behavior anything but pathological; indeed, it may be understood to be adaptive.

Staged self injuries are a perplexing problem, because neither mental health nor correctional staff are particularly comfortable assuming the responsibility for managing inmates who engage in this behavior. Given the risk of liability, the inclination of corrections, understandably, is to want to assign responsibility to mental health professionals. At the same time, mental health professionals grapple with a location problem. That is, is the locus of the problem within the individual, within the correctional environment, or somehow in the relationship between the individual and the environment?[59] Who is the patient, the inmate or the correctional environment? What role should mental health assume?

Staged self-inflicted injury causes problems for mental health staff precisely because its point, frequently, is to further the inmate's position in the power struggle between him and the correctional system or staff. Metzner, in speaking of this power struggle, observes

> *Institutional rules and practices regarding strip searches, noncontact visits, yard time, shower time, and administrative (or punitive) segregation are often made for security purposes, but may reflect control issues—dynamics between correctional staff and inmates. Both inmates and correctional staff will attempt to engage the mental health professional as an ally in these power struggles, especially within administrative segregation units. An understanding of the institutional organization and the inmates' social system will facilitate a reasonable response by the mental health clinician.[60]*

Mental health staff walk a tightrope in managing these behaviors and, to a lesser extent, other disruptive behaviors such as flooding and throwing bodily fluids and waste because treating individuals who engage in these behaviors as if they had mental health problems is fraught with disastrous consequences—disastrous, because as the principles of behavioral conditioning advise, doing so will tend to increase the probability of the behavior's reoccurrence. In the language of learning theory, the strength of a behavior rises in proportion to its likelihood of eliciting a reward.[61, 62] Worse, in instances in which institutional responses may be variable (the typical state of affairs in correctional facilities) where only some inmates affect desired ends some of the time, a difficult problem becomes nearly intractable. Intermittent reinforcement schedules tend to not only increase the likelihood of the undesirable behavior but also intensify the risk-taking associated with it. This state of affairs makes the behavior both more lethal and more difficult to eliminate.[59]

From a behavioral management perspective, the behavior needs to be stopped without being reinforced. The first requirement of a corrections-based behavioral management program is to have sufficient professional mental health staff who can conduct the necessary assessments to distinguish between those individuals who may be a danger to themselves because of mental illness from those who injure themselves for secondary gain. Clearly, these are sometimes difficult to distinguish, but, in most instances, it is not. However, only a qualified mental health professional should make this decision. Of course, individuals who are seen as a danger to themselves because of a mental illness will meet the criteria in most jurisdictions for an immediate transfer to an off-site psychiatric hospital or a facility-based mental health area where patients can be safely monitored under the status of "suicide watch."

The housing of malingering inmates who inflict injury on themselves is complicated. It is desirable to have a designated location where inmates who have been evaluated to be in imminent danger of harming themselves can be observed to ensure their safety while not being given suicide watch status. At the D.C. jail, inmates may be housed in an infirmary area (not the mental health units) where they may be placed on behavioral watch status and closely observed. Establishing a safe setting within which an individual can be prevented from harming themselves will include the construction of a "safe" cell removed of apparatuses, apertures, or appliances that could directly or indirectly be used to cause a self-inflicted injury. A cell constructed for behavioral observation will actually be no different from that used for suicide watches.

What should be distinct are the cell's location and the clinical management ground rules. Such ground rules include not imbuing the observation period with extraneous meaning or social opportunity and not facilitating access to other goods or services. It is important that this period be as emotionally sterile as possible and that clinical encounters be as valence free as possible. The observation period is *only* about ensuring safety.

Although behavioral programs in other than correctional settings strive to establish reinforcement contingencies that reward an individual's production of desired behaviors, the culture of correctional settings makes following this principle ripe for abuse. Too few get too little for most not to realize that engaging in unwanted or undesirable behavior can be a means to accessing desired ends. In correctional settings, withdrawing privileges and predicating their return on the production of desired behavior is more likely to be an effective strategy in mediating behavior. Some facilities have all or some of an administrative segregation unit designated for these purposes.

The point of behavior management is to focus on the elimination of the undesirable behavior.[63] In these interventions, mental health staff can serve an essential liaison function between inmates and correctional staff, while being careful not to ally with either faction. Mental health staff can provide a useful role in interpreting and mediating whatever may be at issue in a dispute.

Special Populations: Women and Juveniles

Women. Another chapter in this volume offers a comprehensive examination of the need for services in jails and prisons that address the needs of women. This chapter will not expound on the treatment needs of incarcerated women, except to note some urgency in developing programs, given the exploding numbers of women in jails and prisons and their relative unlikelihood of receiving services. The female jail inmate population more than tripled between 1983 and 1994 (compared with the figure for men, which doubled). By 1994, the jail census for women was 19% of the total jail census. Figures for prisons indicate that between 1980

and 1994, the number of women in state and federal prisons increased 396% (compared with an increase for men of 214%). By the end of 1995, the women prisoner population had reached 69,028, or 6.3%, of 1,104,074 individuals incarcerated in the nation's prisons.[37]

A recent study conducted by the National Council on Crime and Delinquency[37] found, not surprisingly, that there is a critical paucity of programs that addresses women in correctional settings though the need for services is great. The report, which focused on women in three states, California, Connecticut, and Florida, found that more than 90% of the women surveyed reported significant physical, sexual, or emotional abuse during their lifetime, and 67.5% reported a history of violent victimization as children; that a majority of women were sentenced for petty drug and property crimes; that 80% were single caretakers of minor children; and that a majority experienced one or more medical (51.4%) or mental health (24.5%) problems.[64] These findings are substantiated in study after study.[36, 65–69]

Meeting the needs of this growing population is particularly worrisome because, as a study conducted by Teplin[69] demonstrated, less than one quarter of women who were identified as being in need of services actually received them while in jail. In structured interviews with 1,272 female detainees in the Cook County Jail during a 2-year period, Teplin found that only about 50% of the women with serious mental health illnesses (such as schizophrenia or bipolar disorder) received services. As few as 15% received services for less serious disorders such as depression. Teplin's data further indicated a positive correspondence between women's treatment histories and an increased likelihood of receiving services. This finding is consistent with a previous study that observed this same phenomenon among incarcerated men.[70, 71] Treatment history is obviously a critical indicator of an individual's likelihood of requiring current services; however, many factors besides individuals' need for services often determine whether they are likely to have accessed these previously. As Teplin's data attest, not having received services previously puts individuals at continued risk for not receiving them.

Juveniles. Yet another growing population is juveniles, whose numbers have risen as more and more are waived into adult courts and housed in adult correctional facilities. Like women, this population presents problems because their numbers, relative to adults, are small. Although there are actually fewer youths in jails and prisons today than 20 years ago (roughly 65,000[72] annually, compared with 500,000[73] in 1980), recently, the get-tough policies have resulted in the numbers inching upward again. Most recently, advocates have been attempting to stem the flow by challenging lawmakers' efforts to both lower the age youths may be waived into adult courts and increase the number of crimes for which they may be waived.

Developing programs for youths currently confined in adult facilities is made more complex because what is known about them is, for the most part, based largely on extrapolations of what is known about those who are detained in juvenile facilities. Prevalence data regarding learning disabilities, mental illnesses, and substance abuse disorders reported here are all based on figures previously reported by researchers who examined incidence rates among adolescents in the juvenile system. Further confusing the data, as discussed by Cocozza[74] in his introduction to the monograph, *Responding to the Mental Health Needs of Youth in the Juvenile Justice System*, to the extent that most researchers only associated a single disorder to a particular youth is the fact that data on the incidence of mental illness among juveniles likely underestimate the complexity of the pathologic conditions actually observed, by neglecting to take into account the frequent occurrence of youths with multiple disorders.

In spite of built-in methodological confounds, the prevalence data yield some interesting findings in terms of reported ranges (in percentages):

- Conduct disorder: (the most frequently occurring disorder) 50% to 90%;
- Attention deficit disorder/hyperactivity: 19% to 46%;
- Learning disabilities (17%) and specific developmental disorders (53%);
- Substance abuse and dependence: 25% to 95%;
- Personality disorders: 2% to 46%;
- Mental retardation: 7% to 15%;
- Affective disorders: 32% to 78%;
- Anxiety disorders: 6% to 41%; only one study assessed the incidence of posttraumatic stress disorder (41%;
- Psychotic disorders: 1% to 6%.[75]

Although it seems reasonable to presume that youths who commit more serious offenses, such as murder or rape, are likely to evidence more serious psychopathologic conditions and/or use or abuse of alcohol or other substances, for now, this is a hypothesis in need of confirming data. In a report to the State of Washington on the mental health needs of juveniles, Trupin et al.[76] noted that the level of the pathologic conditions observed among incarcerated youth was nearly indistinguishable from that observed among their psychiatrically hospitalized counterparts (76% of the sample of incarcerated youths were thought to be "severely emotionally disturbed"). Hutchinson described the mental health experience of youth incarcerated in Washington, D.C. in 1989:

> *Of 50 youth referred by the courts for psychiatric assessments in 1989, 10 had a history of psychiatric hospitalization and/or use of psychotropic medications. Diagnoses included major depression, dysthymia, sexual paraphilia, bipolar depression, schizophrenia, obsessive–compulsive disorder, posttraumatic stress disorder, seizure disorders, and organic mood disorders."[77]*

The problem is that juveniles have just as great, if not greater, a need for all the programs and treatments already

discussed, and, although housed in adult facilities, they cannot access adult services. In all but the largest facilities, the relatively small number of adolescents will make it impractical to consider developing an exhaustive array of services. In such instances, designating some or all of a clinician's time to the provision of direct services to juveniles, in addition to serving a liaison and advocacy function to corrections and the courts, will be advantageous. Coordination with community agencies for volunteer programs and services can enhance available resources. Departments of education also continue to be responsible for general and special education program for eligible juveniles. Nevertheless, this is a very difficult area and is likely to get more difficult as state and federal legislative changes are fully implemented during the coming years.

SOME PRINCIPLES FOR STRUCTURING FACILITY SERVICES

Structuring services so that they are accessible and predictable is critical. Steadman makes this point in observing that all the standards established by the professional agencies for mental health services in correctional facilities stress the importance of "health care services [being] delivered in the context of a formal structured program. This is particularly so because mental health service provision has traditionally been very haphazard with services arranged only on an as-needed basis."[78] The program structure gets established by the drafting of policies that define and describe service elements and that stipulate procedural issues such as how inmates will access both emergency and nonemergency services, how communication is to be established between providers of services; and how disparate disciplines can be helped so that their services are coordinated into a more integrated system of care.

Accessing Services

The APA[9] clearly identifies appropriate access to treatment as the yardstick by which mental health care should be evaluated in correctional facilities. Access, the APA notes, is typically measured in time frames.[79] Metzner[34] refers to access as a dynamic concept assessed in terms of inmates' ability to obtain services within "reasonable" time frames. Determining what constitutes reasonable time frames is easiest when determining response times in crisis situations. However, what constitutes reasonable access for nonemergency services is less clear and is likely to be largely predicated on staffing ratios. The more staff a facility has, the more likely it is that services will be made available more quickly. Establishing a tautological tangle, the APA specifically notes that "after extensive consideration [they have] concluded that staffing levels are virtually impossible to set with any objective formula or standard that has general applicability"[79] and, instead, substitute the notion of access to essential services as determinative in evaluating the quality of the program.

Ultimately, reasonable access may be a fluid concept, varying according to the particular inmate and issue and the program's system for scheduling appointments and informing inmates of that schedule. For example, an inmate, in receipt of written notification of a scheduled appointment, may be able to wait a week or more for a nonemergency. On the other hand, inmates left to wonder if or when they will be seen can reach the point of crisis.

As a general matter, clearly, it is undesirable for anyone to have to have an emergency to access services. All nonurgent requests for services should be responded to within 48–72 hours, even if the response is notification that an appointment has been scheduled.

Another issue related to inmates' access to services concerns the development of a formal system for inmates to use in requesting services. Systems that rely on inmates conveying their health needs through correctional staff run the risk of access being thwarted. Developing procedures for the direct communication of inmates' mental health concerns and desires for services to a specially trained, designated mental health triaging agent will be critical in establishing access.

Staffing

It seems reasonable to conclude, as the APA does, that staffing levels need to be assessed by individual institutions after determining the clinical requirements of those mental health services to be provided. Given the possibility that some services may be contracted for from private vendors, determining necessary in-house staffing ratios will be more complicated. However, there are some constants in adequately staffing an outpatient mental health program.

There needs to be adequate psychiatric coverage to initiate and monitor up to 15%–20% of outpatients who require psychoactive medication management. In prisons and with populations with chronic conditions, psychiatric nurses can provide daily or weekly observations and serve a triage function for the psychiatrist, who may see inmates monthly or even, in routine and stable cases, every 6–8 weeks.

Professional organizations' guidelines[9, 10] recommend that staffing levels should be sufficient to provide the same level of care available in the community. Given the remarks made earlier regarding the paucity of community-based services for those with serious mental illnesses being one of the principle causes for their ever-increasing rate of incarceration, establishing standards for correctional settings with reference to what is provided in the community is a dubious yardstick.

Location for the Provision of Services

The location for the provision of mental health services is a very significant issue in terms of the likely success of the program. On the one hand, services delivered in or proximate to housing units afford maximal opportunity for clinical staff to interact with correctional staff regarding their observations of the behaviors of inmates. Metzner speaks to the desirability of establishing this kind of cooperative relationship between correctional and mental health staff, remarking that it "improves the overall environment" of facilities[80] and tends to make issues such as an inmate's movement to designated locations for appointments go more smoothly.

On the other hand, inmates frequently value time spent away from housing units almost as much as they may value the specific services they receive. Trips to a designated mental health area for clinical encounters vary the scene and establish boundaries between the space in which inmates live and that in which they receive services, which contributes to a greater sense of confidentiality around the therapeutic exchange. These issues are particularly severe in what Goffman[29] referred to as "total institutions" where, because residents' authority over their own lives is so minimal, whatever sense of privacy and autonomy mental health services can provide seems desirable.

Service Integration

Within a facility, one of the most important functions mental health outpatient staff can provide is case management. As the conduit for critical information, nurses, psychologists, or social workers can serve a coordinating function among correctional staff and medical and mental health service providers. Typically, inmates receive services from multiple in-house providers who may not communicate directly with each other. The mental health case manager is the one professional who can establish an integrated view of the inmate and his service needs. Obvious examples of this integration include the following: (1) anticipating inmates' release dates for purposes of targeting them for education and training regarding how they are to administer their own medications before their return to the community; (2) in anticipating an individual's release, ensuring that psychiatric staff will time needed medication changes sufficiently in advance of release to monitor possible reactions; and (3) as the holder of information, being sure that legal and psychiatric schedules don't collide.

One of the strategies for providing more coordinated, integrated services among multiple disciplines and service providers is the development of treatment plans. Well-articulated plans function as contracts between individual practitioners and inmates indicating what problem areas are the focus of the therapeutic intervention and what concrete, observable outcomes are being worked toward so that the success of interventions can be evaluated. In addition, treatment plans can provide a useful avenue for communication across disciplines.

The mental health case manager also needs to coordinate with correctional case managers and community service providers for purposes of planning discharges and establishing necessary linkages to community-based agencies for inmates soon to be released.

CONCLUSION

Although there is general agreement on the necessity and desirability of outpatient mental health services in correctional settings, there is relatively little that has been written that specifically identifies the components or structure for such programming. Although this paper attempts to articulate what some of these components might be, it is by no means exhaustive. There are many areas not covered, such as the necessity for cultural sensitivity of mental health programs, the desirability of introducing more effective strategies for intra-agency and interagency information management, strategies for addressing the more political issue of how to move correctional systems toward greater acceptance of a more rehabilitative model, and methods of advocating more effective mental health services in local communities. It is hoped that, in the future, practitioners and clinicians will develop guidelines in these areas.

REFERENCES

1. Steadman HJ, McCarty DW, Morrissey JP: *The Mentally Ill in Jail: Planning for Essential Services.* New York, Gilford, 1989.
2. Monahan J, Steadman HJ: Crime and mental disorders: An epidemiological approach, in Tonry M and Morris N (eds): *Crime and Justice: An Annual Review of Research.* Chicago, University of Chicago, 1983.
3. Steadman HJ (ed): *Effectively Addressing the Mental Health Needs of Jail Detainees.* Seattle, The National Coalition for the Mentally Ill in the Criminal Justice System, 1990.
4. Abram KM, Teplin LA: Co-occurring disorders among mentally ill jail detainees: Implications for public policy. *Am Psychol* 46:1036–1045, 1991.
5. Teplin LA, Pruett NS: Police as streetcorner psychiatrist: Managing the mentally ill. *Int J Law Psychiatry* 15:139–156, 1992.
6. Isaac RJ, Armat VC: *Madness in the Streets: How Psychiatry and the Law Abandoned the Mentally Ill.* New York, Free Press, 1990.
7. Metzner JL: Guidelines for psychiatric services in prisons. *Criminal Behav Ment Health* 3:252–267, 1993.
8. *Standards for Adult Correctional Institutions,* ed 3, College Park, Md, American Correctional Association, 1990.
9. *Psychiatric Services in Jails and Prisons: Report of the Task Force on Psychiatric Services in Jails and Prisons.* Washington, D.C., American Psychiatric Association, 1989.
10. *Standards for Health Services in Jails and Prisons.* Chicago, National Commission on Correctional Health Care, 1992.
11. Torrey EF, Stieber J, Ezekiel J, et al: *Criminalizing the Seriously Mentally Ill: The Abuse of Jails as Mental Hospitals.* Washington, D.C., Public Citizens' Health Research Group and National Alliance for the Mentally Ill, 1992.
12. Dvoskin J: Jail-based mental health services, in Steadman HJ (ed): *Effectively Addressing the Mental Health Needs of Jail Detainees.* Seattle, The National Coalition for the Mentally Ill in the Criminal Justice System, 1990.
13. Gelberg L, Linn L, Leake B: Mental health, alcohol and drug use, and criminal history among homeless adults. *Am J Psychiatry* 145:191–196, 1988.
14. Torrey EF: *Out of the Shadows: Confronting America's Mental Illness Crisis.* New York, John Wiley & Sons, 1997.
15. Teplin LA: The criminalization of the mentally ill: Speculation in search of data. *Psychol Bull* 94:54–67, 1983.
16. Teplin LA: Criminalizing mental disorders: The comparative arrest rates of the mentally ill. *Am Psychol* 39:794–803, 1984.
17. Teplin LA, Swartz J: Screening for severe mental disorders in jails:

18. Jemelka R: The mentally ill in local jails: Issues in admission and booking, in Steadman HJ (ed): *Effectively Addressing the Mental Health Needs of Jail Detainees,* Seattle. The National Coalition for the Mentally Ill in the Criminal Justice System, 1990.
19. Steadman HJ, Morris SM, Dennis DL: The diversion of mentally ill persons from jails to community-based services: A profile of programs. *Am J Public Health* 95:1630–1635, 1995.
20. Zimbardo P, Musen K: *Quiet Rage: The Stanford Prison Experiment.* Harper Collins College Publishers, Stanford University Zimbardo tape, 1992.
21. Zimbardo P: On transforming experimental research into advocacy for social change, in Deutsch M, Hornstein H (eds): *Applying Social Psychology.* Hillsdale, NJ, Erlbaum Press, 1975.
22. Grassian S: Psychopathological effects of solitary confinement. *Am J Psychiatry* 140:1450–1454, 1983.
23. Declaration of Dvoskin J, *Madrid v Gomez,* No. C90-3094-TEH at 27-4443-75, (ND Calif, June 22, 1991).
24. Declaration of Sheff, *Madrid v Gomez,* No. C90-3094-TEH at 25-4115-16, (ND Calif, June 22, 1991).
25. Declaration of Haney C, *Madrid v Gomez,* No. C90-3094-TEH pp 7–56, at 67 (ND Calif, June 22, 1991).
26. Grassian S, Friedman R: Effects of sensory deprivation in psychiatric seclusion and solitary confinement. *Int J Law Psychiatry* 8:49–54, 1986.
27. Toch H: *Mosiac of Despair: Human Breakdowns in Prison.* Washington, D.C., American Psychological Association, 1992.
28. Toch H: *Living in Prison: The Ecology of Survival.* Washington, D.C., American Psychological Association, 1992.
29. Goffman E: *Asylums: Essays on the Social Situation of Mental Patients and Other Inmates.* New York, Anchor Books, 1961.
30. Dubler NN (ed): *Standards for Health Services in Correctional Facilities,* ed 2. Washington, D.C., American Public Health Association, 1986.
31. National Alliance for the Mentally Ill (NAMI) Newsletter. Arlington, Va, May 1997.
32. Steadman HJ: Boundary spanners: A key component for the effective interactions of justice mental health systems. *Law Hum Behav* 16:75–87, 1992.
33. Initial remedial plan for mental health care, medical care and compliance monitoring at the District of Columbia Jail. *Campbell v McGruder,* CA No 1462-71 pp 7–56 (D.C. Cir October 11, 1994).
34. Metzner JL: Prison Draft #1, unpublished manuscript, 1997.
35. Rice ME, Harris GT: Treatment for prisoners with mental disorder, in Steadman HJ, Cocozza JJ (eds): *Mental Illness in America's Prisons.* Seattle, The National Coalition for the Mentally Ill in the Criminal Justice System, 1993.
36. *Double Jeopardy: Persons With Mental Illnesses in the Criminal Justice System.* Rockville, Md, Center for Mental Health Services, Substance Abuse and Mental Health Services Administration, Public Health Service, U.S. Department of Health and Human Services, Report to Congress, 1995.
37. Acoca L, Austin J: *The Crisis: Women in Prison.* Washington, D.C., National Council on Crime and Delinquency, 1996.
38. Herman J: *Father–Daughter Incest.* Cambridge, Mass, Harvard University, 1981.
39. Herman J, Kiss MR: Time-limited group therapy for women with a history of incest. *Int J Group Psychother* 34:605–616, 1984.
40. Finkelhor D: *Child Sexual Abuse: New Theory and Research.* New York, Free Press, 1984.
41. Russell DEH: *The Secret Trauma: Incest in the Lives of Girls and Women.* New York, Basic Books, 1986.
42. Mauer M, Huling T: *Young Black Americans and the Criminal Justice System: Five Years Later.* Washington, D.C., Sentencing Project, 1995.
43. Anno BJ: *Prison Health Care: Guidelines for the Management of an*

The development of the Referral Decision Scale. *Law Hum Behav* 13:1–18, 1989.

Adequate Delivery System. Washington, D.C., U.S. Department of Justice and the National Institute of Corrections, 1991.

44. Peters RH, Hills HA: Inmates with co-occurring substance abuse and mental health disorders, in Steadman HJ, Cocozza JJ (eds): *Mental Illness in America's Prisons.* Seattle, The National Coalition for the Mentally Ill in the Criminal Justice System, 1993.

45. *Treatment of People With Co-occurring Disorders in the Justice System.* Delmar, NY, The National GAINS Center, 1997.

46. Metzner JL: Prison Draft #1, unpublished manuscript, 1997, p 33.

47. Peters R: *In-jail Substance Abuse Treatment Program.* Tampa, Fla, Department of Mental Health Law & Policy, 1997.

48. Bureau of Justice Statistics: *Violence Against Women: Estimate From the Redesigned Survey.* Washington, D.C., U.S. Department of Justice, 1995.

49. *Sex Offender Treatment Program.* St. Paul, Minn, Minnesota Office of the Legislative Auditor, 1994.

50. Bureau of Justice Statistics: *Sex Offenses and Offenders: An Analysis of Data on Rape and Sexual Assault.* Washington, D.C., U.S. Department of Justice, 1997.

51. Alaska Department of Corrections: *Sex Offender Treatment Program: Initial Recidivism Study.* Anchorage, Alaska, Justice Center, University of Alaska, 1996.

52. North Carolina Department of Corrections: *Sex Offender Accountability and Responsibility Program.* Division of Prisons, Mental Health Service, Lillington, NC, 1997.

53. Lotke E: *Sex Offenders: Does Treatment Work?* Alexandria, Va, National Center on Institutions and Alternatives, Research Update, 1997.

54. Williams SM: *A National Strategy for Managing Sex Offenders.* Canada, Correctional Service of Canada Regional Psychiatric Centers, 1997.

55. Winchel RM, Stanley M: Self-injurious behavior: A review of the behavior and biology of self-mutilation. *Am J Psychiatry* 148:3, 306–316, 1991.

56. Carr EG: The motivation of self-injurious behavior. *Psychol Bull* 84:800–816, 1977.

57. Jones A: Self-mutilation in prison: A comparison of mutilators and nonmutilators. *Criminal Justice Behav* 13:3, 286–296, 1986.

58. *Diagnostic and Statistical Manual of Mental Disorders,* ed 4. Washington, D.C., American Psychological Association, 1994.

59. Wapner B, Kaplan B, Cohen SB: An organismic developmental perspective for understanding transactions of men and environments. *Environ Behav* 5:255–289, 1973.

60. Metzner JL: Guidelines for psychiatric services in prisons. *Criminal Behav Ment Health* 3:262, 1993.

61. Skinner BF: *The Behavior of Organisms: An Experimental Analysis.* New York, Appleton–Century–Crofts, 1938.

62. Ullman LP, Krasner E (eds): *Case Studies in Behavior Modification.* New York, Holt, Rinehart & Winston, 1965.

63. Kimm DC, Masters JC: *Behavior Therapy: Techniques and Empirical Findings.* New York, Academic Press, 1974.

64. Acoca L, Austin J: *The Crisis: Women in Prison.* Washington, D.C., National Council on Crime and Delinquency, 1996, pp 6–11.

65. Teplin LA, Abram KM, McClelland GM: The prevalence of psychiatric disorders among incarcerated women: I. Pretrial jail detainees. *Arch Gen Psychiatry* 53:505–512, 1996.

66. Barry E: Pregnant prisoners. *Howard Women's Law J* 12: 189–205, 1989.

67. Shaw NS: Female patients and the medical profession in jails and prisons, in Rafter, Stanko (eds): *Judge, Lawyer, Victim, Thief.* Boston, Mass, Northeastern University, 1982.

68. Immarigeon R: When parents are sent to prison. *Natl Prison Project J* Fall:13–16, 1994.

69. Teplin L, Abram D, McClelland G: Mentally disordered women in jail: Who receives services? *Am J Public Health* 87:4, 604–609, 1997.

70. Teplin LA: Policing the mentally ill: Styles, strategies, and implications, in Steadman HJ (ed): *Effectively Addressing the Mental Health Needs of Jail Detainees.* Seattle, The National Coalition for the Mentally Ill in the Criminal Justice System, 1990.

71. Teplin LA: Psychiatric and substance abuse disorders among male urban jail detainees. *Am J Public Health* 84:290–293, 1994.

72. Austin J, et al: *Juveniles Taken Into Custody.* Washington, D.C., Office of Juvenile Justice and Delinquency Prevention, Department of Justice, Fiscal Year 1993—Statistics Report, September, 1995.

73. Flaherty MG: *An Assessment of the National Incidence of Juvenile Suicide in Adult Jails, Lockups, and Juvenile Detention Centers.* San Francisco, Juvenile Justice Legal Advocacy Project, Office of Juvenile Justice and Delinquency Prevention, Department of Justice, 1980.

74. Cocozza JJ (ed): *Responding to the Mental Health Needs of Youth in the Juvenile Justice System.* Seattle, The National Coalition for the Mentally Ill in the Criminal Justice System, 1992.

75. Otto R, Greenstein J, Johnson M, et al: Prevalence of mental disorders among youth in the juvenile justice system, in Cocozza JJ (ed): *Responding to the Mental Health Needs of Youth in the Juvenile Justice System.* Seattle, The National Coalition for the Mentally Ill in the Criminal Justice System, 1992.

76. Trupin E, Low B, Forsyth–Stephens A, et al: *Washington State Children's Mental Health System Analysis.* Seattle, Washington State Department of Social and Health Services, 1988.

77. Hutchinson J: Mental health issues for incarcerated black youth, in Farrow JA and Jenkins R (eds): *East Coast Scientific Symposium on the Health of the Black Adolescent Male.* Rockville, Md, U.S. Department of Health and Human Services, 1990, pp 19–20.

78. Steadman HJ (ed): *Effectively Addressing the Mental Health Needs of Jail Detainees.* Seattle, The National Coalition for the Mentally Ill in the Criminal Justice System, 1990, p 39.

79. *Psychiatric Services in Jails and Prisons: Report on the Task Force on Psychiatric Services in Jails and Prisons.* Washington, D.C., American Psychiatric Association, 1989, p 6.

80. Metzner JL: Guidelines for psychiatric services in prisons. *Criminal Behav Ment Health* 3:259, 1993.

20

Managing the Patient With an Acute Psychiatric Condition

Roxanne Sanders, M.D.

Anderson Freeman, Ph.D.

Laurie Goldman, M.D.

INTRODUCTION

The intent of this chapter is to provide a guide to managing patients with acute psychiatric conditions in the unique and challenging correctional setting. The American Psychiatric Association task force[1] reports that the recognition and treatment of the those with severe mental illnesses is an essential program priority for jails and prisons. We provide mental health services for a patient population of more than 800 detainees at Cermak Health Services, Cook County Jail in Chicago, Illinois and wish to share what we have learned about managing psychiatric inmates with acute illnesses. This chapter will address the identification and management of patients with acute illnesses in a correctional setting. In addition, some broader health care issues will be discussed.

HISTORICAL PERSPECTIVE

After 200 years of movement in the direction of treating those with mental illnesses in mental health facilities, we are witnessing the re-incarceration of individuals with mental illnesses in jails and prisons. Jails were a primary site for the placement of those with mental illnesses during the colonial period. In 17th-century America, any individual could be jailed for being considered "lunatic and so furiously mad as to render it dangerous to the peace or safety of the good people for such lunatic person to go at large."[2] A Massachusetts statute in 1699 differentiated between rogues and vagabonds, who would be set to work in jails, and the idle and disorderly, who were obliged to work in workhouses. Almshouses, on the other hand, were designed to lodge, feed, and employ the town's needy. Psychiatric historians studying records of this period have concluded that those with mental illnesses were housed in all three of these settings. Quen[3] maintains that those with mental illnesses who were violent and difficult to control were housed in correctional facilities, whereas those who were compliant were treated as if they were merely sane paupers. Beatings and floggings were not uncommon for those with mental illnesses in these facilities for both major and minor offenses. Not until 1807 did the legislature of a state (New York) authorize local officials to contract with a major health care facility (New York Hospital) for the care and maintenance of "pauper" lunatics. Even then, few such individuals were actually admitted to the hospital. Most continued to be cared for in jails or poor houses, were boarded with private families, or were left to roam at large.[4]

In the last decade or two, trends toward the re-incarceration of those with mental illnesses have been noted. Not surprisingly, it is again the poor, minorities, and homeless who are the primary victims. During the early 1980s, Robins and Regier[5] conducted their massive Epidemiologic Catchment Area Study on psychiatric disorders in America. A major part of their procedure was to sample community, outpatient, residential, and inpatient settings, and to describe the incidence and prevalence rates of severe mental disorders. One of their most significant findings was that the prevalence of mental illness in prisoners was two to five times greater than that in the general population. Their study documented that, among inmates, 6.7% had schizophrenia, 21% had an affective disorder, and 28% had an anxiety disorder. Another study, by Bolton,[6] found that in a five-county, combined sample of 1,084 adults in California county jails, 6.7% had psychotic conditions. More recently, Teplin[7] administered highly structured interviews to 728 individuals admitted to the Cook County Jail in Chicago. She found that 6.4% had serious mental illnesses, defined as schizophrenia, mania, or major depression. In a less rigorous but highly suggestive study, Torrey et al.[8] surveyed 1,391 jails across America. One of their key findings was that 1 of every 14 inmates (7.2%) has a serious mental illness. Torrey et al. also found that the jail size was related to the percentage of inmates with serious mental illnesses. Jails with a daily census of 51 to 250 had an average of 4.4% of detainees with serious mental illnesses, whereas jails with a census of 251 to 1,000 had an average of 7.3%. In Cook County Jail, we presently have 8% to 10% of 9,000 as active patients.

Most of the aforementioned statistics reflect mental illness rates for incarcerated men. What little data we have on mental illness among incarcerated women are even more disturbing. The number of women in correctional facilities in the United States is at an all-time high. During the last 10 years, the number of women in our nation's prisons increased by more than 250%. Two recent studies have documented the higher prevalence of psychiatric illnesses in the female correctional population. Teplin's study[9] on incarcerated women found that 70% of jailed women were symptomatic for psychiatric illnesses within the past 6 months. The study by Jordan et al.[10] found women prison inmates to have elevated rates of borderline personality disorder and mood disorders, compared with the general population.

The literature, thus, reveals that the number of jail detainees with acute psychiatric disorders has increased markedly during the last 30 years. We can speculate that this increase has come about as a result of a number of social policy changes. Deinstitutionalization of those with mental illnesses beginning in the 1960s was, theoretically, a move toward community rehabilitation. Unfortunately, many communities lacked the resources to provide adequate care for these individuals. As a result, many who would have previously been treated are now living on the streets, "rotting with their rights on." Untreated mental illness usually compromises judgment, which results in limited coping skills, stressed support systems, and a lack of regard for self-care. Incarceration may result from "crimes of survival" such as criminal trespass, prostitution, and theft, which are primarily nonviolent. Substance abuse may also be considered a coping tool. Many inmates note that it is easier to obtain illicit drugs to obliterate their psychotic symptoms than to obtain an appointment at a mental health clinic.

The increase in the incidence of acute mental disorders in correctional facilities has made on-site mental health assessment and care a necessity. Some of the larger urban jails have developed in-house inpatient units that rival and even surpass community and state mental health facilities in the numbers of patients that they serve. In part, the development of these in-house units is the result of lobbying and legal actions by inmate and health care advocacy groups that stress proper medical treatment for these captive psychiatric populations.

PATIENT EVALUATION

Mental health assessment in a correctional facility should begin as a general evaluation and should be no different than that conducted in other settings. By starting with a broad view, the evaluator is in a better position to later focus on specific problems. All inmates require mental health screening at intake, or shortly thereafter. This reduces the risk of inmates with mental illnesses "falling through the cracks" and not receiving needed care; it also reduces the risk of suicide. Although suicide is a relatively low-frequency event, risk is reduced by screening for depression and agitation. General screening also conveys a concern for inmate welfare that can decrease feelings of isolation. Correctional institutions also need a process for urgent or emergency assessments for the general inmate population. Many acute mental health problems may be identified in an intake screening, but others may arise anytime during incarceration.

A mental health evaluation may be requested by a correctional staff member or health care provider, or via an inmate health request. The referral may be generated because of an inmate's stated problems or, more commonly, because of abnormal or inappropriate behavior. Inmates who express ideas of or plans for harming themselves or others should automatically be investigated further. Threatening comments are not uncommon in the correctional environment. Nevertheless, it does no harm and is likely to be informative as well as therapeutic to ask questions such as, "Do you really want to kill inmate Jones or are you just angry?" Inmates with acute mental illnesses engage in a range of behaviors that may trigger an emergency referral: violent behavior, bizarre behavior, behavior that suggests depression, and so on. In some facilities, inmates are separated from other inmates in an infirmary setting, or they may be in segregation while waiting for an evaluation. Wherever the inmate with an acute mental illness is located, it is imperative that he receive close monitoring.

What Is Acute Psychiatric Illness?

Acute psychiatric illness simply means a mental disorder or condition that is severe. Such conditions may result from recent precipitants (e.g., death of a loved one), worsening of a chronic mental illness, or, as is often the case with incarcerated populations, a combination of pre-existing illness and increased stressors. For example, a stable patient with schizophrenia may experience an increase in intrusive thoughts and hallucinations under the stress of close quarters in jail, or an inmate who was previously functioning well may decompensate when being informed that her child is being placed in a foster home. The management of new onsets of illness and chronic illness may be the same, initially. The primary treatment goals are to prevent harm to self or others (suicide or homicide), then to reduce symptoms. Subsequently, specific treatment plans should be developed to reduce the risk of recurrence, to set future emotional and behavioral goals, and to educate the patient.

Inmates may be referred by correctional officers and evaluated initially by mental health professionals or general medical professionals. When individuals other than a mental health professional perform the evaluations, they must determine whether the inmate with the mental illness is in need of emergency care and then make an appropriate referral. It has been our experience that the process for making such referrals needs to be reviewed with all staff. Most correctional facilities have clear guidelines for handling medical emergencies. Psychiatric emergencies should be handled the same way. If inmates are at risk for harming themselves or others or are not able to take care of basic needs (eating, protecting themselves from harm, or following simple instructions), an immediate mental health evaluation is needed. Severe psychiatric symptoms such as hallucinations, paranoid delusions, and mania may warrant an

emergency evaluation, especially if they are of new onset or the inmate is not known to the staff. These symptoms may be obvious to the observer or expressed verbally by the inmate. Other requests for mental health services should be reviewed daily to look for requests that may indicate an emergency.

In private practice, psychiatric referrals usually follow specific procedures, and the reason for such a referral is communicated. In large institutions, however, the disruption caused by a seriously ill inmate may result in movement of the inmate for an evaluation without sufficient information reaching the evaluator. It is important for the mental health evaluator to communicate with other correctional or civilian staff to obtain as much information as possible.

Case example

An inmate is brought to the sick call nurse by a correctional officer. The officer, who just came on duty, states that his sergeant told him to bring the inmate because he is "acting like a nut." The inmate looks disheveled and has red abrasions on his arms. When asked about the abrasions, he states, "When people push me, I push back." He looks defiantly at the officer and says the staff dislikes him. He attributes the referral to his being involved in an altercation and the officers wanting him off their tier.

The nurse contacted the referring sergeant. He had seen the inmate talking to himself in an angry tone and accusing the correctional staff of using "Gestapo tactics" to control his mind through the air vents and television. The inmate had stated he would make them stop "one way or another," and had lunged toward an officer.

This case exemplifies the importance of collateral information—having it means that relying only on the patient's report of events or symptoms can be avoided. Many patients with mental illnesses minimize or deny their symptoms, which can result in inadequate diagnosis and management.

There are two basic components of a mental health evaluation. The first is the history. It should include present symptoms, a general health history, and information about functional abilities. The other component is the mental status examination, which is the psychiatric counterpart of a physical examination. This includes evaluating physical appearance, behavior, affect or emotional expression, thought organization, speech, and cognition. It is sometimes impossible to evaluate a severely ill patient in a methodical way. However, it is important to attempt to obtain as much clinical information as one can so that the most effective plan of action can be developed.

History

This part of the evaluation includes present as well as past information. It should include present symptoms or relevant problems such as depression, hallucinations, and confusion, as well as current and past treatment, including medication. It is important to document the onset, duration, severity, and presumed causes of the symptoms, as well as what makes them better or worse. It is helpful to know the reason for the incarceration, the sentence or bond (depending on the incarceration setting), and the number of past incarcerations. A inmate with psychosis who has been in prison numerous times may improve relatively quickly with treatment because of his familiarity with the correctional setting and routine, whereas another inmate with a psychiatric history but no prior arrests may impulsively harm himself in reaction to his incarceration.

The history should also include past mental disorders and treatments. It is important to document the names of any medication, as well as the dosages, duration, side effects, and response. The relatively little time it takes to obtain this information will result in a big payoff in terms of efficient management and symptom reduction. It is critical to note any previous suicide attempts. A general medical history must also be taken. Psychiatric disorders may be affected by any number of medical conditions or their treatment, and vice versa. Any known allergies also need to be documented.

It is extremely important when dealing with this population to take a substance-use history. This includes alcohol and illicit drugs and the frequency, amount, and route of usage (IV, nasal, or inhaled). Knowing the most recent use is especially important in emergency evaluations. Inmates in jails who have been recently arrested may be in withdrawal or still intoxicated. Past withdrawal symptoms may forewarn clinicians about impending problems, especially delirium tremens. Some inmates will be actively enrolled in a methadone clinic. In our facility, the pharmacy verifies current enrollment to meet strict dispensing regulations. The inmate then receives a 21-day taper of the methadone.

Female inmates should be asked about their obstetric and gynecologic history. The date of the last menstrual period should be documented. Even when this information is elicited, all women of childbearing age entering a correctional facility need a pregnancy test. The menstrual history may not be reliable, particularly under the stress of incarceration and illness. At Cook County Jail, all women receive pregnancy tests on intake, but because pregnancy tests can only detect a pregnancy 10–14 days after conception, a repeat pregnancy test may be indicated in some clinical situations.

Mental Status Examination

The second part of the assessment is the mental status examination. The mental status examination is a present-state evaluation and should be documented in terms that are objective and consistent with standard psychiatric terminology. This enables the evaluator to develop a clinical record that leads to specific diagnoses and treatment and aids other treating professionals who review the medical record. The *Diagnostic and Statistical Manual of Mental Disorders*, ed 4 (*DSM IV*),[11] provides the generally accepted diagnostic criteria for mental disorders, including symptom terminology. There are also numerous other helpful texts describing interviewing techniques and characteristics of mental disorders.

For the severely ill inmate, the mental status examination may be the only clinical information obtainable. Properly documented, it will provide a lasting description of that inmate at that point in time. Observations begin with the inmate's appearance. An astute mental health professional starts the evaluation the moment the patient enters the room, noting posture, grooming, dress, and hygiene. In a correctional facility, one must consider the limited resources for self-care. Even so, concern (or lack thereof) for appearance is usually noticeable and telling. The general demeanor of the inmate should also be noted. Is he calm and cooperative or agitated, frightened, suspicious, or hostile? Eye contact and general interpersonal relatedness are important to describe. Affect, which is the inmate's facial and physical expression, should be recorded, as should the mood, which is the inmate's self-reported emotional state. Thought processes should be noted: whether there are loose associations, tangential thoughts, or racing ideas, or whether the processes are normal and sequential. Thought content may be logical, or it may include suicidal or homicidal thoughts or psychotic ideas such as delusions or hallucinations. In evaluating the speech, the mental health professional should give consideration to the rate, volume, spontaneity, and rhythm. Finally, the cognitive examination should be performed. This usually, but not always, requires the inmate's cooperation. The evaluator should ask basic questions to determine orientation (person, place, time, and situation), short-term and long-term memory, attention span, concentration, insight, and judgment. Even uncooperative inmates may unknowingly provide detailed information about their knowledge of the date, recent events, their present location, and future plans, which are all clinically relevant.

The importance of documentation and the use of standard terminology cannot be overstated. In the previously mentioned case example, the correctional officer said the inmate was "acting like a nut." This could mean that the inmate was being belligerent and uncooperative with security procedure or that he was exhibiting bizarre behavior suggestive of psychosis. Reporting that an inmate "looks depressed" may enable a slightly faster diagnosis but is not as meaningful as "the inmate was disheveled and exhibited slouched posture, poor eye contact, slow gait, and monotone speech, and he nodded tearfully when asked if he were suicidal." The latter description provides objective clues to the inmate's mental state. This reduces the chances of miscommunication between evaluators from different disciplines. This is especially important in a correctional environment in which inmates may be motivated to either avoid being labeled as a patient with a psychiatric condition or falsify symptoms for personal gain.

PATIENT MANAGEMENT

Correctional institutions have varying access to mental health professionals. Ideally, an inmate with an acute mental illness, once identified, will be transferred to a health care setting staffed by or with good access to a licensed mental health professional. Some facilities, like Cook County Jail, have a psychiatric infirmary with 24-hour staffing. Many detention facilities, however, must rely on psychiatrists who are on site infrequently, or they may transfer the inmate to a local mental health treatment facility. The first goal of the health care professional is always the preservation of life. This may seem self-evident. However in the correctional care setting, security issues (e.g., high escape risk or sentence) or staffing or timing considerations (e.g., change of shift or inmate count time) sometimes supersede needed medical action. Health care professionals must do everything in their power to keep this from happening.

Case example

Inmate Smith had a long history of psychiatric treatment in correctional facilities and in the community. He was being treated with high doses of medication for his long-standing auditory hallucinations, which had remitted. He had a history of minor "suicide attempts," such as superficial wrist-cutting when he wanted to see the visiting psychiatrist. Mr. Smith began experiencing uncomfortable side effects. The psychiatrist gave a telephone order to reduce the medication and scheduled Mr. Smith for an appointment at the next visit in 5 days. Two days after the medication was reduced, inmate Smith ran off his tier during the shift change. As a result, he was placed in administrative segregation and reclassified as a maximum security escape risk. When seen in the mental health clinic, he was withdrawn and hostile, which was uncharacteristic for him, but it was attributed to his being in solitary confinement. At times, he was seen mumbling to himself and rocking and covering his ears. When released from his cell the next day, he jumped over the second story railing, sustaining severe injuries.

It is likely that inmate Smith's care was affected by his security classification and his escape attempt. In this case, the impulsive escape attempt resulted from his psychotic decompensation. He should have been transferred immediately to a supervised clinical setting in which his behavior and medication could have been monitored.

Several types of inmates present special concerns for clinical management in a correctional facility. These include the violent inmate, the inmate with psychosis, the suicidal inmate, the inmate with a substance abuse problem, and the inmate with a severe personality disorder. They pose problems because of their unique needs, vulnerability, dangerousness, or their high and often inappropriate use of staff resources.

The Violent Patient

There is a relationship between mental disorder and violence, whether one is measuring the prevalence of violence among the disordered or the prevalence of disorder among the violent.[12] The majority of individuals with mental disorders are not violent. It is only individuals currently experiencing psychotic symptoms who may be at an increased risk for being violent.[13] Individuals with psychotic disorders (non-paranoid schizophrenia, in particular) may pose the greatest risk for assaultive behavior.

Safety is the primary concern when any patient is violent, aggressive, or physically intimidating to others. Further evaluation and treatment cannot proceed unless the environment is physically safe for inmates and staff. Clinical staff should be in charge, using the assistance of security officers as needed. Staff should be well trained and sufficient in number. If correctional officers are armed, their weapons should be safely stored away from the inmate's access.

Whenever possible, the first action to be taken is to slowly and calmly approach the patient. For mental health treatment, the least restrictive and most effective measures should always be used. All staff need to remain nonthreatening and reassuring. Give the inmate clear directions such as, "Put the chair down and then we can talk this out." Surrounding a violent inmate with staff yelling "Calm down!" is likely to escalate the situation. Unfortunately, many violent inmates are beyond the point of responding to verbal requests, and trained clinical or correctional staff or both must forcibly restrain or seclude the inmate.

As a second step, antipsychotic medication or anxiolytic medication or both can be used either orally or intramuscularly to help the patient become calmer. The clinical effects of antipsychotic medication (e.g., chlorpromazine) generally appear within 30–60 minutes when administered orally, and within about 10 minutes when given via IM injection. It may take as long as 4–6 weeks before the psychotic symptoms (e.g., delusions or hallucinations) improve with antipsychotic medication. Anxiolytics (e.g., diazepam and lorazepam) are rapidly absorbed orally and, with the exception of lorazepam, are poorly absorbed intramuscularly. For an uncontrollable patient with a psychotic condition, frequent, equally spaced doses of an antipsychotic medication, such as haloperidol, should be given every 30–60 minutes until the agitation is under control. Seldom is more than 20–30 mg of haloperidol (or its equivalent) needed. Higher doses increase the likelihood of adverse effects without significantly increasing the benefit. The combination of an antipsychotic medication and a benzodiazepine may be even better for reducing agitation quickly and is generally well tolerated.[14] There are some data to suggest that mood stabilizers and β-blockers may reduce impulsive, aggressive behavior. Medication information should be given at the time of administration. If the inmate is obviously not able to understand the information, the risks and benefits of the medication should be explained when the patient's mental status reverts to normal.

Full leather restraints are a therapeutic intervention used by clinical staff, in an appropriate clinical setting, to prevent inmates from harming themselves or others. The use of full leather restraints is usually regulated by state law. They should be used when other less restrictive interventions are ineffective or when there is an immediate risk of the inmate harming himself or others. Often, full leather restraints are used to gain control of a dangerous situation rapidly and to allow staff to administer treatment safely. The inmate should be searched thoroughly, all belts, pins, and other such objects should be removed, and the inmate should be placed in a gown, if possible.

The staff can then perform and document the assessment and plan. Management of the inmate will depend on whether the violent behavior is the result of a mental illness or condition (e.g., psychosis, intoxication, or a seizure) or is intentional. Underlying medical or psychiatric conditions should be treated aggressively. The inmate should be tested for drug or alcohol intoxication, particularly if recently brought to jail. Of course, there are patients who continue to display intentional or "rational violence," even when stabilized. Reasonable efforts should be made to minimize provocation for these inmates and to provide more appropriate outlets, such as recreation activity. Nevertheless, some inmates continue to display long-term violent behavior and must be separated from others. Because violence is difficult to predict, risk assessments need to be updated and documented regularly.

Case example

Mr. Little is a 30-year-old inmate with above-knee amputation of both legs. He has been arrested many times, and his present charge is assault. He is wheelchair bound but has good upper body strength. Shortly after his arrest, Mr. Little became angry, demanding medication for "his nerves." He removed the arms from his wheelchair and used them to strike at officers. As a result, the wheelchair was taken from him. Mr. Little retaliated by flooding the sink and toilet in his cell. Because he continued to demand medication and threaten staff, he was transferred to the mental health unit. There he was given chlorpromazine, an antipsychotic medication, for his agitation and reported auditory hallucinations. Within 1 week, his agitation and hallucinations improved. Although he continued to provoke officers and inmates occasionally, he was less impulsive, hostile, and destructive.

Case example

Mr. Battle is 25 years old and is incarcerated for attempted murder. His first arrest was at age 13 years, and he has been in correctional institutions for most of the past 10 years. He was referred to mental health services because he had attacked correctional officers on several occasions and had seriously injured one officer. Mr. Battle was powerfully built, and prison administrators were concerned about officer and inmate safety. Although Mr. Battle was evaluated, and there was no evidence of a major mental health disorder, he was exquisitely sensitive to interpersonal slights and went to great lengths to get the staff to like him. He confided to his psychologist that he was getting revenge on a group of officers who had taunted and then assaulted him. He had considered one of them a friend, and it was this officer who had received the most brutal assault. Mr. Battle named the remaining two officers he was planning to "punish for messing with me." The mental health staff were unable to convince Mr. Battle to use more appropriate means to manage his resentment. They also concluded that, although the behavior was extreme, it did not result from delusional ideas. The

psychologist worked with prison administrators to move Mr. Battle to another area, helped Mr. Battle with anger management, and worked with the new correctional staff on conflict resolution techniques. Mr. Battle was allowed to become a worker on his tier, where his physical strength was appreciated. He valued this privilege and had no further incidence of violent behavior.

The Patient With Psychosis

There are a number of definitions for the term *psychosis*. Descriptions in *DSM IV* include delusions, hallucinations, disorganized speech or behaviors, or other severe impairments in reality. Delusions are false beliefs that are a result of misinterpretation of external reality. Hallucinations are distortions of perception that appear to be part of reality, but occur without external stimulation. They can occur in any sensory modality (*i.e.*, auditory, visual, olfactory, tactile, or gustatory). Psychosis can arise as a primary mental disorder, or can result from organic causes such as medication toxicity or head injuries. Inmates exhibiting psychotic symptoms should have a general medical examination as well as a mental health assessment. Psychotic symptoms occurring with signs of medical instability (e.g., a fever, abnormal blood pressure, pupil changes) or other unusual presentations signal a need for urgent medical attention. Hallucinations of taste, touch, smell, or vision strongly suggest a general medical condition or substance use. Alcohol hallucinosis or delirium may not occur until 3–5 days after the last drink.

The more typical psychiatric symptoms are auditory hallucinations, delusions, and disorganized thinking and/or behavior. Psychotic symptoms may result from schizophrenia or related disorders or from a severe mood disorder or traumatic experience. Many individuals with chronic mental illnesses have poor social skills manifested by poor hygiene, strange rituals, and a failure to appreciate personal boundaries. Such symptoms may be viewed with fear or even disbelief by untrained staff and inmates. The inmate with psychosis who wanders aimlessly, laughs inappropriately, and rants about delusional religious beliefs is an easy target for predatory inmates. Correctional staff usually have little tolerance for inmates who don't conform to behavioral rules and increase tension on the tier. Thus, patients with psychotic disorders become "hot potatoes" inside the institution and out. In jail settings, these inmates are frequently found unfit for trial, which delays the resolution of their case. They may be sent to public mental institutions, where they are often stigmatized as "forensic" patients.

Fortunately, there are medications that reduce many psychotic symptoms. These medications have the additional benefit of calming an agitated inmate with psychosis. Traditional antipsychotic medications, such as haloperidol and chlorpromazine, are effective in treating positive symptoms. These are behaviors or thoughts that are distorted or exaggerated, such as delusions, hallucinations, bizarre behavior, and disorganized speech. It may take days to weeks before these symptoms improve. Negative symptoms represent a loss or decrease in functions, such as emotional expression, spontaneous movement, or speech. These symptoms are common in psychosis but may also be seen in patients with depression. If such symptoms are a result of depression, they may respond to antidepressant medication. Newer antipsychotic medications, such as clozapine and olanzapine, have better side effect profiles and offer promise for treating negative as well as positive psychotic symptoms. Benzodiazepines such as lorazepam may be used with antipsychotic medication to decrease anxiety and agitation.

The inmate with psychosis will likely need more than medication to function in the correctional environment. Many inmates with chronic mental illnesses will have residual psychotic symptoms. Correctional and clinical staff should provide clear expectations and goals. As acute psychotic symptoms improve, hygiene and cooperation with correctional rules should be emphasized. Inmates with psychotic disorders frequently need reorientation to the date, to their location and situation, and to basic rules. There are many advantages to housing inmates with mental illnesses together, particularly for large institutions. Clinical staff are centralized and can provide programs efficiently. Correctional officers can be assigned to psychiatric units based on their training and willingness to work with those with mental illnesses. Medication administration and record keeping are also simplified. Creating a mental health unit also allows clinical and correctional staff to evaluate an inmate over time, and to develop and maintain a clinical plan.

Ongoing patient education is important in maintaining compliance with clinical programs and medication. As the inmate's psychotic symptoms improve, it is important to discuss past and present symptoms, benefits and side effects of medications, and long-term treatment goals. This increases inmates' participation in maintaining their health and encourages rapport between the inmates and staff. Medication compliance may be improved by giving long-acting medication or by reducing the frequency of dosing. The more doses to be remembered or delivered, the greater the chance that one will be forgotten. It may still be difficult to maintain compliance with medication. Correctional institutions should have policies for administering involuntary medication in emergency and nonemergency situations. Giving medication while there is an imminent risk of inmates with mental illnesses harming themselves or others is usually straightforward. Inmates with psychotic disorders who display ongoing poor judgment (such as eating out of garbage cans or masturbating publicly), which puts them at risk, may require a judicial or administrative review to receive treatment.[15]

The Suicidal Patient

The suicide rate for men in jail is more than 15 times greater than that for the general population.[16] Prison suicide rates also exceed those in the community, but are lower than those in jails. Most jailed inmates are pretrial detainees and are uncertain about the outcome of their cases. They often come directly from the community or the police lockup and must adjust quickly to the reality of their situation. They may be intoxicated or in drug or alcohol withdrawal. Many new detainees haven't eaten, showered, or spoken with their families. The risk of suicide is the major justification for mental health screening during intake for all correctional institutions.

The relative rarity of suicide makes its accurate prediction in a particular individual difficult. All complaints or reports of suicidal thoughts need to be taken seriously. This can be difficult in the correctional setting because of the volume of inmates who fake illnesses to get medication or better housing or who repeatedly mutilate themselves. Staff members become weary of inmates who use indirect means to achieve their goals; in addition, they may believe that inmates are taking advantage of them. However, every patient who reports suicidal thoughts is asking for help or attention of some kind and deserves a full evaluation. Desperation, impulsiveness, or simple miscalculation by a patient denied the proper evaluation may lead to what would have been a preventable death.

The assessment of the suicidal inmate should focus on both what the inmate reports (subjective) and what the evaluator observes (objective). A malingering inmate may appear depressed and may detail suicide plans to the mental health staff, but then interact jovially with other inmates and correctional staff whenever he believes he is not being watched. Other inmates may "fake good" by smiling and denying any suicidal plans while waiting for an opportunity. Staff should not rely on verbal contracts if they suspect an inmate is suicidal. Such contracts have limited success in the community despite strong patient–therapist bonds and are probably less meaningful for a despondent inmate.

Although depression and aloneness usually arouse concern, signs of anxiety and agitation should not be overlooked. Anxiety and physical agitation have been shown to be a significant risk factor for suicide. It is theorized that the anxiety or agitation may provide the energy to carry out the suicide. Patients with depression who suddenly improve may develop the energy to successfully carry out their suicidal thoughts. Pharmacologic management of anxiety or agitation should be aggressive in any suicidal patient. Treating physicians routinely use benzodiazepines, such as lorazepam, or sedating antipsychotics, such as chlorpromazine. The suicidal inmate should not be left alone. At the very least, high-risk inmates should be in a cell with another inmate or observed by staff every 15 minutes. The frequency of staff checks should be staggered so that the inmate cannot predict the routine.

It is inevitable that some patients will commit suicide or cause themselves serious injury. Emergency medical procedures must be activated, and resuscitation efforts must be initiated despite the inmate's apparent condition. Suicidal inmates who have been hospitalized for self-inflicted injuries are likely to return to the correctional setting. Such inmates may be ashamed of their actions or experience feelings of failure. Health care and correctional staff may be angry at the inmate for the disruption caused or fearful of future attempts. Inmates who have made a serious suicide attempt are especially vulnerable to subsequent attempts in the first few days to weeks after their return to the correctional setting. There should be a written treatment plan including high-risk housing, staff observation, and medications as needed. Inmates should be informed of the plan to assure them that staff members are concerned and that care will be consistent. Such written treatment plans should be easily accessible to staff, easy to read, and, importantly, discussed with correctional staff.

Case example

Mr. Ramos is a 24-year-old in jail for the first time and is charged with manslaughter. He had been in the United States for less than a year and knew few people. He was referred to mental health services after superficially cutting his wrist. The correctional officer noted that he became depressed and withdrawn about 1 week before the referral. Mr. Ramos said he was not "crazy," but wanted to get out of the general population because he was not a "common criminal." He was apologetic about the suicidal gesture, but somewhat aloof with mental health staff. The psychiatrist inquired about Mr. Ramos' ability to cope in jail. Mr. Ramos became tearful and said that his charge resulted from killing his best friend in an automobile accident while he was driving under the influence. He said that he wished for death but did not have the courage. He denied any past psychiatric treatment or serious symptoms. The psychiatrist believed that Mr. Ramos was grieving, but also manipulative and not suicidal. He informed the inmate that he would be returned to the general population. Mr. Ramos appeared terrified and asked to be sent to a different living area. He then reluctantly admitted that he had been sexually assaulted by a group of inmates. He was ashamed, and said that he would kill himself rather than suffer such abuse again. He was referred for medical attention and received suicide watch status.

Suicide prevention programs in correctional facilities should include training for all staff members with inmate contact. Training will help staff target high-risk inmates. It should also review procedures for protecting suicidal inmates and procedures for lifesaving interventions (e.g., cutting down a hanging inmate, cardiopulmonary resuscitation, and applying a pressure bandage). Suicide prevention programs should also include procedures or systems to identify suicidal inmates and medical and/or psychiatric programs to provide supervision and treatment. Correctional facilities need an internal review process, in addition to any outside investigation, not only for staff accountability but also to provide continuous improvement. Correctional facilities, especially jails and mental health units, need to be designed as suicide-proof as possible, with the knowledge that most successful inmate suicides are by hanging.

The Patient With a Substance Abuse Problem

The inmate with a substance abuse problem presents ongoing management concerns for the correctional staff, particularly in jails. They are high volume and high risk in the correctional setting. Inmates abusing substances are at greater risk for harming themselves. There is also overlap between some acute psychiatric symptoms and severe drug withdrawal and intoxication. The majority of our patients with psychotic disorders have coexistent substance abuse problems. It is difficult to determine whether delusions or hallucinations are a result of intoxication, withdrawal, or a primary psychiatric illness during a single evaluation. Severe withdrawal symptoms will usually begin within a week after the last use of the drug. Thus, a symptomatic inmate needs to be under the care of an experienced health professional during this time. Psychotic symptoms that persist beyond 2 weeks are likely primary or a result of an organic injury (including brain damage from drugs) and should be treated as chronic.

Inmates abusing substances may be intoxicated at the time of arrest, which may make them more impulsive and less cooperative with intake procedures. The inmate who is intoxicated may be unable to give important information. For example, an inmate was intoxicated and incoherent for 2 days before remembering that her young child was left unattended at home. Intoxication can be serious, and the inmate needs to be checked regularly. The inmate may have taken an overdose of illicit or prescription medication that could be lethal. Central nervous system depressants like alcohol or narcotics may cause confusion, a staggering gait resulting in falls, stupor, or possibly vomiting and asphyxiation. Stimulants like cocaine and speed can cause agitation, changes in blood pressure and heart rhythms, delirium, and brain damage.

Intoxication may quickly give way to withdrawal. Some drugs of abuse have severe and even life-threatening withdrawal syndromes. Alcohol withdrawal can be complicated by seizures, hallucinations, and delirium tremens up to 5 days after the last drink. Benzodiazepine withdrawal is similar to that of alcohol withdrawal. Barbiturate withdrawal is particularly dangerous and can occur with abrupt withdrawal or dose reduction. Mild symptoms like anxiety usually begin within 12–48 hours and can progress to unremitting seizures, a severe fever, and death. Any inmate with a history of abusing these drugs needs close supervision and, if severely symptomatic, needs hospitalization. Opiates or narcotics are common drugs of abuse. Withdrawal symptoms may begin within hours of the last use for short-acting drugs (e.g., morphine and heroin) or longer for long-acting drugs. The withdrawal symptoms are usually not life-threatening and include tearing, a runny nose, sweating, and an increased blood pressure and pulse. These may progress to vomiting, diarrhea, and joint pain. The inmate could be at risk for dehydration, and many facilities treat opiate withdrawal with methadone or clonidine. Opiate abusers are notoriously manipulative and drug seeking.

Stimulant withdrawal is associated with intense psychiatric symptoms such as paranoia, hallucinations (including tactile ones), irritability, and depression, which can lead to suicidal thoughts and actions. There may also be coughing, muscle aches, nightmares, headaches, and, rarely, seizures.

Hallucinogens such as lysergic acid diethylamide (LSD) were popular in the 1960s and 1970s, and are probably not as prevalent in the correctional population. They induce psychotic experiences and feelings of unreality. Intoxication usually brings signs of physical arousal such as an increased heart rate, sweating, and dilated pupils. Chronic psychosis may develop, but flashbacks are more common. Phencyclidine (PCP, or angel dust) is a popular drug of abuse and is particularly dangerous because it can produce severe assaultiveness. Other symptoms of intoxication include high blood pressure, rigidity, unstable gait, and nystagmus (jerking eye movements). Intoxication usually peaks within an hour, but severe reactions may require the short-term use of an antipsychotic.

Most correctional staff are aware of the existence of illicit drugs within their institutions. It is important to consider the possibility of intoxication whenever an inmate is seen with a sudden change in behavior or a change in mental status. Inmates with past substance abuse histories may seek drugs, but the stress or boredom of incarceration may tempt the novice as well.

The Patient With a Personality Disorder

Personality disorders are persistent, maladaptive traits affecting behavior, perception of the environment, and relationships with others. These maladaptive traits are of a severity that significantly impairs functioning and/or causes distress. These disorders are evident by the age of 18 years. Most of us recognize the difficulty in changing our attitudes, habits, and expectations; thus, it is not surprising that it is difficult to change the patient with a personality disorder. There are several types of personality disorders; however, patients with borderline, narcissistic, and antisocial disorders tend to display the most troublesome behavior. In a correctional setting, inmates with acute personality disorders may present severe problems. These inmates have a unique ability to produce intense emotions in the individuals around them. A team approach is best when managing inmates with personality disorders. This encourages "collective problem solving" and minimizes inconsistency in the treatment plan.

These inmates are often seen because of behavior that is harmful to themselves or others. Inmates with severe personality disorders are notorious for setting fires, mutilating themselves, flooding cells, and fighting. The precipitants for the behavior may be internal, such as feelings of isolation and emptiness. This makes their behavior unpredictable, because many of these patients have long-standing difficulties with interpersonal closeness and the management of unpleasant emotions. Often, destructive behavior is brought on by minor slights from others or inconveniences that are inevitable in the correctional setting. An example is an inmate who set a fire because he was not given a second food tray. He believed that the inmate worker and officer were not showing him proper respect. Other inmates also received one tray, but that was not significant to the patient. He felt enraged and emotionally abandoned.

Most inmates with severe personality disorders and destructive behavior become well known to correctional and health care staff. Management should include evaluation and treatment of any injuries. These inmates may hurt themselves directly or by provoking others to harm them. A mental health evaluation should explore possible primary disorders, including depression and psychosis. There is a high incidence of co-occurring psychopathologic conditions in patients with personality disorders. Inmates with severe personality disorders may be seen with extreme agitation, despite minimal apparent provocation. Agitation may be relieved by sedative medication, usually for short periods. Some patients with personality disorders benefit from mood-stabilizing medication such as valproic acid. Such medical treatments should be managed by an experienced psychiatrist who should consider the risk of patient noncompliance and the level of supervision available in the facility. No cures exist, although these inmates are often transferred between facilities or housing units as a "therapeutic" solution for staff. Management of the patient with a personality disorder should focus on consistency as much as possible. Clear and, preferably, written plans to manage behavior should be established. An example may be to specify the amount of time that the inmate will spend in the infirmary when admitted and to schedule routine, short, supportive therapy sessions. Initiating treatment plans requires staff effort and cooperation but, over time, will reduce conflict and chaos. Treatment plans are especially effective when combined with a contract developed with and signed by the patient. This gives the patient a sense of control and responsibility, and may reduce resistance to the treatment plan.

UNIT MANAGEMENT ISSUES

Small correctional facilities may have linkages with community health care providers for the evaluation and treatment of small numbers of inmates. Large facilities may be faced with providing care on site to reduce unnecessary and costly transport or as a result of court mandates. Correctional mental health units or infirmaries may rival those in state mental hospitals in terms of staffing and patient volume. Because of the prevalence of severely ill and high-risk inmates, many correctional facilities must address health care unit management in the unique correctional environment.

Staffing

Providing acute care begins with having staff in sufficient quantity and with appropriate experience and training. Some facilities use correctional staff for intake screening. Although this is not preferable, these officers should have special training to identify mental disorders and to make referrals as necessary. Ideally, correctional officers assigned to work with inmates with mental illnesses do so voluntarily with the approval of mental health staff.

There is no formula for determining the appropriate level of professional staffing. However, there are some basic considerations. Severely ill inmates need to be evaluated, and necessary treatment needs to be started as quickly as possible. There should be 24-hour-a-day access to mental health professionals. This may range from on-site nurses to an around-the-clock physician-staffed unit. If this is not possible, procedures should be developed to obtain services in the community. Psychiatric emergencies rarely confine themselves to business hours.

Most inmates with acute mental illnesses will need medication. These inmates may not be able to take medication reliably on their own. Nurses should be available in any acute care unit to administer medication and to monitor vital signs, at the very least. Licensed psychologists can evaluate patients and develop treatment plans. Any licensed physician can prescribe medication; however, psychiatrists are trained to treat mental illnesses specifically. Our facility has several psychiatrists and psychologists, a 24-hour-a-day emergency room, and male and female acute care psychiatric nursing units. In addition to providing evaluation and treatment, the health care professionals improve security. They can recognize and rapidly stabilize severely ill inmates. They also manage the difficult task of detecting malingering and return inmates who are not ill to the general population. This allows staff resources to be used more efficiently.

The role of the correctional officers should not be overlooked, as they are a consistent presence. Correctional officers play an important role in supporting the efforts of psychiatric staff. They provide security for the clinical staff and inmates. Psychiatric staff must be safe so that they can do their jobs, and staff safety must be a primary aspect of unit management. Correctional officers assist with emergency interventions, such as restraining and secluding violent patients. They also provide valuable clinical observations.

Milieu Management

The goal of milieu management is to foster a therapeutic atmosphere that, in turn, supports the acute care goal of patient stabilization and symptom reduction. Milieu management involves structuring the unit's physical plant, promoting a team approach to care, and facilitating patient participation. Milieu management activities support medical autonomy by making it obvious that the unit is a therapeutic area. Structuring a mental health unit in a correctional environment can be a challenging process. A secure but private space must be allocated for evaluations. Restraint and seclusion rooms must be separate from other living areas. Patients in restraints are particularly vulnerable. Restraint beds should be highly visible to correctional and nursing staff. Shatterproof glass doors and windows offer visibility with additional protection. Fire- and smoke-resistant materials should be used for restraints, bed frames, and bedding. Seclusion rooms must be suicide-proof, adequately ventilated and heated, and allow for good observation of patients.

Cooperation benefits the staff as well as the patients, yet it is difficult to achieve. Correctional mental health unit personnel are often stressed by high-risk patients, inadequate staffing, and an unattractive work environment. Inadequately trained staff may verbalize or act out antitherapeutic attitudes toward patients. This may result from a failure to appreciate mental illness as genuine and not under the control of the inmate. Such behavior, particularly from correctional officers, creates a dangerous environment and undermines morale. Medical autonomy, a necessity for managing acute care clinical situations, is threatened when correctional officers prevent access to inmates, provoke patients, or otherwise compromise the therapeutic atmosphere.

Clinical staff must, in turn, respect the function of the correctional staff. Security procedures, like room searches and count time, should be viewed as a necessary part of the program. Communication between staff members may be facilitated by having regular meetings to discuss the inmates' conditions and treatment plans. It may be helpful to have correctional officers present to give their clinical observations as well as to be informed about the program. All staff should also receive continuing education about treatment issues and unit policies.

Policy Development for Acute Care Patients

Correctional institutions were developed to protect society by isolating and rehabilitating criminals. They now serve the additional purpose of providing health care to rapidly expanding numbers of chronically ill, indigent inmates. Policies and procedures for the efficient and consistent delivery of health care services are necessary. One goal of such policies is to develop standards for appropriate mental health staffing and training. For example, all correctional officers who have contact with inmates should be considered part of the suicide prevention program. It is important for correctional and clinical administrators to work together to develop policies that conform to institutional needs and that are enforceable. Many policies are artfully written, but bear no resemblance to the actual daily practices of the personnel.

When developing policies for acute psychiatric care in a correctional facility, one should first review established standards for mental health care developed by governmental and sanctioning bodies. Correctional institutions are regulated by numerous governmental and private agencies, and there is no need to "reinvent the wheel" when developing new policies or updating old ones. There are health care standards for correctional institutions developed by the National Commission on Correctional Health Care, the National Institute of Mental Health, the American Correctional Association, and the American Public Health Association. These standards usually provide detailed descriptions of basic health care requirements for inmates. For example, the National Commission on Correctional Health Care has standards for intake screening, suicide prevention, medical record keeping, and the response to victims of sexual assault, to name a few.

Most states also have codes for mental health treatment in health care facilities. Some of these mental health codes are relevant to the correctional environment. In Illinois, the codes of the department of mental health define procedures for therapeutic seclusion, the use of restraints, and involuntary treatment.

In addition to guidelines developed for institutions, most professional organizations, such as the American Psychiatric Association, also publish standards for practicing clinicians. State licensing boards may have standards for clinical practice specific to correctional institutions.

The policy development process should begin with a review of functions needed to provide care for the inmate with an acute illness. For small institutions, this may be as simple as training officers to detect illness and having procedures to refer high-risk inmates out of the facility. For facilities providing care on site, the basic standards of care must be defined. This includes admission criteria for the mental health unit, the frequency of staff evaluations, the medication available, and other issues. The standard of care is often based on community practices, and it may be helpful to network with local health care facilities or other correctional institutions. Policies should be practical and written in simple language. All disciplines affected by the policy should be involved in its development. This may seem obvious, but many good plans are undermined when there is a failure to consult all relevant parties. This can be avoided by having correctional and clinical administrators and managers sign joint policies before they are implemented. Clinical policies that involve the participation of correctional officers must be reviewed, approved, and signed by the correctional administrator. Among other things, this assures that correctional staff are not being asked to perform duties for which they are not trained, and that may be in conflict with their job guidelines. Involvement of correctional administrators in policy development also serves to educate them about mental health care issues and standards of care for the inmates under their charge. It also provides an opportunity for clinical staff to better understand the correctional perspective and to address obstacles to clinical care in a proactive manner.

REFERENCES

1. APA Task Force on Psychiatric Services: *Position statement on psychiatric services in jails and prisons. Am J Psych* 146(a): 1244, 1989.
2. Deutsch A: *The Mentally Ill in America: A History of Their Care and Treatment from Colonial Times.* New York, Columbia University, 1937.
3. Quen J: Learning from history. *Psychiatry Ann* 5:15–31, 1975.
4. Grob G: *The State and the Mentally Ill: A History of Worchester State Hospital in Massachusetts, 1830–1920.* Chapel Hill, NC, University of North Carolina, 1973.
5. Robins L, Regier D: *Psychiatric Disorders in America: The Epidemiologic Catchment Area Study.* New York, The Free Press, 1980.
6. Bolton A: *A Study of the Need for and Availability of Mental Health Services for Mentally Disordered Jail Inmates and Juveniles in Detention Facilities.* Sacramento, Calif, California Department of Health, 1976.
7. Teplin L: Detecting disorder: The treatment of mental illness among jail detainees. *J Consult Clin Psychol* 58:233–236, 1990.
8. Torrey E, Stieber J, Ezekiel J, et al: *Criminalizing the Seriously Mentally Ill: The Abuse of Jails as Mental Hospitals.* Washington, D.C., Public Citizen's Health Research Group and National Alliance for the Mentally Ill, 1992.
9. Teplin L: The prevalence of psychiatric disorder among incarcerated women. *Arch Gen Psychiatry* 53:505–512, 1996.
10. Jordan B, Schlenger W, Caddell J, et al: Etiological factors in a sample of convicted women felons in North Carolina, in Zanarini MC (ed): *Role of Sexual Abuse in the Etiology of Borderline Personality Disorder.* Washington, D.C., American Psychiatric Press, 1997.
11. *Diagnostic and Statistical Manual of Mental Disorders,* ed 4. Washington, D.C., American Psychiatric Association, 1994.
12. Monahan J: Mental disorders and violence, another look, in Sheilagh (ed): *Mental Disorders and Crime.* Newbury Park, Calif, Sage, 1993.
13. Link B, Andrews H, Cullen F: The violent and illegal behavior of mental patients reconsidered. *Am Sociological Rev* 57(3): 275–293, 1992.
14. Andreasen N, Black D: *Introductory Textbook of Psychiatry.* Washington, D.C., American Psychiatric Press, 1995.
15. *Washington v Harper,* 110 SCt 1028 (1989).
16. Gunn J, Taylor P: *Forensic Psychiatry: Clinical, Legal, and Ethical Issues.* Oxford, England, Linacre House, 1993.

21

Suicide Prevention in Correctional Facilities: An Overview

Lindsay M. Hayes, M.S.

Hundreds of inmates commit suicide in local jails and state and federal prisons each year. Despite increased general awareness of the problem, research that has identified precipitating and situational risk factors, emerging correctional standards that advocate increased attention to suicidal inmates, and demonstration of effective strategies, prevention remains piecemeal and inmate suicides continue to pose a serious public health problem within correctional facilities. An overview of inmate suicide and a discussion of effective prevention techniques are offered below.

JAIL SUICIDE

Suicide is a leading cause of death in jails across the country,[1] where over 400 inmates take their lives each year.[2] In some urban jail facilities, AIDS-related deaths slightly outnumber deaths by suicide.[3] The only national research conducted to date calculated that there were 107 county jail

suicides per 100,000 inmates, a rate that was approximately nine times greater than that of the general population.[2] This same research, representing findings from jails of all types and sizes (e.g., rural and urban county jails, city jails, and police department lockups), found that most victims were young white males arrested for non-violent offenses and intoxicated upon arrest. Many were placed in isolation and were dead within 24 hours of incarceration. The overwhelming majority of victims were found hanging by either bedding or clothing. Most victims were not screened for potentially suicidal behavior upon entrance into the jail.[2, 4] Jordan et al. reported similar findings regarding the presence of intoxication, non-violent offenses, and length of incarceration prior to suicide.[5] Research on suicides in urban jail facilities provides certain disparate findings. Most victims of suicide in urban facilities had been arrested for violent offenses,[6–9] and were dead within 1 to 4 months of incarceration.[7, 9] Intoxication is normally not the salient factor in urban jails as it is in other types of jail facilities. Suicide victim characteristics such as age, race, gender, method, and instrument remain generally consistent in both urban and non-urban jails.

Of course, demographic victim profiles are not predictive of suicide risk and jail officials have been previously warned that their use should be limited to sensitizing correctional personnel to the general risk of suicide for those in custody.[2] As aptly stated by Farmer and colleagues:

> *In predicting who will be at risk over time, factors such as mental disorders, prior psychiatric hospitalizations, prior suicidal and self-destructive acts, substance abuse, and ongoing stressors may eventually prove to be more useful danger signals than demographic variables such as age, race, and gender.*[10]

Indeed, the risk factors of history of suicidal behavior and/or psychiatric treatment have been reported in the jail suicide literature.[6, 7, 9, 10]

The precipitating factors of suicidal behavior in jail are well established.[11, 12] It has been theorized that there are two primary causes for jail suicide—first, jail environments are conducive to suicidal behavior, and the inmate is facing a crisis situation. From the inmate's perspective, certain features of the jail environment enhance suicidal behavior: fear of the unknown, distrust of authoritarian environment, lack of apparent control over the future, isolation from family and significant others, shame of incarceration, and dehumanizing aspects of incarceration. In addition, there are certain factors often found in inmates facing a crisis situation that could predispose them to suicide: recent excessive drinking and/or use of drugs, recent loss of stabilizing resources, severe guilt or shame over the alleged offense, current mental illness, history of suicidal behavior, and approaching court date.[2] Marcus and Alcabes reported that 50% of jail suicides occurred within 3 days of a court appearance.[9] Bonner has offered the stress vulnerability model, the theory that suicide should be viewed in the context of a process by which an inmate is (or becomes) ill-equipped to handle the common stresses of confinement.[11] As the inmate reaches an emotional breaking point, the result can be suicidal ideation, attempt, or completion. During initial confinement in a jail, these stressors can be limited to fear of the unknown and isolation from family, but over time (including stays in prison) may become exacerbated and include loss of outside relationships, conflicts within the institution, victimization, further legal frustration, physical and emotional breakdown, and problems of coping within the jail environment.

The general suicidology literature has also identified various risk factors to suicidal behavior, including current degree of suicidal ideation and previous attempts, dysfunctional assumptions, dichotomous (all-or-nothing) thinking, problem-solving deficits and view of suicide as the desirable solution, psychiatric disorders, substance abuse, and

availability of method.[13] Such factors, in combination or interaction with the common stresses of confinement, may break down coping ability and create the emotional avenue for suicidal behavior. However, with few exceptions,[14-16] these factors have not been empirically tested in a correctional setting. Although research has not sufficiently addressed the psychosocial process of inmate suicide, as will be discussed later, court decisions and developing national standards have, to a degree, filled the void by advocating the view that suicide is a process that typically displays observable signs of maladaptive coping and suicidal intention. If identified in time, the process can be reversed or prevented in most cases.[11]

PRISON SUICIDE

While suicide is recognized as a critical problem within jails, the issue of prison suicide has not received comparable attention — primarily because the number of jail suicides far exceeds the number of prison suicides. Suicide ranks third, behind natural causes and AIDS, as the leading cause of death in prisons.[17] A recent study documented 158 inmate suicides in state and federal prisons during 1993, and calculated a suicide rate of 17.8 per 100,000 inmates, a number and rate considerably lower than in jails but almost 50% greater than the general population.[18] Some observers are simply unimpressed with prison suicide rates and are not convinced that the issue bears significant attention.[19] These same observers assume that, while the risk of suicide looms large in jail among inmates facing the initial stages of confinement, such risk dissipates over time in prison as individuals become more comfortable or tolerant of their predicament and develop coping skills to effectively handle life behind bars. This assumption, of course, has not been empirically studied, is far too simplistic, and ignores both the process and individual stressors of confinement as offered by Bonner.[11]

Most research on prison suicide has found that the vast majority of victims were convicted of personal crimes, housed in single cells, and had histories of suicide attempts and/or mental illness.[20–22] Salive et al. found higher suicide rates among white prison inmates and those aged 25 to 34, convicted of personal crimes, and housed in a maximum security facility.[23] In addition, while the length of actual time served by inmates who committed suicide varied widely, few victims had sentences under 8 years, and almost a quarter were serving life sentences. Similar findings regarding sentence and suicide were reported by White and Schimmel, who also found that although pretrial inmates and Mariel Cuban detainees represented only 6% and 4% of the total federal prison population, respectively, these two groups combined accounted for the majority of all suicides.[22]

Two states with large prison populations—California and New York—have recently analyzed data on inmate suicides within their respective systems. In a review of 15 suicides that occurred in its prison facilities during 1990, the California Department of Corrections found that 60% of victims had been diagnosed with a serious mental disorder, and that 53% had a history of substance abuse.[24] All but one of the victims were housed in a single cell, with 40% confined in administrative segregation units. The New York State Department of Correctional Services analyzed 52 suicides in its prison facilities between 1986 and mid-1994, and compared the data with that of the general inmate population.[25] White inmates represented 18% of the prison population, but 42% of suicides, whereas black inmates represented 50% of the prison population but only 20% of suicides. Further, although inmates convicted of a violent felony represented 56% of the prison population, they accounted for 80% of the suicides. Regarding length of incarceration, 64% of all victims committed suicide within 2 years of entering the prison system, and 66% of victims had mandatory minimum sentences of at least 4 years, with 23% serving life sentences.

White and Schimmel found that new legal problems, marital or relationship difficulties, and inmate-related conflicts were possible precipitating factors in prison suicides[22]; while Anno found that almost all the victims' medical records contained various behavioral and verbal cues that should have alerted staff to the impending suicide: "In some cases, the inmate told someone he had been thinking of suicide. In others, it was noted that the individual had just received some bad news (e.g., death of a family member). In still other instances, there were notations in the record of bizarre behavior or withdrawn, depressed behavior or expressions of extreme shame and remorse regarding their crime."[20]

Haycock has written that several recent developing characteristics of prisons suggest higher suicide rates in the future: emerging mandatory sentencing laws, dramatic increases in death penalty and life sentences, overcrowded prison systems, increased cases of AIDS, and the "graying" of inmate populations (inmates 55 years and older represent the fastest-growing age group) could instill despair and hopelessness in inmates.[26] Observers also suggest that overcrowded prisons have paralyzed correctional budgets, straining both medical and mental health services. As such, future prison suicides will "represent causalties of the era of mushrooming penitentiaries, harsher mandatory sentencing, and lengthening death rows."[26]

SELF-INJURY AND SUICIDE ATTEMPTS

A discussion of inmate suicide would be incomplete without a few words regarding self-injury and suicide attempts. In a study of self-injury among prison inmates, Thorburn found that acts of self-mutilation often signify increased tension in the inmates' lives caused by situations they sensed were beyond their direct control.[27] LeBrun found that county jail inmates with a history of suicidal behavior and suffering from a serious mental disorder were more

likely to attempt suicide, often in response to negative events (such as relationship losses and court dates).[28] A study of parasuicide (or nonfatal self-harm) among prison inmates found that young age, psychiatric history, and suicidal behavior of significant others (e.g., close family and relatives) were the best predictors of intentional self-harm.[15, 16] Liebling found that, compared with the regular inmate population, inmates who attempted suicide had an inability to cope, felt more vulnerable, grew increasingly bored during incarceration, and were unable to make constructive use of their time in confinement.[29]

It is not uncommon for acts of self-injurious behavior to be perceived by staff as manipulative behavior.[30] As offered in a later section of this chapter, however, it would be dangerous for staff to either ignore or punish this behavior. And, although the majority of inmates that engage in self-injurious behavior do not go on to commit suicide, a history of such behavior places them at greater risk of suicide.[16, 30] In any event, at a minimum, *all* acts of self-injury can be said to reflect personal breakdowns resulting from crises of self-doubt, poor coping and problem-solving skills, hopelessness, and fear of abandonment.[31]

NATIONAL CORRECTIONAL STANDARDS FOR SUICIDE PREVENTION

Beginning in the early 1960s and continuing today, various legislative bodies and agencies have examined correctional systems in an effort to fashion standards for the efficient operation of their jail and prison facilities. From these efforts, two basic types of standards have emerged to measure the adequacy of conditions of confinement: 1) the minimum standards of constitutional decency developed and refined by federal courts in decisions challenging the conditions of confinement, and 2) the growing body of self-regulatory standards and accreditation procedures promulgated by professional and federal agencies to stimulate facility improvement through voluntary, administrative action.[32]

Aside from recent enactment of the Prison Litigation Reform Act of 1996, courts have traditionally taken an active role in measuring the adequacy of a correctional system. Although correctional standards in general are not legally binding and do not set constitutional requirements,[33] the U.S. Supreme Court has stated that such standards have the ability to serve as guidelines or benchmarks in assessing the "duty of care" or "reasonable conduct."[34] Correctional standards have become a yardstick for measuring conditions of confinement. As noted several years ago, "The new judicial activism has added a sense of urgency to the development of increasingly *specific self-regulatory standards* by executive and professional organizations. In turn, the availability of these standards promises to introduce a new level of objectivity to litigation challenging the conditions of confinement."[32]

A recent study to determine the impact of the American Correctional Association's (ACA) correctional standards on court rulings found that 1) courts often consult ACA standards when attempting to determine appropriate expectations in a correctional setting, 2) courts sometimes cite ACA standards as the basis for establishing a court standard or a requirement in a decision, and 3) courts have sometimes used ACA standards and accreditation as a component of a continuing order or consent decree.[35] Not all courts use standards (ACA or otherwise) to measure conditions of confinement, however, because, in "many instances, a lower requirement is adopted consistent with the court's view of the constitutional or statutory requirement. In others, a higher standard might be established by the court given the circumstances of the case. And often the court prefers to take a totality of conditions perspective instead of relying on specific standards."[35]

In attempting to manage a correctional facility, the administrator is faced with two dilemmas: what constitutes sound correctional practices and what represents "state of the art." Correctional standards, whether state-regulated or offered nationally, can provide guidance for the administrator. When devising a strategy to reduce liability, for example, the administrator can cite compliance with national and/or state regulated standards as part of a good faith defense. Because standards reflect the state-of-the-art, they provide reasonable and minimal guidelines on which the administrator can base policies and procedures. As aptly stated in the preface of one state's jail standards: "It is intended for the standards to serve as a catalyst for sheriffs and jail administrators to reexamine existing policies, procedures, and practices, and to aid in policy planning, development, modification, and/or validation. The standards may also assist jail officials: a) to create greater uniformity in the operation and management of facilities, b) by serving as a resource for internal audits, and c) as a guide to developing lesson outlines for training."[36]

During the past 20 years, numerous organizations have promulgated national standards for use in correctional facilities (e.g., American Correctional Association, American Medical Association, American Psychiatric Association, American Public Health Association, Commission on Accreditation for Law Enforcement Agencies, Joint Commission on Accreditation of Healthcare Organizations, and National Commission on Correctional Health Care). However, the infusion of suicide prevention provisions into these standards is a fairly recent phenomenon, with great variation as to its specificity. In fact, several standards (e.g., from the American Psychiatric Association and the Joint Commission on Accreditation of Healthcare Organizations) have failed to even address the issue of suicide prevention. The most widely recognized and respected correctional standards are those promulgated by both the American Correctional Association and National Commission on Correctional Health Care.

Beginning in 1977, the American Correctional Association has published standards that contain a primary emphasis on the operation and administration of jails. It was not until 1984 that ACA standards included a requirement that correctional facilities maintain a suicide prevention program. Currently, both the ACA's jail and prison standards contain the same suicide prevention requirements:

There is a written suicide prevention and intervention program that is reviewed and approved by a qualified medical or mental health professional. All staff with responsibility for inmate supervision are trained in the implementation of the program.
Comment: The program should include specific procedures for intake screening, identification, and supervision of suicide-prone inmates.[37, 38]

Correctional standards of the National Commission on Correctional Health Care (NCCHC) provide the most comprehensive and practical guidelines for suicide prevention. First promulgated in 1987, both of the NCCHC's current jail and prison standards not only require correctional facilities to develop a written suicide prevention plan, but list the essential components for such a program: identification, training, assessment, monitoring, housing, referral, communication, intervention, notification, reporting, review, and critical incident debriefing.[39, 40] In addition, the appendices of the NCCHC standards offer several sample suicide prevention screening forms, and a multiple-level suicide prevention protocol for the housing and observation of suicidal inmates. Depending on the degree of suicide risk, housing options include suicide-resistant cells, infirmary rooms, and general population; whereas supervision levels include constant observation, 5- to 10-minute checks, and 10- to 30-minute checks.

Historically, national correctional standards have been viewed with some skepticism, referred to as too general or vague, lacking in enforcement power, and often politically influenced.[41] And, formal adoption of national standards by a correctional system does not necessarily ensure that individual facilities have put those procedures into operation. There are numerous examples of "accredited" facilities that have been found liable for inadequate conditions of confinement. In addition, most of the national standards were developed as recommended procedures rather than regulations that measured *outcome*. For example, the ACA standards require correctional facilities to maintain a "written suicide prevention and intervention program," but offer no guidance as to what components should be included in such a program.[37, 38] The potential result, of course, is that two correctional systems could be in compliance with this standard yet have dramatically different procedures.

The National Center on Institutions and Alternatives has conducted several national surveys to determine the degree to which the issue of suicide prevention is reflected in state jail standards and state prison policies and procedures.[42-44] The most recent survey found that 32 states had standards regulating county and local jails, with 24 mandatory and eight voluntary programs.[43] Of the states with jail standards, only a third required suicide prevention policies, and only one state (Texas) required county jails to maintain procedures regarding six critical prevention components (staff training, intake screening, communication, housing, supervision, and intervention). Three other states had jail standards that required procedures addressing all but one of the critical components. In regard to suicide prevention policies in state and federal prison systems, a recent survey found that, although 41 of 52 departments of correction (including the Federal Bureau of Prisons and District of Columbia) had a suicide prevention policy, only 15% of these agencies had procedures that contained either all, or all but one, critical component of suicide prevention.[44]

Despite slow progress within states, the relationship between suicide prevention and national correctional standards has progressed significantly in recent years. Several national organizations and other influential bodies have recognized that, because suicide remains a leading cause of death in correctional facilities, standards needed to be promulgated and revised to address the specific area of suicide prevention. Once a footnote in medical care standards, suicide prevention is now addressed separately and distinctly in many national standards. Perhaps as best exemplified by the NCCHC standards, national guidelines for suicide prevention have provided the opportunity and framework for both jail and prison systems to create and build upon their policies and procedures for the prevention of suicides.

KEY COMPONENTS OF A SUICIDE PREVENTION PROGRAM

As exemplified by the national standards, general awareness of suicide prevention in correctional facilities has greatly expanded during the past several years and programmatic accomplishments have resulted in the identification of essential elements that practitioners believe can dramatically reduce the incidence of inmate suicide. Although comprehensive suicide prevention programming has not been institutionalized consistently throughout the country, the literature has highlighted numerous jail and prison systems that have developed effective suicide prevention programs.[18, 22, 45–47] New York continues to experience a significant drop in the number of jail suicides following the implementation of a statewide comprehensive prevention program.[9, 48, 49] Texas has seen a 50% decrease in the number of county jail suicides, as well as almost a sixfold decrease in the rate of these suicides from 1986 through 1996, much of it attributable to increased staff training and a state requirement for jails to maintain suicide prevention policies.[43] Felthous reported no suicides during a 7-year period in a large county jail after the development of suicide prevention policies, based on the following principles: screening; psychological support; close observation; removal of dangerous items; clear and consistent proce-

dures; and diagnosis, treatment, and transfer of suicidal inmates to the hospital as necessary.[50]

All correctional facilities, regardless of size, should have a comprehensive suicide prevention policy that addresses the key components noted below.

Staff Training

The essential component to any suicide prevention program is properly trained correctional staff, who form the backbone of any jail or prison facility. Very few suicides actually are prevented by mental health, medical, or other professional staff because suicides usually are attempted in inmate housing units, and often during late evening hours or on weekends, when they are generally outside the purview of program staff. These incidents, therefore, must be thwarted by correctional staff who have been trained in suicide prevention and have developed an intuitive sense about the inmates under their care. Correctional officers are often the only staff available 24 hours a day; thus, they form the front line of defense in preventing suicides.

All correctional staff, as well as medical and mental health personnel, should receive 8 hours of initial suicide prevention training, followed by 2 hours of refresher training each year. Training should include why correctional environments are conducive to suicidal behavior, potential predisposing factors to suicide, high-risk suicide periods, warning signs and symptoms, and components of the facility's suicide prevention policy. In addition, all staff who have routine contact with inmates should receive standard first aid and cardiopulmonary resuscitation (CPR) training. All staff should also be trained in the use of various emergency equipment located in each housing unit. In an effort to ensure an efficient emergency response to suicide attempts, "mock drills" should be incorporated into both initial and refresher training for all staff.

Intake Screening/Assessment

Screening and assessment of inmates when they enter a facility are critical to a correctional facility's suicide prevention efforts. Although the psychiatric and medical communities disagree about which factors can be used to predict suicide in general, there is little disagreement as to the value of screening and assessment to the increased likelihood of preventing suicide.[51] Intake screening for all inmates and ongoing assessment of inmates at risk is critically important, because prior research has consistently reported that at least two-thirds of all suicide victims communicate their intent some time before death and that any individual with a history of one or more suicide attempts is at a much greater risk for suicide than those who have never made an attempt.[52]

Intake screening may be contained within the medical screening form or as a separate form, and should include inquiry regarding: past suicidal ideation and/or attempts; current ideation, threat, plan; prior mental health treatment/hospitalization; recent significant loss (job, relationship, death of family member/close friend, etc.); history of suicidal behavior by family member/close friend; suicide risk during prior confinement; and arresting/transporting officer(s) belief that inmate is currently at risk. The process should also include referral procedures to mental health and/or medical personnel for assessment. Following the intake process, should any staff hear an inmate verbalize a desire or intent to commit suicide, observe an inmate making a suicidal gesture, or otherwise believe an inmate is at risk for suicide, a procedure should be in place that allows that staff member to take immediate steps to ensure that the inmate is continuously observed until appropriate medical, mental health, and/or supervisory assistance is obtained.

Communication

Certain behavioral signs exhibited by the inmate may be indicative of suicidal behavior and, if detected and communicated to others, can prevent a suicide. There are essentially three levels of communication in preventing inmate suicides: between the arresting/transporting officer and correctional staff; between and among facility staff (including medical and mental health personnel); and between facility staff and the suicidal inmate.

In many ways, suicide prevention begins at the point of arrest. During *Level 1*, what an individual says and how they behave during arrest, transportation to the jail, and at booking are crucial to detecting suicidal behavior. The scene of arrest is often the most volatile and emotional time for the arrestee. Arresting officers should pay close attention to the arrestee during this time; suicidal behavior may be manifested, and previous behavior can be confirmed by onlookers such as family and friends. Any pertinent information regarding the arrestee's well-being must be communicated by the arresting/transporting officer to correctional staff. During *Level 2*, effective management of suicidal inmates often comes down to communication among correctional officers and other professional staff. Because inmates can become suicidal at any point during incarceration, correctional officers must maintain awareness, share information, and make appropriate referrals to mental health and medical staff. During *Level 3*, facility staff must use various communication skills with the suicidal inmate, including active listening, staying with the inmate if they are in immediate danger, and maintaining contact through conversation, eye contact, and body language. Correctional staff should trust their own judgment and avoid being misled by others (including mental health staff) into ignoring signs of suicidal behavior. A common factor found in the review of many inmate suicides has been the communication breakdown between correctional, medical, and mental health personnel.[18, 20, 21, 53]

Housing

In determining the most appropriate housing location for a suicidal inmate, correctional officials (with concurrence

from medical and/or mental health staff) often tend to physically isolate and sometimes restrain the individual. These responses might be more convenient for all staff, but they are detrimental to the inmate, since the use of isolation escalates the inmate's sense of alienation and further removes the individual from proper staff supervision. To every extent possible, suicidal inmates should be housed in the general population, mental health unit, or medical infirmary, located close to staff. Further, removal of an inmate's clothing (excluding belts and shoelaces) and the use of physical restraints (e.g., leather straps, straitjackets, etc.) should be avoided whenever possible, and used only as a last resort when the inmate is physically engaging in self-destructive behavior. Handcuffs should never be used to restrain a suicidal inmate. Housing assignments should be based on the ability to maximize staff interaction with the inmate, not on decisions that heighten depersonalizing aspects of incarceration.

All cells designated to house suicidal inmates should be suicide-resistant, free of all obvious protrusions, and provide full visibility.[5, 54, 55] These cells should contain tamper-proof light fixtures and ceiling air vents that are protrusion-free. Each cell door should contain a heavy gauge Lexan (or equivalent grade) glass panel that is large enough to allow staff a full and unobstructed view of the cell interior. Each cell housing a suicidal inmate should not contain any electrical switches or outlets, bunks with open bottoms, towel racks on desks and sinks, radiator vents, or any other object that provides an easy anchoring device for hanging. Finally, each housing unit in the facility should contain various emergency equipment, including a first aid kit, pocket mask or face shield, Ambu-bag, and rescue tool (to quickly cut through fibrous material). Correctional staff should ensure that such equipment is in working order on a daily basis.

Levels of Supervision

Medical experts warn that brain damage from strangulation caused by a suicide attempt can occur within 4 minutes, and death often within 5 to 6 minutes.[56] In jail and prison suicide attempts, the promptness of the response is often driven by the level of supervision afforded the inmate. Standard correctional practice requires that "special management inmates," including those housed in administrative segregation, disciplinary detention, and protective custody, be observed at intervals that do not exceed every 30 minutes, with mentally ill inmates observed more frequently.[37, 38] Inmates held in medical restraints and "therapeutic seclusion" should be observed at intervals that do not exceed every 15 minutes.[39, 40] Consistent with national correctional standards and practices, two levels of supervision are generally recommended for suicidal inmates: close observation and constant observation. *Close observation* is reserved for the inmate who is not actively suicidal, but expresses suicidal ideation (through verbalization or behavior) and/or has a recent history of self-destructive behavior. Staff should observe such an inmate at staggered intervals not to exceed every 15 minutes (e.g., 5, 10, 7 minutes, etc.). *Constant observation* is reserved for the inmate who is actively suicidal, either threatening or engaging in the act of suicide. Staff should observe such an inmate on a continuous, uninterrupted basis. Other aids (e.g., closed-circuit television, inmate companions or watchers, etc.) can be used as a supplement to, but never as a substitute for, these observation levels. Finally, mental health staff should observe, assess, and interact with suicidal inmates on a daily basis.

Intervention

Following a suicide attempt, the degree and promptness of the staff's intervention often foretell whether the victim will survive. National correctional standards and practices generally acknowledge that a facility's policy regarding intervention should be threefold. *First*, all staff who come into contact with inmates should be trained in standard first aid procedures and cardiopulmonary resuscitation (CPR). *Second*, any staff member who discovers an inmate attempting suicide should immediately survey the scene to ensure the emergency is genuine, alert other staff to call for medical personnel, and begin standard first aid and/or CPR as necessary. *Third*, staff should never presume that the inmate is dead, but rather should initiate and continue appropriate life-saving measures until relieved by arriving medical personnel. In addition, medical personnel should ensure that all equipment used in responding to an emergency within the facility is in working order on a daily basis.

Reporting

In the event of a suicide attempt or suicide, all appropriate correctional officials should be notified through the chain of command. Following the incident, the victim's family should be immediately notified, as well as appropriate outside authorities. All staff who came into contact with the victim prior to the incident should be required to submit a statement as to their full knowledge of the inmate and incident.

Follow-up/Administrative Review

An inmate suicide can be extremely stressful for staff. They may also feel ostracized by fellow personnel and administration officials. Following a suicide, misplaced guilt is sometimes displayed by the officer who wonders: "What if I had made my cell check earlier?" When crises occur and staff are affected by the traumatic event, they should receive appropriate assistance. One form of assistance is Critical Incident Stress Debriefing (CISD). A CISD team, comprising professionals trained in crisis intervention and traumatic stress awareness (e.g., police officers, paramedics, fire fighters, clergy, and mental health personnel), provides affected staff an opportunity to process their feelings about

the incident, develop an understanding of critical stress symptoms, and develop ways of dealing with those symptoms.[57, 58] For maximum effectiveness, the CISD process or other appropriate support services should occur within 24 to 72 hours of the critical incident.

Every completed suicide, as well as serious suicide attempt (i.e., requiring hospitalization), should be examined through an administrative review process. (If resources permit, clinical review through a psychological autopsy is also recommended.) Ideally, the administrative review should be coordinated by an outside agency to ensure impartiality. The review, separate and apart from other formal investigations that may be required to determine the cause of death, should include: 1) critical review of the circumstances surrounding the incident; 2) critical review of jail procedures relevant to the incident; 3) synopsis of all relevant training received by involved staff; 4) pertinent medical and mental health services/reports involving the victim; and 5) recommendations, if any, for change in policy, training, physical plant, medical or mental health services, and operational procedures.

CONTROVERSIAL ISSUES IN SUICIDE PREVENTION

In the quest to prevent inmate suicides, various interventions sometimes spark controversy—because of their unconventional nature, quick-fix philosophy, or concern for liability.[59] A sampling of several controversial approaches, including the use of inmate aides or companions to conduct suicide watch, is offered below.

No-suicide Contracts

Various mental health agencies develop contracts with potentially suicidal inmates, seeking assurances that their clients will not engage in self-injurious behavior. Correctional agencies will, in turn, request that each incoming inmate sign a standard letter as an apparent shield against liability; for example:

> *I promise not to harm myself while incarcerated at the Smith County Jail. If I should have any tendency to harm myself, I will immediately alert the staff.*

In truth, however, most legal experts opine that a no-suicide contract is simply a self-serving sheet of paper that does *not* provide a correctional agency or mental health worker with any legal protection.

While there may be many positive therapeutic aspects to no-suicide contracts, most clinicians agree that once an inmate becomes acutely suicidal, their written or verbal assurances are no longer sufficient to counter suicidal impulses.[60] As Clark and Kerkhof noted:

> *We do not think that one can reason reliably with persons in severe suicidal crisis, any more than one can reason with a person who believes God is sending them personal mes-*

sages via advertising billboards, or with someone who is convinced (medical evidence to the contrary) that a tumor is going to result in death ... there is no harm associated with 'suicide contracts' so long as the therapist does not succumb to the illusion that the contract is likely to prevent a suicide.[61]

Stripping Potentially Suicidal Inmates Naked

Some correctional facilities, regardless of an inmate's suicidal lethality, automatically strip potentially suicidal inmates of all their clothes and house them in an isolation cell. From the inmate's perspective, this practice is very degrading and increases feelings of depression. Although paper gowns and/or blankets are sometimes provided to inmates stripped of their clothing, these measures are still insufficient without proper staff observation. More appropriate measures should include constant observation or close supervision, placement in a suicide-resistant room or cell, and prompt intervention by mental health staff. As one observer noted:

> *Less attention should be paid to physically restricting him from suicide by removal of all potential suicide implements, and more attention should be paid to providing essential human interaction with staff or other inmates, to hopefully provide alternative solutions and services.*[62]

Using Closed Circuit Television Monitoring as an Alternative to Staff Observation

Used predominantly in small jail facilities that lack adequate staffing, closed circuit television (CCTV) is a popular yet deadly form of inmate supervision. There are numerous examples of inmates committing suicide in full view of CCTV equipment. Although facilities that use CCTV often limit the number of hours that any one officer can view a monitor, it is not unusual for correctional staff to suffer from monitor hypnosis or burnout during their assignment. Other serious problems include fuzzy or distorted CCTV reception, equipment breakdowns, and officers being distracted from monitor viewing by other responsibilities. Despite its intended use, CCTV does not *prevent* a suicide, it only *records* a suicide attempt in progress. In fact, the mere presence of CCTV may encourage suicidal or other acting-out behavior, particularly from manipulative inmates. Most experts agree that CCTV should be used only as a supplement (not as a substitute) for staff observation, and an officer should not be assigned to view a monitor for more than 1 hour without being relieved by another staff member.

Dealing With Manipulative Inmates

Few issues challenge correctional staff more than the management of manipulative inmates. It is not unusual for inmates to call attention to themselves by threatening suicide or even feigning an attempt to avoid a court appearance, bolster an insanity defense, be relocated to a different cell, be transferred to the facility's infirmary or local hospital, receive preferential staff treatment, or seek compassion from a previously unsympathetic spouse or other family member. As stated previously, manipulative behavior and suicide attempts can also be provoked by the presence of CCTV—wherein the inmate believes he has an attentive audience.

Although the prevailing theory is that any inmate who would go to the extreme of threatening suicide, or even engaging in self-injurious behavior, is suffering from at least an emotional imbalance that requires special attention, too often correctional officials (with the support of mental health staff) conclude that the inmate is not dangerous and simply attempting to manipulate his environment. They often suggest that such behavior be ignored and not reinforced through intervention. In fact, it is not unusual for mental health professionals to resort to labeling, with inmates engaging in deliberate self-harm termed manipulative or attention seeking; and truly suicidal inmates seen as serious and crying for help.[63] Clinicians routinely differentiate behavior they regard as genuine suicide attempts from other self-injurious behavior labeled as self-mutilation, suicidal gestures, parasuicide, manipulation, or malingering.[30] Such labeling, however, may reflect more upon the clinician's reaction to self-injurious behavior or the inmate rather than the inmate's risk of suicide.[60] Haycock has suggested that all (correctional, medical, and mental health) staff relinquish the tendency to view self-injurious behavior by inmates according to expressed or presumed intent.

> *There are no reliable bases upon which we can differentiate 'manipulative' suicide attempts posing no threat to the inmate's life from those 'true, non-manipulative' attempts which may end in death. The term 'manipulative' is simply useless in understanding, and destructive in attempting to manage, the suicidal behavior of inmates (or of anybody else).*[64]

Other clinicians would disagree and argue that self-injurious behavior displayed by truly suicidal and manipulative inmates should result in different interventions. For suicidal inmates, intervention that promotes close supervision, social support, and access to or development of psychosocial resources is crucial. For manipulative inmates, intervention that combines close supervision with behavior management is crucial in preventing or modifying such behavior.[11] Historically, the problem has been that manipulative behavior was ignored or resulted in punitive sanctions, including isolation. Often, manipulative inmates escalate their behavior and die, either by accident or miscalculation of staff's responsiveness. Therefore, the problem is not in how we label the behavior, but how we react to it—and the reaction should not include punitive measures such as isolation.

Policy of Never Entering a Cell Without Backup

The policy of many correctional facilities is that an officer should never enter a cell or room without backup support. From the standpoint of officer safety, few could argue with the soundness of this policy, although other correctional administrators support a more flexible policy that allows officers to use their judgment in asking themselves—Is the inmate faking and planning an escape? If the alleged victim is hanging with his feet off the floor and appears to be in distress, there is little doubt that the scene is genuine. If, however, the inmate is sitting or kneeling on the bottom bunk, it could be a different situation and the inmate could be feigning an attempt. Staff should always be instructed, however, not to be misled into believing that hanging attempts only occur when the body and/or feet are off the cell floor. Numerous successful suicides occur in the sitting and/or kneeling position.

What happens in many police department lockups where only *one* dispatcher/jailer is on duty? Does the individual wait 5 to 10 minutes for backup support from the patrol officer to arrive from the streets? In these small jails, with the inmate hanging on the front of the cell bars, can a dispatcher/jailer at least check the victim's vital signs and begin limited life-saving measures (e.g., loosening/removing the noose) from outside the cell before arrival of backup staff? What of another controversial intervention—policies that authorize correctional staff to act quickly, lock down all but one or two trusted inmates to assist in the rescue attempt?

The issue of whether or not staff should enter a cell area to rescue an inmate in the midst of a suicide attempt without proper backup support is indeed a difficult decision that continues to stir controversy. It is, however, also illustrative of a facility that lacks adequate staffing to protect the health and safety of both officers and inmates.

When No Vital Signs Exist, Don't Presume That Death Has Occurred

There have been a number of incidents when, without the victim displaying any vital signs (i.e., pulse and breathing), life-saving measures were never initiated. Those staff apparently did not realize that the sole purpose of CPR was to assist in reestablishing vital signs. Many inmates once presumed to be dead are alive today because CPR was started immediately. There are other instances in which CPR was not started because staff feared the victim might also suffer from an infectious disease, including AIDS. Beyond the need for additional training to educate reluctant staff, all housing units should be equipped with pocket masks or face shields, latex gloves, and other appropriate infectious disease equipment. Of course, only a physician, emergency medical service personnel, or other professionals as designated by state law, can pronounce an individual dead. Until such time, standard first aid and CPR should be initiated and continued until staff are relieved by qualified medical personnel.

Protecting the Scene of the Crime

Too many correctional facilities continue to maintain antiquated policies that treat the scene of an alleged suicide as a crime scene and require that it be preserved. Associated with the crime scene perception is the conclusion that the body should not be touched. Literal application of this belief can lead to the absurdity of leaving a person hanging, when they might otherwise be alive. In one recent example from Alaska, the first officer on the scene of a police lockup suicide attempt chose not to grab the CPR mask hanging on the corridor wall. Instead, he grabbed a camera and began making an historical record of the incident. The victim remained in a hanging position until paramedics arrived more than 10 minutes later. When paramedics began to connect a defibrillator to the victim, the officer intervened and requested that the body be disturbed as little as possible.[65]

Needless to say, preserving life should always be the first priority, and correctional officials who place preserving-the-scene-of-the-crime policies first can be expected to garner a high degree of liability. In fact, the decision not to cut down a hanging victim upon the belief that the crime scene was to be preserved may persuade a fact-finder that staff were indifferent or lacked training.

Use of Inmates to Conduct Suicide Watch

In early October 1991, Mike Robertson and Richard Greene (pseudonyms) were cellmates in a county jail located in northern New Jersey.[65] They had met approximately 6 weeks earlier at a county psychiatric hospital, where both were being treated as a result of unrelated suicide attempts. Robertson and Greene were now housed in the jail's mental health unit and, based upon their continued suicidal threats and ideation, had been placed under the highest level of suicide watch—constant observation by an inmate observation aide and checks by a correctional officer at 15-minute intervals. Housed together, these two inmates frequently talked about suicide. On several occasions, Robertson told Greene that he wanted to go back to the county hospital and thought a feigned suicide attempt would guarantee his chances of transfer. Greene, on the other hand, was genuinely despondent about life, saw little positive value in his future, and frequently contemplated "hanging up".

In the late afternoon of October 4, Richard Greene tied one end of his bed sheet to a ceiling vent and the other end to his neck. Stepping onto the sink, Greene turned to his cellmate and asked him not to interfere. He stepped off the sink and, before losing consciousness, heard Robertson yelling for assistance. Shortly thereafter, officers responded to the scene and initiated life-saving measures to Greene. At the same time, Mike Robertson walked though the open cell door into the corridor, where he was met by Kurt Bernard (a pseudonym), the inmate observation aide assigned to Robertson and Greene. The aide was sitting on a chair dutifully recording Greene's suicide attempt in his log as required by jail policy. As Robertson walked past Bernard toward the shower area, the aide asked where he was going. Robertson responded that he needed to make a telephone call. Bernard, apparently not noticing that Robertson was clutching a white shoelace in his right hand, continued writing in his log. Approximately 20 minutes later, another inmate began yelling for assistance from the shower area. Bernard quickly responded and observed Mike Robertson hanging from a shower fixture by the white shoelace. As the aide began to lift the inmate's body, an officer arrived and cut the ligature. Robertson was placed on the floor and, although CPR was promptly initiated, the inmate, once viewed as manipulative, was later pronounced dead at the local hospital.

Why were two suicidal inmates housed together under suicide watch in a cell with an exposed ceiling vent, access to shoelaces, and allegedly under the constant surveillance of an inmate observation aide? Not surprisingly, litigation was filed as a result of Mike Robertson's suicide.

In contrast, inmate observation aides are selected according to written guidelines and receive extensive training at various correctional facilities in New York City. They are paid for their services and are deployed in several special housing areas. Aides are instructed to promptly inform correctional officers or mental health staff when they believe an inmate poses a risk of suicide, presents an immediate danger of suicide, or is engaging in bizarre behavior.[66] A buddy system has demonstrated long-term success in one county jail.[47] In another state, trained inmate aides have an expanded role as peer counselors and befrienders of potentially suicidal inmates.[55] Their duties include: 1) reaching inmates before they become suicidal risks, 2) befriending inmates who are depressed and alert mental health or medical staff to a developing crisis, 3) listening to inmates' problems, 4) asking relevant questions to potentially suicidal inmates to assess their suicidal risk, and 5) informing new arrivals of what to expect in prison in regard to daily routine (rules, visitation privileges, telephone calls, etc.) and where to get help.

Currently, there are no national correctional standards that address the issue of using non-staff resources in the supervision of suicidal inmates, and only a small percentage of local jurisdictions throughout the country use inmate observation aides to observe suicidal inmates, most in an effort to supplement staff observation at 15-minute intervals and to avoid use of staff for constant supervision. West Virginia and the Federal Bureau of Prisons appear to be the only prison systems that authorize use of inmate observation aides in lieu of *any* staff supervision of suicidal inmates.[44]

The controversy surrounding use of inmates to conduct suicide watch is perhaps best exemplified by the Federal Bureau of Prisons (FBOP). Assigned to 4-hour shifts and paid on a performance basis, inmate companions are required to continuously observe suicidal inmates.[22] They

are not placed in a clinical or therapeutic role, and are trained in basic aspects of suicidal behavior, communication, and procedures necessary to summon staff assistance. What is most interesting about the program is that it is not uniformly used across the federal prison system. According to an early survey of FBOP chief psychologists, 70% of respondents used the option of inmate companions, yet warned that no other issue so clearly appears to generate a strong opinion one way or the other.[67] In a more recent survey, it was found that 65% of FBOP facilities used inmate companions, and 72% of all suicide watch hours in these facilities during 1992 were performed by inmate companions.[22] Of the 35% of responding chief psychologists who did not use companions, most cited philosophical or ethical problems, liability concerns, or security and logistical issues at their particular facility. One chief psychologist voiced specific concerns of accountability for clinicians and potential violations of confidentiality in his reluctance to use inmate companions.[68]

Suicide watchers, observation aides, inmate companions, or buddies; by whatever name, the *informal* use of other inmates to prevent suicides can have various positive attributes, such as having an extra set of eyes watching suicidal inmates, and providing needed companionship to alleviate despair and the loneliness of single-cell isolation. On the other hand, ethical and legal concerns accompany the *formalized* use of inmate observation aides. And, despite promises to the contrary, use of other inmates to conduct suicide watch can result in relaxation of staff responsibilities for inmate safety and treatment. In addition, some jurisdictions even rationalize its formalized use by insisting that observation aides eliminate the need to automatically restrain or strip potentially suicidal inmates of their clothing. However, when used strictly as an alternative to staff supervision of actively suicidal inmates, observation aides are simply a budgetary rationalization for inadequate staff coverage.

While some may argue that no-suicide contracts, CCTV, stripping inmates, protecting the crime scene, and inmate companions are no more than typical controversial issues in suicide prevention, these interventions simply and collectively exemplify further separation of correctional, mental health, and medical staff from suicidal inmates.

CONCLUSION

Despite appearances of protected environments that offer regular observation, restriction of movement, and varying levels of health care services, inmates continue to commit suicide in correctional facilities at rates far greater than those in the community. While often lacking the ability to accurately predict if and when an inmate will commit suicide, correctional facilities and their personnel maintain an obligation to be in the best position to identify, assess, and treat potentially suicidal behavior. As one distinguished clinician once noted:

Suicide .... is not a bizarre and incomprehensible act of self-destruction. Rather, suicidal people use a particular logic, a style of thinking that brings them to the conclusion that death is the only solution to their problems. This style can be readily seen, and there are steps we can take to stop suicide, if we know where to look.[69]

And, while not all inmate suicides are preventable, most are if correctional facilities are determined to "know where to look" and intervene accordingly.

REFERENCES

1. Bureau of Justice Statistics: *Jails and Jail Inmates 1993-94.* Washington, D.C., U.S. Department of Justice, 1995.
2. Hayes LM: National study of jail suicides: Seven years later. *Psychiatric Q* 60:7-29, 1989.
3. Camp GM, Camp CG: *The Corrections Yearbook.* South Salem, NY, Criminal Justice Institute, 1993.
4. Hayes LM: And darkness closes in .. national study of jail suicides. *Crim Justice Behavior* 10:461-484, 1983.
5. Jordan FB, Schmeckpeper K, Strope M: Jail suicides by hanging: An epidemiological review and recommendations for prevention. *Am J Forensic Med Pathol* 8:27-31, 1987.
6. Copeland AR: Fatal suicidal hangings among prisoners in jail. *Med Sci Law* 29:341-345, 1989.
7. DuRand CJ, Burtka GJ, Federman EJ, et al: A quarter century of suicide in a major urban jail: Implications for community psychiatry. *Am J Psychiatry* 152:1077-1080, 1995.
8. Frost R, Hanzlick R: Deaths in custody: Atlanta City Jail, and Fulton County Jail, 1974-1985. *Am J Forensic Med Pathol* 9:207-211, 1988.
9. Marcus P, Alcabes P: Characteristics of suicides by inmates in an urban jail. *Hosp Commun Psychiatry* 44:256-261, 1993.
10. Farmer KA, Felthous AR, Holzer CE: Medically serious suicide attempts in a jail with a suicide-prevention program. *J Forensic Sci* 41:240-246, 1996.
11. Bonner RL: Isolation, seclusion, and psychological vulnerability as risk factors for suicide behind bars, in Maris R, Berman AL, Maltsberger JT, et al (eds): *Assessment and Prediction of Suicide.* New York, Guilford Press, pp 398-419, 1992.
12. Winkler GE: Assessing and responding to suicidal jail inmates. *Commun Mental Health J* 28:317-326, 1992.
13. Weishaar ME, Beck AT: Clinical and cognitive predictors of suicide, in Maris R, Berman AL, Maltsberger JT et al (eds): *Assessment and Prediction of Suicide,* New York, Guilford Press, pp 467-483, 1992.
14. Bonner RL, Rich AR: Cognitive vulnerability and hopelessness among correctional inmates: A state of mind model. *J Offender Rehab* 17:113-122, 1992.
15. Ivanoff A: Background risk factors associated with parasuicide among male prison inmates. *Crim Justice Behavior* 19:426-436, 1992.
16. Ivanoff A, Jang SJ, Smyth NJ: Clinical risk factors associated with parasuicide in prison. *Int J Offender Ther Comp Criminol* 40:135-146, 1996.
17. Bureau of Justice Statistics: *Correctional Populations in the United States, 1991.* Washington, D.C., U.S. Department of Justice, 1993.
18. Hayes LM: Prison suicide: An overview and guide to prevention. *Prison J* 75:431-456, 1995.
19. Payson HE: Suicide among males in prison - why not? *Bull Am Acad Psychiatry Law* 3:152-161, 1975.
20. Anno BJ: Patterns of suicide in the Texas Department of Corrections, 1980-1985. *J Prisons Jail Health* 5:82-93, 1985.
21. Jones D: *Study of Inmate Suicides.* Frankfort, KY: Kentucky Corrections Cabinet, 1986.
22. White TW, Schimmel DJ: Suicide prevention in federal prisons: A suc-
cessful five-step program, in Hayes LM (ed): *Prison Suicide: An Overview and Guide to Prevention.* Washington, D.C., National Institute of Corrections, U.S. Department of Justice, pp 46-57, 1995.
23. Salive ME, Smith GS, Brewer TF: Suicide mortality in the Maryland state prison system, 1979 through 1987. *JAMA* 262:365-369, 1989.
24. California Department of Corrections: *Suicide Prevention in the California Department of Corrections: Annual Report - 1990.* Sacramento, CA, 1991.
25. New York State Department of Correctional Services: *Characteristics of Suicide Victims in NYSDOCS Between 1986-1994.* Albany, NY, 1994.
26. Haycock J: Crimes and misdemeanors: A review of recent research on suicides in prison. *Omega* 23:81-94, 1991.
27. Thorburn KM: Self-mutilation and self-induced illness in prison. *J Prison Jail Health* 4:40-51, 1984.
28. LeBrun LD: Characteristics of male suicide attempts in the Sacramento county jail, 1985-1987. *Jail Suicide Update* 2(4):1-4, 1989.
29. Liebling A: Vulnerability and prison suicide. *Br J Criminol* 35: 173-187, 1995.
30. Haycock J: Manipulation and suicide attempts in jails and prisons. *Psychiatric Q* 60:85-98, 1989.
31. Toch H: *Men in Crisis: Human Breakdowns in Prison.* Chicago, Aldine Publishing, 1975.
32. National Institute of Justice: *American Prisons and Jails, Volume 1: Summary Findings and Policy Implications of a National Survey.* Washington, D.C., U.S. Department of Justice, 1980.
33. *Rhodes v Chapman,* 452 US 337 (1981).
34. *Bell v Wolfish,* 441 US 520 (1979).
35. Miller R: Standards and the courts: An evolving relationship. *Corrections Today* 54(3):58-60, 1992.
36. Utah Sheriff's Association: *Utah Jail Standards.* Santa Clara, UT, 1995.
37. American Correctional Association: *Standards for Adult Local Detention Facilities* ed 3, Laurel, MD, ACA, 1991.
38. American Correctional Association: *Standards for Adult Correctional Facilities,* ed 3, Laurel, MD, ACA, 1990.
39. National Commission on Correctional Health Care: *Standards for Health Services in Jails,* ed 3, Chicago, NCCHC, 1996.
40. National Commission on Correctional Health Care: *Standards for Health Services in Prisons,* ed 2, Chicago, NCCHC, 1992.
41. Anno BJ: *Prison Health Care: Guidelines for the Management of an Adequate Delivery System.* Washington, D.C., National Institute of Corrections, U.S. Department of Justice, 1991.
42. Hayes LM: National standards of jail suicide prevention. *Jail Suicide Update* 2(2):1-6, 1989.
43. Hayes LM: Jail standards and suicide prevention: Another look. *Jail Suicide/Mental Health Update* 6(4):1-11, 1996.
44. Hayes LM: National and state standards for prison suicide prevention: A report card. *J Correctional Health Care* 3(1):5-38, 1996.
45. Hayes LM: Model prevention programs. *Jail Suicide Update* 3(1-4), 1990.
46. Hopes B, Shaull R: Jail suicide prevention: Effective programs can save lives. *Corrections Today* 48(8):64-70, 1986.
47. Manning R: A suicide prevention program that really works. *Am Jails* 3(1):18-24, 1989.
48. Cox JF, Landsberg G, Paravati MP: The essential components of a crisis intervention program for local jails: The New York local forensic suicide prevention crisis service model. *Psychiatric Q* 60:103-117, 1989.
49. New York State Commission of Correction: Medical review board's statistical breakdown of inmate mortalities by type of facility and manner of death, (1977-1995), Albany, NY, NYCC, 1996.
50. Felthous AR: Preventing jailhouse suicides. *Bull Am Acad Psychiatry Law* 22:477-488, 1994.

51. Hughes DH: Can the clinician predict suicide? *Psychiatric Services* 46:449-451, 1995.

52. Clark DC, Horton-Deutsch SL: Assessment in absentia: The value of the psychological autopsy method for studying antecedents of suicide and predicting future suicides, in Maris R, Berman AL, Maltsberger JT, et al (eds): *Assessment and Prediction of Suicide,* New York, Guilford Press, pp 144-182, 1992.

53. Appelbaum K, Dvoskin J, Geller J, et al: *Report on the Psychiatric Management of John Salvi in Massachusetts Department of Correction Facilities,* 1995-1996. Worcester, MA, University of Massachusetts Medical Center, 1997.

54. Atlas R: Reducing the opportunity for inmate suicide: A design guide. *Psychiatric Q* 60:161-171, 1989.

55. Lester D, Danto BL: *Suicide Behind Bars: Prediction and Prevention.* Philadelphia, PA, The Charles Press, 1993.

56. Emergency Cardiac Care Committee and Subcommittees, American Heart Association: Guidelines for cardiopulmonary resuscitation and emergency cardiac care. *JAMA* 268:2172-2183, 1992.

57. Mitchell JT, Everly GS: *Critical Incident Stress Debriefing: An Operations Manual for the Prevention of Traumatic Stress Among Emergency Services and Disaster Workers,* ed 2. Ellicott City, MD, Chevron Publishing, 1996.

58. Meehan B: Critical incident stress debriefing within the jail environment. *Jail Suicide/Mental Health Update* 7(1):1-5, 1997.

59. Rowan JR, Hayes LM: *Training Curriculum on Suicide Detection and Prevention in Jails and Lockups,* ed 2. Mansfield, MA, National Center on Institutions and Alternatives, 1995.

60. Thienhaus OJ, Piasecki M: Assessment of suicide risk. *Psychiatric Services* 48:293-294, 1997.

61. Clark DC, Kerkhof AJ: No-suicide decisions and suicide contracts in therapy. *Crisis* 14:98-99, 1993.

62. Denoon KS: *BC Corrections: A Study of Suicides, 1970-1980.* British Columbia, Canada, Ministry of Attorney General, Corrections Branch, 1983.

63. Franklin RK: Deliberate self-harm: Self-injurious behavior within a correctional mental health population. *Crim Justice Behavior* 15: 210-218, 1988.

64. Haycock J: Listening to 'attention seekers': The clinical management of people threatening suicide. *Jail Suicide Update* 4(4):8-11, 1992.

65. Hayes LM: Use of inmates to conduct suicide watch and other controversial issues in jail suicide prevention. *Jail Suicide/Mental Health Update* 6(1):1-6, 1995.

66. Rakis J, Monroe R: Monitoring and managing the suicidal prisoner. *Psychiatric Q* 60:151-160, 1989.

67. Schimmel D, Sullivan J, Mrad D: Suicide prevention: Is it working in the federal prison system? *Fed Prisons J* 1:20-24, 1989.

68. Bonner RL: Letter to the editor. *Jail Suicide/Mental Health Update* 6(2):8, 1995.

69. Shneidman E: At the point of no return. *Psychology Today* March: 55-58, 1987.

Public Health

22

Preventive Health Issues for Individuals in Jails and Prisons

John P. May, M.D.

William E. Lambert, Ph.D.

Ill health, injury, and premature death are often preventable. A study in the early 1990s found that approximately half of the deaths occurring in the United States can be directly attributed to preventable causes.[1] Many inmates engage in behaviors or come from environments that place them at risk for these preventable deaths. A correctional medicine program should emphasize prevention to be most comprehensive and effective.

While clinicians intuitively understand the value of prevention, inmates do not always appreciate it. Often, their lives are so unpredictable and uncertain that the idea of investing efforts to prevent anything that is not an immediate threat or to gain some possible future benefit by altering an established behavior seems meaningless. Despite their many years of destructive or unhealthy behaviors, they have survived. Convincing them that change is necessary does

not come easy. They also carry many obstacles to change with them, and traditional prevention messages are frequently irrelevant. Furthermore, any positive behaviors that might be learned within the jail or prison become difficult to sustain when they return to different environments, particularly if those areas are filled with violence, poverty, or reduced opportunities. A successful preventive medicine program must address the risks most relevant to the correctional population, address the many barriers to behavioral change, and prepare the inmate to maintain the changes in different environments.

PREVENTABLE DEATHS

In the United States, the number one cause of preventable deaths is tobacco, which contributes significantly to various cancers, cardiovascular disease, lung disorders, low birth

Table 22-1. Actual causes of death in the United States, 1990

Cause	Estimated number of deaths	Percent of total deaths
Tobacco	400,000	19
Diet/activity patterns	300,000	14
Alcohol	100,000	5
Microbial agents	90,000	4
Toxic agents	60,000	3
Firearms	35,000	2
Sexual behavior	30,000	1
Motor vehicles	25,000	1
Illicit use of drugs	20,000	< 1
TOTAL	1,060,000	50

weights, burns, and more. Other preventable causes of death involve diet and activity patterns, which contribute to cardiovascular diseases and cancers; alcohol causes death through unintentional injuries, liver diseases, and cancers; infectious agents, which could be avoided through vaccinations or behavioral change; toxic agents from occupational or environmental exposures, which result in respiratory diseases or malignancies; firearms, which cause death from intentional or unintentional injuries; sexual behavior, which transmits human immunodeficiency virus or hepatitis B, or leads to cervical cancer; motor vehicle crashes, which kill passengers and pedestrians; and illicit use of drugs, which causes overdoses, unintentional injuries, and infections. Table 22-1 demonstrates how these factors contributed to half of the 2,148,000 deaths in the general population of the United States in 1990.

These conditions, products, agents, and behaviors exact a great toll among the correctional population. A 1983 jail study found that 84% of the detainees use tobacco, 74% use alcohol, and 24% use illicit drugs.[2] Sexually transmitted diseases, hepatitis, and human immunodeficiency virus are all more common in the correctional population.[3] They also have an extraordinary amount of injuries from firearms and other violence-related events. For example, studies at Cook County Jail in Chicago[4] and the Central Detention Facility in Washington, D.C.[5] both found that one in four male detainees entering the institutions had been shot at least one time. Most were shot by strangers while out in the streets.

Added to the risk from prisoners' unhealthy behaviors and environments are their educational and economic experiences. Approximately 60% of inmates have not completed 12 years of education, and most are poor.[6] Health studies found that death rates for undereducated persons are nearly threefold higher than rates for those who have completed 12 or more years of education, and impoverished families are fivefold more likely to have poor health than wealthy families.[7] Being aware of all of these conditions

and risks is important in developing an effective prevention program.

PREVENTION WITHIN THE CORRECTIONAL SETTING

Successes are possible within the correctional setting. The health of inmates can improve during incarceration, reducing their risk of death. Institutions can shelter and protect inmates from many of the environmental and behavioral forces that had been so destructive in their lives. In essence, incarceration often stabilizes health.

Excluding deaths from HIV disease, the death rate for inmates is much lower than an age-matched group of the general population. This lower death rate is because deaths from leading causes of death for younger adults—firearms and motor vehicle crashes—are almost nil, which illustrates how environment contributes to ill health. Additionally, the suicide rate is decreased in prison. Even for individuals with HIV infection, in those facilities with quality medical services, life expectancy can increase because of better access to health care and medications. Furthermore, incarceration is time away from reckless lifestyles on the streets. The regular prison routines of sleep, meals, and exercise enables many inmates to gain weight, strength, and healthy habits.

Because of the higher prevalence of pre-existing HIV infection in persons entering prisons, however, the overall death rates for inmates compared to a cohort group in the general population is nearly equal. This is demonstrated in Table 22-2. For the purpose of the comparison, the general population age group 15 to 54 years (95% of incarcerated persons are within this age group[8]) is matched to death rates for incarcerated persons of all ages (because age-specific death rates are unavailable for the correctional population). Injury-related deaths are markedly reduced by factors of up to 15 in males and 10 in females, while AIDS deaths are increased by a factor of 2 in males and 8 in females. Deaths from smoking-related diseases, such as malignancies or cardiovascular disease, would be expected to be higher in the incarcerated population since inmates smoke at higher rates than the general population. Data, however, on specific causes of death in older, incarcerated persons are unavailable for the comparison, and most persons are released from prison before they reach an age at which smoking-related illnesses would likely manifest.

PREVENTION BEYOND INCARCERATION

While the risk of death is reduced during incarceration, persons released from prison have a much higher death rate than either the incarcerated population or the general population. (Table 22-2.) The death rate for parolees increases nearly fourfold, and any gains for improving health that were made during the incarceration seem to be lost. This is due in part to the environment to which an inmate returns after incarceration. While the majority of the excess deaths

Table 22-2. Rates of death, 1994

	All causes	AIDS	Suicide	Unintentional injury	Homicide*
General population males, ages 15–54	295.1	40.6	23.9	51.0	24.2
Sentenced males, all ages	301.9	92.8	15.8	3.3	7.0
General population females, ages 15–54	134.2	7.1	5.5	16.6	5.3
Sentenced females, all ages	204.8	58.3	6.6	1.7	1.7
Male parolees,† all ages	1200.0	**	**	**	**
Female parolees,† all ages	700.0	**	**	**	**

*Includes all deaths caused by other inmates or correctional staff, excluding sanctioned executions.
†Data from 1992, specific causes of death not available nationally.
(Reprinted by permission of the U.S. Department of Justice, from Bureau of Justice Statistics, 1995; National Center for Health Statistics, 1995; and Centers for Disease Control and Prevention.)

are firearm homicides, deaths from AIDS and smoking-related illnesses also contribute significantly.

The large increase in the preventable deaths upon release speaks for intervention. It also demonstrates the need for prevention strategies that are effective beyond incarceration. While it is not easy to alter inmates' home environments, they can be given the tools for recognizing high-risk situations and making appropriate choices. Prevention should not stop when incarceration stops.

THE BIG THREE: HIV, VIOLENCE, SMOKING

The following sections focus on three leading causes of morbidity and mortality for the incarcerated population: HIV disease, violence, and smoking-related illnesses. Each section discusses the impact of the condition of the correctional population and suggests interventions for prevention. If success were to be achieved in reducing the incidence of these three conditions, then many premature deaths of incarcerated persons would be eliminated.

Human Immunodeficiency Virus

By 1994, AIDS had become the leading cause of death for young adult men and women in the United States between the ages of 25 and 44.[9] By that time, AIDS had already become the leading cause of death for incarcerated persons in most prison systems. In 1994, death from AIDS accounted for nearly 60% of all inmate deaths in Connecticut, New York, and Florida, and 35% of inmate deaths overall.[10] The prevalence of HIV seropositivity in sentenced inmates, based on the best available reporting data, was 2.3% in 1994, yet varies widely depending on location.[11] This is more than eightfold higher than the estimated prevalence of 0.3% in the general population.[12]

Persons entering jails and prisons have multiple risk factors for HIV infection. Approximately one-quarter of state prisoners report having used a needle to inject drugs at some time in their lives.[13] While sharing of injection equipment is a well-documented mode of HIV transmission, the use of other illicit drugs, particularly crack cocaine, is also

an associated risk factor for the disease. This is due, in part, to the exchange of sex for drugs or money by some drug users to support their habits and their higher number of sex partners.[14] In 1994, over one third of male and female arrestees in more than 20 major cities had positive test results for cocaine, thus presenting another high-risk group for HIV infection.[15] Commercial female and male sex workers comprise another group commonly found in jails and prisons who are at high risk for HIV through their sexual activity and frequently associated drug use. Additionally, persons entering jails have higher rates of sexually transmitted diseases than the general population and bring further opportunities for co-infection with HIV.[16]

Incarcerated women, in general, have a higher rate of HIV seroprevalence than incarcerated men. Incarcerated women are more likely to be drug users than incarcerated men, and have more associated risks such as economic dependency, physically abusive partners, or histories of childhood sexual abuse.[17] A study of incarcerated women in Massachusetts found that those who had a history of sexual abuse were more likely to have HIV infection, to have been a sex worker or an injection drug user, and to have abnormal Papanicolaou smear results than women without a history of abuse.[18]

Concern and misconceptions exist among inmates, staff, and the general public about the transmission of HIV within jails and prisons. Based on the best estimates, the events that could lead to HIV transmission, such as sexual activity, injection drug use, or blood exposure, occur less frequently within the controlled correctional environment than in the general population. But when these events do occur, and since protective measures are unavailable, the exposure risk can be much greater, based on a higher prevalence of infected persons in prison and the circumstances of the behavior.

Most correctional institutions have implemented policies to reduce the risk of blood exposures to staff. The practice of universal precautions and the wide availability of gloves significantly reduce the risk. As of 1994, no job-related cases of HIV infection among correctional officers have been reported to the Centers of Disease Control and Prevention.[19] Occupational exposures to bloodborne pathogens in the over 100,000 correctional health care workers has not been well characterized, but some suggest that the risks are higher than those in other health care settings.[20] This results from not only higher patient prevalence rates, but also problems relating to staffing, equipment, supplies, amount of safety training, and lack of in-house health programs.

The risk for inmates, however, is much higher than that for staff. Transmission of HIV has occurred among inmates, although the true incidence is unknown. A prospective study of HIV transmission among prison inmates was done at the Illinois Department of Corrections in 1988. Researchers enrolled 2,459 male inmates for HIV testing upon entry into the prison system after being at a county jail for a minimum of 90 days, and then repeated the testing 10–15 months later as part of a yearly physical examination. Of the 80 (3.25%) who had positive test results, eight had had negative test results at entrance. Thus, at least eight (0.33%) HIV seroconversions were observed.[21] The 90-day incarceration minimum prior to the initial testing was designed to eliminate any conversions that may have occurred during the window phase, yet such occurrences could not be completely ruled out. Another study in Florida during 1991 found 18 long-term inmates, who had been incarcerated since at least 1977, to be infected with HIV.[22] If HIV was not present in the general population prior to 1977, then it was argued that these infections occurred within the correctional setting. Additionally, several anecdotal reports have confirmed the transmission of HIV within prisons related to sexual transmission and injection drug use.[23]

Reliable information on the occurrence of high-risk behaviors for HIV transmission within jails and prisons is difficult to obtain. The data on sexual activity within prison are inconsistent and vary widely. Variations result from factors such as reporting accuracy, terminology, definitions, sample selections, age of participants, length of sentences, security classification, location, and methods of the survey. Most studies find, however, that the preponderance of sexual activity is consensual rather than rape, and that both events occur less often than commonly believed by the general population. In one study of a Delaware prison in 1994, only 2% of male inmates reported sexual encounters with other males; fewer than 1% reported attempted rapes; less than 25% reported ever witnessing consensual sex in prison; while 11% claimed to have had sexual encounters with other females (i.e., visitors, correctional officers, or female inmates).[24] A study of Ohio prisoners in 1989 found nearly 20% reporting sexual contact with at least one other inmate while in prison, and less than 10% claimed ever being forced or threatened into a sexual act.[25] Of particular concern, however, is when a sexually promiscuous inmate

engages in activities with multiple persons, sometimes for money or other goods. The multiple exposures with multiple individuals increase the risk of HIV transmission among all involved.

As with data on sexual activity, data on syringe use of illicit drugs within prisons vary.[26] Nevertheless, anecdotal reports confirm that it occurs with regularity, including deaths of inmates from injection drug overdoses. A study of Tennessee inmates in 1982 found 28% used an intravenous drug while incarcerated.[27] A 1988 study of six South Carolina correctional institutions found that more than 40% of inmates reported knowledge of needle-sharing among certain inmates in the past year.[28] Importantly, because syringes are relatively difficult to find in jail or prison, they are almost always shared.[29] A survey of Canadian inmates found that more than 80% believed bleach should be available to prisoners because of their knowledge of needle-use patterns within the system.[30] Similar to an inmate who is being sexually promiscuous, a single needle can make the rounds to many individuals, creating a high-risk situation.

Even though most persons are aware of the major transmission risks for HIV, the behavior of some persons entering and leaving prisons suggest that a certain level of risk is acceptable to them. A study of detainees entering the St. Louis jail found that only one-quarter used recommended safe-sex practices, such as consistently using a condom, having only one partner, or being celibate. Almost one third took no steps to protect themselves from HIV infection, while others believed that they could avoid HIV by choosing healthy or clean-looking partners, assessing a partner's job or social status, insisting that the partner washes before sex, and other practices. For many, if the partner was involved in another primary relationship, such as the spouse of another, then he or she was considered safe.[31]

Another study found that incarcerated juveniles in Los Angeles had knowledge, attitude, and beliefs about AIDS that put them at much higher risk than other youth their age. The study measured responses about AIDS among four groups of adolescents: urban public high school students, suburban private school students, gay teenagers in a youth organization, and incarcerated juveniles. The incarcerated juveniles possessed the least knowledge about HIV transmission, had the least perceived threat of AIDS, felt the least personal efficacy in avoiding AIDS, and believed the norm of their peers was least likely to use a condom or practice safe sex.[32] Fortunately, the prevalence of HIV infection in adolescents is relatively low, and a higher prevalence has not been clearly observed in samples of incarcerated juveniles.[33] Nevertheless, given the much higher rate of HIV infection in incarcerated adults, it is these attitudes and beliefs that likely cause infection.

But educational deficits, cultural patterns, or perceived invulnerability do not explain fully why persons continue high-risk behaviors for HIV. Intravenous drug users, for example, show a high degree of awareness of HIV risk in general, but tend to minimize their risk over the chance to get high. Some individuals resist safe-sex practices because a condom is perceived to threaten the primary sexual relationship by conveying a lack of trust in or respect for the intimate partner. For certain women, the use of condoms has been linked to an increased risk of violence from an abusive partner. For women who are HIV-infected, the expectation of a violent response from their partner might cause them to resist notifying the partner of the infection.[34] For some young people, unprotected sex and pregnancy are means to obtain something tangible in lives filled with violence and uncertainty.[35] People at high risk for HIV have no less an interest than others in initiating and sustaining intimate sexual relationships and creating life accomplishments. Failure to reconcile these powerful desires with risky behaviors can leave a person susceptible.[36]

For prevention to be effective, it must address all of the attitudes, behaviors, and environmental conditions that increase an inmate's risk for HIV infection. Information alone is not sufficient to induce permanent changes in the deeply ingrained or addictive behaviors that place a person at risk. Ingredients of an effective program should include training on basic information, access to materials for implementing safe behavior, and addressing the complex emotional, interpersonal, and cultural context in which high-risk behaviors occur and persist. Strategies should include communication face to face in understandable language, an engaging delivery of messages, working to change peers' attitudes toward sex and drug use, imparting social and recovery skills, and continuously assisting persons to avoid relapses into unsafe behavior.[37] Such prevention strategies should begin within the institution, and the knowledge and tools to prevent HIV infection should follow the inmate when he returns to the community. Prevention strategies would benefit from the following components.

Educational sessions about HIV. Although most people are probably better informed about HIV than they were during the 1980s, areas of uncertainty and misinformation remain. This is particularly true with many persons within jails and prisons. For some inmates, incarceration might be their first opportunity to receive accurate risk-reduction information. Basics on HIV disease, including the modes of transmission, the shift in incidence rates to drug users and heterosexuals, the cleaning of drug paraphernalia, proper use of condoms and lubricants, and the most risky practices, need continuous reinforcement. Myths about identifying potentially infected persons based on appearance or status must be discussed. The education can be accomplished through lectures, pamphlets, videos, workbooks, and other learning materials, but learning is most enhanced with input and questions from the inmates. Care should be given so that instructions are culturally sensitive, interesting, and at the appropriate education level. Another issue to be taken seriously is the extent to which certain groups, particularly minority populations, believe that HIV was deliberately introduced into the population for genocidal purposes. This belief makes it important to have HIV education programs presented by persons with credibility among inmates who are able to develop rapport with the audience.[38]

Peer education. Some of the most effective learning programs come from the language and experiences of inmates themselves. Typical pressures and beliefs of inmates are best understood by other inmates. Programs delivered by carefully selected and trained peer educators may be more meaningful for inmates since peers can speak in terms relevant to them. Peer educators are able to do substantial informal one-on-one outreach and support throughout the facility, as well as conducting formal education, counseling, and support groups. Peers living with HIV who are willing to openly discuss their situation can be particularly powerful. Such revelations can penetrate the sense of invulnerability found in many persons.

Substance abuse treatment. Given the close association of HIV transmission and substance abuse, programs to overcome chemical addictions and alcohol or drug misuse is an essential piece of HIV prevention. The effectiveness of substance abuse treatment varies widely according to the quality of the program. Counseling alone would not be expected to sustain risk reduction behavior. Most drug-using offenders generally have lifestyles characterized by hedonistic, self-destructive, and antisocial behaviors. They also have problems related to poor social skills, the absence of job training, and dependence on others. To be effective, a program must address these issues. The most success has been found in programs where funding is at least adequate, personnel are well-trained and emotionally involved, and the treatment programs are carefully planned and implemented.[39]

HIV testing. Persons at risk for HIV infection should be encouraged to have HIV antibody testing. The testing process provides an opportunity for risk assessment and prevention education. For persons who have negative test results, proper counseling can motivate safer behavior for future activities. Sometimes even the anxiety that can accompany the test will serve as a behavior modifier in itself. For persons who are identified as being infected with HIV, comprehensive counseling should be offered that includes education about reducing the risks of reinfection or transmission to others. Several studies do provide convincing evidence that risk behavior is reduced in many who are found to be HIV positive and appropriately counseled.[40] Nevertheless, single pre-test and post-test counseling sessions should not be expected to cause sustained behavioral changes in all individuals. Several sessions, as well as a variety of additional interventions, are required to achieve substantial behavioral risk reduction.

Condoms and bleach. Because activities known to transmit HIV occur with some frequency within a correctional environment, and because these activities are often riskier than if practiced on the outside because of higher concentrations of infected persons, many have advocated for condoms and bleach or needles for inmates. Most correctional officials, however, do not provide these materials to inmates. Part of the concern is that, since sexual activity and injection drug use are prohibited within the institutions, providing protective items might be perceived as condoning those behaviors. Another part of the concern is that the items might be used as weapons or to conceal drugs or other contraband.

A few institutions have made condoms available for inmates. At present, only three prison systems (Mississippi, Washington, D.C., and Vermont) allow inmates to have condoms. Four jail systems (San Francisco, Philadelphia, New York, and Washington, D.C.) also make condoms available. As an example, the Washington, D.C. jail offers condoms free of charge to inmates during HIV pre- or post-test counseling, during health education classes, and when requested privately in sick call. No security-related problems have occurred as a result of the condoms. The practice is quietly and widely accepted by the staff, inmates, and administration. While the demand for condoms is not large, a small number of requests do occur regularly.

On the other hand, no system officially provides bleach for inmates. At least two jail systems, (San Francisco and Houston) however, have bleach available in the institutions. The Canadian prison system makes small quantities of bleach easily accessible to inmates, and a Swiss prison has a needle exchange program. In systems where bleach is available, very few security problems have been reported.[41]

Integration with community resources. Most communities have public or private agencies that provide HIV prevention information and support services for those living with HIV. State and local health departments provide HIV counseling and testing services in hundreds of correctional institutions in the United States. Joining forces with such agencies can be an effective means to expand HIV prevention and services to inmates. Often, the agencies have not been invited to provide services to the incarcerated population but would be excited to have the opportunity. Several federally funded HIV prevention programs are even required to collaborate with juvenile and adult correctional systems.[42]

Needle exchange programs. Needle exchange programs exist in many cities as a means to reduce the risk of HIV transmission among injection drug users. Much evidence has accumulated to show that needle exchange programs significantly reduce the transmission of HIV among injection drug users without stimulating increased use among nonusers.[43] In addition to providing access to sterile injection equipment, community outreach has been shown to be important in maintaining low HIV seroprevalence in populations of drug users.[44] Given the high likelihood that many, if not most, injection drug users in a community will pass through the correctional system, providing informa-

tion about local needle exchange programs is critical in making the program successful.

Referrals for inmates being released. Inmates being released from jail or prison often return to environments and behaviors that put them at high risk for HIV. Even some who had the best of intentions while incarcerated find old habits too difficult to leave, once given new freedom and absence of structure. Others find building a new life too difficult or uncomfortable and find solace in familiar environments and behaviors. Providing community contacts for inmates can assist them in making a safer and healthier transition. For example, some inmates will benefit from alcohol or drug rehabilitation centers. Female inmates should be made aware of resources to which they can turn, if they find themselves in abusive relationships that might put them at risk for HIV.

Information on HIV prevention may be provided to inmates upon discharge from their facilities. These packets might include condoms and lists of service agencies, such as needle exchange programs or HIV testing centers. This process is done in some facilities with a high degree of acceptance.

Discharge planning for inmates with HIV. Assistance should be offered to inmates with HIV infection to develop a plan for accessing services upon their release. Connections should be made to medical care, housing, employment training, drug treatment, and support groups. Without such interventions, the health of many might deteriorate and some might return to behaviors that transmit HIV. In a 1993 study of 55 HIV-infected drug users paroled in New York, 67% relapsed into drug use even though most had participated in a drug treatment program in prison. Post-relapse was found to be associated with poor housing status, limited social support, lack for drug treatment, and less frequent visits with case managers.[45]

Post-exposure prophylaxis. Although taking proper precautions to avoid exposure is the primary means of preventing HIV infection, responding appropriately to a distinct and significant exposure may reduce the likelihood of infection. A typical scenario would be a needle-stick injury after drawing blood from an HIV-infected person. The average risk of infection from all types of percutaneous exposures to HIV-infected blood is 0.3%. However, significant variability exists with individual exposures. An exposure involving a large blood volume or blood from a patient with higher titers of HIV would greatly exceed 0.3%. The risk of HIV seroconversion is higher for exposures involving deep injuries, visible blood on the device causing the injury, a hollow-bore needle that had been in the source patient's vein or artery, and a source patient who dies of AIDS within 60 days of the exposure.[46]

The Centers for Disease Control and Prevention has issued provisional recommendations for chemoprophylaxis immediately following occupational percutaneous exposure to HIV-infected blood.[47] The recommendations are provisional because they are based on limited data regarding efficacy and toxicity of the drug regimen. Furthermore, changes in the regimen might be appropriate depending on the antiretroviral drug resistance profile of the source patient, potential drug toxicity in the recipient, concurrent drug therapies, or advances in antiretroviral therapies. In summary, the recommendations following exposure are:

1) Chemoprophylaxis is recommended after high-risk exposures. For lower risks, the potential benefits should be weighed with the uncertain efficacy and potential toxicity of the drugs. Post-exposure prophylaxis is not justified for exposures with a negligible risk.

2) Retrovir should be considered for all chemoprophylaxis regimens, usually with 3TC. A protease inhibitor, preferably indinavir, should be added for high-risk exposures.

3) The post-exposure prophylaxis should be initiated within 1 to 2 hours after exposure. Initiating therapy after a longer interval (even 1 to 2 weeks) may be considered for the highest risks. The optimal duration of treatment is unknown, but usually 4 weeks.

4) If the source patient's HIV status is unknown, prophylaxis should be made on a case-by-case basis.

5) Exposed persons should have HIV antibody tests at baseline, and periodically for at least 6 months after exposure. Drug toxicity monitoring, including base line complete blood cell counts, and renal and hepatic function tests at baseline should be done along with follow-up medical evaluations and counseling.

6) Persons receiving post-exposure prophylaxis are encouraged to enroll in an anonymous registry to assess toxicity by calling 888-737-4448. Institutions should prepare protocols for such occurrences in advance. Having prepackaged starter kits of the chemoprophylaxis medications available would avoid delays in initiating treatment.

Recommendations for initiating post-exposure prophylaxis after a sexual exposure, such as rape, have not yet been issued. The decision to provide such treatment should be based on a risk assessment of the exposure, including the serostatus of the other person, the type of exposure (anal, vaginal, oral, or ejaculation), and the nature of any physical injuries.[48]

Violence

Contrary to popular belief, a person is more likely to be killed in the streets than in prison. Homicide rates in the general population, 9.7 per 100,000 in 1994,[49] are higher than homicide rates in prisons, 4.7. This low rate of inmate-on-inmate homicide is remarkable, considering that prisons presumably have the highest concentration of society's violent persons. Furthermore, the general population homicide rate extends to all ages, races, and genders, whereas the prison rate is drawn from a population disproportionately consisting of the age, race, and gender groups at highest risk for homicide. That is not to say, however, that violence is less in prison, only that lethal non-sanctioned violence is less. One of the most important explanations for this discrepancy is that 70% of homicides in the United States occur with firearms.[50] Since inmates are not allowed to possess firearms, many violent events that might have been otherwise lethal are not.

Nevertheless, the potential for violence within jails and prisons is continuous. Crowded spaces, past and current rivalry and retaliation, exploitation, extortion, positioning, same-gender tensions, psychological behavioral disorders, boredom, frustration, minimized consequences, peer pressure, fear, intimidation, inequalities, power plays, dehumanization, and more conditions kindle violence within the crucible of jails and prisons. Whereas in the community, a person might have an opportunity to escape a violent environment or feel safer by establishing security measures, inmates are generally unable to do so. Consequently, many live with fear, apprehension, and anxiety. Many feel the need to maintain constant vigilance. Even the institutions or the persons meant to protect them can be threatening or harmful.

Many forms of violence occur against prisoners; some sanctioned and some not. In recent years, nearly the same number of inmates has been killed by correctional staff or through capital punishment as killed by other inmates.[51] Legally sanctioned executions are occurring with increasing frequency in the nation's prisons. Some have believed that these executions can have detrimental effects rather than reducing or deterring crime by imparting a devalued sense of human life and legitimizing lethal violence. Studies have shown, in fact, that in some states with capital punishment, certain patterns of homicide have increased following executions.[52] Within the small prison community, an execution impacts each person and is a difficult time for both the staff and inmates. Several institutions conduct trauma and stress management courses for members of the execution team because of the extreme emotion often associated with the death.[53] Little programming is routinely done for the surviving inmates. The potential for increasing an environment of violence must be considered.

The low rate of inmate-on-inmate violence-related deaths within prisons is a credit to the majority of correctional staff who perform well to maintain order and security within frequently adverse and difficult environments. Most officers do not misuse force, yet it does occur with regularity.[54] Legal instruments commonly used for controlling inmates include teaser guns, pepper spray and mace, stun guns, rubber bullets, K-9s (canines), .37 mm gas guns projecting wood blocks or rubber pellets, birdshot, side-handle batons, and stun shields. These can be easily misapplied. The policy of the American Correctional Association authorizes the use of force only when no reasonable alternative is possible, and permits only the minimal force necessary. It prohibits the use of force as a retaliatory or disciplinary measure. Lethal force is generally reserved for instances where there is an imminent threat to human life or threat to public safety that cannot be reasonably prevented by other means.[55] Yet over a 5-year period in California, more than two dozen inmates were shot and killed by correctional officers breaking up fights, a figure three times higher than all other states combined. This led to a state regulation in 1995, which struck the words "physically assaultive behavior," a reference to unarmed fights, from an official list of justifiable reasons for using firearms.[56] The irony is that the use of force and violence, which is what brought many persons to be incarcerated in the first place, is acceptable and reinforced within prison.

Assault injuries by inmates upon correctional employees also occur regularly, including occasional homicides. Fewer employees, however, are killed by inmates than inmates killed by employees. Over a 10-year period, starting in 1983, the rate of occupational homicide among correctional officers was 1.5 per 100,000 workers, compared to a rate of 0.7 per 100,000 for workers of all occupations. Many other occupations have higher homicide risks, including bartenders, barbers, and stock handlers. The occupational homicide risk for taxicab drivers is tenfold higher than that for correctional officers.[57] The occupational homicide risk for health care professionals is generally low,[58] and no data yet exist for health care workers within correctional institutions.

Medical resources are heavily used to respond to intentional injuries caused by other inmates or correctional staff. A study at Cook County Jail in Chicago in 1994 found that nearly one third of patients sent to an outside hospital were referred because of an intentional injury. Intentional injuries that occur within the institution, however, are not always the primary source of expenditures. The Cook County study examined more than 400 inmates accessing sick call and found that one in five had a complaint of a violence-related injury. The majority of the injuries (62%) occurred prior to the incarceration and involved gunshot wounds. Fifteen percent of the intentional injuries occurred at the time of their arrest, and only 23% occurred within the jail. The injuries that occurred prior to incarceration were associated with three times more complications than those occurring in the jail, attesting to the more serious nature, in general, of these injuries. Fifteen percent of the patients with violence-related complaints had permanent disabilities resulting from their injury, such as the loss of an eye or hearing, seizure disorders, or neurologic impairments.

Life in the streets has a much higher violent death risk than life in prison. Homicide rates are lower within prison, but change considerably when the person is released. Homicide is the leading single cause of premature death for young persons paroled from prison. A study of nearly 4,000 youths paroled from the California Youth Authority during

the 1980s found that 181 died within 10 years of parole, 54% from homicides. For these youth, their rate of homicide increased more than fivefold over similar youth matched within the same high-risk age and race groups.[59] The Illinois Department of Corrections found that homicide was the cause of death for 50% of parolee deaths in the early 1990s.[60] In large urban areas in the United States, reports have found that 44%–67% of homicide victims have prior criminal records or were on parole.

The reason for the increased risk of homicide in persons released from jail or prison is a matter of conjecture. No study has carefully examined this phenomenon. Some homicides might be related to the former inmate's original offense or consequences of events that occurred during the incarceration. Other explanations might include the application of risky attitudes and behaviors acquired in prison that reward aggression, power, and strength. Persons released from jail or prison often find themselves disconnected from their communities, uprooted from meaningful relationships, and unaccepted by the majority of society. Their opportunities have been reduced, and assimilation is difficult. Many face obstacles in obtaining meaningful employment; in fact, many laws, licensing restrictions, and civil service rules exclude them from many types of jobs.[61] The interplay of these factors with the easy availability of firearms in the community likely increase their homicide risk.

Involvement in the criminal justice system may be the single best predictor of the probability that a person becomes injured or killed through violence.[62] In the California youth study, higher probability of death for parolees was observed in youths with a history of gang involvement, institutional violence, and a history of drug arrests. Similar risk factors were observed in a study of adolescent assault-related firearm injuries in Richmond, Virginia, where court-involved adolescents had a firearm injury prevalence more than 13 times greater than their non–court-involved peers.[63] Detainees of Cook County Jail who had prior gunshot wounds were three times more likely to have been in jail before than those who had never been shot.[64] Surveys of assault victims found that violent offenders were much more likely to be victims of assault themselves than non-violent offenders.[65]

In many ways, violence behaves as a chronic disease with an ominous prognosis. One study found that, among patients admitted to a trauma center for assault-related injuries, 20% died over the next 5 years. A history of violence-related injuries signals a person at high risk for future injuries. Given the extraordinary histories of violence among the incarcerated and their high risk of violence-related death upon parole, attention needs to be given to appropriate prevention strategies and interventions.

The potential for a violent event is omnipresent within jails and prisons. Preventing a violent disturbance is a top priority of jail and prison officials. While corrections play a central role anticipating, minimizing, controlling, and responding to violence, medical services have a role beyond their traditional tertiary response to the wounded. The notion of preventing violence through a public health model gained momentum in the 1980s. Since that time, numerous programs and interventions have emerged to identify and respond to the many factors that precipitate violent events. The prevention of violence can be accomplished in several ways.

Data collection. Data are an important starting point. Collecting data on events or conditions such as the prevalence of prior injuries in patients, the occurrence of in-house injuries, or resources used to respond to violence-related injuries can be useful in developing prevention strategies. Discovering a paucity of data on intentional injuries, the National Research Council of the National Academy of Sciences recommended in 1992 that high priority be placed on expanding statistical information for "counts and descriptions of violent events that are receiving considerable public attention but are poorly counted by existing measurement systems. These include . . . jails and prisons."[66] Without understanding the factors contributing to violence-related events, prevention would be less effective.

Few institutions presently track injuries, whether intentional or unintentional, yet delineation of the precipitating factors for these injuries is essential for prevention. In 1994, the Michigan Department of Corrections began to monitor the number of inmates with acute unintentional injury (occurring during recreational, occupational, and other activities) and acute intentional injuries (assault and self-inflicted). While the number of unintentional injuries was nearly fourfold greater than that for intentional injuries, temporal studies found the assault injuries to be closely correlated to the timing of recreational injuries, suggesting that some inmates reported an assault injury as a recreational injury to avoid official investigation or retribution by a perpetrator.[67] The Hawaii Department of Public Safety and Correctional facilities similarly found higher rates of unintentional injuries versus assault-related injuries, yet their overall injury rates were less than half of those occurring in Michigan.[68] This illustrates the multifactorial basis to injury-related events, and suggests that if injuries can be prevented in one system, they could be reduced in another.

Documentation of in-house injuries. Violence-related injuries within institutions should be monitored and documented. This can be done with a typical risk management model. Information on the type of injury, method, category of assaulter (such as inmate, correctional officer, or other staff), location, and circumstance can be useful. Maintaining an accurate account of violence-related injuries serves many purposes. Often patterns or trends in the injuries become apparent and then prevention strategies can be developed. For example, an investigation of frequent fights in one particular area of the institution might find

overcrowded conditions, which could then be remedied. Intentional injuries from staff might even be reduced by the very act of documenting the occurrences.

Documentation of prior violence-related injuries. Often, medical records do not reflect a history of violence-related injuries. A common finding would be the chart of a young woman who appears to be in good health, but makes no mention of an arm fracture that occurred earlier at the hands of her boyfriend; or the chart of a young man which describes him as in good health, but failed to note a gunshot wound that occurred some time ago. Failure to document violence-related injuries ignores a significant risk factor for future violence-related injuries and diminishes the significance of those events. Inquiries of prior violence-related injuries should be made of all patients. Even the discussion of the event can be therapeutic for some or provide an opportunity to discuss prevention messages for others. The findings should be noted in the chart so that they can serve as a prompt for practitioners to continuously screen and address risks of future violence-related injuries.

Support during treatment of injuries. An opportunity for secondary prevention occurs when patients are being treated for a violence-related injury. Care must be given to avoid inappropriate or offensive comments, rather, words should be nonjudgmental and supportive. Practitioners should recognize the opportunity to convey essential messages. For some patients, the injury might have forced them to face the potential for their own mortality for the first time. This might be the time they are most receptive to reassuring and reasonable advice. Within hospitals or infirmaries or emergency departments, case managers, social workers, peer counselors, or other trained individuals can meet with patients to discuss the circumstances of their injury and how subsequent injuries might be prevented. Traumatic event counseling, of the sort traditionally offered for rape victims, could be available for anyone recovering from an intentional injury.

In a survey of 364 male and female detainees in Chicago who had been hospitalized at any time for violence-related injuries, only 41% recalled anything said by their doctor or nurse. Of those, only 23% recalled any reassuring words, such as, "Do you have a safe place to stay?", while others recalled negative comments, such as, "Stop complaining that it hurts!"[69]

During wound cleaning, bandaging, or suturing of a wound, practitioners can provide helpful and important information to patients. A useful mnemonic to guide responses during treatment of an intentional injury utilizes the word "suture":

-S: Reassure the patient that he is now SAFE and will be okay.

-U: Be certain to UNDERSTAND the circumstances of the injury.

-T: TEACH about the risks for violence-related injuries.

-U: URGE nonviolent resolutions to conflict.

-R: Inquire about and discourage thoughts of violent RETALIATION.

-E: Provide EMPATHY about the event, and ENCOURAGE safer options.

Services for victims of violence. Persons who have been victims of violence can carry psychological as well as physical scars. Often, perpetrators of violence have been previously victimized themselves. The trauma of witnessing violent events can also impact a person's life. Children who are exposed to violence, either as a victim or by witnessing a violent injury or death, can develop post-traumatic stress syndrome.[70] Violent victimization can diminish a person's sense of self, reduce hope for the future, and impair the ability to form trusting interpersonal relationships. Many youth, especially boys, who witness violence turn to weapon carrying for protection.[71]

This creates a cycle of violence. Breaking the cycle requires support and counseling services for those victims of violence. A variety of treatments can be offered, depending on the exact nature of the problem. These might include group discussions, individual psychotherapy, role-playing exercises, art or poetry therapy, spiritual counseling, and more. Personalized interventions are the best because, for many, the trauma of violence victimization is debilitating and their coping mechanisms can be fragile.

Identification of high risks. Screening can be useful for identifying those patients at highest risk for violence-related injuries. The screening should be appropriate for the population and with knowledge of the greatest risk factors. Women, often the victims of domestic violence, and young men, often the victims of street violence, can have different risk factors for and circumstances of victimization.

Domestic violence is often unrecognized and unaddressed in the clinical setting. For most women, the greatest risk of physical, emotional, and sexual violation will be from a man they have known and trusted, often an intimate partner. In the United States, more than 50% of women who are murdered are killed by male intimates.[72] Still, many health care practitioners do not feel comfortable asking women about violence for fear of being personally or professionally overwhelmed by the responses. Failing to do so, however, can leave a patient open for continuing injury.[73] Routine screening, recognizing, and treating manifestations of domestic violence for women is increasingly becoming a standard of care in medicine.

Use of the acronym "RADAR" has been suggested as a practical tool in clinical settings.[74] This includes

-R: Remember to ask about violence and victimization in the course of the routine patient encounter.

-A: Ask directly, "Have you been hit, kicked, punched, or otherwise hurt by someone within the past year? If so, by whom?"

-D: Document findings in the medical record.

-A: Assess safety.

-R: Review options and refer as appropriate.

Using these questions about physical injuries in the emergency department has been shown to detect a majority of women who have a history of physical partner violence.[75]

Screening young men for risk of violence includes inquiring about prior fights, injuries, and lifestyles. Most men are victimized by other men, and the characteristics of persons most at risk for violent crime are shared by the incarcerated population: young, poor, undereducated, and male.[76] The risks increase for those using alcohol and illicit drugs, trafficking drugs, gun carrying, and having prior exposure to violence.[77] It has been suggested that the risks for a gunshot injury are even more specific for this population. A study of detainees at Cook County Jail found five factors more common in men who had been shot[78]: 1) previously been in jail, 2) seen someone get shot sometime before high school, 3) prior sexually transmitted disease, 4) gang-related tattoo, and 5) easy access to a semiautomatic weapon.

These factors were significantly associated with prior gunshot wounds and could be used to identify the young men at highest risk for firearm injuries.

Counseling about firearms. The United States' excessive homicide rate relative to other countries is predominately consisting of firearm deaths.[79] The majority of young adult homicides and suicides are the result of gunshot wounds. Young adults in the United States are more likely to die from firearms than all natural causes combined.[80] Children in the United States are 12 times more likely to die from firearms than children in at least 25 other industrialized countries.[81] Guns have become the leading health risk for young people in the United States.

Many juvenile and adult inmates came from environments where guns and gunfire are commonplace. The health risk of the gun becomes minimized for many inmates by its potential to gain power and respect, however ill-fated. Participants in the illicit drug industry are especially likely to carry guns. In these settings, guns are used largely as an instrument of dispute resolution. Also, for some young people, arming themselves is a way to build status. Consequently, and given the recklessness and bravado often characteristic of young people, many of the fights that would otherwise have taken place and resulted in no arrests or serious injury can turn into a crime and substantial injury or death because of the presence of a gun.[82] Had many youth not had access to a firearm, jails and prisons would be less crowded, and hospitals and morgues would be less busy.

Reducing a patient's risk for firearm injury or death includes imparting knowledge on the health consequences of keeping guns. Instead of providing protection, the medical literature has shown that a gun increases the risk of injury or death. Homes with guns are five times more likely to be sites of a suicide, three times more likely to be sites of a homicide, and the victim of the homicide is 18 times more likely to be a member of the household than a stranger.[83] A study of detainees at Cook County Jail found that those who had easy access to a semiautomatic weapon were twice as likely to have been shot than those who did not have such access.[84] For many young people, a message from a health care professional that a gun can increase their risk of injury or death is welcomed. One study found that counseling about guns was the preventive health issue that patients remembered more than any other issue.[85]

While effecting a change in the environment to which an inmate is being released is more difficult, addressing behaviors and attitudes pertaining to firearms is a place to start in reducing firearm deaths. Counseling patients about firearms includes assessing the risk and providing appropriate advice on reducing that risk. Using the mnemonic "GUNS,"[86] where each letter of the word prompts a question, can assist in guiding the discussion:

-G: Do you keep a GUN?
-U: Are you around USERS of alcohol or other drugs?
-N: Do you feel a NEED to protect yourself?
-S: Do any of these SITUATIONS apply:
Seen, or been involved in, acts of violence?
Sadness, depression, or mental illness?
School-aged children at home?

Affirmative answers to any of the questions in "GUNS" indicate significant risk for firearm injuries or deaths. Patients should be advised of the risks in these situations and ways to overcome them without firearms.

Create an environment supportive of violence alternatives. For violence prevention to be meaningful and effective within an institution, the entire staff, medical and non-medical, must embrace the goal of reducing violence. This includes an atmosphere where verbal or sexual harassment is not tolerated, physical altercations are shunned, the use of force is monitored and justified, victims are supported, and perpetrators are investigated and appropriately corrected. Violent altercations should not be a source of entertainment or jokes. Creating an environment that is supportive of violence prevention can also include displaying posters, brochures, and other materials with violence prevention messages. A broad campaign of violence prevention using lectures, educational videos, and resource manuals can sensitize staff and inmates to the importance of the issue.

Cooperation with correctional staff. Because a primary responsibility of the correctional staff is to maintain security, medical staff should be mindful of policies and procedures established to prevent violent occurrences. Medical staff must also be careful to not inadvertently precipitate violent events by issuing devices that can readily be used as weapons. This is especially a concern for health care workers providing only episodic care to inmates.[87] Medical staff can also communicate concerns or suspicions of impending violence with correctional staff. Upon treating patients with intentional injuries, inquiries should be made of the correctional staff's plan to protect the patient from future harm.

Education on violence prevention. Educating inmates about violence, risks factors, and prevention strategies can be done with programming modeled after other health education issues. Many institutions have initiated programs teaching conflict resolution, anger management, firearm risks, and peer mediation. Resources such as videos, slides, brochures, and posters are available and can be helpful. Because many of the materials and approaches are new, comprehensive or long-term evaluations have not been completed to measure effectiveness. Short-term evaluations, however, have shown some success with these strategies; yet, whether such success can be maintained has yet to be determined.[88]

Smoking

Cigarette smoking has been linked to a variety of adverse health outcomes, including heart disease, stroke, chronic obstructive pulmonary disease, low birth weights, and lung and other cancers. For decades it has been recognized to be the single most preventable cause of disease and death in our society.[89] Even for nonsmokers, exposure to environmental tobacco smoke (ETS) has been shown to cause chronic cardiac and respiratory diseases in adults, and asthma and acute respiratory infections in children.[90, 91]

The health impacts of smoking and ETS are a particularly important concern in correctional institutions, since this single-most cause of preventable death is one of the most common behaviors among inmates. While the prevalence of smoking in the general population is approximately 23%, the prevalence of smoking among inmates may exceed 80%—nearly fourfold higher.[92] The higher prevalence may be attributed to differences in demographic characteristics of prison and jail inmates vs. the general population, but also to the confinement and prison culture itself. Historically, the attitudes of jail and prison administrators toward cigarette smoking have been very tolerant.[93] Administrators have generally regarded smoking as one of prisoners' basic rights, and they have accepted the associated negative aspects of smoking, such as fights among prisoners over cigarettes, fires, littering of butts and ashes, and smuggling of contraband in cigarettes and their packaging. To further legitimize smoking, cigarettes are often an unofficial currency of institutions. At Cook County Jail, a pack of cigarettes is the pay for a day's work in the kitchen. Other institutions actually manufacture cigarettes as their industry product.[94] Tobacco is distributed at no cost or at greatly reduced prices in some prisons, and used as a reward for good behavior or subtle manipulation in others. For prisoners, the nicotine can stimulate or relax, reduce tension, and alleviate boredom.

While it is not possible to judge the precise health impact of cigarette smoking in prisons and jails based on current evidence, heart disease and lung cancer are leading causes of death among older, long-term prisoners.[95] Cigarette smoking contributes greatly to these deaths. The impact of ETS exposures by nonsmoking prisoners and corrections workers has not been studied, but its immediate effects are illustrated by asthma exacerbations and sinus-related problems. Exposures to ETS are substantial in many correctional facilities, and increased by the combination of the high prevalence of smokers, overcrowding, and old buildings with inadequate ventilation. An environmental air quality survey in a medium-sized New Mexico jail found respirative particulate levels more than three times the federal health standard and nicotine levels five times higher than a smoking section of a restaurant. Soon after these findings, the jail became smoke free.[96] Obviously, the opportunity for adverse health effects among nonsmokers in jails or prisons is large.

In recent years, the awareness of the health impacts of smoking has increased. Resolutions and statements in support of the implementation of no-smoking policies were adopted in 1990 by the American Jail Association and in 1993 by the American Correctional Health Services Association. Change has also been forced by clean indoor air regulations enacted by local and state authorities for publicly-owned buildings, and by workplace smoking standards.[97] Lawsuits brought by nonsmoking inmates against state and federal prison authorities to obtain separate living areas have provided impetus for change.[98] As the scientific evidence for the hazards to health from ETS has accumulated, and the societal standards on the provision of no-smoking areas have changed, the courts have considered these suits more seriously.[99] Involuntary and continuous exposure to high ETS conditions were argued to be cruel and unusual punishment under the Eighth Amendment. In September 1993, the United States Supreme Court, in *Helling v. McKinney,* ruled that inmates have a constitutional right be free from unreasonable risks to future health problems from exposure to environmental smoke.[100] On the other hand, prisoners seeking protection from the courts for the right to smoke have had little or no success.[101]

Change to restrict smoking in correctional facilities, however, has not come easily. This is partly because, relative to other institutions, jails and prisons have unique constraints. For example, reduction of exposure to ETS by separating smokers and nonsmokers is often impractical because of overcrowding and severe space limitations. Furthermore, while separation within the same air space might reduce exposures of nonsmokers to ETS, it might not completely eliminate their exposure, because substantial amounts of ETS may be recirculated by mechanical ventilation systems throughout buildings.[102] Large reductions in ETS pollution inside buildings can, in most cases, only be achieved by establishing separately ventilated spaces that are directly exhausted to the outside. Retrofitting or constructing new buildings with separate ventilation systems is very expensive.

Clearly, the most effective policy is to go entirely smoke free, and a growing number of jails and prisons are doing so. By early 1997, at least 13 state prison systems were either making the transition to be smoke free, or were entirely smoke free, including the two largest systems, California and Texas.[103] A smoke-free environment is what many inmates might actually prefer, but are unlikely to admit. A survey of more than 400 detainees entering the Washington, D.C. jail found that while two thirds smoke, 69% had previously tried to quit and 78% wanted to quit.[104]

But many jail and prison administrators are reluctant to accept smoke-free recommendations from their medical personnel for fear of discontent and violence, yet this is not widely observed.[105] A study in the Texas Department of Criminal Justice found that, during implementation of its tobacco-free policy in 1995, stress, tension, and assaults did increase somewhat, but this was also during a time of tremendous expansion of the inmate population, and so it cannot be said that these increases were due to the tobacco-free policy. On the other hand, several benefits to the department including cleaner facilities, cleaner air, healthier environments, and fewer medical problems were noted by the wardens.[106] The available anecdotal evidence suggests that smoking restriction policies are often implemented without protest, and that in addition to the benefits of improved indoor air quality and cleanliness, there are substantial improvements in fire safety and health.[107] After implementation of its smoke-free policy, the Oregon Department of Corrections noted marked reductions in intentional fires, including none during a major disturbance for an unrelated issue.[108] The medical staff of Utah Department of Corrections found a 20% reduction in respiratory complaints including sinusitis and bronchitis 1 year after its facilities became smoke free.[109]

Information on ways to implement smoke-free policies in corrections facilities is sparse and scattered, but the National Institute of Corrections (Longmont, Colorado), the American Jail Association (Hagerstown, Maryland), and the U.S. Department of Justice (Washington) collect information from local and state organizations and distribute it upon request. Review of these materials from corrections systems that have successfully made the transition to smoke-free policies suggests a common approach: 1) educate policymakers on benefits of change; 2) present policymakers with realistic transition plan; 3) seek input on the plan for change from prisoners and staff; 4) set a time line for gradual reduction of cigarette sales to prisoners; 5) provide clear notice of intent in advance to staff and prisoners; 6) provide smoking-cessation training to staff; 7) offer smoking-cessation materials to prisoners; 8) adjust prisoners' meals, snacks, and recreation to support efforts to quit; and 9) clearly establish and document operations procedures for maintenance of the tobacco-free policy.

The adoption of a smoke-free policy represents a drastic change, and a successful transition requires commitment from the top levels of the administration down through all operational elements. Administrators and other decision makers need to be educated about the health and safety benefits associated with elimination of smoking, the reduced health care costs, and the legal liabilities gained through change. Full endorsement of the need for change must be clearly communicated from the administration to operations. Once the directive for change is announced, planning for implementation should begin with input from staff and prisoners. Again, education of mid-level administration, operations, and prisoners on the reasons for change will be needed to increase acceptance. The time spent on education will engage the stakeholders, solidify commitment, and provide an opportunity for participation, which will, in turn, generate constructive ideas for crafting the plan for transition.

A typical timeline for the phase-out of smoking is provided in Table 22-3. Incremental restriction of cigarette sales over a 30-day period has been most frequently used, although periods of up to 90 days have been used with success. With advance notice of restriction on the volume of cigarettes sold, inmates can mentally prepare themselves for acceptance of the change. In a series of steps, the number of packs of cigarettes are repeatedly cut in half, until finally, 1 week before cigarettes are declared contraband, all sales are stopped. Correspondingly, the distribution of lighting materials and matches are restricted without notice 1 to 2 weeks in advance of the end of cigarette sales to prevent hoarding of matches and reducing the opportunity for fires to be started in protest of the ban on smoking. Floor officers need to be provided with lighters to assist those still smoking who no longer have matches. On the last day to possess, searches of property are usually not necessary because prisoners will soon smoke all available cigarettes.

To provide an environment that is supportive of prisoners' efforts to quit smoking, adjustments are usually made in snacks, meals, and recreation. Preferences for snacks and favorite foods can be sought from prisoners during the planning process. In this way, canteen orders and meal planning can begin in advance of the change. A strategy of providing additional fluids (e.g., water, fruit juices), snack foods (e.g., popcorn, crackers), and hard candies has been universally used with success. Changes in television viewing, library privileges, and recreation schedules vary with institutional preferences and practical aspects of prisoner management, but can be effective outlets for stress reduction and coping with nicotine withdrawal. Distribution of literature on smoking cessation, and individual and group counseling by medical staff on ways to quit may be useful, although at the early stages of the transition most prisoners will not take advantage of this information.

Officers and all other staff, regardless of level of contact with prisoners, should receive smoking-cessation training early in the transition. This should include an understanding of the stages of behavioral change. The stages of change

Table 22-3. Example of a schedule to phase out smoking in a jail

Date	Action
January 2	Notice of intent: 30-day advance notice of intent to phase out smoking
February 1	Limit of 5 packs per weekly canteen order
February 8	Limit of 3 packs per weekly canteen order
February 15	Limit of 2 packs per weekly canteen order. With no advance notice to prisoners, matches are no longer distributed by the canteen
February 22	Limit of 1 pack per weekly canteen order. Cigarettes no longer sold by the canteen after this date
February 29	Last day to possess: Cigarettes and lighting materials are considered contraband after this date

consist of precontemplation (belief that the benefits far outweigh any negative effects of a behavior), contemplation (ambivalence about the positive and negative effects of a behavior), preparation (committing to change of behavior), action (the behavior is changed), and maintenance (interventions to prevent relapse).[110] Everyone should appreciate that the institutional elimination of smoking forces smokers to move abruptly into the action phase with little time for contemplation, which may heighten anxieties.

Increasing the awareness of the benefits of quitting should also be part of in-service training, along with developing sensitivities to the difficulties associated with nicotine withdrawal. Lessons on the physiologic aspects of withdrawal will allow personnel to appreciate the value of additional fluids or the need to adjust recreation schedules to accommodate efforts by prisoners to cope with changes in their bodies. Role playing will help staff anticipate issues that might occur during the transition and later as the policy is enforced among incoming prisoners. Smoking cessation training can build skills in medical staff, social workers, clergy, and counselors whose encouragement and assistance may be sought by prisoners who are anticipating the impending challenges of quitting. In short, all staff having contact with prisoners should be provided with basic skills in smoking cessation and problem solving, because prisoners can be expected to seek help from the most available person at the time of their particular need during withdrawal.

Although expensive, some jails and prisons also provide nicotine replacement to inmates. Transdermal nicotine, nicotine gum, and nasal sprays have been demonstrated to be efficacious treatments to assist patients to stop smoking.[111] Patches can be particularly useful in the correctional setting because of their ease of distribution. When the state of Utah became smoke free, special contracts were arranged with manufacturers of nicotine patches. These were made available to inmates at a reduced price through a doctor's prescription. The Oregon Department of Corrections Health Services Division assisted its inmates in going smoke free by offering the patches at half price. Both programs had good acceptance.

Most smoke-free policies established in jails and prisons totally prohibit the possession of cigarettes and lighting materials by prisoners. Tobacco products and lighting materials, if discovered, are handled in the same fashion as other contraband and are confiscated and destroyed. Tobacco products discovered at the time of booking are considered property, logged, and returned to prisoners upon release. Procedures must be developed to prevent opportunities to obtain cigarettes during the special situations of facility transfer, participation in work release and road crews, and during visitation. Prominent signs and the incorporation of tobacco policies into staff training and prisoner handbooks are usually used. The strategy of restriction of smoking to outdoor recreation areas has been less commonly used in jails and prisons because of the impracticalities of distributing cigarettes and lighting materials, personal searches, and limited surveillance.

No-smoking policies in some institutions are not applied to staff and officers. In these cases, tobacco products and lighting materials are only prohibited in secure areas of the facility. Designated smoking areas where staff may smoke and leave their smoking materials are provided and identified by signs. Ideally, however, the no-smoking policy should extend to the entire institution. Smoke-free policies should be of special interest to unions, because one of their objectives is to protect the health and safety of their members. However, smoking can be politically challenging for labor unions since they represent both smokers and non-smokers. Moreover, in some instances, public policies and political agendas are influenced by tobacco industry monies and strategies making certain positions less attractive for unions.[112] It may be advisable to include all officially recognized employee organizations in formulating the policy. Reducing occupational health hazards is a primary objective of labor unions, and failure to provide such protection could later expose the employer to claims of negligence by nonsmokers.

Physicians, dentists, nurses, and medical section staff are uniquely positioned to assist patients who smoke, and the importance of clinical intervention is widely accepted.[113] Despite this opportunity for effective intervention even with brief advice, many clinicians are not consistent in confronting cigarette smoking.[114] Success might seem less obtainable within the correctional environment because of prison-culture influences, yet the history of quit attempts for prisoners often mirror those of smokers in the general population. A health practitioner's advice to quit may be an important motivator for attempting to stop. Health care personnel must be vocal and persistent advocates for smoke-free environments, provide support for individuals seeking to quit, and encourage all others to live without tobacco.

Smoking can be a chronic behavior maintained by strong psychologic and biologic forces, supported by a variety of different social, physical, and emotional cues linked to cigarettes. Health care practitioners serve as an important catalyst for the patient's progression through the stages of change toward cessation.[115] Jail and prison health care services can identify smokers for intervention, provide primary care clinicians with training on individual-to-individual counseling strategies that can be delivered within the time constraints of short clinic visits, provide self-help smoking cessation materials to prisoners at the time of routine physician and dentist visits, and provide follow-up assessment, since repeated attempts to quit will be necessary before permanent abstinence is achieved. Extensive guidance developed for practice in the general population is available,[116, 117] and many aspects can be applied to jail and prison populations.

REFERENCES

1. McGinnis JM, Foege WH. Actual causes of death in the United States. JAMA 270:2207-2212, 1993.
2. Raba JM, Obis CB: The health status of incarcerated urban males: Results of admission screening. J Prison Jail Health 3(1):6-24, 1983.
3. Hammett TM: 1994 update: HIV/AIDS and STDs in correctional facilities. National Institute of Justice; Oct 1995. NCJ-156832.
4. May JP, Ferguson MG, Ferguson R, et al: Prior nonfatal firearm injuries in detainees of a large urban jail. J Health Care Poor Underserved 6(2):162-176, 1995.
5. May JP, Zabeheian V, Oen R: Unpublished data. Central Detention Facility Health Services, Washington, D.C., 1997.
6. Reiman J: The Rich Get Richer and the Poor Get Prison. New York, Macmillan, 1990, p 114.
7. National Center for Health Statistics: Health, United States, 1995. Hyattsville, MD: Public Health Service 1996; Tables 35 & 62.
8. Maguire K, Pastore AL, eds: Sourcebook of Criminal Justice Statistics, 1995. Washington, D.C., US Dept of Justice, Bureau of Justice Statistics, USGPO, 1996, Table 6.31.
9. Singh GK, Kochanek KD, MacDorman MF: Advance report of final mortality statistics, 1994. Monthly vital statistics report: 45(3) Suppl. Hyattsville, MD: National Center for Health Statistics, 1996.
10. Maguire...Table 6.71.
11. Maguire...Table 6.69.
12. Karon JM, Rosenberg PS, et al: Prevalence of HIV infection in the United States, 1984-1992. JAMA 276(2):126-131, 1996.
13. Beck A, Gilliard D, Greenfeld L, et al. Survey of state prison inmates, 1991. Washington, D.C., US Dept of Justice, National Institute of Justice, March 1993, NDC-136949.
14. Polonsky S, Kerr S, et al: HIV prevention in prisons and jails: Obstacles and opportunities. Public Health Rep 309(5):615-625, 1994.
15. Maguire...Table 4.32.
16. Glaser JB, Greifinger RB: Correctional health care: A public health opportunity. Ann Intern Med 118(2):139-145, 1993.
17. Hammett...p 11.
18. Stevens J, Zierler S, et al: Prevalence of prior sexual abuse and HIV risk-taking behaviors in incarcerated women in Massachusetts. J Correctional Health Care 2(2):137-149, 1995.

19. Hammett TM, Widom R, et al: 1994 update: HIV/AIDS and STDs in correctional facilities. U.S. Dept of Justice; Dec 1995. NCJ- 156832.

20. Gershon RRM, Vlahov D, et al: Infectious diseases in prison-based health care workers. Unpublished manuscript. Personal communication. Baltimore, Johns Hopkins University School of Public Health, March 1997.

21. Castro K, Shansky R, Scardino V, et al: HIV transmission in correctional facilities. Centers for Disease Control, Abstract for Seventh International Conference on AIDS. Florence, Italy. June 1991.

22. Mutter RC, Grimes RM, Labarthe D: Evidence of intraprison spread of HIV infection. Arch Intern Med 154:793-795, 1994.

23. Tayor A, et al: Outbreak of HIV infection in a Scottish prison. Presentation at the 9th International Conference on AIDS, Yokohama, Japan, August 1994.

24. Saum CA, Surratt HL, et al: Sex in prisons: Exploring the myths and realities. Prison J 75(4):413-430, 1995.

25. Tewksbury R: Measure of sexual behavior in an Ohio prison. Sociol Soc Res 74:34-39, 1989.

26. Brennan M: Prisoners in desire. POZ Magazine. Feb 1997, pp 80-96.

27. Decker MD, Vaughn WK: Seroepidemiology of hepatitis B in Tennessee prisoners. J of Infectious Disease 150(3):450–459, 1984.

28. Monroe MC, Colley-Niemeyer BJ, Conway GA: Report of studies of HIV seroprevalence and AIDS knowledge, attitudes, and risk behaviors in inmates in the South Carolina Department of Corrections. Dec 1988, p 9-13.

29. Mahon N: New York inmates' HIV risk behaviors: The implication for prevention policy and programs. Am J Public Health 86(9): 1211-1215, 1996.

30. Jurgens R: HIV/AIDS in prisons. Correctional Services Canada, Feb 1994.

31. Decker SH, Rosenfeld: My wife is married and so is my girlfriend: Adaptations to the threat of AIDS in an arrestee population. Crime Deliquency 41(1):37-53, 1995.

32. Nader PR, Wexler DB, et al: Comparison of beliefs about AIDS among urban, suburban, incarcerated, and gay adolescents. J Adolesc Health Care 10(5):413-418, 1989.

33. Baker CJ: HIV seropositivity in incarcerated adolescents in Los Angeles county. The Forgotten Child in Health Care: Children in the Juvenile Justice System. Washington, D.C., U.S. Dept of Health and Human Services, National Center for Education in Maternal and Child Health, 1991, pp 91-97.

34. North RL, Rothenberg KH: Partner notification and the threat of domestic violence against women with HIV infection. N Engl J Med 16:1194-1196, 1993.

35. Dash L. When children want children: The urban crisis of teenage childbearing. New York: William Morrow and Co., 1989:65.

36. Decker and Rosenfeld. 1995.

37. Hammett...p 23.

38. Hammett...p 24.

39. Anglin MD, Maugh TH: Ensuring success in interventions with drug-using offenders. Ann Am Acad 521:66-90, 1992.

40. Higgins DL, Galavotti C, et al: Evidence for the effects of HIV antibody counseling and testing on risk behaviors. JAMA 266(17): 2419-2429, 1996.

41. Hammett...p. 39.

42. CDC: HIV prevention in the U.S. correctional system, 1991. MMWR 41(22):389-397, 1992.

43. Watters JK, Estilo MJ, et al: Syringe and needle exchange as HIV/AIDS prevention for injection drug users. JAMA 271(2): 115-120, 1994.

44. DesJarlais DC, Hagan H: Maintaining low HIV seroprevalence in populations of injecting drug users. JAMA 274(15):1226-1231, 1994.

45. Mayer J, et al: Drug relapse among recently paroled HIV+ individuals. Abstract No. PO-D12-3693. Presented at the 9th International conference on AIDS, Berlin, June 6-11, 1993.

46. Ippolito G, Puro V, et al: Prevention, Management, and Chemoprophylaxis of Occupational Exposure to HIV. Charlottesville, University of Virginia, International Health Care Worker Safety Center, 1997.

47. CDC. Update: Provisional public health service recommendations for chemoprophylaxis after occupational exposure to HIV. MMWR Jun 7, 1996; 45(22):468-72.

48. Gostin LO, Lazzarini Z, et al: HIV testing, counseling, and prophylaxis after sexual assault. JAMA 271:1436-1444, 1994.

49. National Center for Health Statistics... Table 52.

50. Maguire... Table 3.114.

51. Maguire... Table 6.73.

52. Thompson E. Deterrence versus brutalization. Homicide Studies. May 1997;1(2):110-128.

53. Vasquez D: Helping prison staff handle the stress of an execution. Corrections Today 55:70-72, 1993.

54. Weinstein C. Violence: The crucible of jail and prison. Presentation to Am Public Health Assn. San Diego, CA; Oct 1995.

55. American Correctional Association: Public correctional policy on use of force. Lanham, MD, Jan 1985.

56. Report from Prisoners Rights Union, Pelican Bay Information Project. San Francisco. 1995.

57. Jenkins L: Violence in the workplace: Risk factors and prevention strategies. Washington, D.C., National Institute for Occupational Safety and Health, June 1996.

58. Goodman RA, Jenkins EL, Mercy JA. Workplace-related homicide among health care workers in the United States, 1980 through 1990. JAMA. Dec 7, 1994;272(21):1686-88.

59. Lattimore PK, Linster RL: Risk of death among serious young offenders. Presentation to the Homicide Research Working Group, Santa Monica, CA, June 1996.

60. Coe J: Institutional population deaths. Internal report. Ill Dept of Corrections. 1993.

61. Richards SC, Jones RS: Perpetual incarceration machine: Structural impediments to postprison success. J Contemp Crim Justice 13: 4-22, 1997.

62. Rosenfeld R, Decker S: Where public health and law enforcement meet: Monitoring and preventing youth violence. Am J Police 1993;12(3):11-57.

63. McLaughlin CR, Reiner MS, Waite DE, et al: Firearm injuries in juvenile offenders: A public health crisis. Abstract presentation. Am Public Health Assoc Nov 1996.

64. May and Ferguson

65. Rivera FP, Shepard JP, Farrington DP, et al: Victim as offender in youth violence. Ann Emerg Med 26:609-614, 1995.

66. National Research Council, Reiss A, Roth J (eds): Understanding and preventing violence. Washington, D.C., National Academy Press, 1993, p 336.

67. CDC Injury surveillance in correctional facilities—Michigan, April 1994–March 1995. MMWR. 1996;45:69-72.

68. Thorburn KM: Violence is a public health concern: Interdiction in the correctional setting. Presentation to the American Correctional Health Services Association, Philadelphia, April 1997.

69. May JP. Addressing the gun violence epidemic. Presentation to the 18th National Conference of the National Commission on Correctional Health Care, San Diego. Sept 1994.

70. Pynoos RS, Nader K: Psychological first aid and treatment approach to children exposed to community violence: Research implications. J Traumatic Stress 1:445-473, 1988.

71. Jenkins EJ: Violence exposure, psychological distress, and risk behavior (in a sample of inner-city youth). Paper presented at the Homicide Research Working Group, CDC National Center for Injury Prevention and Control and Emory University, Atlanta, GA, June 1994.

72. Brown A: Violence against women: Relevance for medical practi-

tioners. Council on Scientific Affairs Report. JAMA. 1992; 267:3184.

73. Warshaw C: Domestic violence: Challenges to medical practice. J Women's Health 2:73-79, 1993.

74. Alpert EJ: Violence in intimate relationships and the practicing internist: New "disease" or new agenda? Ann Intern Med 123: 774-781, 1995.

75. Feldhaus KM, Koziol-McLain J, et al: Accuracy of 3 brief screening questions for detecting partner violence in the emergency department. JAMA 277:1357-1361, 1997.

76. Bureau of Justice Statistics. Criminal victimization in the United States, 1991. Washington, D.C.: U.S. Dept of Justice, Dec 1992:18. NCJ-139563.

77. U.S. Preventive Services Task Force: Guide to Clinical Preventive Services, ed 2. Baltimore, Williams & Wilkins, 1996, pp 687-698.

78. May and Ferguson.

79. Fingerhut LA, Kleinman JC: International and interstate comparisons of homicide among young males. JAMA 263:3292-3295, 1990.

80. Fingerhut LA. Firearm mortality among children, youth, and young adults 1–34 years of age, trends and current status: United States, 1985–90 Advance data from vital and health statistics; no 231. Hyattsville, MD: National Center for Health Statistics. 1993.

81. CDC. Rates of homicide, suicide, and firearm-related death among children–26 industrialized countries. Feb 7, 1997;46(5):101-05.

82. Blumstein A: Youth violence, guns, and the illicit-drug industry. J Crim Law Criminol 86:10-36, 1990.

83. Kellermann AL, Rivara FP, et al: Suicide in the home in relation to gun ownership. N Engl J Med 327:467-472, 1992.

84. May and Ferguson.

85. May JP, Martin KL. A role for the primary care physician in counseling young African American men about homicide prevention. J of Gen Int Med. 1993;8:380-82.

86. May JP, Christoffel KK, Sprang ML: Counseling patients about guns. Chicago Med 97:13-16, 1994.

87. Hayden JW, Laney C, Kellermann AL: Medical devices made into weapons by prisoners: An unrecognized risk. Ann Emerg Med 26:739-742, 1996.

88. Bell CC, Jenkins EJ: Violence prevention and intervention in juvenile detention and correctional facilities. J of Correctional Health Care. Spring, 1995;2(1):17-38.

89. Department of Health and Human Services: The Health Benefits of Smoking Cessation. A Report of the Surgeon General. Rockville, MD, U.S. Department of Health and Human Services, Public Health Service, Centers for Disease Control, Center for Disease Prevention, Office on Smoking and Health, DHHS Publication No. (CDC) 90-8416, 1990.

90. Department of Health and Human Services. *The Health Consequences of Involuntary Smoking. A Report of the Surgeon General.* U.S. Department of Health and Human Services, Public Health Service, Centers for Disease Control, Center for Health Promotion and Education, Office on Smoking and Health, Rockville, MD. DHHS Publication No. (CDC) 87-8398, 1986.

91. Environmental Protection Agency: Respiratory Health Effects of Smoking: Lung Cancer and other Disorders. Washington, D.C.: U.S. Environmental Protection Agency, Office of Research and Development, Office of Air and Radiation, EPA Publication No. EPA/600/6-90/006F, 1992.

92. Romero CA, Connell FA: A survey of prison policies regarding smoking and tobacco. J Prison Jail Health 7(1), 1988.

93. Skolnick A: Jails lead prisons in smoking bans. JAMA 264:1514, 1990.

94. Skolnick A: Tobacco foes attack ads that target women, minorities, teens, and the poor. JAMA 264:1505-1513, 1990.

95. Salive ME, Smith GS, Brewer TF: Death in prison: Changing mortality pattern among male prisoners in Maryland, 1979-87. Am J Public Health 80:1479-1480, 1990.

96. Lambert WE: 'Ain't nothing to do in here but smoke': Establishing a smoke-free policy in a county jail. Presentation to ASSIST Information Exchange Training, National Cancer Institute, Washington, D.C., April 16, 1997.

97. Centers for Disease Control: State tobacco prevention and control activities: Result of the 1989–1990 Association of State and Territorial Health Officials (ASTHO) Survey final report. MMWR 40(No. RR-11):1-41, 1991.

98. Himelstein L: Supreme Court plans to consider prisoners' right to smoke-free cell. Legal Times, July 6, 1992, p 13.

99. Iowa: Inmate Requests Transfer Due to Prison Smoke. USA Today, August 2, 1995, p A8.

100. Vaughn M, del Carmen R: Smoke-free prisons: Policy dilemmas and constitutional issues. J Crim Justice 151-171, 1993.

101. Prisoners plan to fight for the right to smoke. Washington Times, June 15, 1995, p C5.

102. DHHS, 1986.

103. National Institute of Corrections, Longmont, CO. Personal communication, March 1997.

104. May JP, Zabeheian V, Oen R: Characteristics of detainees entering an urban jail. Unpublished survey. Central Detention Facility, Washington, D.C.: 1997.

105. Skolnick.

106. Garner JM: The impact of the new tobacco-free policy in the Texas Department of Criminal Justice. Report for the Texas Department of Criminal Justice. Aug 5, 1995.

107. Centers for Disease Control. Cigarette smoking bans in county jails–Wisconsin, 1991. MMWR. 1992;41:101-03.

108. Thompson SF: Smoke-free prisons. Presentation to the ASSIST Information Exchange Training. Washington, D.C., National Cancer Institute, Apr 16, 1997.

109. Jones R: Personal communication. Utah Department of Corrections. 1997.

110. Botelho RJ, Skinner H: Motivating change in health behavior: Implications for health promotion and disease prevention. Primary Care: Clinics in Office Practice, Prevention in Practice, Dec 1995; 22(4):565-589.

111. Henningfield JE: Nicotine medications for smoking cessation. N Engl J Med 333:1196-1203, 1995.

112. Kansas Department of Corrections. Creating smoke-free correctional facilities. Discussion paper.

113. Department of Health and Human Services: Smoking Cessation. Clinical Practice Guideline Number 18. Washington, D.C., U.S. Department of Health and Human Service, Agency for Health Care Policy and Research, Centers for Disease Control and Prevention. AHCPR Publication No. 96-0692, 1996.

114. Gilpin EA, Pierce JP, et al: Physician advice to quit smoking: Results from the 1990 California tobacco survey. J Gen Intern Med 8: 549-553, 1993.

115. Fisher EB, Bishop DB, et al: Implications for the practicing physician of the psychosocial dimensions of smoking. Chest 93:69S-78S, 1988.

116. Department of Health and Human Services: Tobacco and the Clinician. Interventions for Medical and Dental Practice. Washington, D.C., U.S. Department of Health and Human Services, Public Health Service, National Institutes of Health, NIH Publication No. 94-3693, 1994.

117. DHHS 1996.

23

The Treatment of Alcohol and Other Drug Abstinence Syndromes

H. Blair Carlson, M.D., M.S.P.H.
Jane A. Kennedy, D.O.

Alcohol and other drug (AOD) withdrawal syndromes are seen frequently by health care workers in correctional settings. This is so because there is a high prevalence of AOD problems in the offender population, and the sudden interruption of alcohol or other drug use, or both, occurs regularly when an individual is taken into custody. The ability to anticipate problems through the identification of individuals at risk, to assess the likelihood of a major abstinence syndrome, and to treat appropriately, early in the course of withdrawal, are the responsibilities of health care providers. Besides the fact that accurate diagnosis and treatment are humane acts, the avoidance of major withdrawal disorders can be lifesaving and can also provide for a smooth intake process that is free of disruptive emergent events. The goal of treating withdrawal from alcohol and other drugs is the safe and effective management of a

serious medical problem. The objectives of treatment in accomplishing this goal are the relief of symptoms, the prevention or treatment of delirium or seizures, or both, and the prevention or treatment of associated medical conditions. Also, with motivational counseling throughout the withdrawal process,[1] the patient may see this treatment as the first step in a potential long-term recovery. This chapter is written in the hope that correctional health care personnel will be able to add to their understanding of the nature and treatment of the withdrawal syndromes.

Generally, the signs and symptoms of drug abstinence are opposite to the signs and symptoms of drug use. For example, the opiates are constipating, so when an opiate-dependent individual becomes abstinent, diarrhea usually occurs. Similarly, alcohol is a depressant, so it is not surprising to find that, when individuals are withdrawing from alcohol, they are often anxious and agitated. The severity of the withdrawal depends on how heavy the AOD use had been and for how long, although other factors come into play as well. The focus here will be on alcohol, other depressants, and opiates, because these drugs cause most of the problems from a health care perspective. However, stimulants, cannabis, inhalants, and hallucinogens will also be discussed briefly.

Supportive care is critical in attending to patients withdrawing from AOD. Asking questions, confirming their discomfort, providing reassurance, letting them know when they are doing well, and showing them their progress, for example, by letting them see their flow chart, are all means of tangible support that encourage recovery. When possible, a quiet place that is not too brightly lit can help to quiet their often overstimulated nervous systems by reducing unnecessary sensory input. Finally, there is no substitute for a careful assessment for identifying medical, psychiatric, and emotional issues that may play a role in the withdrawal signs and symptoms.

ALCOHOL AND ALCOHOL ABSTINENCE
Background and Pathogenesis

Before the 1950s, no one had a clear picture of what happened when a chronic drinker abruptly stopped or reduced drinking, or even knew if there were such a thing as an abstinence syndrome. Some thought that drinking, rather than abstinence, caused what we now know as the withdrawal syndrome.[2] In 1953, however, Victor and Adams published the results of a careful analysis of 266 consecutive admissions to the Boston City Hospital over a 60-day period "with obvious alcoholic complications." Included in the analysis were observations accurately describing the clinical events that followed abrupt abstinence in alcoholics.[3] Later, two experimental studies on correctional volunteers confirmed that a set of predictable events takes place when heavy drinkers stop or even reduce their drinking.[4, 5] Health care providers are frequent witnesses to these phenomena in two fairly common circumstances: when patients are hospitalized and when individuals are taken into custody. In either case, there is an unexpected interruption of daily drinking that may or may not be recognized at intake. Mildly intoxicated individuals or those who have gone 6–8 hours since their last drink may seem quite fit, only to be found delirious and unmanageable 2–3 days later. Physical dependence on alcohol is measured most accurately, in retrospect, by the intensity of the withdrawal.[6] Forecasting withdrawal intensity, however, can be roughly accomplished through careful history taking, which will be discussed shortly.

Recent research directed at the cause of physical dependence on alcohol has focused on the major inhibitory and excitatory neurotransmitter systems, the gamma-amino butyric acid (GABA) system and the *N*-methyl-D-aspartate (NMDA) subtype of the glutamate receptor, respectively.

An adaptive downregulation of the inhibitory system follows long-term stimulation of the GABAergic neurons by alcohol. In addition, there is an upregulation of the neuroexcitatory system that follows inhibition of the glutamate system by the long-term use of alcohol. As a result, the brain is left in a hyperexcitable state when alcohol is reduced or removed.[6–8] The upregulated glutamate system and subsequent abrupt removal of alcohol is now believed to be related to alcohol withdrawal seizures and also to excitotoxic neuronal cell death. Thus, repeated alcohol withdrawals and related neurotoxicity may be responsible for some of the cognitive deficits found in individuals with chronic alcoholism.[7] At any rate, it is clear that the adaptation of the brain to alcohol leaves it in a physically dependent state that is not apparent in the presence of alcohol but is unmasked, in sometimes dramatic fashion, with alcohol abstinence.[6]

Clinical Features

Alcohol abstinence symptoms begin 6–8 hours after the last drink and often begin before the blood alcohol level reaches zero in individuals with tolerance.[1, 8] Tremors are common and may be severe enough to interfere with an individual's gait and ability to eat. Mild to moderate elevations in pulse, blood pressure, and temperature may occur. The patient becomes agitated, irritable, and anxious. Gastrointestinal symptoms occur and may include nausea, vomiting, and diarrhea. Sweating is common and can be profuse. Patients often find it difficult or impossible to sleep. There is a heightened sensitivity to light and sound, peculiar sensations in the skin, and problems with concentration. Hallucinations that occur are usually visual but may also be auditory, tactile, or, rarely, olfactory. Small animals such as mice, rats, snakes, and bugs are common visual hallucinations. Usually, by 48 hours, the symptoms have first intensified, then diminished, and are slowly abating. The common syndrome just described does not include confusion. By contrast, the major withdrawal syndrome, referred to as delirium tremens or DTs, is accompanied by delirium, disorientation, and agitation severe enough to require restraints. It may be accompanied by hyperpyrexia and often is associated with a worsening of many of the symptoms and signs found in the earlier syndrome, such as a marked increase in autonomic activity with profuse sweating and elevation in vital signs. Delirium tremens may appear to begin "out of the blue" at 72–96 hours after the last drink if earlier symptoms have gone unnoticed. The syndrome, if untreated or treated too late, may last a week or more. It is far more satisfactory to recognize the likelihood of a major withdrawal syndrome and prevent it than to attempt to treat it after it has been established, because available pharmacotherapy is less effective in the later stage. Furthermore, there is often a problem recognizing and treating co-morbid medical conditions when the patient is combative, disoriented, and restrained. Delirium tremens can be fatal, although the current practice of adequate drug treatment and supportive nursing care has reduced the mortality rate to an estimated 2% or less.[1] Seizures occur in the setting of alcohol abstinence in 5%–15% of patients after heavy daily drinking, and they are nearly always generalized tonic-clonic (grand mal) seizures; only 5% experience focal seizures.[3, 9–11] They are usually single or in a set of two or three, and status epilepticus is uncommon. In one series, 86% occurred in the first 72 hours,[9] and in another series, 99% occurred by 72 hours.[10] However, seizures sometimes occur later than 5 days after the last drink; when they do, either the ingestion of a sedative drug with the alcohol or a co-morbid brain disorder should be suspected. Individuals with epilepsy, head injuries, and other causes of seizures may also be seen with alcohol withdrawal, so taking a careful history is important in properly classifying seizures in this population.

Assessment of Withdrawal Potential

Because the prevalence of heavy drinking in individuals admitted to detention facilities is fairly high, adequate screening at intake is needed to anticipate problems and to respond appropriately. This section might be labeled "giving it your best guess," for here you are asked to forecast the withdrawal potential of a drinking individual who may not be able to give an accurate history of the drinking or who may not be a credible historian. The severity of an alcohol abstinence syndrome can be estimated roughly as the product of the blood alcohol level multiplied by time,[1, 12] that is, how much for how long? The first question to be asked is, "Have you been drinking?" Next, some creative questioning may arrive at a reasonable estimate of how much for how long. The questioning should be accompanied by an explanation of its purpose, that is, "We need to get an idea of how much you have been drinking, because you might need some medication to avoid getting sick now that you won't be drinking for awhile." Providing this information is likely to get you some help in estimating the intensity and duration of an individual's drinking problem. If drinking has only occurred over a day or two, then major withdrawal is unlikely. If drinking has occurred on a daily basis for weeks, and in amounts equivalent to more than 6 oz of ethanol, then a significant withdrawal becomes more likely. Still, some drinkers can drink much more than this and have only minor symptoms on withdrawal, and some have serious withdrawal problems after drinking less than 6 oz of ethanol a day. Therefore, although it is not possible to predict precisely who will have a major withdrawal, other factors can help to fine-tune an estimate. A demonstration of tolerance can alert the health care worker to potential problems because tolerance and physical dependence, although not the same thing, develop in a somewhat parallel fashion.[6, 13–16] For example, an individual taken into custody who behaves normally with a blood alcohol concentration of 200–300 mg/dL or greater clearly has a

tolerance for alcohol, and this tolerance is likely to be accompanied by physical dependence as well. Further, tolerance leads to increasing alcohol intake as the alcoholic drinks more to get the same effect. Younger individuals can drink more and have a less severe withdrawal, whereas individuals in their 40s and 50s or older with a long drinking history are likely to be susceptible to more withdrawal problems.

Individuals with alcoholism who have had many debauches and many episodes of withdrawal are more likely to have seizures or a major withdrawal syndrome, because their brains may have undergone a sensitizing process known as *kindling*.[17] Taking a cue from an earlier work demonstrating that repeated stimulation sensitized animal brains, which then became hyperexcitable,[18] Ballenger and Post[17] reviewed the records of 200 male heavy drinkers and postulated that multiple episodes of CNS stimulation (in this case, alcohol withdrawal episodes as the stimulant) led to changes in the brain that made it more susceptible to seizures and to more severe withdrawal syndromes. They suggested that, in individuals who had been drinking daily for years, there were not only major withdrawal experiences but also regular daily withdrawals before the next day's drinking began. The term *kindled* is used to describe a brain that has been sensitized in this manner, and research has supported this kindling hypothesis in laboratory animals and in women as well as in men.[19, 20] For example, an individual who has been drinking daily in amounts of a pint or more of spirits, and who has a long drinking history of 15 or more years, should be watched more carefully and treated early for alcohol withdrawal as it arises. A previous history of severe withdrawal or seizures also makes the likelihood of severe symptoms much greater.

Treatment

Mild withdrawal from alcohol requires only supportive care. Some inner shakiness, irritability, and a headache may be all there is to withdrawal, particularly in young people. In ideal situations in which maximum supportive care is available, even moderate alcohol withdrawal may respond without medication if staff are available to provide adequate support.[21, 22] Medication can be administered easily in an infirmary, dispensary, or even a holding cell, when health care workers are at hand and available to monitor the course of the withdrawal. If assessment suggests that a major withdrawal is likely, early treatment with adequate doses of benzodiazepines is indicated to prevent delirium, seizures, and other manifestations of a severe withdrawal syndrome. Delirium, once it occurs, should be treated in a hospital environment, preferably in an ICU.

As withdrawal symptoms develop and progress, it is important to be able to monitor accurately what is happening, including the response to treatment if medications are administered. The Clinical Institute Withdrawal

Assessment—Alcohol, Revised (CIWA-Ar, Fig. 23-1) has become a widely used instrument for this purpose.[23-28]

Its validity and reliability are established, and after some practice, it is simple to use. It is valuable in monitoring the individual who has major withdrawal potential and can receive medication in time to prevent this catastrophe. It is also useful in determining when medication is not needed in withdrawal. The CIWA (pronounced "seewaa") scale permits symptom-triggered rather than around-the-clock medication administration. There are 10 domains that are measured on a seven-level Likert scale, except for the last domain, which has four levels. A maximum theoretical score would, therefore, be a score of 67, but the useful detoxification range is commonly from 0 to 30. Measured domains are nausea and vomiting, tremors, diaphoresis, anxiety, agitation, orientation, headaches, and three domains of perceptual distortions (visual, auditory, and tactile). An individual who scores less than 10 on the scale would receive no medication, whereas 10 or greater indicates a need for increasing levels of pharmacotherapy, which will be described below.

The benzodiazepines have been shown to be effective in treating alcohol withdrawal when medications are needed in addition to supportive care.[1, 8, 9, 25-27, 29, 30] Those benzodiazepines with long-acting metabolites, such as diazepam, clorazepate, and chlordiazepoxide, are useful because their long half-lives of perhaps 100 hours[31] allow for a self-taper after the medication is discontinued.[25, 30, 32] Clorazepate is a prodrug with long-acting metabolites and has the relative disadvantage of having no parenteral preparation. Oxazepam and lorazepam have no active metabolites and have shorter half-lives; therefore, they may clear more rapidly than is sometimes optimal.[30] Nonetheless, they may be safer drugs to use in instances in which there is severe liver disease because metabolism by the liver is not necessary. All of the benzodiazepines already mentioned are rapidly absorbed orally, so this route is preferred unless there is vomiting or the patient can take nothing by mouth for other reasons, in which case the IV route can be used. The bioavailability of benzodiazepines, after IM administration, is unpredictable, although they are often successfully used in this fashion when there is vomiting and IV use is not feasible. Because the benzodiazepines exhibit cross-tolerance to alcohol, fairly large doses are often necessary to manage alcohol withdrawal. Further, it has been found efficacious to "front load" with medication until a withdrawal syndrome is under control, in much the same manner that digitalis is "loaded" in a patient with atrial fibrillation or steroids are loaded in a patient with an asthmatic crisis. In all these situations, it makes no sense to administer the medication in small increments over time, when larger and earlier loading doses can be expected to bring the event under control. The wide margin of safety of benzodiazepines facilitates the use of the loading technique.

Figure 23-2 schematically describes how loading doses are used to achieve a cumulative pharmacologic effect so that control is gained of the signs and symptoms of alcohol withdrawal. In this schematic from Naranjo and Sellers,[32] they describe a hypothetical major alcohol withdrawal syndrome, the effect of benzodiazepines (diazepam or chlordiazepoxide or both), and their median dose of diazepam when give in a symptom-triggered, front-loaded fashion. Using the CIWA-Ar scale, a score of 10 or less indicates that no medication is necessary, a score of more than 10 but less than 20 would suggest a dose of 50 mg of chlordiazepoxide or its equivalent, and a score of greater than 20 would suggest a dose of 100 mg of chlordiazepoxide or its equivalent. In this example, chlordiazepoxide at 100 mg is used as the equivalent of 20 mg of diazepam in the symptom-triggered treatment of a hypothetical alcohol withdrawal syndrome depicted in Figure 23-2 *C*. However, one finds variability in these equivalencies. For example, some use 40 mg of diazepam as the equivalent of 100 mg of librium.[31] The wide margin of safety, a symptom-triggered method of administration, and frequent monitoring minimize the differences in dose equivalents. In the front-loading process, the patient is assessed every $1/2$ to 1 hour and treated every 1–2 hours with a dose that is appropriate to the CIWA-Ar scores. When the score drops below 10, no treatment is given, unless the score rises again; thus, over-sedation is avoided. Less benzodiazepine is given by this method than by a set-schedule format.[26, 27]

Accurate assessment of withdrawal status using the CIWA-Ar or some other instrument of measurement must be accompanied by attention to the patient's medical status. This should include the identification and treatment of coexistent medical disorders, including the state of hydration and nutrition, and the compilation of a history of psychiatric problems that are likely to affect the withdrawal status. Whenever possible, oral fluids are preferred over IV solutions. Thiamine in a single IM injection of 100 mg is adequate to repair a presumed deficiency of this vitamin and may prevent Wernicke's disease. When glucose administration is contemplated, the thiamine should be given first. Magnesium deficiency is common in individuals with alcoholism and can be corrected. Although individuals with alcoholism regularly recover from alcohol withdrawal without magnesium replacement, the importance of the Mg^{2+} ion should not be underestimated, even though its precise role in the alcohol withdrawal syndrome is not clear.[1, 33, 34] Multivitamin administration over a period of several days may also be useful, particularly when adequate nutrition has been lacking. β-blockers can be used to control tachycardia and elevated blood pressure in patients who have a persistent elevation in vital signs, despite evidence that their withdrawal is otherwise under control.[35] Supportive care should not be overlooked in favor of medication. Ten minutes each hour should be devoted to assessment, reassurance, reality orientation, and general nursing care.[22, 24]

Date_____/_____/_____   Time_____:_____

Patient_____   Blood Pressure ____/____ Pulse ____/minute

NAUSEA AND VOMITING Do you feel sick to your stomach? Have you vomited? Observation

_____

0 no nausea and vomiting
1 mild nausea, no vomiting
2
3
4 intermittent nausea and dry heaves
5
6
7 constant nausea, frequent vomiting and dry heaves

TREMOR Arms extended and fingers spread apart

_____

0 no tremor
1 not visible, but can be felt fingertip to fingertip
2
3
4 moderate with patient's arms extended
5
6
7 severe, even without arms extended

PAROXYSMAL SWEATS Observation

_____

0 no sweat visible
1 barely perceptible sweat visible, moist palms
2
3
4 beads of sweat obvious on forehead
5
6
7 drenching sweats

ANXIETY Do you feel nervous? Observation

_____

0 no anxiety, at ease
1 mildly anxious
2
3
4 moderately anxious or guarded
5
6
7 equivalent to acute panic states as seen in delirium or acute schizophrenic reactions

AGITATION Observation

_____

0 normal activity
1 somewhat more than normal activity
2
3
4 moderately fidgety and restless
5
6
7 paces back and forth during most of the interview or constantly thrashes about

This scale is not copyrighted and may be used freely.

TACTILE DISTURBANCES Have you any itching, pins and needles sensations, any burning, any numbness, or do you feel bugs crawling on or under your skin? Observation

_____

0 none
1 very mild itching, pins and needles, burning, or numbness
2 mild itching, pins and needles, burning or numbness
4 moderately severe hallucinations
5 severe hallucinations
6 extremely severe hallucinations
7 continuous hallucinations

AUDITORY HALLUCINATIONS Are you more aware of sounds around you? Are they harsh? Do they frighten you? Are you hearing anything that is disturbing to you? Are you hearing things you know are not there? Observation

_____

0 not present
1 very mild harshness or ability to frighten
2 mild harshness or ability to frighten
3 moderate harshness or ability to frighten
4 moderately severe hallucinations
5 severe hallucinations
6 extremely severe hallucinations
7 continuous hallucinations

VISUAL DISTURBANCES Does light appear to be too bright? Is its color different? Does it hurt your eyes? Are you seeing anything that is disturbing to you? Are you seeing things you know are not there? Observation

_____

0 not present
1 very mild sensitivity
2 mild sensitivity
3 moderate sensitivity
4 moderately severe hallucinations
5 severe hallucinations
6 extremely severe hallucinations
7 continuous hallucinations

HEADACHE, FULLNESS IN HEAD Does your head feel different? Does it feel like there is a band around your head? Do not rate for dizziness or lightheadedness. Otherwise, rate severity.

_____

0 not present
1 very mild
2 mild
3 moderate
4 moderately severe
5 severe
6 very severe
7 extremely severe

ORIENTATION AND CLOUDING OF SENSORIUM What day is this? Where are you? Who am I?

_____

0 oriented and can do serial additions
1 cannot do serial additions or is uncertain about date
2 disoriented about date by no more than 2 calendar days
3 disoriented about date by more than 2 calendar days
4 disoriented about place and/or person

Total CIWA-Ar Score _____ Rater's Initials _____

Fig 23-1. Addiction Research Foundation Clinical Institute Withdrawal Assessment for Alcohol, Revised (CIWA-Ar) (From Sullivan JT, Sykora K, Schneiderman J, et al: Assessment of alcohol withdrawal: The revised clinical institute withdrawal assessment for alcohol scale (CIWA-Ar). *Br J Addict* 84:1353–1357, 1989.)

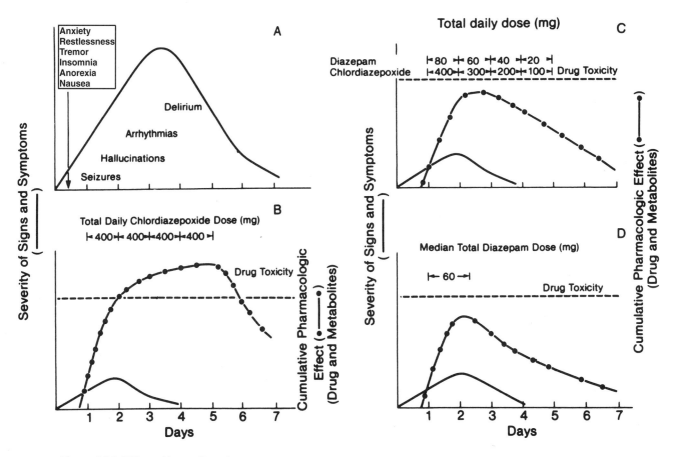

Figure 23-2. Effect of benzodiazepine therapy on the clinical course of alcohol withdrawal. **A**, clinical features of the alcohol withdrawal syndrome. **B**, cumulative pharmacologic effect of chlordiazepoxide and its active metabolite, desmethylchlordiazepoxide, during repeated daily administration of the same daily dose. Because of cumulation of parent drug and active metabolite, excessive sedation occurs. **C**, cumulative pharmacologic effect of diazepam or chlordiazepoxide or both during repeated administration of daily doses reduced gradually. This procedure is effective and avoids excessive sedation, but requires administration of the drug for several days. **D**, cumulative pharmacologic effect of diazepam and its active metabolite, desmethyldiazepam, when the loading dose technique is used. This procedure is simple and very effective, and because total dose of drug is smaller and titrated to patient's response, excessive sedation is avoided. (From Naranjo CA, Sellers EM: Clinical assessment and pharmacotherapy of the alcohol withdrawal syndrome, in Galanter M (ed): *Recent Developments in Alcoholism, vol 4.* New York, Plenum, 1986, p 268, with permission.)

BENZODIAZEPINE WITHDRAWAL
Backgound, Pathogenesis, Clinical Features

The depressant drug withdrawal syndromes are discussed separately from the alcohol withdrawal syndrome, even though the clinical features, pathophysiologic characteristics, and treatment are similar. This is necessary because significant differences remain.[36] It is clear that the long-term use of benzodiazepines is accompanied by physical dependence,[37–39] which is likely a result of receptor downregulation and/or reduced coupling between GABA-A receptor–chloride channel gating and benzodiazepine receptor binding.[40] The symptoms may be mild in some cases and may include anxiety, malaise, headaches, and sleep interference. However, at high doses (e.g., 30 mg/day or greater of diazepam or its equivalent, taken over many months), the

symptoms may include dysphoria, perceptual distortions, psychosis, and seizures. The longer the half-life of the drug used, the greater the likelihood of physical dependence; however, the shorter the half-life, the earlier the onset of the withdrawal and the more severe the symptoms are likely to be.[37] This is so because the longer half-life benzodiazepines have a self-tapering kinetic that allows for neuroadaptation to the absence of the drug. Because the half-lives of some benzodiazepines (and their active metabolites) may be 100 hours or more, regular dosing results in accumulation of the drug such that smaller doses may ultimately result in fairly high blood levels over time.[31] Benzodiazepines can be taken therapeutically without the development of physical dependence, although physical dependence can develop with long-term therapeutic use. They can be abused in a binge-like fashion without the development of physical dependence. However, when abused over the long term, often in conjunction with alcohol or other drugs seen in an addict population, there is likely to be physical dependence, which may require treatment.[36, 41] Drug abusers are said to prefer diazepam and alprazolam over other benzodiazepines, and are more likely to find benzodiazepines to be reinforcing than would non–drug abusers.[42]

Treatment

When an individual is taken into custody and gives a history of long-term benzodiazepine abuse over several months and at daily levels of use equivalent to 30 mg of diazepam or greater, some preventive treatment is in order. At lesser amounts or over a shorter time period, observation is indicated and treatment should be instituted only if necessary. Withdrawal from benzodiazepines can be accomplished using a long-acting drug such as diazepam, chlordiazepxide, or phenobarbital. Phenobarbital has the advantage of being less reinforcing; thus, it is less likely to engender drug seeking. An assessment or estimation of the scale of daily drug use is obtained from the patient, then 30 mg of phenobarbital is substituted for each 10 mg of diazepam or the equivalent (25 mg chlordiazepoxide, 1 mg alprazolam, 15 mg chlorazepate, 2 mg lorazepam, etc.) in whatever benzodiazepine was being used up to a maximum of 500 mg of phenobarbital per day. The daily dose of phenobarbital is then decreased by 30 mg/day. If phenobarbital intoxication (nystagmus, slurring of speech, obvious sedation) takes place, indicating less tolerance than at first assumed from the history, the dose is then decreased by 50% and the 30-mg/day taper is continued.[42]

BARBITURATE AND OTHER DEPRESSANT DRUG WITHDRAWAL
Background, Pathogenesis, Clinical Features

With barbiturates, the abstinence syndrome appears a bit later after last use than it does with alcohol, and the clinical presentation is less predictable. The most common barbiturates that are accompanied by a withdrawal syndrome are the oxybarbiturates: secobarbital (Seconal, "reds"), pentobarbital (Nembutal, "yellows"), amobarbital (Amytal, "blues"), amobarbital–secobarbital in combination (Tuinal, "rainbows or tooies"), and butalbital in various combinations.[43] For long-term prescribed use, these drugs have largely been replaced by the benzodiazepine preparations that have a wider margin of safety, with the exception of butalbital, which is still used as therapy for headaches. The use of butalbital continues in spite of the fact that, according to Sullivan and Sellers, "there are no controlled studies demonstrating the specific benefits of the barbiturates in combination therapy for tension headache or migraine."[36] The barbiturates remain drugs of abuse, however, with the exception of phenobarbital, which has little abuse potential and is widely used for the treatment of withdrawal symptoms and as an

anticonvulsant. When abused, phenobarbital is not without withdrawal problems, however.[44] The shorter-acting barbiturates mentioned above are abused, although not as frequently as in the past; in fact, less than 3% of the arrestees in the Drug Use Forecasting (DUF) study[45] in 1992 tested positive for barbiturates, compared with 48% to 85% that tested positive to "any drug." Furthermore, barbiturates are not mentioned in the 1994 DUF study.[46] For a review of the barbiturates, see the fifth edition of *Goodman and Gilman*.[47]

Although barbiturates are not abused to the same extent as in years past, they have not totally disappeared and, thus, deserve discussion. The symptoms and signs of barbiturate withdrawal resemble those of alcohol withdrawal and include tremors, nausea, vomiting, anxiety in the early and milder form followed by hallucinations (usually visual), perceptual distortions, and delirium. Seizures, commonly multiple, occur regularly and are grand mal in nature. As mentioned earlier, the symptoms begin somewhat later than in alcohol withdrawal, and minor symptoms begin between 8 and 36 hours, reach a maximum at an average of 40 hours, then decline over the next 2–15 days. A major withdrawal is characterized by confusion, much like in alcoholic delirium, that may last for several days.[36, 48,] Based on a human experiment on volunteer prisoners,[49] it is possible to predict who is likely to have a major withdrawal, in that a daily dose of 900 mg or greater over 30 days or more of either pentobarbital or secobarbital resulted in delirium or seizures, or both, in 18 of 18 research subjects. With 600–800 mg/day over 35–57 days, 2 of 18 patients had seizures and 9 had significant minor symptoms; with only 400 mg/day, there were little or no symptoms. Based on these data, all patients who give a history of barbiturate use that exceeds 400 mg of pentobarbital, secobarbital, or the equivalent over 30 days or more should be carefully observed and treated prophylactically, especially if they have histories of severe barbiturate withdrawal. It would seem prudent to treat all individuals who have histories of long-term use of 800 mg or more for more than 30 days.[36, 49]

Treatment

A reasonable approach, suggested by Sullivan and Sellers,[36] provides an assessment of the degree of dependence and begins the pharmacotherapy at one and the same time. If the individual is not intoxicated or in withdrawal, but gives a history of heavy regular barbiturate use, a loading dose of 1.7 mg/kg of phenobarbital is given orally each hour until any three of the following effects occur: nystagmus, drowsiness, ataxia, dysarthria, or emotional lability. If the patient is in withdrawal, the loading can be stopped when the withdrawal signs and symptoms disappear. Before each hourly dose, patients are assessed for intoxication or withdrawal. Based on this regimen, patients requiring less than 7 mg/kg are not physically dependent enough to require further treatment. In treating heavy barbiturate users, Sullivan and Sellers found the median dose of phenobarbital in this protocol to be 1,440 mg and the mean loading dose to be 23.4 ± 7.1 mg/kg. Given the prolonged half-life of phenobarbital in these patients abusing barbiturates (38–240 hours; median, 90 hours), no further medication is given because the tapering kinetics introduced by the long half-life are judged to be sufficient to prevent a reemergence of the withdrawal syndrome.[36] Withdrawal from glutethemide, ethylchlorvinyl, methaqualone, methyprylon, and meprobamate may be managed in this fashion as well. When these drugs are used on a long-term basis at levels of more than 1.0–2.5 g/day, Sullivan and Sellers[36] consider them "approximately equal to 600 mgm of secobarbital and treatment is indicated."

OPIOIDS

Background

Criminal activity has long been associated with heroin dependence; an estimated 50 million crimes are committed per year to support daily heroin habits.[50] There are approximately 500,000–600,000 heroin addicts in the United States, and about 20% are receiving opioid maintenance treatment.[50] Because of the improved purity and availability of heroin, its use is increasing, and the number of individuals taken into custody who are withdrawing from heroin can be expected to increase as well. Also, although methadone maintenance treatment is strongly associated with decreased criminal activity, individuals currently receiving methadone may be incarcerated on past charges or after a new crime and have withdrawal symptoms when incarcerated. Thus, even though it is most likely that inmates seen with opioid abstinence syndrome are withdrawing from heroin, there also may be individuals who have abruptly discontinued methadone or prescription opioid analgesics.

Clinical Features

As with alcohol, the severity of opioid withdrawal correlates with the amount and duration of the recent regular use of opioids. With mild dependence or intermittent use, there is minimal withdrawal. However, there is a significant abstinence syndrome that occurs with the abrupt cessation of opioids; the time of onset and duration depends on the elimination half-life of the opioid. When the short-acting opioids are involved (heroin or the prescription analgesics such as oxycodone or hydromorphone), symptoms begin within 8–12 hours, peak at 48–72 hours, and persist for 5–7 days. When the longer acting drugs such as methadone or *l*-—acetylmethadol (LAAM) are involved, symptoms begin from 36 to 48 hours, peak at 4–6 days, and persist for at least 14 days.[51] The acute symptoms that follow abrupt cessation of opioids include restlessness, irritability, anxiety, nausea or anorexia, abdominal cramps, myalgias, and sleep disturbance. Objective signs of withdrawal that a clinician can identify include rhinorrhea, lacrimation, piloerection ("cold turkey"), yawning, sneezing, dilated pupils, sweat-

ing, chills, a low-grade fever, diarrhea, vomiting, tachycardia, hypertension, myoclonus ("kicking"), ejaculation, and, sometimes, assuming of a fetal position.[52] Seizures are so rarely associated with opioid withdrawal that the occurrence of a seizure may indicate other drug withdrawal or a co-morbid medical condition. Withdrawal from the long-acting opioids may be less severe, but the longer duration of withdrawal is seen by addicts as worse than the shorter heroin withdrawal. There is some evidence that a protracted abstinence syndrome lasting as long as 6 months may occur, which is characterized by anxiety, insomnia, drug craving, and cyclic change in pupil size, weight, and respiratory center sensitivity.[53]

Treatment

Opioid withdrawal is known to be very unpleasant for patients, but is not generally associated with life-threatening complications. Perhaps because opioid withdrawal has been described as a "flu-like" syndrome, the severity of the discomfort may be underestimated and patients may suffer unnecessarily.

The most researched method for the treatment of opioid withdrawal is the substitution of methadone for the narcotic being used, which allows for gradual withdrawal over time. However, federal regulations require a special license to administer narcotics for the purpose of maintenance or detoxification of narcotic addicts,[54] and correctional institutions are not usually licensed for narcotic addiction treatment. Licensing of correctional institutions to administer methadone is feasible in most (but not all) states and requires a state agency, the Drug Enforcement Administration, and the Food and Drug Administration (FDA) to be involved in the approval process.[55] Jails have been known to allow the administration of methadone to inmates who have been involved with a methadone maintenance program when the local clinic assumes responsibility and delivers and administers the methadone at the jail.[56] The Key Extended Entry Program (KEEP) at Rikers Island, the New York City central jail facility, has become a model program for treatment of addicts in a correctional institution and is operated by Montefiore Medical Center's Rikers Island Health Services. Opioid addicts who had been receiving methadone maintenance or who wished to begin a methadone program, and whose stay was to be brief, were treated with methadone while incarcerated and were guaranteed a treatment slot in the community on release. Initial results were mixed and indicated problems in funding, administration, and other systems, especially those regarding outpatient follow-up.[57] Currently, however, 80% of KEEP patients report to their assigned programs in the community. Prisoners who will remain incarcerated and those who do not want community methadone maintenance are detoxified using methadone; in 1996, 18,644 patients received outpatient opiate detoxification services at Rikers Island. If appropriate licensing or an affiliation with a licensed narcotic treatment program is obtained, methadone treatment of withdrawal can be very helpful. However, physicians are advised to not only seek training in the use of methadone, but also be well acquainted with the risks and benefits of such treatment.

Federal regulations require evidence of physiologic dependence,[58] so signs and symptoms of opioid withdrawal must be present before methadone may be given. It is difficult to estimate tolerance by the self-reported amount of heroin that an addict is using, so the goal is to give enough methadone to suppress withdrawal without risking an overdose.[59] Because even a 40 mg dose of methadone has been known to be lethal in an individual without tolerance for the drug,[60] the starting dose should be 10–30 mg, and the first day's dose should not exceed 30–40 mg unless the dose and enrollment in a methadone program can be verified. Methadone has an average half-life of 24 hours and accumulates over the first 5 days before a steady state is achieved; thus, doses should be increased slowly to avoid the risk of an overdose.[59] For short-term withdrawal, patients can usually be stabilized on 30–40 mg, then the daily dose can be decreased by 10%–20% per day. In KEEP, heroin-dependent prisoners are given a 12-day taper with methadone; those coming from methadone maintenance treatment programs receive a lengthened withdrawal depending on dosage. Usually the dose is decreased 10 mg every 3 days until 40 mg is reached, then the dose is decreased 5 mg every 3 days. Prisoners in Switzerland[61] who were withdrawing from opioids were given methadone detoxification with starting doses of 25–40 mg, and the daily dose then decreased 5 mg/day; the authors suggest that symptom relief and reducing the risk of continued drug use and HIV risk while incarcerated justify inmate methadone detoxification. In the community, relapses would be likely with such rapid reduction of methadone; however, in a closed setting, this protocol may be more successful. Health care providers should be aware that the relapse rates of opioid addicts who have undergone detoxification are extremely high[62]; therefore, if the inmate will return to the community relatively soon, providers are encouraged to refer the addict to narcotic maintenance treatment. For individuals heavily involved with opioid drugs, methadone maintenance has repeatedly been shown to have the most favorable outcomes in terms of reduced drug use, reduced criminal activity, improved health, decreased HIV transmission, and improved social and occupational functioning.[63] Another long-acting opioid, LAAM, now approved by the FDA, can be administered every 2–3 days because of its long half-life.[64, 65] In addition, buprenorphine, a partial opiate agonist, will soon be available for opioid maintenance treatment.[66] Withdrawal symptoms after cessation of buprenorphine are significantly less than with methadone and LAAM, and buprenorphine shows promise in the treatment of opioid withdrawal as well.[67, 68] Some opioid addicts can benefit from opioid

antagonist treatment with naltrexone, an oral opioid antagonist, to block the effects of continued opioid use, although it does not block craving or protracted withdrawal symptoms.

Clonidine hydrochloride, an α_2-adrenergic agonist, is a drug used for hypertension that also has been used as a nonnarcotic opioid withdrawal agent[69] (Table 23-1). Opioids suppress the noradrenergic neurons in the locus ceruleus, so withdrawal results in disinhibition and increased adrenergic activity. Clonidine helps relieve the autonomic symptoms of opioid withdrawal by acting on presynaptic noradrenergic neurons, but is not very helpful in alleviating the craving, muscle aches, or insomnia. Side effects include sedation, a dry mouth, and hypotension. Blood pressure should be monitored for an hour after the first dose of 0.1 mg, then subsequently to avoid a fall in blood pressure that would result in syncope. Patients should be cautioned about getting up quickly, and Kleber[52] suggests that a dose be held if the blood pressure falls below 85/55. The hypotensive effect makes clonidine less useful for women, because they generally have lower blood pressures than men. Usually, the need for clonidine follows the same curve as the severity of the withdrawal symptoms. Maximum doses for outpatients should not exceed 1.2 mg daily, but doses up to 2.5 mg/day have been used in inpatients when vital signs could be closely monitored. Larger doses than those used in outpatients could be used when there is a holding cell near a medical unit with adequate staff to monitor appropriately. Transdermal patches can be used, but some control is lost; additionally, oral clonidine must be used anyway for the first 2 days until blood levels from the patch become effective. Clonidine should not be used during pregnancy, in patients who have recently used tricyclic antidepressants, in those with psychotic conditions, and if there is a risk of cardiac arrhythmia. Although there have not been reports of rebound hypertension with the use of clonidine in this population, it is advisable to taper as noted in Table 23-1.

A more rapid opioid detoxification can occur when clonidine is combined with naltrexone, a long-acting oral opioid antagonist.[70] The patient is pretreated with clonidine (0.1–0.3 mg three to four times per day), then given small doses of naltrexone (12.5 mg, day 1; 25 mg, day 2; 50 mg, day 3 and thereafter), which, if given alone, would generate severe symptoms of withdrawal. Withdrawal is induced by naltrexone and treated with clonidine as already described. The addition of short-acting benzodiazepines, such as lorazepam or oxazepam, antiemetics, and nonsteroidal anti-inflammatory drugs, will help with withdrawal symptoms not covered by clonidine. Although the overall withdrawal duration is shorter with the clonidine–naltrexone combination protocol, patients will require more frequent monitoring. Lofexidine, another nonopioid α_2-adrenergic agonist, has been shown in randomized, double-blind studies in Britain[71] to work well for opioid detoxification. It causes

Table 23-1. Clonidine detoxification schedules

Type of patients	Total dose per day in three divided doses of clonidine (mg)
Offenders who have been on methadone	
Outpatients	
Day 1	0.3
2	0.4–0.6
3	0.5–0.8
4	0.5–1.2
5–10	Maintain on above dose
11 to completion	Reduce by 0.2 mg/day; give in two or three divided doses; the nighttime dose should be reduced last. If the patient complains of side effects, the dose can be reduced by one half each day; not to exceed 0.4 mg/day
Inpatients	
Day 1	0.4–0.6
2	0.6–0.8
3	0.6–1.21
4–10	Maintain or increase if any withdrawal signs occur
11 to completion	Reduce 0.2 mg/day or by one half each day; not to exceed 0.4 mg/day
Offenders who have been on heroin, morphine, oxycodone HCl, meperidine HCl, or levorphanol	
Outpatient/inpatient	
Day 1	0.1–0.2 mg orally every 4 hours up to 1 mg
2–4	0.1–0.2 mg orally every 4 hours up to 1.2 mg
5 to completion	Reduce 0.2 mg/day; given in divided doses; the nighttime dose should be reduced last or reduce by one half each day; not to exceed 0.4 mg/day

Modified from Kleber HD: Opioids: Detoxification, in Galanter M, Kleber HD (eds): *Textbook of Substance Abuse Treatment.* Washington, D.C., American Psychiatric Press, 1994, p 203, with permission.

significantly less hypotension, sedation, and lethargy than clonidine, but is not yet available in the United States.

Pregnancy and Opioid Dependence

Opiate addicts who are pregnant present a special problem because abrupt opiate withdrawal may endanger the fetus; there is a risk of miscarriage in the first trimester and premature labor in the last trimester. It is better, of course, that mothers be abstinent throughout pregnancy. Current thinking suggests that opiate-dependent mothers should be stabilized on methadone, then slowly and carefully withdrawn during the second trimester, by only a few milligrams per week if the mother is stable.[72] In the KEEP on Rikers Island, pregnant women are informed of the dangers of detoxification to the fetus and are allowed the option of methadone maintenance treatment.[73] If the mother is maintained with methadone during the pregnancy, higher doses may be needed in the third trimester as a result of increased fluid space and altered drug metabolism.[72]

STIMULANT WITHDRAWAL
Background

Cocaine is the most frequently found drug in the urine of adult female and male arrestees.[46] There is also frequent use of amphetamines in the many regions of the United States. Thus, many offenders will have abruptly discontin-

ued stimulants when taken into custody. However, it is unlikely that stimulant withdrawal will require any medical treatment.

Clinical Features

The abrupt withdrawal of stimulants results in symptoms that are both psychological and physical. Sporadic use of cocaine or amphetamines does not produce significant withdrawal symptomatology; however, a "run" or "binge" of heavy use over days at a time may end in a "crash" that lasts hours or several days.[74] Because the half-life of amphetamines is longer than that of cocaine, the withdrawal can be expected to last longer but be less severe. Gawin et al.[74] have proposed stages of cocaine withdrawal beginning with depression, agitation, anorexia, and craving, followed by anergia, fatigue, and insomnia accompanied, by an intense desire to sleep. In the later stages of the crash, there is exhaustion, hypersomnolence, hyperphagia, and no craving. Suicide is a risk when dysphoria and depression are severe. For several weeks after the cessation of heavy stimulant use and the crash, there may be a period of withdrawal that includes variable craving, anhedonia, anergia, anxiety, protracted dysphoria, and a high susceptibility to conditioned cues that precedes entry into recovery, if that is to happen.[74] Others have described a greater severity of withdrawal in the first week, followed by a gradual and consistent lessening of craving, as well as sleep and mood disturbances, over several weeks.[75]

Treatment

Treatment should be supportive, although sedation may be helpful if agitation and anxiety are severe. The course of withdrawal after a stimulant binge should be monitored so that suicide can be prevented, and the monitoring process is itself a supportive therapy. Substance-induced psychosis has been associated with stimulant intoxication, and although not a symptom of stimulant withdrawal, the condition may persist after drug use has been discontinued. Patients who are still intoxicated as a result of stimulants and who are psychotic should be managed in a hospital environment. Antipsychotic medication may be helpful in those with acute or chronic stimulant-induced psychosis.

CANNABIS WITHDRAWAL

The use of marijuana is quite common among male and female arrestees, ranging from 20%–44% in adult males and 7%–28% in adult females, to 16%–66% in young adults aged 15–20 years, as measured at 23 sites across the United States.[46] Although cannabis-precipitated psychotic episodes, anxiety, and panic attacks may occur in some individuals, usually with the heavy use of potent cannabis products, the abrupt cessation of cannabis use results in no such severe symptomatology. However, a withdrawal syndrome has been reported in animals and humans after as little as 7 days of tetrahydrocannabinol (THC) administration.[76–78] Rats injected with THC for 4–6 days showed immediate and profound withdrawal after being given a THC receptor antagonist.[79] In humans, 120 research subjects living on a research ward for 2–6 weeks were administered oral doses of THC under double-blind conditions. Stopping the THC resulted in insomnia, irritability, nausea, anorexia, and restlessness, as well as sweating, tremors, and increased salivation.[76] Most symptoms resolved within 24 hours, although some research subjects reported disturbed sleep for up to a few weeks. Marijuana withdrawal was also reported in a female research subject allowed to smoke high doses of marijuana for 21 days, followed by abrupt cessation; she experienced similar symptoms as well as lateral gaze nystagmus and exaggerated deep tendon reflexes—symptoms peaked at 48 hours.[80] Treatment, for the most part, should be supportive only, unless sedation is indicated because of unusually severe agitation and restlessness.

HALLUCINOGENS

The most commonly abused hallucinogen, lysergic acid diethylamide (LSD), is used most frequently by adolescents and young adults.[81] Tolerance to the euphoria and perceptual experiences occurs rapidly with daily use (within a few days), and most users report that they must wait several days between "trips" because of the tolerance. Users rarely report compulsion or loss of control with LSD use. Persistent hallucinogen-associated psychosis may be substance-induced or an unmasking of an underlying psychotic disorder and may be relieved by antipsychotic medication.[82] A withdrawal syndrome has not been identified, and animal studies show that LSD is not a reinforcing drug. Posthallucinogen perceptual disorder (flashbacks) is most frequently visual and may respond to benzodiazepines.[82]

PHENCYCLIDINE

Phencyclidine (PCP, angel dust, sherm, embalming fluid) is seen more frequently in major cities such as New York, Washington, D.C., St. Louis, and Los Angeles. Usually, cigarettes (tobacco, marijuana, mint, oregano) are dipped in PCP and smoked, but it may be taken orally, by the IV route, or by nasal insufflation. A drug-induced psychosis that lasts from 24 hours to several weeks may occur and can be treated with antipsychotic medication after the acute intoxication has subsided. Because PCP has anticholinergic qualities, anticholinergic neuroleptics such as chlorpromazine should be avoided. A severe withdrawal syndrome has been seen in monkeys and includes diarrhea, piloerection, somnolence, tremors, and seizures; however, no such syndrome has been described in humans.[83]

INHALANTS

Volatile substances such as gasoline, glue, spray paint, solvents, and lighter fluid are inhaled ("sniffed" or "huffed"), inexpensive, easily accessible, and legal.[81] There has not been a withdrawal syndrome described that is associated with inhalants.

CONCLUSION

Withdrawal syndromes that follow the abrupt cessation of drug use are medical events that require medical attention. Different drugs are characterized by different abstinence phenomena that vary in their degree of risk and intensity. These phenomena are acute events in the chronic disease of addiction, and we, as health care personnel, have much to offer our addict-patients. We, and most medical professionals, have received too little education in the disease of addiction to drugs during our schooling and early careers. We find it necessary to continue to teach and learn from our colleagues to maintain expertise in a growing and demanding field, made even more demanding by the vast number of addicts who now find themselves incarcerated. It is hoped that this chapter will contribute to this incredibly important venture.

REFERENCES

1. Schultz TK: Alcohol withdrawal syndrome: Clinical features, pathophysiology, and treatment, in Miller NS (ed):*Comprehensive Handbook of Drug and Alcohol Addiction.* New York, Marcel Dekker, 1991, pp 1091–1112.

2. Piker P: On the relationship of the sudden withdrawal of alcohol to delirium tremens. *Am J Psychiatry* 93:1387–1390, 1937.

3. Victor M, Adams RD: The effect of alcohol on the nervous system. *Res Public Assoc Res Nerv Ment Dis* 32:526–623, 1953.

4. Isbell H, Fraser HF, Wikler A, et al: An experimental study of the etiology of "rum fits" and delirium tremens. *Q J Stud Alcohol* 16:1–33, 1955.

5. Mendelson JH, LaDou J: Experimentally induced chronic intoxication and withdrawal in alcoholics. *Q J Stud Alcohol* (Suppl) 2:1–39, 1964.

6. Deitrich RA, Radcliffe R, Erwin VG: Pharmacologic effects in the development of physiological tolerance and physical dependence, in Begleiter H, Kissin B (eds): *The Pharmacology of Alcohol and Alcohol Dependence.* New York, Oxford University, 1996, pp 431–476.

7. Hoffman P, Grant KA, Snell LD, et al: NMDA receptors: Role in ethanol withdrawal seizures. *Ann NY Acad Sci* 654:52–60, 1992.

8. Anton RF, Becker HC: Pharmacology and pathophysiology of alcohol withdrawal, in Kranzler HR (ed): *Handbook of Experimental Pharmacology, vol 114: The Pharmacology of Alcohol Abuse.* New York, Springler–Verlag, 1995, pp 315–353.

9. Earnest MP: Neurologic complications of drug and alcohol abuse: Seizures. *Neurol Clin* 11:563–575, 1993.

10. Victor M, Brausch C: The role of abstinence in the genesis of alcoholic epilepsy. *Epilepsia* 8:1–20, 1967.

11. Devinsky O, Porter RJ: Alcohol and seizures: Principles of treatment, in Porter RJ, Mattson RH, Cramer JA, et al (eds): *Alcohol and Seizures: Basic Mechanisms and Clinical Concepts.* Philadelphia, F.A. Davis, 1990, pp 253–264.

12. Goldstein D: Relationship of alcohol dose to intensity of withdrawal signs in mice. *J Pharmacol Exp Ther* 186:203–215, 1972.

13. Ritzmann RF, Tabakoff B: Dissociation of alcohol tolerance and dependence. *Nature* 263:418–419, 1976.

14. Snell LD, Gyula S, Tabakoff B, et al: Gangliosides reduce the development of ethanol dependence without affecting alcohol tolerance. *J Pharmacol Exp Ther* 279:128–136, 1996.

15. Tabakoff B, Hoffman P: Alcohol addiction: An enigma among us. *Neuron* 16:909–912, 1996.

16. Kalant H, LeBlanc AE, Gibbins RJ: Tolerance to, and dependence on, some non-opiate psychotropic drugs. *Pharmacol Rev* 23:135–191, 1971.

17. Ballenger JC, Post RM: Kindling as a model for alcohol withdrawal syndromes. *Br J Psychiatry* 133:1–14, 1978.

18. Goddard GV, McIntyre DC, Leech CK: A permanent change in brain function resulting from daily electrical stimulation. *Exp Neurol* 25:295–330, 1969.

19. Lechtenberg R, Worner TM: Relative kindling effect of detoxification and non-detoxification admissions in alcoholics. *Alcohol Alcohol* 26:221–225, 1991.

20. Maier DM, Pohorecky LA: The effect of repeated withdrawal episodes on subsequent withdrawal severity in ethanol-treated rats. *Drug Alcohol Depend* 23:103–110, 1989.

21. Whitfield CL, Thompson G, Lamb A, et al: Detoxification of 1024 alcoholic patients without psychoactive drugs. *JAMA* 239:1409–1410, 1978.

22. Naranjo CA, Sellers EM, Chater K, et al: Nonpharmacologic intervention in acute alcohol withdrawal. *Clin Pharmacol Ther* 34:214–219, 1983.

23. Sullivan JT, Sykora K, Schneiderman J, et al: Assessment of alcohol withdrawal: The revised clinical institute withdrawal assessment for alcohol scale (CIWA-Ar). *Br J Addict* 84:1353–1357, 1989.

24. Shaw JM, Kolesar GS, Sellers EM, et al: Development of optimal treatment tactics for alcohol withdrawal: I. Assessment and effectiveness of supportive care. *J Clin Psychopharmacol* 1:382–387, 1981.

25. Sellers EM, Naranjo CA, Harrison M, et al: Diazepam loading: Simplified treatment of alcohol withdrawal. *Clin Pharmacol Ther* 34:822–826, 1983.

26. Wartenberg AA, Nirenberg TD, Liepman MR, et al: Detoxification of alcoholics: Improving care by symptom-triggered sedation. *Alcohol Clin Exp Res* 14:71–75, 1990.

27. Saitz R, Mayo-Smith MF, Robert MS, et al: Individualized treatment for alcohol withdrawal. *JAMA* 272:519–523, 1994.

28. Sullivan JT, Swift RM, Lewis DC: Benzodiazepine requirements during alcohol withdrawal syndrome: Clinical implications of using a standardized withdrawal scale. *J Clin Psychopharmacol* 11:291–295, 1991.

29. Kaim SC, Klett CJ, Rothfeld B: Treatment of the acute alcohol withdrawal state: A comparison of four drugs. *Am J Psychiatry* 125:54–60, 1969.

30. Fuller RK, Gordis E: Refining the treatment of alcohol withdrawal (editorial). *JAMA* 272:557–558, 1994.

31. Kaplan H, Sadock BJ: *Pocket Handbook of Psychiatric Drug Treatment.* Baltimore, Md, Williams and Wilkins, 1993.

32. Naranjo CA, Sellers EM: Clinical assessment and pharmacotherapy of the alcohol withdrawal syndrome, in Galanter M (ed): *Recent Developments in Alcoholism,* vol 4. New York, Plenum, 1986, pp 265–281.

33. Altura BM, Altura BT: Peripheral and cerebrovascular actions of ethanol, acetaldehyde, and acetate: Relationship to divalent cations. *Alcohol Clin Exp Res* 11:99–111, 1987.

34. Altura BM, Altura BT: Magnesium in cardiovascular biology. *Scientific American* May/June:28–37, 1995.

35. Linnoila M, Mefford I, Nutt D, et al: Alcohol withdrawal and noradrenergic function. *Ann Intern Med* 107:877–880, 1987.

36. Sullivan JT, Sellers EM: Treating alcohol, barbiturate, and benzodiazepine withdrawal. *Ration Drug Ther* 20:1–8, 1986.

37. Busto U, Sellers EM, Naranjo CA, et al: Withdrawal symptoms after long-term therapeutic use of benzodiazepines: A randomized, double-blind, placebo-controlled trial (Abstract). *Clin Pharmacol Ther* 37:185, 1985.

38. Tyrer P, Owen R, Dawling S: Gradual withdrawal of diazepam after long-term therapy. *Lancet* 1:1402–1406, 1983.

39. Busto U, Sellers EM: Pharmacologic aspects of benzodiazepine tolerance and dependence. *J Subst Treat* 8:29–33, 1997.

40. Schoch P, Moreau JR, Martin JR, et al: Aspects of benzodiazepine receptor structure and function with relevance to drug tolerance and dependence. *Biochem Soc Symp* 59:121–134, 1993.

41. Kleber H: The nosology of abuse and dependence. *J Psychiatr Res* 24:S57–S64, 1990.

42. Wesson DR, Smith DE, Seymour RB: Sedative-hypnotics and tricyclics, in Lowinson JH, Ruiz P, Millman RB, et al (eds): *Substance Abuse: A Comprehensive Textbook.* Baltimore, Md, Williams and Wilkins, 1992, pp 271–279.

43. Wilford BB: Major drugs of abuse. in Wilford BB (ed): *Drug Abuse: A Guide for the Primary Physician.* Chicago, American Medical Association, 1981, pp 21–84.

44. Gersema LM, Alexander B, Kunze KE: Major withdrawal symptoms after abrupt discontinuation of phenobarbital. *Clin Pharm* 6:420–422, 1987.

45. National Institute of Justice: *Drug Use Forecasting: 1992 Annual Report.* Washington, D.C., Office of Justice Programs, 1993.

46. National Institute of Justice: *Drug Use Forecasting: 1994 Annual Report.* Washington, D.C., Office of Justice Programs, 1995.

47. Harvey SC: Hypnotics and sedatives, the barbiturates, in Goodman LS, Gilman A (eds): *The Pharmacological Basis of Therapeutics,* ed 5. New York, Macmillan, 1975, pp 102–123.

48. Isbell H: Addiction to barbiturates and the barbiturate abstince syndrome. *Ann Intern Med* 33:108–121, 1950.

49. Fraser HF, Wickler A, Essig CF, et al: Degree of physical dependence induced by secobarbital or pentobarbital. *JAMA* 166:126–129, 1958.

50. Nurco DN: Drug addiction and crime: A complicated issue. *Br J Addict* 82:7–9, 1992.

51. Jaffe JH: Opiates: Clinical aspects, in Lowinson JH, Ruiz P, Millman

RB (eds): *Substance Abuse: A Comprehensive Textbook.* Baltimore, Md, Williams & Wilkins, 1992, pp 186–194.

52. Kleber H: Opioids: Detoxification, in Galanter M, Kleber HD (eds): *Textbook of Substance Abuse Treatment.* Washington, D.C., American Psychiatric Press, 1994, pp 191–208.

53. O'Brien CP: Drug addiction and drug abuse, in Hardman J, Limbird L, Molinoff P (eds): *Goodman and Gilman's The Pharmacological Basis of Therapeutics,* ed 9. New York, McGraw-Hill, 1996, pp 568–577.

54. Drug Enforcement Administration: *Physician's Manual: An Informational Outline of the Controlled Substances Act of 1970.* Washington, D.C., U.S. Department of Justice, 1990.

55. McArthur LC, Goldsberry Y: *Approval and Monitoring of Narcotics Treatment Programs.* Rockville, Md, Department of Health and Human Services, CSAT, 1994.

56. Payte JT, Chairman, Methadone Maintenance Committee, American Society of Addiction Medicine (ASAM). Personal communication, 1997.

57. Magura S, Rosenblum A, Lewis C, et al: The effectiveness of in-jail methadone maintenance. *J Drug Issues* 23:75–99, 1993.

58. Food and Drug Administration: *Drugs Used for the Treatment of Narcotic Addicts.* Washington, D.C., 291.505–21 CFR, 1993.

59. Drummer OH, Opeskin K, Syrjanen M, et al: Methadone toxicity causing death in ten subjects starting on a methadone maintenance program. *Am J Forensic Med Pathol* 13:346–350, 1992.

60. Reisine T, Pasternak G: Opioid analgesics and antagonists, in Hardman J, Limbird L, Molinoff P (eds): *Goodman and Gilman's The Pharmacological Basis of Therapeutics,* ed 9. New York, McGraw-Hill, 1996, pp 521–555.

61. Jeanmonod R, Harding T, Staub C: Treatment of opiate whithdrawal on entry to prison. *Br J Addict* 86:457–463, 1991.

62. Ball JC, Ross A: *The Effectiveness of Methadone Maintenance Treatment: Patients, Programs, Services, and Outcomes.* New York,Springer-Verlag, 1991.

63. Zweben JE, Payte JT: Methadone maintenance in the treatment of opioid dependence. *West J Med* 152:588–599, 1990.

64. Ling W, Klett CJ, Gillis RD: A cooperative study of methadyl acetate. *Arch Gen Psychiatry* 35:345–353, 1978.

65. Marion IJ: *LAAM in the Treatment of Opiate Addiction.* Rockville, Md, U.S. Department of Health and Human Services, Center for Substance Abuse Treatment, D.H.H.S. Publication No (SMA) 95-3052, 1995.

66. Strain EC, Stitzer ML, Liebson IA, et al: Comparison of buprenorphine and methadone in the treatment of opioid dependence. *Am J Psychiatry* 151:1025–1030, 1994.

67. Fudala PJ, Jaffe JH, Dax EM, et al: Use of buprenorphine in the treatment of opioid addiction: II. Physiologic and behavioral effects of daily and alternate-day administration and abrupt withdrawal. *Clin Pharmacol Ther* 47:525–534, 1990.

68. Nigam AK, Ray R, Tripathi BM: Buprenorphine in opiate withdrawal: A comparison with cloniodine. *J Subst Abuse Treat* 10:391–394, 1993.

69. Gold MS, Pottash A, Sweeney DR, et al: Opiate withdrawal using clonidine. *JAMA* 243:343–346, 1980.

70. O'Connor PG, Waugh ME, Schottenfield RS: Ambulatory opiate detoxification and primary care: A role for the primary care physician. *J Gen Intern Med* 7:532–534, 1992.

71. Kahn A, Mumford J, Rogers GA, et al: Double-blind study of lofexidine and clonidine in the detoxification of opiate addicts in hospital. *Drug Alcohol Depend* 44:57–61, 1997.

72. Finnegan LP, Kandall SR: Maternal and neonatal effects of alcohol and drugs, in Lowinson JH, Ruiz P, Millman RB (eds): *Substance Abuse: A Comprehensive Textbook.* Baltimore, Md, Williams & Wilkins, 1992, pp 628–645.

73. Glick AJ, Bellin E, Oquendo S, et al: *Opiate Addiction Treatment: A Manual for Interdisciplinary Opiate Addiction Treatment at Rikers Island.* New York, Montefiore Medical Center, 1995.

74. Gawin FH, Khalsa ME, Ellinwood E: Stimulants, in Galanter M, Kleber HD (eds): *Textbook of Substance Abuse Treatment.* Washington, D.C., American Psychiatric Press, 1994, pp 111–139.

75. Miller NS, Summers GL, Gold MS: Cocaine dependence: Alcohol and other drug dependence and withdrawal characteristics. *J Addict Dis* 12:25–35, 1993.

76. Jones RT, Benowitz NL, Herning RI: Clinical relevance of cannabis tolerance and dependence. *J Clin Pharmacol* 21(8–9 Suppl): 142S–152S, 1981.

77. Wiesbeck GA, Schuckit MA, Kalmijn JA, et al: An evaluation of the history of a marijuana withdrawal syndrome in a large population. *Addiction* 91:1469–1478, 1996.

78. Millman RB, Beeder AB: Cannabis, in Galanter M, Kleber HD (eds): *Textbook of Substance Abuse Treatment.* Washington, D.C., American Psychiatric Press, 1994, pp 91–109.

79. Tsou K, Patirck SL, Walker M: Physical withdrawal in rats tolerant to delta-9-tetrahydrocannabinol precipitated by a cannabinoid receptor antagonist. *Eur J Pharmacol* 280:R13–R15, 1995.

80. Mendelson JH, Mello NK, Lex BW, et al: Marijuana withdrawal syndrome in a woman. *Am J Psychiatry* 141:1289–1290, 1984.

81. Dinwiddie SH: Abuse of inhalants: A review. *Addiction* 89:925–939, 1994.

82. Abraham HD, Aldridge AM: Adverse consequences of lysergic acid diethylamide. *Addiction* 88:1327–1334, 1993.

83. Zukin SR, Zukin RS: Phencyclidine, in Lowinson JH, Ruiz P, Millman RB (eds): *Substance Abuse: A Comprehensive Textbook,* ed 2. Baltimore, Md, Williams and Wilkins, 1992, pp 290–302.

24

Desmoteric Medicine and the Public's Health

Robert B. Greifinger, M.D.
Jordan B. Glaser, M.D.

"... he knew that the tale he had to tell could not be one of a final victory. It could be only the record of what had to be done, and what assuredly would have to be done again in the never-ending fight against terror and its relentless onslaughts, despite their personal afflictions, by all who, while unable to be saints but refusing to bow down to pestilences, strive their utmost to be healers."

Albert Camus, 1948[1]

Houses of incarceration are components of a larger criminal justice system, a system whose mission is to protect public safety. One piece of public safety is the protection of the public's health. Thus, it is a natural extension for desmoteric medicine (health services for the incarcerated) to reach beyond personal medical care to matters of public health in the broader community. Although inmate medical care has improved in the past two decades, with expanded access and better organized systems of care, there is more to accomplish.

One opportunity for improvement is the protection of the workforce, and another is the prevention of communicable disease transmission to the communities to which the inmates inexorably return. Public health efforts by correctional health care staff make a difference. Properly achieved, they are cornerstones of the public protection we seek from our criminal justice system.

Public health agencies have worked quietly to stem widespread illnesses, attack health-related environmental issues, and contain potential epidemics such as AIDS.[2]

Although public health efforts have been funded separately and operated in parallel to personal health systems, public funding for the federal agencies that work on public health has been reduced.[3]

Unfortunately timed to the decreased funding for public health, old scourges such as tuberculosis (TB) are increasing their presence, and newly recognized microorganisms, such as HIV and hepatitis B and C viruses, are more prevalent. It has only been since the appearance of AIDS among the incarcerated and the dramatic increase in TB in prisons and jails that the paths of personal and public health systems have crossed.[4] The success of these joint efforts points to a new opportunity to extend the benefits of desmoteric medicine beyond the walls of the institutions to the communities to which most inmates will return.

The potential for public health interventions during the period of confinement is both large and compelling. We can serve individuals, the workforce, and our communities by preventing disease or moderating the risk of transmission of communicable diseases.[5] Funding for these efforts comes through prudent public policy. This public policy must be sensitive to demographic and social changes that influence the number of inmates, sentencing structure, and services available to those inmates. Correctional systems can further stratify their population in terms of risk. Different subgroups have unique risks for communicable diseases, thereby posing different infection control challenges. Each system can tailor its programs to the unique population in its custody.

Other chapters in this volume include excellent discussions on screening for communicable diseases and treatment for HIV and TB. These are good disease-specific resources, but they cannot be used in a vacuum. We have to answer questions such as, how do we deal with special populations such as the elderly or the foreign born? what is the health care agenda for juveniles? what are the special needs of women, whose numbers are increasing at rates beyond men's? how do we create linkages with public health authorities? how do we provide continuity of care on release? and how do we package public health efforts so that they get appropriate attention?

INFLUENCE OF DEMOGRAPHICS ON HEALTH CARE PRIORITIES

The prison and jail population continues to rise. At midyear 1996, there were an estimated 615 incarcerated individuals per 100,000 U.S. residents, two thirds of whom were in the custody of states and the federal government and one third of whom were in local jails. This represents an annual growth rate of 7.7% in prisons and 4.2% in jails since 1990. This increase is disproportionate by sex and by race. At midyear 1996, women accounted for 6.3% of all prison inmates nationwide (69,000), which is up from 4.1% in 1980 and 5.7% in 1990. The female population in local jails reached 10.8% (55,700).[6]

Forty-one percent of all inmates are black (non-Hispanic), and 15.6% are Hispanic.[6] Although the lifetime risk of confinement in a state or federal prison is 5.1%, it is higher for blacks and Hispanics than for whites. At current levels, a black male in the United States today has greater than a 1 in 4 chance of going to prison during his lifetime, and a Hispanic male has a 1 in 6 chance, as compared with a 1 in 23 chance of serving time for a white male.[7]

The incarcerated population is increasing disproportionately among minorities, and there is an increase in foreign-born inmates, both citizens and noncitizens. The risk status is high. Many inmates have a history of alcohol or substance abuse. Most are poor and come from poor communities. There is a high prevalence of infection with TB and diseases transmitted by sex or injection drug use in incoming inmates.[8]

Although there is a high burden of illness among inmates, there are opportunities for important interventions and meaningful improvements in health. Correctional systems provide good access to a large number of individuals at risk for vaccine-preventable conditions. More than 10 million inmates are released per year in the United States. Each release offers a new opportunity for a public health intervention. With their higher rates of injection drug use, they are predisposed to hepatitis virus infection (A, B, and C). They are underimmunized, as the systems for immunizing both children and adults in poor communities are not as good as in other communities.[9, 10] They have high rates of HIV infection, TB infection, and sexually transmitted disease.

Their institutionalized status in a confined environment predisposes prisons and jails to outbreaks of vaccine-preventable diseases such as rubella, measles, and varicella. Inmates are not the only ones who are susceptible. Workers are also susceptible and can bring prison-acquired infections to their homes. Outbreaks are costly and may lead to disruption of orderly activities and time lost from work for correctional personnel. They have the potential to threaten security because of fears of contagion. The successful implementation of inmate vaccination programs has long-term benefits for public health.

Various factors may hinder the optimum use of immunization programs by correctional systems. More than $5.8 billion was spent on correctional health care in the United States in 1990, and is likely higher now.[11] There are pressures on health care spending, not the least of which are litigation, the aging prisoner population, AIDS, TB, and other communicable diseases.[12] Efforts to provide vaccines requiring a series of doses (e.g., hepatitis B vaccine) may be hindered by the relative short duration of incarceration subgroups, such as jail inmates, or by the frequent transfers of inmates in some prison systems.

Correctional jurisdictions should be vigorous in their attention to immunization programs, as inmates are at greater risk for vaccine-preventable illnesses than is the free world population. Immunization programs show better evidence of cost-effectiveness than virtually any other health care intervention. The programs can be tailored to risk status and to predicted length of stay. Automated systems can be developed to not only track primary and secondary prevention opportunities throughout an incarceration period, but also to bridge several periods of confinement.

PRIMARY PREVENTION THROUGH IMMUNIZATION
Hepatitis B

Hepatitis B virus (HBV) infection remains a tremendous public health burden in the United States. There are approximately 300,000 new infections each year, and deaths are from both acute infection (250) and HBV-associated cirrhosis or hepatomas (6,200). There is a national goal to achieve universal vaccination, beginning with children and those with a high occupational risk. Because of their high rates of injection drug use, inmates are in an especially high-risk category.

Decker and co-workers[13] studied HBV among male prison inmates. They reported that 37% of inmates studied had injected drugs before incarceration, 7% had engaged in homosexual activity before incarceration, and 18% had engaged in homosexual activity during incarceration. Similarly, Nacci and Pane[14] reported that 39% of incarcerated federal prisoners engaged in homosexual activity. There is a high prevalence (19% to 44%) of HBV serologic markers among the general inmate population.[15–17] Although these latter data are old, there is no recent suggestion of any reduction in the presence of such serologic markers among inmates. Indeed, with an increasing proportion of sentences for drug offenses, it is likely that infection rates for hepatitis viruses are at least as high as had been previously.

Interestingly, according to these studies of the 1980s, the incidence of new HBV infections among inmates, although incarcerated, is low. This does not rule out new infection on release, however, as many inmates resume high-risk behavior soon after release. Those at especially high risk within the prison include inmates who inject drugs while incarcerated and those serving unusually long sentences.

Inmates as a group can be categorized as high risk for hepatitis B. The potential for infection in those with high-risk behavior is high, and the chance of transmitting this infection in the community is likewise high. Further, the chronicity rate for hepatitis B is 5% to 10%, manifested as a carrier state without apparent liver disease or as mild-to-severe chronic hepatitis. The latter may progress to cirrhosis and primary hepatocellular carcinoma.[18]

Selective screening and vaccination for HBV in high-risk, susceptible inmates have been recommended for the past several years.[5] Hepatitis B virus immunization programs for inmates are beneficial, not only at the time when individuals are directly at risk, but also after their release.[19] Successful HBV vaccination programs have been imple-

mented among juveniles in Oregon[20] and for adult prison inmates on a regular basis in the Michigan prison system.

The Michigan HBV program is offered to all inmates in the general prison population and to new entrants. Seventy percent of inmates without a history of vaccination or imminent parole received one or more doses. In the Michigan prison system example, it was not cost-effective to perform preimmunization HBV marker testing in view of the relatively low overall prevalence of HBV in Michigan inmates, low vaccine acquisition cost, and high laboratory and indirect costs.

Prescreening may be cost-effective for systems with a high prevalence of HBV markers. Pregnancy should not be considered a contraindication to HBV immunization. Infection with HIV is associated with suboptimal antibody response to plasma-derived HBV, and determination of antibody levels after vaccination in inmates with HIV seropositive status may be warranted.[21] On the other hand, immunity may be present without high antibody titers, and additional doses may not confer additional immunity.

The National Commission on Correctional Health Care has a position statement on hepatitis B that includes, among other things, a recommendation that "treatment and prevention programs should be developed to detect and prevent the spread of hepatitis B virus."[22] All recommendations have been, at the least, for high-risk individuals. High risk in this case included those who inject drugs while incarcerated and those serving long sentences. In addition, those with a history of injection drug use or previous jaundice, hepatitis, or transfusions, were included in the list.

More recently, as use of the vaccine has become more widespread, the annual incidence of HBV has declined by 62% since 1986.[23] This success has spurred public health officials to expand the definition of high risk. The Centers for Disease Control recommends hepatitis B vaccine for high-risk adults and long-term inmates.[24] The U.S. Preventive Services Task Force recommends hepatitis B vaccine for all children and young adults not previously immunized and for all susceptible adults in high-risk groups, including injection drug users and their sexual partners, among others.[25]

There are a growing number of cases of HBV in the correctional environment, a high recidivism rate, and a high cost of HBV infection treatment. As the disease is preventable, there are both financial and public health incentives to advising full immunization for inmates in prisons. Because of high risk and the opportunity for a complete series, hepatitis B vaccine is recommended for all inmates with terms exceeding 1 year.

Hepatitis A

It is unclear whether selective screening is useful for inmate vaccination against hepatitis A virus (HAV). This virus causes an estimated 80,000–130,000 cases per year of acute hepatitis in the United States, which result in 100 deaths and cost approximately $200 million.[26] A history of injection drug use is commonly identified (11%) as a risk factor for HAV and is often associated with fulminating disease. There are two preparations available for use.

The Advisory Committee on Immunization Practices does not currently recommend routine immunization for HAV, but they suggest that such a program will be recommended as soon as studies are completed on children younger than 2 years of age.[27] There is currently no basis for a recommendation for routine vaccination of inmates against HAV. It should be considered in those at highest risk, including inmates with chronic liver disease and men who have sex with men.

Rubella

Rubella outbreaks have been described in the prison setting.[28, 29] The American College of Physicians reports that 6%–11% of nonincarcerated young adults remain susceptible to rubella.[10] Preventing fetal infection and consequent congenital rubella syndrome is the primary objective of rubella immunization. The rubella vaccine is recommended for adults, particularly women in their childbearing years, unless there is proof of immunity (documented rubella vaccination on or after their first birthday, or a positive serologic test) or unless the vaccine is specifically contraindicated, as in pregnancy or in instances in which individuals have severe neomycin allergies.

The rubella vaccine should be given to all juveniles and nonpregnant women and should be considered for all male inmates. The combined measles, mumps, and rubella (MMR) vaccine is, however, indicated for individuals infected with HIV older than 15 months of age.[30] The combined vaccine is indicated when individuals are likely to be susceptible to more than one of the vaccine's components.

Rubeola

Measles outbreaks have been described in the correctional setting.[31] This is a concern because measles-related deaths, usually from pneumonia or encephalitis, occur more often among adults.[32] Measles during pregnancy may result in premature labor, spontaneous abortion, and maternal death.[33, 34] Severe cases of measles have also been reported among individuals infected with HIV.[35]

Seronegativity to measles is high (11.8%) among inmates infected with HIV, but would be expected to be lower among those born before 1957 because of naturally acquired immunity. One small study, however, revealed that 3 of 32 inmates infected with HIV born before 1957 had seronegative status for measles.[36] The rate of seronegativity among nonincarcerated Hispanic male military recruits (19%) is similar to the rate among whites (22.4%), but greater than blacks (9.5%).[37, 38] Military recruits have similar demographics to inmates incarcerated for the first time.

Individuals are considered to be immune to measles only if they have documentation of (1) adequate immunization with live measles vaccine, (2) physician-diagnosed measles, or (3) laboratory evidence of measles immunity. The measles vaccine is contraindicated during pregnancy, for those inmates with a history of anaphylaxis after egg ingestion or receipt of neomycin, and for individuals with immunosuppression. As previously mentioned, the MMR vaccine is, however, indicated for individuals infected with HIV older than 15 months of age.[30] The combined vaccine is indicated when individuals are likely to be susceptible to more than one of the components of the vaccine.

The combined MMR vaccine is recommended for all juveniles and nonpregnant women. The combined vaccine should be considered for all men.

Varicella

Varicella (chickenpox) outbreaks have been described in the correctional setting.[39] Among military recruits, rates of seronegativity among nonincarcerated black (13.6%) and Hispanic (10.7%) males are greater than that for white (6.5%) recruits; rates are even higher among recruits enlisting from the island nations and territories.[37] Adults who contract varicella are at an increased risk for pulmonary and CNS complications. Pregnancy and immunocompromised states are also associated with an increased severity of illness.[40, 41]

The varicella vaccine is recommended for individuals living in closed environments with a high risk for varicella-zoster virus transmission and for nonpregnant women of childbearing age. Vaccination of this group reduces the risk for perinatal or congenital varicella.[42]

There are no formal recommendations for the immunization of inmates against varicella-zoster. The live, attenuated vaccine is contraindicated in pregnant women and in individuals infected with HIV. Based on the experience with measles immunity among inmates and the usefulness of histories in predicting varicella among nonincarcerated individuals,[43] inmates with reliable histories may be assumed to be immune.

In a vaccination program, serologic testing before vaccination of inmates without reliable histories of varicella and without HIV risk behavior is probably not cost-effective. In the course of a contact trace, a history of the disease can be assumed to be valid, and the decision to immunize susceptible contacts according to the lack of a history of the disease or according to antibody testing should be driven by the timing and costs involved.

There is no current recommendation for widespread varicella vaccination of inmates.

Tetanus and Diphtheria

Although tetanus and diphtheria are no longer common in the United States, this is true in large part because of effective immunization programs. In 1996, the U.S. Preventive Health Services Task Force affirmed the Advisory

Committee on Immunization Practices recommendation for periodic tetanus and diphtheria (Td) vaccination for adults.[25] Although the interval for a booster dose is not established, 10 years has been a long-standing recommendation. Inmates are at a higher risk for tetanus than is the general population, because of a limited access to health care before incarceration (presuming a low immunization rate) and a high rate of injury among inmates.[44, 45] The vaccine is contraindicated for inmates with histories of a neurologic or hypersensitivity reaction after a previous dose. Booster doses confer protection in 83% of individuals infected with HIV with CD4+ lymphocyte counts of less than 100/mL and in 100% of individuals infected with HIV with CD4+ lymphocyte counts of greater than 300/mL.[46]

Adult Td vaccination is recommended on admission for inmates who do not have reliable histories of current vaccination, and is also recommended every 10 years.

FOREIGN-BORN INMATES

A survey of state prison inmates in 1991 revealed that 4% were not U.S. citizens.[47] In the New York State prison system, the number of inmates born in the United States increased 2.5 times the rate of inmates born outside the United States and its territories. By the end of 1993, foreign-born inmates represented 12% of the New York prison population.[48] Other correctional systems (federal, Texas, Florida, and California) have had increases in the foreign born.[49, 50] For the purposes of this section, a foreign-born inmate is defined as any incarcerated noncitizen, including legal immigrants, amnesty recipients, refugees, and undocumented individuals. In 1990, there were 11.8 million foreign-born noncitizens in the United States.[51]

Tuberculosis

Tuberculosis is the leading cause of death by infection in the world.[52] About one third of the world's population is latently infected with *Mycobacterium tuberculosis.* More than 8 million cases of active disease and nearly 3 million deaths occur each year. The global cumulative number of individuals co-infected with HIV and TB was estimated to be 4.4 million.[53] The proportion of individuals in the United States reported to have TB who were foreign born increased to 30% by 1993. During this period, most foreign-born patients with TB were from Latin America, especially Mexico and Southeast Asia. The incidence of active TB among foreign-born individuals is almost quadruple the rate for native residents. Fifty-five percent of immigrants with TB had the condition diagnosed in their first 5 years in the United States.[54]

Although the incidence of active TB among foreign-born inmates is unknown, their rate of tuberculin skin test reactivity is higher than among inmates born in the United States. In April 1994, for example, 24.2% of New York State inmates had positive Siebert purified protein deriva-

tive of tuberculin (PPD) tests. In that cohort, the range of positivity varied by region of birth from 30% in U.S. possessions to 36% in Canada and Mexico, to 55%–60% in South America, Central America, and the Caribbean.[55] Primary drug resistance is more common among foreign-born than U.S.-born nonincarcerated individuals.[56] Foreign-born inmates are at higher risk for having active TB than U.S.-born inmates.

Hepatitis B

Foreign-born inmates are at a high risk of being chronic carriers of HBV. Selected programs that screened all incoming refugees arriving in the United States from various countries revealed that the crude prevalence rates of hepatitis B surface antigen were highest among refugees from countries in Southeast Asia (range, 11.7%–15.5%) and intermediate among refugees from Africa (range, 7.1%–9.4%).[57] Twenty-five percent of adolescent Fugian Chinese boat refugees were chronic carriers, and 95% had HBV serologic markers. Prevalence rates of hepatitis B surface antigen among residents of the Caribbean and Central and South America are also high.[58]

There is a high prevalence of HBV serologic markers among the general inmate population, as described earlier in this chapter. The rate of hepatitis B surface antigen positivity is higher among inmates who have been involved in violent offenses.[59] Foreign-born inmates are more likely to be convicted of more serious felonies than are inmates born in the United States.[47] Foreign-born inmates are at higher risk for HBV infection than are U.S.-born inmates.

Other Infections

Other viral infections. Foreign-born inmates are at increased risk for having hepatitis C virus (HCV). There are minimal data on the overall prevalence of HCV among the general inmate population. Strong anecdotal reports from California, New Mexico, and Canada, however, indicate that the inmate HCV rate approaches 50%. There is a high rate among female inmates infected with HIV. Hepatitis C virus is especially prevalent among individuals from Southeast Asia.[60]

Human T-cell lymphotropic virus type-I (HTLV-I) occurs among injection drug users and individuals from the Caribbean.[61] It is associated with asymptomatic infection, adult T-cell leukemia, and HTLV-I–associated myelopathy. Recent studies have demonstrated the efficacy of zidovudine for adult T-cell leukemia.[62] Human T-cell lymphotropic virus type-II is also associated with these conditions and is found among injection drug users.[63, 64]

Bacterial infections. *Salmonella* is distributed worldwide. Inmates from Mexico, Columbia, and Vietnam are at an increased risk for typhoid fever. It is unknown whether *Salmonella typhi* produces more complications in HIV infection. Nontyphoidal species may cause recurrent bacteremia, which requires suppressive therapy in patients with AIDS.[65, 66]

Brucellosis, predominately caused by *Brucella meliten-sis,* may be associated with asymptomatic, localized, or chronic infections. Affected inmates may complain of anorexia, loss of weight, headaches, fever, myalgia, and sweats. It may manifest with hepatosplenomegaly or lymphadenopathy. Localized infection may lead to osteomyelitis, pulmonary disease, abscesses, or endocarditis. Chronic infection may persist with nonspecific complaints for longer than 1 year.

Brucellosis has evolved as an important health concern, especially at the U.S.-Mexican border. It has become a disease of the Hispanic population. Inmates with a history of migration from these countries may remain asymptomatic or have nonspecific symptoms. A history of fever, myalgia, and hepatosplenomegaly and ingestion of raw milk products may aid in the early diagnosis and treatment.

Affecting more than 11 million individuals, leprosy (Hansen's disease) is a major health problem in many regions of the world. The burden is greatest in southern and Southeast Asia, Africa, and Latin America.[67] Southeast Asia, Mexico, the Caribbean, and Central America account for the majority of cases.

Fungal infections. Histoplasmosis and coccidiomycosis are fungal infections with focal geographic distributions, associated with reactivation among immunocompromised hosts, including those with HIV infection.[68, 69] Histoplasmosis has been reported from all continents; however, coccidiomycosis is found in parts of Mexico and Central and South America. Clinical manifestations include a prolonged fever, weight loss, generalized lymphadenopathy, hepatosplenomegaly, and a skin rash. The diagnosis can often be made by direct microscopic examination and culture of the fungus from skin and lymph node specimens.

Inmates originating from southern China and parts of Southeast Asia, such as Thailand, may be seen with fevers, marked weight loss, anemia, and molluscum contagiosum-like skin lesions. These are consistent with a *Penicillium marnaffeii* infection. The organism most commonly affects patients who are immunocompromised or those infected with HIV.[70]

Parasitic infections. A variety of parasites acquired before immigration may manifest themselves among foreign-born inmates. Malaria is widespread. *Plasmodium fal-ciparum* predominates in Africa, Haiti, and New Guinea. *Plasmodium vivax* is common in the Indian subcontinent and Central America. Both species are found in Southeast Asia, South America, and Oceania. *Plasmodium malariae* is widespread, and *Plasmodium ovale* is limited mainly to Africa. Most cases of infection with *P. falciparum* develop within 1 month of arrival in the United States, but infection with *P. vivax* can take much longer. *P. falciparum* infection must be distinguished because of chloroquine resistance and the potential for high-grade parasitemia with massive hemolysis and renal failure, cerebral malaria, or noncardiogenic pulmonary edema.[71]

Entamoeba histolytica, the agent of amebiasis, is widespread and highly endemic in Mexico. Inmates may have asymptomatic stool carriage or may be seen with colitis or liver abscesses. *Giardia lamblia* is common in mountainous regions. Patients may have asymptomatic stool carriage or may be seen with acute diarrhea with abdominal cramps, bloating, flatulence, weight loss, or chronic diarrhea with malabsorption.

Cysticercosis as a result of *Taenia solium* (pork tapeworm) is endemic in areas such as Mexico, South America, and parts of Africa, and can manifest after years of U.S. residence.[72] Inmates with a history of recent immigration from Southeast Asia, Africa, South America, or the Caribbean may have manifestations of filariasis, such as a fever, chills, lymphangitis, and lymphadenitis of the extremities and external genitalia. Persistent and chronic lymphatic obstruction may result in elephantiasis. Diagnostic peripheral blood smears should be drawn at night because of the nocturnal period of the microfilariae.

Foreign-born inmates with HIV infection may also be at risk for chronic protozoal infections. Cryptosporidium is the most frequently identified cause of chronic diarrhea among patients with AIDS in tropical and developing countries.[73] This may result in malnutrition, wasting, and increased susceptibility to other infections.

OLDER INMATES AND INMATES WITH CHRONIC DISEASES

Older inmates are a small but increasing part of the confined correctional population. In 1994, the state prison population of older inmates was 19,160, which is a 44% increase over 1990.[74] This is already more than 3% of the population in federal and state prisons. With baby boomers reaching 50 years of age, with increasing rates of incarceration, and with longer terms of incarceration, this proportion will increase over time.

An aging population has increased morbidity from chronic diseases, including diabetes, cardiovascular disease, renal disease, and pulmonary disease. Older prisoners are disproportionately heavy consumers of health care services. Approximately 31% of all personal health care expenditures nationwide are for individuals 65 years of age and older.[75] In prisons, "older" inmates are commonly considered to be 50 years of age or older, because the average health status of inmates is comparable with that of individuals 10 years older and never incarcerated.[76]

Black adults have a three to five times higher incidence of pneumococcal bacteremia than do comparably aged whites.[10] Nonwhite males, the predominant inmate group, have a higher rate of diabetes mellitus, a condition that predisposes to invasive pneumococcal disease. Inmates with diabetes mellitus, as well as all elderly inmates and those with chronic cardiopulmonary disorders, metabolic diseases, hemoglobinopathies, immunosuppression, or renal dysfunction, should receive a pneumococcal vaccine.[20]

Chronic cardiopulmonary disorders probably occur at a higher rate among the incarcerated, as inmates have higher rates of hypertension and smoking than those not incarcerated.[44, 77, 78] These studies report that 85% of inmates admitted to prisons or jails are smokers, as compared with 36.5% of nonincarcerated men older than 17 years of age. Although these are old data, there is no reason to believe that they have changed in the past 15 years.

Adult inmates are particularly susceptible to a variety of other pathogens that spread within institutions.[79] Current levels of immunization against influenza among nonincarcerated populations are 30%–37% for individuals 65 years of age or older and 9%–13% among those 18–64 years of age with high-risk conditions.[9, 80]

Pre-incarceration immunization rates are likely to be low. For example, a review of Medicare reimbursement data for 1993 revealed that the influenza vaccination rate for blacks (17%) was less than half that of whites (37%).[81] Importantly, the antibody titer response to the influenza vaccine is reduced in proportion to the CD4+ lymphocyte count among individuals infected with HIV, although this is not a reason for withholding the vaccine.[82]

Correctional systems are likely to reduce hospitalizations for pneumonia and influenza with a simple annual immunization program. All inmates older than age 65 years and all those with HIV immunosuppression, hemoglobinopathies, metabolic diseases—including diabetes, chronic cardiovascular disease, renal dysfunction, pulmonary disease, and hepatic dysfunction—should receive a pneumococcal vaccine at least once and an influenza vaccine annually.[83] Inmates receiving long-term aspirin therapy should also be vaccinated, as they risk contracting Reye's syndrome if they become infected with influenza.[10] The influenza vaccine is contraindicated for inmates with a history of anaphylactic hypersensitivity to eggs. So that the antibody response is optimized, immunization should be given during the early phases of HIV infection, or at least 1 month after the initiation of antiretroviral therapy for inmates with advanced HIV disease.[84]

Primary prevention of influenza through immunization is recommended by the Centers for Disease Control, the U.S. Preventive Services Task Force, and national professional organizations. Both the pneumococcal and influenza vaccines are inexpensive and have high cost–benefit ratios.[85, 86] The influenza vaccine should be given annually to elderly and high-risk inmates. The pneumococcal vaccine should be given to elderly and high-risk inmates once. Revaccination with a pneumococcal vaccine is indicated in the elderly if the vaccine was given more than 5 years before, and if the patient was younger than age 65 years at the time. Revaccination is also indicated for individuals who are immunocompromised, including those with early HIV infection, if 5 years have elapsed since the receipt of the first dose.

KITCHEN WORKER SCREENING

Screening kitchen workers is a common practice in prisons and jails. This can be a valuable activity if the program is rational about who is screened and for what diseases. In the food service area, we are mostly concerned with diseases that are transmitted by indirect contact through the food. The two most common concerns within this category are hepatitis A and certain bacterial pathogens.

All potential kitchen workers should have a clinical evaluation for acute hepatitis before being allowed to work in the kitchen. An inspection of the skin and scleras for jaundice, along with a palpation of the abdomen for liver tenderness or enlargement, should suffice. Although there is no need to do any further physical or laboratory examination, there may be state or local requirements for further laboratory testing.

Any kitchen worker in whom an acute illness or jaundice develops should be restricted from food service until the problem is diagnosed and the condition is resolved. Hand washing before and after handling food is a very important preventive measure.

Direct-contact transmission involves a body surface–body surface contact, with physical transfer of microorganisms between an infected or colonized individual and a susceptible host. This is more likely at a basketball game than in a kitchen. Nevertheless, all prospective kitchen workers should have their skin evaluated for impetigo before handling food. Hand washing before and after handling food is sufficient to prevent direct contact transmission.

Hepatitis B is not a foodborne illness, so the presence of the hepatitis B surface antigen is not a contraindication to food handling. Human immunodeficiency virus is not transmitted by direct or indirect contact, and is not a contraindication to food handling.

If there are cases of gastrointestinal illnesses that are clustered in time, an investigation of the possibility of a foodborne illness should be initiated. This is the only circumstance when stool cultures might be appropriate for *Escherichia coli*, *Salmonella*, or *Shigella* species. These investigations should always be done in conjunction with public health authorities.

There is no firm recommendation for the routine use of hepatitis A vaccine for nonimmune food handlers. However, if there is an outbreak, it is time to consider a hepatitis A vaccine. The most important preventive technique in the food service area is the teaching of a good hand washing technique and continual reinforcement of its necessity; soap and running water are essential items. Food handlers should be instructed to use friction on all skin surfaces for at least 10 sec while working up a lather. Hands should be rinsed and dried with a disposable paper towel.

RESPONDING TO BLOOD AND BODY FLUID EXPOSURES
Percutaneous and Permucosal Blood Exposures

Every correctional institution should have a clear and rational policy for the response to body fluid exposures, especially those involving percutaneous or permucosal contact with blood. An exposure to blood in the workplace should set a complex chain of events into motion, involving biological, emotional, and institutional responses. These should apply to staff and inmates alike. The policies that drive these activities should conform to current medical thinking and Occupational Safety and Health Administration requirements for the potential exposure to bloodborne pathogens.

A medical determination should be made as to whether a significant exposure has occurred. The risk of seroconversion for HIV after documented significant exposure is low but present at an estimated 0.3%.[87] The rate is higher for hepatitis B and C, approaching 15%. Significant exposures are considered to be exposures of blood or potentially infectious body fluid to the blood, mucous membranes, or nonintact skin. Blood has the most risk, although semen, vaginal secretions, CSF, and other body fluids might be considered significant risks in instances in which it is difficult or impossible to differentiate between body fluids. The exposure of mucous membranes to fluids such as feces, urine, saliva (outside of a dental procedure), and sweat are not significant exposures.

As part of the consideration of the risk of significant exposure, the medical record of the source individual should be evaluated for any documentation of HIV, syphilis, hepatitis B, or hepatitis C. In some areas, the communication of this information may be restricted by laws on confidentiality, although it is usually acceptable to the source to share the information. If this is not possible, the practitioner at least can use informed professional judgment as to the follow-up testing and care.

Seroconversion usually occurs 3–6 weeks after exposure, but a follow-up period of at least 6 months with a physician or HIV clinic is recommended. Baseline testing for HIV, syphilis, and hepatitis B and C should be performed. An example of an emergency protocol for blood exposures is found in Box 24-1.

Prophylaxis should be considered for both HIV and hepatitis B exposure, depending on the significance of the exposure and the risk status of the source.[88] A convergence of indirect evidence strongly suggests that chemoprophylaxis with zidovudine is effective. Treatment with zidovudine after percutaneous exposure appears to reduce the odds of infection by almost 80%. Most AIDS specialists supplement this with a second antinucleoside and a potent protease inhibitor. This treatment should be initiated immediately, or as soon after the exposure as possible.[88]

If he is not already vaccinated, the exposed individual should be offered the entire series of hepatitis B vaccine, beginning soon after the injury. If baseline testing demonstrates current immunity, then the later two doses of the series can be canceled. If the source individual is positive for hepatitis B antigen, or if the source is high risk, the exposed individual should be given a single dose of

---

Box 24-1. Protocol for Blood Exposures

1. Wash the wound first.
2. Proceed immediately to the facility health unit.
3. Manage the wound.
4. Assess whether the exposure was significant.
5. Assess the risk status of the source for HIV, syphilis, hepatitis B, and hepatitis C.
6. Begin counseling on risks.
7. Begin emotional support.
8. Refer for immediate baseline testing for HIV, syphilis, hepatitis B, and hepatitis C.
9. Consider chemoprophylaxis for HIV and vaccination for hepatitis B.
10. Begin prophylaxis immediately.
11. Make emotional support available, as well as counseling for family members.
12. Analyze the event to determine steps for preventing further similar episodes.

---

hepatitis B immune globulin, if this can be given within 7 days.[89]

In addition to wound management, assessment, and prophylaxis, the exposed individual needs emotional support beginning immediately after the injury. This support should be made available for as long as necessary, at least until a 6-month follow-up examination can confirm that no transmission of HIV occurred.

Finally, the injury episode should be analyzed for opportunities for improvement in technique or procedure. Most significant exposures to blood or body fluids can be prevented.

Human Bites

On occasion, correctional staff are intentionally bitten by inmates. When this occurs, routine medical and surgical therapy should be implemented as soon as possible, including an assessment of tetanus vaccination status. Such bites frequently result in infection with organisms other than HIV and HBV (see the Emergency chapter for treatment).

Bite victims should be evaluated for significant exposure to blood, as previously mentioned in the Blood Exposure section. Hepatitis B antigen-positive saliva has been shown to be infectious in human bite exposures. It is not known to be infectious when applied to mucosal surfaces.[89] Human immunodeficiency virus is unlikely to be transmitted by mucosal exposure, although there has been one recent case in which infection may have occurred from deep-kissing a patient with HIV-positive status and gingivitis.

Sexual Assault

Sexual assaults are not infrequent events in prisons and jails. They are high-risk events in terms of emotional complications, communicable diseases, and, in women, pregnancy.[90] Inmates have a high prevalence of HIV and sexually transmitted diseases (STDs). Victims of assault by inmates should be considered to be at very high risk for infection. It is estimated that 0.5%–3% of male inmates are sexually assaulted.[91] Victims may have a heterosexual, homosexual, or bisexual orientation before incarceration. One reported cohort of inmates infected with HIV who were homosexual or bisexual before incarceration demonstrated a high rate (44%) of coexistent injection drug use.[92] However, sexual assault among incarcerated men does not necessarily involve assailants who were gay before incarceration.[93]

Recommendations in this section are limited to the identification and treatment of sexually transmitted infections and conditions commonly identified in the management of such infections. Additional documentation may be necessary for forensic purposes. In women, pregnancy testing should be done at the initial examination to establish a baseline, then in a follow-up examination to determine whether the assault may have resulted in a conception. Emotional support is a critical element of a response to any sexual assault and should be provided to the victim.

In 1993, the Centers for Disease Control issued recommendations for the evaluation of sexually transmitted infections in sexual assault victims.[94] The initial examination should include cultures for *Neisseria gonorrhoeae* and *Chlamydia trachomatis* from any sites of penetration or attempted penetration. A serologic test for syphilis should be performed. Women should have a wet mount and culture of a vaginal swab specimen for *Trichomonas vaginalis* infection. Because the prevalence of HIV and hepatitis B are so high in inmates, it is recommended that baseline screenings be done for both viruses in sexual assault victims in prisons and jails.

There are no data on the prevalence of HIV infection among those who assault, so it is difficult to predict risks for HIV transmission in terms of deciding whether to use postexposure prophylaxis for HIV. If the source individual is known to be infected with HIV, or is at high risk for infection, many infectious disease specialists recommend postexposure prophylaxis, just as it is given for those who have had a significant exposure to blood (see Blood Exposure section). Most patients would benefit from prophylaxis for hepatitis B and antimicrobial therapy, with an empirical regimen for chlamydial, gonococcal, and trichomonal infections.

The examination for sexually transmitted infection should be repeated 2 weeks after the assault. This allows time for acquired infectious agents to produce sufficient concentrations of organisms to result in positive tests. An additional follow-up examination should be done 12 weeks after the assault with serologic tests for syphilis and HIV. If positive, the results should be compared with the results collected on the day of the assault.

THE USE OF ISOLATION FOR CONTAINMENT

Respiratory isolation is part of the armamentarium to reduce the risk of transmission of airborne microorganisms. Airborne transmission occurs by dissemination of either airborne droplet nuclei (5 mm or smaller) or evaporated droplets containing microorganisms that remain suspended in the air. Microorganisms carried in this manner can be dispersed widely by air currents; therefore, special handling of the air and ventilation are required to prevent airborne transmission.

The diseases in this category are TB and the rubeola and varicella viruses. The principles of isolation for each of these conditions are the same. Anyone with suspected or confirmed TB, measles, or chickenpox should be put into isolation as soon as the indication for it is recognized, and should remain in isolation until the disease is ruled out or until they are no longer contagious.

The patient should be the sole occupant of the isolation room, and there should be a visible sign posted indicating respiratory cautions. Patients should not leave the room, except for medical treatment unable to be provided within the room. Patients should wear a regular surgical mask if they do leave the room for medical treatment.

The isolation room should have negative pressure, be ventilated directly to the outdoors, be more than 25 ft from an air intake, and the air exchanges of the room should exceed 8 per hour. An anteroom is advisable. Public health authorities should be consulted regarding the design of isolation rooms, especially the ventilation requirements.

Anyone who enters the isolation room with a patient in respiratory isolation should wear a mask. There are strong public health recommendations for the type of mask to be worn by all contacts with the patient. In 1995, the National Institute of Occupational Safety and Health (NIOSH) revised their certification requirements to a mask that is be rated at least N95, which means that it has 95% efficiency. There are masks that are more efficient, such as high-efficiency particulate air filter respirators; however, they are uncomfortable and, therefore, less likely to be worn properly without breaching the seal. N95 masks should be available in any correctional health care facility for use with patients in respiratory isolation.[95]

Occasionally, patients in respiratory isolation need to be transferred. This should only be for medical reasons. If the transfer must occur, anyone likely to share the same breathing space with a patient in isolation should be informed of the patient's status. The patient should be wearing a surgical mask, and all transport staff should be wearing N95 masks. Vehicle ventilation systems should be set on the nonrecirculating cycle, and staff should be encouraged to keep the vehicle's windows open.

For TB, respiratory isolation should be continued until the patient has appropriate therapy for 2 weeks, or, in the case of known or suspected multidrug-resistant TB, until the patient has received a minimum of two drugs to which the organism is sensitive or that the patient has never taken before. In addition, the patient must be clinically improving and have three consecutive sputum smears negative for acid-fast bacilli.

Alternately, if all sputum smears are negative and the symptoms improve, or therapy directed toward another disease (e.g., pneumonia, pneumocystis pneumonia) results in a cure, then the patient may be released without TB therapy.

MANAGING OUTBREAKS OF COMMUNICABLE DISEASE

Contagious diseases spread more rapidly within institutions than outside. This is no surprise, as the mode of transmission is most often by direct contact or airborne. The more individuals in a confined space, the more likely the spread. There are dozens of diseases that may occur in a correctional facility, and sometimes these spread within the walls. Outbreaks have been reported for vaccine-preventable diseases such as varicella, measles, and rubella. These are described earlier in the chapter. Other unusual but possible culprits include meningococcus.

Several years ago, in the course of a community investigation of meningococcal disease, a strong association with staff or inmate status at one county jail in Los Angeles County was recognized. Nearly half of the community residents with the disease had contact with individuals who had been in a county jail, and the high rate of carriage among recidivists and released inmates suggested that the men became meningococcal carriers while in the jail.[96] This particular investigation revealed carriage of *Neisseria meningitidis* serogroup B into the community and back, while there was coincident outbreak of disease caused by serogroup C, which was limited to the facility.

The lesson from this investigation, once again, is that the walls of prisons are permeable to disease caused by microorganisms. Infections behind the walls can get out and vice versa. In correctional health care, the practitioner has a critical public health role in the prevention of transmission of disease.

Outbreaks of serogroup C meningococcal disease have been occurring more frequently during the past few years, and the use of vaccines to control these outbreaks has increased.[97]

Outbreaks also occur with serotypes A, Y, and W-135. Any case of acute infection with *N. meningitidis* should be thoroughly investigated in conjunction with local public health authorities. At this point, decisions can be made about vaccination or chemoprophylaxis to reduce the risk of transmission of disease.

Linkages with public health departments are the most important; each facility should have contacts at the county department of health and state department of health. When a patient is seen with symptoms of a reportable disease, the local health officials should be notified promptly.

If there are additional cases of patients with symptoms of a communicable disease, the health authorities should be asked to come on site to assist in the investigation. This includes airborne diseases such as TB, rubeola, and varicella. It also includes contact diseases, such as those involving HAV and meningococcus, and foodborne diseases, such as those involving *E. coli, Salmonella,* and *Shigella.* More unusually, but just as important, are diseases that are elusive in their diagnosis, such as hemorrhagic fever, legionnaires' disease, and plague. These conditions are sufficiently uncommon that the diagnosis may be difficult for most prison health staff. An infectious disease consultation may be necessary for treatment decisions, and a public health consultation should be requested for an investigation and the implementation of systemic remedies.

ECTOPARASITES

Pediculosis and Phthiriasis

Infestation by head lice *(Pediculus humanus* ssp *capitis)* can occur on the hair, eyebrows, and eyelashes. Infestation by body lice *(P. humanus* ssp *corporis)* is less common; however, crab lice *(Phthirus pubis)* are common in the pubic area. Inmates are at high risk for infection with these parasites at reception. If there is not universal prophylactic treatment on reception, there is a risk of outbreaks at any time during incarceration. All inmates should be thoroughly inspected on reception for the presence of these organisms and should be treated appropriately. The inmates should be kept in a single cell until treatment is completed, and their clothing should be washed with high-temperature water.

Many correctional systems routinely treat incoming inmates for lice with repellents on a preventive basis. Outbreaks are common in institutions, especially in groups with poor hygiene. The mode of transmission for head and body lice is direct contact with an infested individual or objects used by them. Crab lice are most frequently transmitted through sexual contact.

In these systems, the frequency of outbreaks is much lower than in those that do not use prophylaxis. If there are outbreaks of lice in institutions, correctional facilities should strongly consider universal application of louse repellents. Lice are treated with 1% permethrin cream topically or 0.5% malathion.[18] There are alternative agents.

Scabies

Scabies is caused by a mite, *Sarcoptes scabiei.* The lesions can be papules, vesicles, or burrows. They are prominent around finger webs, anterior surfaces of the upper extremities, belt lines, thighs, and external genitalia in men. In women, the area of the nipples, abdomen, and lower buttocks are more commonly affected. All inmates should be thoroughly inspected on reception for the presence of these organisms and should be treated if they are present. Inmates should be kept in a single cell until treatment is completed.

This is a widespread infection that is common in institutions. The transmission, like other ectoparasites, is by direct contact. The mite does not survive long on bedding or clothing and is less likely to be transmitted in this way than lice. Mites are treated with 5% permethrin topically or by an alternate agent.[18]

CONCLUSION

The period of incarceration is a unique opportunity for prevention. Primary prevention through vaccination is a cost-effective method to avert morbidity and mortality among inmates themselves. It is a further opportunity to avert transmission to workers, their families, and their communities.

Various strategies have been proposed to enhance the delivery of vaccines to adult populations. Inmates should be informed about and offered indicated vaccines (Box 24-2). Correctional facilities should establish and maintain immunization records in view of the high rate of recidivism. These data should be linked with other medical information, including serostatus for HIV and TB data recall systems.

Inmates should be provided with a record of immunization and serologic status, along with a schedule of required booster doses, at the time of release. A few states have developed postrelease aftercare programs for inmates infected with HIV.[98] Vaccine programs should be linked to public health agencies, ambulatory care clinics, and managed care organizations.

Vaccination is only one part of primary prevention. Education on risk factor reduction for bloodborne pathogens and STDs should balance the primary prevention efforts. The next layer of activity is secondary prevention, which involves the early detection of infections or diseases through screening programs. Because of their demographics and risk behaviors, inmates have high rates of infection

with pathogenic organisms. The risk for specific infections should be assessed systemwide, and targeted screening programs should be developed that are consistent with the risk status of the local incarcerated population. Individuals within any system may have symptoms or risk status for a wide variety of communicable diseases. These risk factors should be considered in the diagnosis and treatment.

Tertiary prevention is the prevention of avoidable morbidity and mortality among those with chronic diseases. With communicable diseases, this includes, among others, the chronic manifestations of TB, HIV, syphilis, and chlamydia, which all have a high prevalence in correctional populations. There is an evidence-based treatment regimen for each of these conditions, and they reduce morbidity or improve survival or both.

Public health and community medical care linkages on release are critical components of such care. There should be particular care to prevent interruptions of treatment, as these predispose to the development of resistance. The transmission of a resistant organism becomes a much more difficult public health challenge. Breaches in continuity of care on release are dangerous for the patients themselves and likewise for the community. Each correctional system should have clear and open relationships with public health agencies and community health care resources.

REFERENCES

1. Camus A: *The Plague.* New York, Random House, 1948, p 278.
2. Thrush G: *Empire State Report* January:35–39, 1996.
3. Iglehart JK: Politics and public health. *N Engl J Med* 334:203–207, 1996.
4. Hammett TM, Harrold L: *Tuberculosis in Correctional Facilities.* Washington D.C., National Institute of Justice, 1994.
5. Glaser JB, Greifinger RB: Correctional health care: A public health opportunity. *Ann Intern Med* 118:139–145, 1993.
6. Gilliard DK, Beck AB: *Prison and Jail Inmates at Midyear 1996.* Washington, DC, Bureau of Justice Statistics, US Department of Justice, NCJ-162843, January 1997.
7. Bonczar TP, Beck AJ: *Lifetime Likelihood of Going to State or Federal Prison.* Washington, D.C., Bureau of Justice Statistics, U.S. Department of Justice, NCJ-160092, March 1977.
8. Institute of Medicine: *The Hidden Epidemic: Confronting Sexually Transmitted Diseases.* Washington, D.C., National Academy Press, 1997.
9. Gardner P, Schaffer W: Immunization of adults. *N Engl J Med* 328:125–127, 1993.
10. ACP Task Force on Adult Immunization and Infectious Diseases: *Guide for Adult Immunization,* ed 3. Philadelphia, American College of Physicians, 1994.
11. Anno BJ: *The Cost of Correctional Health Care: Results of a National Survey.* Chicago, National Commission on Correctional Health Care, August 24, 1990.
12. McDonald DC: *Managing Prison Health Care and Costs.* Washington D.C., National Institute of Justice, NCJ-152768, 1995.
13. Decker MD, Vaughn WK, Brodice JS, et al: The incidence of hepatitis B in Tennessee prisoners. *J Infect Dis* 152:214–217, 1984.
14. Nacci PL, Pane L: *Sex and Sexual Aggression in Federal Prisons: Progress Report.* Washington D.C., U.S. Department of Justice, 1982.

15. Decker MD, Vaughn WK, Brodice JS, et al: Seroepidemiology of hepatitis B in Tennessee prisoners. *J Infect Dis* 150:540–549, 1984.

16. Hull HF, Lyons LH, Mann JM, et al: Incidence of hepatitis B in the penitentiary of New Mexico. *Am J Public Health* 75:1213–1214, 1985.

17. Anda RF, Perlman SB, D'Allesio DJ, et al: Hepatitis B in Wisconson male prisoners: Considerations for serologic screening and vaccination. *Am J Public Health* 75:1182–1185, 1985.

18. Mandell GL, Bennett JE, Dolin R: *Principles and Practice of Infectious Diseases.* New York, Churchill Livingstone, 1995, pp 428, 1153–1159.

19. Decker MD, Schaffner W: Should prisoners be immunized against hepatitis B? *Am J Public Health* 75:1134–1135, 1985.

20. Gilbert JL: Give teens a shot: Establishing a hepatitis B immunization program in juvenile correctional facilities. Hepatitis Foundation International.

21. Collier AC, Corey L, Murphy VI, et al: Antibody to human immunodeficiency virus and suboptimal response to hepatitis B vaccination. *Ann Intern Med* 109:101–105, 1988.

22. National Commission on Correctional Health Care: Position statement. *J Correctional Health Care* 5:91–95, 1996.

23. Centers for Disease Control: Summary of notifiable diseases, United States 1995. MMWR 45:73, 1996.

24. Centers for Disease Control: Update: Recommendations to prevent hepatitis virus transmission—United States. *MMWR* 44:574–575, 1995.

25. U.S. Preventive Services Task Force: *Guide to Clinical Preventive Services,* ed 2. Baltimore, Md, Williams & Wilkins, 1996, pp 796–814.

26. Kane MA: Perspectives on the control of hepatitis A by vaccination. *Vaccine* 10(Suppl 1):S59–S62, 1992.

27. Advisory Committee on Immunization Practices: Prevention of hepatitis A through active or passive immunization. *MMWR* 45 (RR-15): 1–30, 1996.

28. Centers for Disease Control: Rubella outbreaks in prisons—New York City, West Virginia, California. *MMWR* 34:615–618, 1985.

29. Chisolm SA: Infection control in correctional facilities: A new challenge. *Am J Infect Control* 16:107–113, 1988.

30. Centers for Disease Control: Recommendations of the Advisory Committee on Immunization Practices (ACIP): Use of vaccine and immune globulins for persons with altered immunocompetence. *MMWR* 42:1–12, 1993.

31. Sprauer M, Markowitz L, Dules L, et al: Evaluation of measles and rubella vaccination among HIV infected adults. Presented at the VI International Conference on AIDS, Abstract No ThB542, San Francisco, June 20–23, 1990.

32. Centers for Disease Control: Measles prevention: Recommendations of the Advisory Committee on Immunization Practices (ACIP). *MMWR* 38:1–18, 1989.

33. Atmar RL, Englund JA, Hammill H: Complications of measles during pregnancy. *Clin Infect Dis* 14:217–226, 1992.

34. Gazala E, Karpus M, Liberman JK, et al: The effect of maternal measles on the fetus. *Pediatr Infect Dis* 4:203–204, 1985.

35. Krasinski K, Borkowsky W: Measles and measles immunity in children infected with human immunodeficiency virus. *JAMA* 261:2512–2516, 1989.

36. Glaser JB, DeCorato DR, Greifinger R: Measles antibody status of HIV infected prison inmates (letter). *J Acquir Immune Defic Syndr* 4:540–541, 1991.

37. Struewing JP, Hyams KC, Tueller JE, et al: The risk of measles, mumps and varicella among young adults: A serosurvey of U.S. Navy and Marine Corps recruits. *Am J Public Health* 83:1717–1720, 1993.

38. Williams W, Hickson MA, Kane M, et al: Immunization policies and vaccine coverage among adults: A serosurvey of U.S. Navy and Marine Corps recruits. *Ann Intern Med* 109:348, 1988.

39. Centers for Disease Control: Varicella outbreak in a women's prison—Kentucky. *MMWR* 38:635–642, 1989.

40. Harris RE, Rhoades ER: Varicella pneumonia complicating pregnancy: Report of a case and review of the literature. *Obstet Gynecol* 25:734–740, 1965.

41. Morens DM, Bregman DJ, West CM, et al: An outbreak of varicella-zoster virus infection among cancer patients. *Ann Intern Med* 93:414–419, 1980.

42. Gardner P, Eickhoff T, Poland GA, et al: Update: Adult immunizations. *Ann Intern Med* 124:35–40, 1996.

43. Alter SJ, Hammond JA, McVey CJ, et al: Susceptibility to varicella-zoster virus among adults at high risk for exposure. *Infect Control* 7:448–451, 1986.

44. Fitzgerald EF, D'Atri DA, Kasl SV, et al: Health problems in a cohort of male prisoners at intake and during incarceration. *J Prison Jail Health* 4:61–76, 1984.

45. Krupp LB, Gelberg EA, Wormser GP: Prisoners as medical patients. *Am J Public Health* 77:859–860, 1987.

46. Kroon FP, van Dissel JT, Labadie J, et al: Antibody response to diphtheria, tetanus and poliomyelitis vaccines in relation to the number of CD4+ T lymphocytes in adults infected with human immunodeficiency virus. *Clin Infect Dis* 21:1197–1203, 1995.

47. *Survey of State Prison Inmates, 1991.* Washington, D.C., Bureau of Justice Statistics, U.S. Department of Justice, NCJ-136949, March 1993.

48. State of New York Department of Correctional Services: *The Impact of Foreign-born Inmates.* Albany, New York, Division of Program Planning, Research and Evaluation, March 1994.

49. Criminal Justice Policy Council: *Alien Offenders in the Texas Correction System* (draft). FY 1990–1994.

50. The Urban Institute: *Fiscal Impacts of Undocumented Aliens: Selected Estimates for Seven States.* September 1994.

51. Census Bureau CH. L98 Table 3.

52. Murray CJL, Styblo K, Rouillon A: Tuberculosis in developing countries: Burden, intervention, and cost. *Bull Int Union Tuberc Lung Dis* 65:6–24, 1990.

53. Snider DE Jr, LaMontagne JR: The neglected global tuberculosis. *J Infect Dis* 169:1189–1196, 1994.

54. McKenna MT, McCray E, Onorato I, et al: The epidemiology of tuberculosis among foreign-born persons in the United States 1968–1993. *N Eng J Med* 332:1071–1076, 1995.

55. Unpublished data, personal communication, New York State Department of Correctional Services.

56. Riley LW, Arathoon E, Loverde VD: The epidemiologic patterns of drug-resistant *Mycobacterium tuberculosis* infections: A community based study. *Am Rev Respir Dis* 139:1282–1285, 1988.

57. Screening for hepatitis B virus infection among refugees arriving in the United States 1979–1991. *MMWR* 40:784–786, 1991.

58. Sobeslavsky O: Prevalence of markers of hepatitis B virus infection in various countries: A WHO collaborative study. *Bull WHO* 58:621–628, 1980.

59. Kibby T, Devine J, Love C: Prevalence of hepatitis B among men admitted to a federal prison. *N Engl J Med* 306:175, 1982.

60. Mansell CJ, Locarini SA: Epidemiology of hepatitis C in the East. *Semin Liv Dis* 15:15–32, 1995.

61. Blattner WA, Blayney DW, Robert-Guroff M, et al: Epidemiology of human T-cell leukemia/lymphoma virus. *J Infect Dis* 147:406–416, 1983.

62. Gill PS, Harrington W Jr, Kaplan MH, et al: Treatment of adult T-cell leukemia-lymphoma with a combination of interferon alfa and zidovudine. *N Eng J Med* 332:1744–1748, 1995.

63. Hjelle B, Appenzelher O, Mills R, et al: Chronic neurodegenerative disease associated with HTLV-II infection. *Lancet* 339:645–646, 1992.

64. Ehrlich GD, Glaser JB, Lavigne K, et al: Prevalence of human T-cell leukemia/lymphoma virus type II infection among high-risk individu-

als: Type-specific identification of HTLVs by polymerase chain reaction. *Blood* 74:1658–1664, 1989.

65. Glaser JB, Morton-Kute L, Berger SR, et al: Recurrent *Salmonella typhimurium bacteremia* as an AIDS-associated process. *Ann Intern Med* 102:189–193, 1985.

66. Sperber SJ, Schleupner CJ: Salmonellosis during infection with human immunodeficiency virus. *Rev Infect Dis* 9:9225–9234, 1987.

67. Mastro TD, Redd SC, Breiman RF: Imported leprosy in the United States, 1978–1988: An epidemic without secondary transmission. *Am J Public Health* 82:1127–1130, 1992.

68. Graybill JR: Histoplasmosis and AIDS. *J Infect Dis* 158:623–626, 1988.

69. Bronnimann DA, Adam RD, Galgiani JN, et al: Coccidiomycosis in the acquired immunodeficiency syndrome. *Ann Intern Med* 106:372–379, 1987.

70. Supporatpinyo K, Chiewchanvits S, Hirunsni P, et al: *Penicillium marneffei* infection in patients with human immunodeficiency virus. *Clin Infect Dis* 14:871–874, 1992.

71. Bjorkman A, Philips-Howard PA: The epidemiology of drug-resistant malaria. *Trans R Soc Trop Med Hyg* 84:177–180, 1990.

72. Scharf D: Neurocysticercosis: Two hundred thirty-eight cases from a California hospital. *Arch Neurol* 46:77, 1989.

73. Malebranche R, Arnoux E, Guerin JM, et al: Acquired immunodeficiency syndrome with severe gastrointestinal manifestations in Haiti. *Lancet* 2:873–877, 1983.

74. *Sourcebook of Criminal Justice Statistics 1995.* Washington D.C., Bureau of Justice Statistics, U.S. Department of Justice, NCJ-158900, 1996, p 565.

75. U.S. Senate Special Committee on Aging, American Association of Retired Persons, Federal Council on Aging, and Administration on Aging: *Aging America: Trends and Projections,* ed 1989–1996. Rockville, Md, U.S. Department of Health and Human Services, 1986.

76. Falter RG: Selected Predictors of Health Services Needs of Inmates Over Age 50 (Ph.D. dissertation). Walden University, 1993, p 17.

77. King LN, Whitman S: Morbidity and mortality among prisoners: An epidemiologic review. *J Prison Jail Health* 1:7–29, 1981.

78. Raba JM, Orbis CB: The health status of incarcerated urban males: Results of admission screening. *J Prison Jail Health* 3:6–24, 1983.

79. Greenberg SB, Couch RB, Kasel JA: An outbreak of an influenza type A variant in a closed population: The effect of homologous and heterologous antibody on infection and illness. *Am J Epidemiol* 100:209–215, 1974.

80. Centers for Disease Control: Race-specific differences in influenza vaccination levels among Medicare beneficiaries—United States 1993. *MMWR* 44:24–27, 33, 1995.

81. Centers for Disease Control: Prevention and control of influenza: Recommendation of the Advisory Committee on Immunization Practices. *MMWR* 46(RR-9): 1–25, April 25, 1997.

82. Kroon FP, van Dissel JT, de Jong JC, et al: Antibody response to influenza, tetanus and pneumococcal vaccines in HIV-seropositive individuals in relation to the number of CD4+ lymphocytes. *AIDS* 8:469–476, 1994.

83. Centers for Disease Control: Prevention of pneumococcal disease: Recommendation of the Advisory Committee on Immunization Practices. *MMWR* 46(RR-8):1–24, April 4, 1997.

84. Glaser JB, Volpe S, Aguire A, et al: Zidovudine improves response to pneumococcal vaccine among persons with AIDS and AIDS-related complex. *J Infect Dis* 164:761–764, 1991.

85. Nichol KL, Margolis KL, Wuorenma J, et al: The efficacy and cost effectiveness of vaccination against influenza among elderly persons living in the community. *N Engl J Med* 331:778–784, 1994.

86. Gross PA, Hermogenes AW, Sacks HS, et al: The efficacy of influenza vaccine in elderly persons: A meta-analysis and review of the literature. *Ann Intern Med* 123:518–527, 1995.

87. Gerberding JL: Prophylaxis for occupational exposure to HIV. *Ann Intern Med* 125:497–501, 1996.

88. Centers for Disease Control: Guidelines for management of occupational exposure. *MMWR* 45:22, June 7, 1996.

89. Centers for Disease Control: Post-exposure management. *MMWR* 38:S6, June 23, 1989.

90. Glaser JB, Hammerschlag MR, McCormack WM: Sexually transmitted diseases in victims of sexual assault. *N Engl J Med* 315:625–627, 1986.

91. Moss C, Hosford R, Anderson W: Sexual assault in prison. *Psychol Rep* 44:823–828, 1979.

92. Bastadjian S, Greifinger RB, Glaser JB: Clinical characteristics of male homosexual/bisexual HIV-infected inmates. *J AIDS* 5:744–745, 1992.

93. Davis AJ: Sexual assaults in the Philadelphia prison system and sheriff's vans. *Transaction* 6:8-16, 1968.

94. Centers for Disease Control and Prevention: 1993 sexually transmitted diseases treatment guidelines. *MMWA* 42(RR-14):1–102, 1993.

95. Hospital Infection Control Practices Advisory Committee: Part II. *Recommendations for Isolation Precautions in Hospitals.* Atlanta, Ga, Centers for Disease Control, Document 250135, June 1995.

96. Tappero JW, Reporter R, Wenger JD, et al: Meningococcal disease in Los Angeles County, California, and among men in the county jails. *N Engl J Med* 335:833–840, 1996.

97. Centers for Disease Control: Control and prevention of serogroup C meningococcal disease: Evaluation and management of suspected outbreaks: Recommendations of the Advisory Committee on Immunization Practices. *MMWR* 46(RR-5): February 14, 1997.

98. Dixon PS, Flanigan TP, DeBuono BA, et al: Infection with the human immunodeficiency virus in prisoners: Meeting the health care challenge. *Am J Med* 95:629–635, 1993.

25

Mortality in Prisons and Jails

Jack Raba, M.D.

To investigate the causes of death, to examine carefully the conditions of organs, after such changes have gone on in them as to render existence impossible, and to apply knowledge to the prevention and treatment of disease, is one of the highest objects of the Physician ...

William Osler, 1991[1]

INTRODUCTION

The goal of all health care delivery systems, including correctional health care programs, is the improvement and maintenance of the health and prevention of illnesses and complications of diseases in the population served. Deaths, especially preventable or avoidable deaths, are important indicators of the quality and effectiveness of a health care program. Mortality data for incarcerated populations, accurately collected and astutely analyzed, can result in the formation and implementation of policies, procedures, and programs that decisively influence the causes and rates of death. The systemic collection of epidemiologic mortality data must be an essential component of an adequate prison or jail program.

IMPACT OF A DEATH IN A CORRECTIONAL FACILITY

The death of a detainee or a prisoner has tremendous impact on all aspects of correctional populations and systems. Death evokes significant emotional responses in all societies. The sense of loss and the need for bereavement impacts on the family, friends, and acquaintances of the deceased in every community. The death of an individual in legal custody is accompanied by all the expected mourning of family and friends. However, the impact of each individual death in prison or jail ripples far beyond the immediate circle of an inmate's family. The death of an incarcerated man or woman has an immediate and, at times, disrupting institutional, systemic, and legal effect.

It is difficult for the family of a deceased detainee or prisoner to accept the announcement of an inmate's death comfortably. Families commonly are hesitant to believe that everything possible had been done to treat the inmate's medical condition or to prevent the circumstances that led to the death. Family members generally have had little, if any, previous or ongoing communication with the correctional medical staff providing the primary and secondary care in the correctional facility. This lack of an established relationship with the inmate's physician or health team eliminates a basis of trust between the provider and the family. Multiple class action litigations have shown that inmates complain most often about food services and health care. It would not be surprising to find that inmate's communications with their families may not have extolled the quality of the correctional health care services, even if it was fully accredited and might even exceed the care available in the inmates' communities of origin. The family's lack of established communication with the correctional health care team and the correctional institution and the potential for displaced anger may result in families initiating legal action, even when there were no clearcut medical errors or deficiencies in the emergency response to the moment of death.

Families of detainees who die in local jails or lock-ups also feel a sense of guilt in that they had been unable or unwilling to post the bond necessary to secure an accused individual's release pending his trial. This guilt may be converted to anger directed at the correctional institution.

In addition, the correctional institution will often feel the impact of the death of an inmate or detainee. Other inmates housed in the facility will be saddened, depressed, or outraged by the death of a fellow inmate. There is a dreaded and quite understandable fear among most inmates concerning dying behind the walls of a prison or jail, distant and separated from the comfort of family and friends.

Deaths in correctional facilities have resulted in riots and the initiation of class action law suits. Deaths have even resulted in other deaths. There is evidence that a death by suicide may trigger a series of suicide attempts and gestures within a correctional institution.[1–3]

Correctional officers spend a significant amount of their workday in direct contact with incarcerated men and women. It is natural that the officers develop certain levels of relationships with inmates. Generally, this officer-inmate relationship is solely professional, yet over time, especially in long-term correctional facilities, a bond of respect and even friendship may develop. Correctional officers and officials and members of the health care team will feel the loss of an inmate through death.

Preventable deaths weigh heavily on the correctional and medical staff who respectively guarded or cared for an individual. Staff striving to fulfill their assigned duties with diligence and competence are impacted negatively by the death of an individual in their charge. They question whether they had done everything to fully protect and treat the deceased. They grieve and mourn and critique the death and, on occasion, may even suffer from reactive depression.

Correctional institutions and systems also are affected administratively by the death of an incarcerated man or woman. Deaths prompt internal and external reviews. Quality improvement and death review committees investigate the circumstances surrounding a death, and policies and procedures are re-evaluated. The training programs of staff are modified, revised, and expanded. Media and political attention can be elicited following a death or a series of deaths in a correctional institution or system. Both malpractice and civil litigation can result from the death of an incarcerated individual. All deaths of men and women in custody are automatically deemed coroner's cases and, consequently, deaths in correctional facilities result in a much higher rate of autopsy than that in the general community. The medical examiner who has a correctional facility within his jurisdiction will be involved with each and every death of an inmate or detainee.

MORTALITY DATA IN PRISONS AND JAILS

Although the overlap between prisons and jails is extensive, a steady river of men and women are being transferred or shipped from jails to prisons, and a smaller stream of inmates are returned to local correctional facilities for retrials and appeals. The data on mortalities in prisons and in jails will be presented separately.

Mortality in Prisons

In 1981, King and Whitman noted the considerable lack of published data on mortality experiences in correctional populations.[4] Because their exhaustive search of the literature in 1980 to 1981 revealed only a single publication of mortality statistics in a prison system, they encouraged correctional health leaders to document and publish mortality data for their respective institutions.

Although most large correctional health programs currently maintain data on mortalities, this information is kept internally and is rarely available for evaluation and comparison with other systems. Seven studies on mortality in prisons were obtained; four of which were published in the literature. The four published reports used statistical tools (mortality rate, SMR, actual vs. predicted deaths) that allowed the comparison of the incarcerated mortality rates with the rates for the general, non-incarcerated population.

Tennessee. The deaths in the Tennessee (USA) Department of Corrections in 1972 were reported by Jones.[5] There were 16 deaths during the calendar year and 20 deaths during the Tennessee fiscal year of 1972. Six (38%) of the deaths were homicides; one (6%) was due to an accidental or external cause. There were no suicides in the Tennessee prisons in 1972. The 1972 death rate for Tennessee prisoners was 20 times higher than that of the general USA population. The 33% variance in deaths between these two overlapping 12-month periods suggests a possible large variation in year-to-year rates.

Coupled with the relatively limited number of deaths, previous authors advised that the Tennessee prison system data be interpreted with caution.[4] This is the only published comparative study that suggested that overall death rates for prisoners were higher than the rates for the general U.S. population.

France. Clavel et al. compared the 1977 to 1983 mortality rate for male prisoners in France with that of the gen-

Table 25-1. Comparison of mortality among male prisoners with that among men in the French population from 1977 to 1983 for major causes of death

Causes of death*	Observed	Expected	SMR†	p
All Causes	286	310.2	92	NS
Infective and parasitic diseases (001-139)	4	3.5	116	NS
Malignant neoplasms (140-208)	32	58.8	54	< 0.0005
Endocrine, nutritional, and metabolic diseases (240-279)	3	2.8	106	NS
Mental disorders (290-319)	5	6.2	81	NS
Diseases of the nervous system and sense organs (320-389)	7	6.3	110	NS
Diseases of the circulatory system (390-459)	61	40.1	152	< 0.001
Diseases of the respiratory system (460-519)	8	1.0	114	NS
Diseases of genitourinary system (580-629)	2	1.1	180	NS
Symptoms and ill-defined conditions (780-799)	13	22.6	58	< 0.05
External causes (E800-E999)	138	134.7	102	NS
Accidents, poisoning, and violence (E800-ZE949, E960-E999)	34	101.5	34	< 0.0001
Suicides (E950-E959)	104	33.2	313	< 0.0001

*9th ICD revision.

†Standardised mortality ratio (compared to 100).

eral French population.[6] They found that the overall mortality rate was lower among prisoners (Table 25-1). The study specifically noted that deaths from malignant neoplasms, accidents, and poisonings were significantly lower among the incarcerated population, while suicides and diseases of the respiratory and circulatory system were much higher than expected. The overall mortality and specifically mortality from cancers, diseases of the circulatory system, and suicides fell with the increasing duration of incarceration. Clavel et al. conjectured that the decreased mortality rate for prisoners was attributable to a variety of factors: those with serious illnesses are less likely to commit crimes and, if charged, are more likely to be released, access to health care services might be enhanced within the prison system especially for lower social classes, and the lifestyle of the prison, including decreased access to alcohol and drugs, might lead to improved physical health. Clavel et al. also made a controversial hypothesis that the lower incidence of cancer may be related to the high use of tranquilizers in the prison population. He quoted references which theorized that tranquilizers had anti-tumor effects.[6]

Michigan. A review of the 162 male and female deaths in the Michigan Department of Corrections from 1973 to 1983 was performed by Faiver.[7] The all-cause mortality rate of 190.5 was lower that for the U.S. general population. Natural causes accounted for 63.6% of the deaths, suicide 22.2%, homicide 11.7%, and accidents 2.5%. Heart disease was the leading individual cause of mortality, followed by suicide, then cancer. Two-thirds of the 24 cancers causing death originated in the lung. The rates for suicide and homicide varied dramatically according to the race of the prisoner. Suicide was 2.1 times higher for prisoners than would be expected for the same age-race cohorts of the U.S. population. For white prisoners in the Michigan Department of

Table 25-2. Homicides, by method: Michigan Department of Corrections, 1977-1983

Method	Frequency	Percentage
Stabbing	15	78.9
Beating	2	10.5
Hanging	1	5.3
Suffocating	1	5.3
All Methods	19	100.0

Corrections, the suicide rate was 2.9 times the U.S. rate and for African-Americans, 1.4 times.

Although homicide was the third-leading cause of death of Michigan prisoners during this period, the rate was only three-tenths the U.S. rate. The method of homicide was predominantly by stabbing (Table 25-2). It is important that black prisoners had one-fourth the homicide mortality compared with blacks of similar age who were not incarcerated, while the homicide rate was the same for incarcerated and non-incarcerated whites. Faiver hypothesized that the decreased mortality rate for blacks was due to the omnipresence of security in the prison system and the absence of guns within the prison.[7]

Maryland. Salive et al. reviewed all deaths in the State of Maryland prison system from 1979 through 1987.[8] Prisoners had a lower all-cause mortality than the general population of Maryland. However, significant elevations of suicide and infection deaths were noted. They observed that, although there were no infectious disease deaths until 1984, by 1987 infectious diseases, predominantly AIDS, had become the leading cause of mortality in Maryland

Table 25-3. Mortality for leading causes of death United States, 1992

Rank	Cause of death	Number of deaths	Death rate per 100,000 population*	Percent of total deaths
	All Causes	2,175,613	679.6	100.0
1	Heart Diseases	717,706	214.1	33.0
2	Cancer	520,578	172.2	23.9
3	Cerebrovascular Diseases	143,769	41.1	6.6
4	Chronic Obstructive Lung Disease	91,938	28.4	4.2
5	Accidents	86,777	30.6	4.0
6	Pneumonia & Influenza	75,719	20.9	3.5
7	Diabetes	50,067	15.9	2.3
8	HIV Infection	33,566	10.6	1.5
9	Suicide	30,484	10.8	1.4
10	Homicide	25,488	9.5	1.2
11	Diseases of Arteries	25,337	7.7	1.2
12	Cirrhosis of Liver	25,263	9.0	1.2
13	Nephritis	22,162	6.5	1.0
14	Septicemia	19,667	5.8	0.9
15	Atherosclerosis	16,831	4.5	0.8
	Other & ill-defined	290,261	91.8	13.3

*Age-adjusted to the 1970 U.S. standard population.

Table 25-4. Illinois Department of Corrections institutional deaths, 1981-1990

	Total
1. Diseases of Heart and Blood Vessels	77
2. Cancer	47
3. Suicide	38
4. Other	33
5. AIDS	30
6. Homicide	29
7. Respiratory	21
8. Accidental	14
9. Unknown	6
10. Execution By Lethal Injection	1

prisons. Cancer, circulatory diseases, and external cause mortalities were lower than those of the non-incarcerated population of Maryland.

In a companion study of suicides, it was observed that the suicide rate for Maryland prisoners during the same time was higher than that of the general U.S. population (39.6 vs. 18.4).[9]

Oregon. Kamara et al. reported on the epidemiology of unnatural deaths (suicide, homicide, and accidental) in the Oregon State Prisons from 1963 to 1987.[10] Forty of the 52 unnatural deaths in the 25 years were caused by suicide. The unnatural prisoner death rates for 1983 through 1992 were compared with the rates for noninstitutionalized citizens of Marion County, a large county in Oregon. Prisoner deaths caused by suicide exceeded the noninstitutionalized rates for suicide (30.3 vs. 13.0) and homicide (5.1 vs. 3.2). Deaths caused by accidents had a much lower rate for the incarcerated (5.1 for prisoners vs. 29.7). The higher accidental death rate outside the prison was mostly attributed to motor vehicle mortalities. It is easily understood that incarcerated populations will spend significantly less time in vehicles and will, accordingly, have lower motor vehicle-related fatalities.

Illinois. The Illinois Department of Corrections (IDOC) has been tracking mortalities in its prison system for more than 16 years. The census of men and women housed in the IDOC grew from 14,711 in 1981 to 38,882 in 1996. During this 16-year period, there were 813 deaths, with an overall mortality rate of 222.1 (personal communication; Schuman H, Coe J; March 1997). As anticipated due to the relatively young age of the IDOC prisoners (92% to 93% of the IDOC inmate population is 45 years of age or younger), this rate is significantly lower that the 1992 U.S. all-age mortality rate of 679.6 (Table 25-3).[11] The death rate for inmates under 45 years was 166.5, which is lower than the 1988 City of Chicago mortality of 278 for 25- to 45-year-olds. The lower mortality rate for prisoners, especially for the younger age groups, is, in part, attributed to the decreased rate of homicide and accident deaths within the prison system in comparison to the non-incarcerated age-matched population.

The homicide rate in the IDOC was 12.6, compared with the U.S. rate for 25- to 34-year-olds of 14.7 (1985) and the City of Chicago rate for non-whites of 68.4.[12] The accidental death rate for IDOC prisoners was less than one-half the

Table 25-5. Cause-specific death ratios (%) in Florida correctional institutions: 1987 through 1992

Cause of death	1987 (n = 75)	1988 (n = 83)	1989 (n = 97)	1990 (n = 93)	1991 (n = 123)	1992 (n = 130)
AIDS	34.7	38.6	41.1	42.7	48.0	52.3
Cardiac arrest	18.7	15.7	13.7	16.7	18.7	13.1
Cancer	13.3	22.9	21.1	20.8	16.3	13.1
Neurological	4.0	1.2	0	4.1	2.4	3.1
Meningitis	0	0	0	2.1	0	0.7
Respiratory	1.3	2.4	3.2	1.0	2.4	3.1
Asthma	2.7	1.2	1.1	0	0	2.3
Tuberculosis	1.3	0	0	0	0.8	0
Hepatic-related	0	4.8	5.3	5.2	2.4	3.8
Renal failure	0	2.4	1.1	0	0.8	0
Septicemia	4.0	0	2.1	0	0.8	0
Vascular	1.3	0	3.2	0	0	0
Postoperation complications	0	2.4	1.1	0	0	0
Bleeding	1.3	0	0	0	0	0
Diabetes complications	0	0	0	0	2.4	0
Gastrointestinal disease	0	0	0	0	0	2.3
Suicide	8.0	2.4	4.2	2.1	2.4	4.6
Accidents	2.7	1.2	2.1	2.1	3.3	1.5
Homicide	6.8	4.8	1.1	3.1	1.6	0

Note: These percentages are based on the number of deaths each year that occurred in Florida's major institutions and that were subject to mortality review by the Bureau of Health Services. Florida Department of Corrections.
Source: Ratios are based on data from the Florida Department of Corrections Health Services. Quality Management Program, 1993.

rate for the U.S. non-incarcerated 25- to 34-year-old population. Over this 16-year period, the leading causes of death were 1) diseases of the heart and blood vessels, 2) AIDS, 3) cancer, and 4) suicide (Table 25-4).

Heart disease was the leading annual cause of death for the 11 years prior to 1992. However, since the first AIDS mortality in the IDOC in 1986, AIDS deaths have steadily increased and from 1993 on, AIDS has become the leading annual cause of death in the IDOC (personal communication, Schuman H and Coe J, March 1997). The IDOC data revealed that the older (more than 46 years of age) segment of the prison population that comprised only 7% to 8% of the census accounted for 30.6% of all mortalities. White inmates also had a higher percentage of death than would have been expected. While 28%–29% of the IDOC population is white, 38% of the system's mortalities were in this group. Blacks and Hispanics in the IDOC had fewer deaths than would be anticipated, based on their percentages of the incarcerated population. The data did not allow further analysis of the reasons for the disproportionate rates of death for the different racial groups.

Florida. The Florida Department of Corrections houses one of the largest inmate populations in the USA, with an average daily census of over 56,000 in 1994 and an annual turnover of 32,000.[13] Table 25-5 reflects the cause-specific death ratios for the Florida Department of Corrections from 1987 to 1994.[14] Acquired immunodeficiency syndrome has clearly become the dominating cause of mortality among

prisoners in Florida. Figure 25-1 indicates the steady increase in the gross number of AIDS deaths over this 8-year period. Cancer mortality exceeded cardiovascular mortality during this period. The reason for this was not explained.

The Florida DOC has effectuated a steady decrease in both the percentage and the actual number of homicides among the prison population. There were 13 homicides from 1987 to 1990 and only 7 from 1991 to 1994, despite a significant increase in the system's average daily census.[13]

MORTALITY IN JAILS

Jails are short-term correctional facilities that house detainees while they are awaiting the completion of their trials or serving sentences of less than 1 year. The average length of stay in jails is generally measured in weeks to months, but may vary widely from institution to institution. Nonetheless, jails consistently have a moderate portion of their detainee population who spend over a year in their facilities while complicated court cases and appeals are litigated. While prison populations turn over from one to two times annually, jails turn over 10 to 20 times per year with a discernible percentage of the admissions being recidivists. Jails admit newly arrested men and women who enter the facility directly from the community. Many enter with untreated, undiagnosed, or neglected medical conditions. Significant numbers are admitted with active substance use histories and are under the influence of legal or illegal

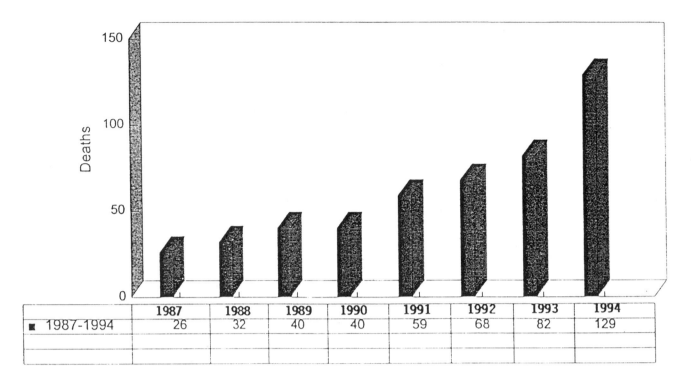

Figure 25-1. Acquired Immunodeficiency Syndrome Deaths, Florida Department of Corrections.

drugs. Jails historically have a population with a younger average age when compared to prison populations.

The dissimilar demographics between jail and prison populations must be considered when evaluating the epidemiology and rates of mortalities, especially if an attempt is made to compare jails and prisons. As with prisons, there are few published or publicly reported sets of data on mortality statistics in jails. The mortality data from four correctional systems, three urban jails in the USA, and a review of police custody deaths from Australia will be discussed.

New York City

Even in the nineteenth century, jails were known to track the numbers and causes of death. The report of the Chief Physician to the New York City Board of Commissioners of Public Charities and Correction dated January 1, 1886 reported 19 deaths in 1885 in the City Prison of New York City. With 39,616 "commitments" to the jail in 1885, there was one death for every 2,085 admissions in 1885. The causes of death were dominated by substance abuse–related diagnoses, including "exhaustion from intemperance and delirium tremens" (Box 25-1), with at least one-half of the deaths presumably caused either directly or indirectly by alcohol use.

In 1978, Novick and Remmlinger published a study of 128 deaths occurring in the New York City correctional facilities between 1971 and 1976.[15] Seventy-one (55%) of the deaths were due to "external causes and accidents" with

suicide the overwhelming cause (52) of deaths in this category and the overall leading cause. In comparison with the male New York City population of similar age ranges, mortality rates for suicide were significantly greater among detainees (Table 25-6).[15] The authors found that whites and Hispanics had disproportionately high suicide rates, while the rates for black prisoners were low.

Twenty-one (16%) of the deaths were attributed to cardiovascular disease, even though the mean age of all inmates who died was only 34 years. Death rates in the New York jails for nonviolent causes and homicide were lower in almost all age groups than in comparable nonincarcerated New York City populations.[15]

Unpublished mortality data from the New York City correctional facilities for 1986 to 1990 revealed a dramatic shift in the causes of detainee death (personal communication, Delone M, 1991). By 1988, AIDS had become the leading annual cause of death in New York City jails. Between 1986 and 1990, 52.4% of all detainee deaths were caused by AIDS. Of notable additional importance was the dramatic decrease in both the incidence and percentage of suicide deaths.

During this 5-year period, there were a total of 17 suicides, accounting for only 4.8% of the deaths. This striking improvement in the suicide rates, when compared with the rate in 1971 to 1976 when suicide accounted for over 40% of all deaths, was in large part attributed to comprehensive changes in both the funding and organization of mental health services and the development and implementation of

Box 25-1. Sample Mortality Report from the Nineteenth Century

PHYSICIAN'S REPORT

CITY PRISON, HALLS OF JUSTICE,

NEW YORK, *January 1st,* 1866.

To the Honorable the Board of Commissioners of Public Charities and Correction

GENTLEMEN—I respectfully lay before you my sixth Annual Report of the medical Department of the City Prison, and its three branches, showing its statistics for the year 1865.

The total number of commitments to this institution during the past year was thirty-nine thousand six hundred and sixteen (39,616), and the number of deaths nineteen (19), from the following causes, viz.:

Exhaustion from Intemperance	9
Apoplexy	1
General Debility	2
Congestion	3
Suicide by Hanging	1
Delirium Tremons	1
Tuberculosis	1
Ascites	1
	19

Table 25-6. Age specific suicide rates (per 100,000) for males, NYC And NYC correctional facilities, 1971-75

Age	NYC correctional facilities[1]	NYC[1]
15-24	76	10
25-34	103	18
35-44	194	13
45-54	49	15
55-64	0	1

Note: Rates are based upon 52 suicides and approximately 51,000 "prisoner-years."
[1]Novick and Remmlinger, 1978.

rigorous mental health standards within New York City correctional facilities.[16]

Wayne County, Detroit

Smialek and Spitz studied all deaths in Wayne County Michigan Jail and in 40 local lockups in the county in 1976 and 1977.[17] These facilities housed over 1,000 detainees on a daily basis, with an average of 941 in the Wayne County Jail. There were 25 deaths during this period. "Of the 25 deaths, 20 were suicides, with one accident, one homicide, one of natural cause, and two of undetermined cause. The deaths of undetermined cause were drug-related." The authors noted that suicide rates in jails and local detention facilities were significantly higher than those in prisons. The age of the inmates who died ranged from 17 to 43 years with a median age of 21 years. Eight of the 20 suicide victims had been arrested on minor charges and nine of the suicide victims were found to have alcohol and/or drugs in their systems. Nineteen of the suicides were by hanging. An astounding 24 of the 25 deaths occurred within the first 24 hours of incarceration. Smialek and Spitz presented a series of astute recommendations concerning the investigation of all deaths in jails and local detention facilities, including a mandatory, thorough autopsy, detailed history of the circumstances of arrest with particular attention to altercations, the position and examination of the body when discovered, and toxicologic examination of the blood, urine,

bile and stomach contents. They also strongly advised the immediate identification of new admissions at risk for suicide and the critical need for observation in the first 24 hours of detention.

Australia

McDonald and Thomson reported on all deaths in police custody in Australia from 1980 to 1989.[18] Of the 199 deaths, 87 were deemed to be self-inflicted (suicide and overdose), 35 other injuries (accidents and overdoses), 20 diseases of the circulatory system, and 3 homicides. The risk for self-inflicted injury and accidental death far exceeded the expected risk, when compared with both non-incarcerated populations and prisoners in Australia. The authors concluded that, as part of a comprehensive plan to prevent jail mortalities, "imprisonment be used as only a sanction of last resort."[18]

Chicago

From 1981 through 1990, there were 85 deaths at the Cook County Department of Corrections (CCDOC) in Chicago, a short-term correctional facility housing at that time 7,000 detainees.[1] Almost all the admissions to this facility had spent a number of hours in local police lockups before being transferred to the custody of the jail. Only 5% of the population was female. Autopsy reports were available on over 70% of the deaths. Eighty-two deaths were male, 3 female. Fifty-three percent of the deaths occurred at nearby Cook County Hospital following referral from the jail. The average age of death was 37.8 years, more than 10 years older that the jail inmate's average age. Men were found to be 1.6 times more likely to die than women detainees. In a facility that was overwhelmingly minority (75% black, 12.5% Hispanic), white detainees had death rates that were, respectively, 3.2 and 2.3 times the rate for blacks and Hispanics. Substance abuse (intravenous drug use, illicit oral drugs, and alcohol) was a contributing factor in 40% of the deaths. The six leading causes of death during 1981 to 1990 were 1) suicide, 2) infectious diseases (including

Table 25-7. Disease-specific mortality rate, Cook County Department of Corrections mortalities, 1981-1990

Male rank	Cause of death (ICD-9)	Number %	Rate	USA rate[1] 1988	USA rank
1	Suicide (E953-959)	19 (23.2%)	38.6	11.7	8
2	Infectious Disease (001-139)	18 (22%)	36.5		
	Acquired Immunodeficiency (043)	14 (17.1%)	28.4	9.7	15
3	Diseases of the heart (390-98, 402, 404-437)	14 (17.9%)	28.4	314.2	1
4	Alcoholism including cirrhosis and delirium tremens (303.9, 291, 591.2)	8 (9.8%)	16.2		
5	Malignant Neoplasms (140-208)	7 (8.5%)	14.2	197.5	2
6	External Causes	7 (8.5%)	14.2		
	Accidental (E800-949)	2 (2.4%)	4	38.7	4
	Overdose (465.01)	2 (2.4%)	4		
	Legal Intervention and	2 (2.4%)	4	8.6	12
	Homicide (E963, E970, E976)	1 (1.2%)	2		
7	Circulatory Diseases	4 (4.9%)	8.1		
	Pulmonary Embolism (415.1)	2 (2.4%)	4		
	SAH (430)	1 (1.2%)	2		
	Ruptured Aortic Aneurysm (441)	1 (1.2%)	2		
8	Respiratory Diseases (490-496)	3 (3.6%)	6.1	18.7	5
	Asthma (493)	2 (2.4%)	4		
	COPD (492)	1 (1.2%)	2		
9	Endocrine and Metabolic (250)	1 (1.2%)	2	16.1	7
	Cardio-pulmonary arrest of undetermined etiology	1 (1.2%)	2		
		82 deaths			

Female rank	Cause of death (ICD-9)	Number %	Rate	USA rate	
1	Suicide (E953)	1 (33%)	35.5	2.5	
1	Infectious Diseases (001-139)				
	SBE, Peritionitis, IBD	1 (33%)	35.5		
1	Cardio-pulmonary arrest etiology undetermined	1 (33%)	3	35.5	
		3 deaths			

1CDC, MMWR 1989; 38 (8) 117-118.

AIDS), 3) cardiac disease, 4) alcoholism, 5) malignant neoplasm, and 6) external causes (Table 25-7). The crude death rates for all categories of death (except for suicide and AIDS) were lower than the overall USA and City of Chicago crude and age-specific rates (Table 25-8).[1]

As also noted in the discussion of deaths in the New York City Department of Corrections, the suicide rates at the CCDOC steadily decreased between 1981 and 1990. The 1988 to 1990 rate (11.3) actually dropped below the USA non-incarcerated rate (11.7) (Table 25-9). Seventeen of the 20 suicides were by hanging and three by ingestion (doxepin: 1, shaving powder: 2). An epidemic in 1990 to 1991 of "copycat" suicide attempts from the ingestion of barium sulfide containing shaving powders causing fatal hypokalemia resulted in the removal of this substance from the institution's commissary.[3] Multiple institutional policy changes enacted after mortality reviews may have resulted in this welcome decrease in suicides. The highest risk for suicide in this detainee population was noted to be Hispanic and white males with a history of psychiatric illness who were in their first weeks of incarceration. Blacks tended to commit suicide at a lower rate than their white and Hispanic counterparts, although the rate still exceeded the USA suicide rate for blacks (Table 25-10). Black detainees tended to commit suicide after 3 or more months of incarceration, and generally subsequent to a negative court outcome.

The CCDOC's evaluation of the epidemiology of suicide deaths resulted in the intensification of intake psychiatric assessment of new admissions and the initiation of a program to reassess all detainees who had been found guilty following a court proceeding.

From 1986 and on, AIDS was the leading cause of death at the Cook County Department of Corrections. Intravenous drug users accounted for 70% of the 14 AIDS

Table 25-8. Age and gender specific mortality rates Cook County Department of Corrections, (per 100,000 patient years), 1981-1990

	CCDOC	City of Chicago 1988	USA 1985
Age			
15-24	25	124	95.9
25-44	148	178	123-207
45-64	634	1211	516-1282
65-84	3333	469	2938-6445
All ages	163	991	873
Male	166		
Female	106		

Raba, 1991

Table 25-9. Decreasing suicide rates over decade of survey, Cook County Department of Corrections, 1981-1990

	Suicide number	Rate: ADM	Rate: 100,000 ADM	Rate: 100,000
1981-85	12	1:23248	4.3	50.3
1986-90	8	1:34494	2.8	29
1988-90	2	1:100,227	1.1	11.3

Raba, 1991

Table 25-10. Suicide (E953-E959) rates gender and race specific, Cook County Department of Corrections, 1981-1990

	Rate per admissions	Rate per 100,000 admissions	Rate per 100,000 patient years	USA rate (1985)
Male	1/27,983	3.6	38.6	19
Female	1/48,652	2.1	34.5	5
Black (M)	1/39,663	2.5	29.7	10.8
White (M)	1/13,292	7.5	81.0	21.5
Hispanic (M)	1/16,615	6.0	64.8	11.0

Raba, 1991

Table 25-11. External cause (E-800-E949) mortality rate, Cook County Department of Corrections, 1981-1990

External causes (E-800-E949)	Rate (male)	USA rate (Ages 25-34)	Chicago rate non-white (ages 25-44)
Accidents (non-MVA)	2	4.0	15.0	48.4
Illicit drug overdose	2	4.0	-.-	8.4
Homicide (E-960-78)	1	2.0	14.7	59.8

Raba, 1991

mortalities while, during this time frame, in the USA intravenous drug use was associated with less than 30% of all AIDS cases.

Coronary artery disease, alcohol-related (cirrhosis, delirium tremens), and malignancy-related deaths occurred in older detainees. White detainees had higher incidences of coronary artery disease and alcohol-related deaths. It was also found that detainee-patients receiving oral anticoagulation treatment were at high risk for death; this information resulted in the housing of detainees on warfarin in units where they could be closely monitored and could not be transferred without medical clearance.

Deaths from external causes (accidents, inadvertent overdoses, legal intervention, homicide) were dramatically lower when compared to the age-specific, non-incarcerated population of Chicago (Table 25-11).

There was only a single inmate-on-inmate homicide among the 600,000 admissions during this 10-year period. This homicide was caused by suffocation with a pillow. (There was also one inmate who died from gunshot injuries during an escape attempt.) Based on age- and race-matched data, one would have predicted over 40 homicide mortalities at the jail during this 10-year period. The lower rates of accidental deaths can be only partially explained by the absence of firearms and motor vehicles within the walls of the jail.

Nearly 40% of the Cook County Department of Corrections' deaths were judged to be preventable, including the suicides and deaths from external causes, asthma, and pulmonary embolus.

DEATH DATA OVERVIEW

The summaries of mortality data from seven prisons and four jails and police lockups revealed clear trends. With the exception of suicide and AIDS, the overall and specific disease category death rates for detainees and prisoners in all but one of the correctional systems were lower than the rates for the general non-incarcerated population. The reasons for the decreased risk of death in correctional facilities are multivariate.

As incongruous as it may seem, the environment and lifestyle patterns in correctional facilities may actually be safer and healthier than those in inmates' communities of origin (personal communication, Shansky R, April 1997).[2, 6, 7, 8, 10]

Institutionalized men and women are provided with three meals a day. Their regimented schedule may allow for a routine of exercise. The availability of alcohol and illegal drugs, although not zero, is certainly diminished within correctional systems. Even though the clustering of significant numbers of men and women accused or convicted of violent crimes creates the potential for incidences of aggressive and assaultive behavior, the presence of security and the absence of firearms appears to decrease the potential for lethal consequences of violent interactions. Incarcerated populations in prisons, and less so in jails, participate in work activities; however, the exposure to toxic chemicals and fumes and other industrial and occupational hazards is thought to be significantly less than that in the community at large. An important factor in the decreased mortality rates in correctional facilities may be the enhanced access to medical care and the mandatory annual or biannual medical examinations that all inmates are offered. It has been repeatedly stated by correctional health experts that the availability of primary and secondary health care services in correctional facilities exceeds that in many inmate's home communities, given that many incarcerated men and women come from low income neighborhoods, many of which are officially designated health manpower shortage areas (HMSA) by the Department of Health and Human Services. The mortality data concerning prisons and jails indicate that these pro-health aspects of correctional systems are counterbalancing, if not overcoming, the significant unhealthy and morbidity producing impact of overcrowding and tobacco use, and a population that enters the correctional system with unhealthy lifestyles and inadequate prior access to medical care.[19]

MORTALITY REVIEW PROCESS

The ultimate goal of a mortality review processes is to identify aspects of the medical care delivery system that can be improved. Some correctional health systems have elaborate guidelines that delineate each step of the mortality review process. Others provide a general framework in which the mortality review committee is to operate but allow a wide range of flexibility in the process and the report. One nationally respected correctional health expert simply requires that the mortality report submitted by his staff answer three questions: 1) Were there any opportunities for improvement in the events immediately surrounding the death? 2) Are there any opportunities for improvement in the care provided during the decedent's incarceration that might have changed the outcome or prevented the mortality? and 3) Independent of the cause of death, are there any opportunities for improvement in the care provided to the deceased individual? (personal communication, Shansky R, April 1997).

Mortality review should be an established indicator in the quality improvement and quality assurance programs of all correctional institutions and systems. The comprehensive evaluation of an individual death can provide important information on the status of the health care delivered within a correctional facility. Although each institution and system will develop mortality review procedures that will be uniquely tailored to the demographics and environment of the population served, the review process should contain certain key components:

- The uniform collection of individual mortality information
- The inclusion of autopsy reports
- The maintenance and tracking of mortality data using statistical measures that allow for comparison with local and national death rates and with other correctional systems
- Written policies and procedures that direct the mortality review process
- An established mortality review committee that functions under the auspices of the facility's quality improvement and assurance program
- An ongoing process that monitors the implementation of recommendations for improvement made by the mortality review committee and ongoing compliance with these recommendations

Collection of Mortality Data

It is extremely important that accurate data on mortalities in correctional health settings be gathered and maintained for individual deaths to be investigated adequately, mortality trends to be analyzed, and corrective and preventive interventions instituted. The actual data to be compiled concerning the death of an inmate must be modified constantly to reflect the unique needs of the incarcerated population and the correctional institution. At the minimum, the data should include the decedent's name, date of birth, gender, ethnicity, duration of incarceration, housing unit, immediate location of death (tier, cell, medical unit, hospital, etc.), medical diagnoses and current medications, cause of death, and autopsy report. The cause of death, officially determined after the completion of a thorough autopsy, should be assigned an International Classification of Diseases number (ICD #) that will enhance the ability of mortality data in different systems and even different countries to be compared. The data gathered for suicides, homicides, traumatic deaths, and accidents should also include an inspection of the site of death by an experienced observer (physician, nurse, medical examiner) in addition to the assessment performed by police and correctional authorities. The circumstances of arrest should be determined if the death occurs within the first 2 weeks of incarceration. In the case of suicide deaths, "the position of the body when found, the time the body was found, the time the victim was last seen, what articles were present around the body and where those articles were found, how the body was handled, and whether any injuries resulted from such handling."[17] The injuries resulting from the handling of the body are of particular importance in hangings—the most common cause of suicide mortality in correctional facilities. The first person on the scene of a hanging will commonly cut the victim down to initiate resuscitation. If the body hits the floor with much force, it may sustain lacerations, bruises, and even fractures. It is vitally important for the observer to know that bruises can occur after death and, depending on the posture of the body, may even enlarge.[17]

The data gathered about the death should be detailed in an official mortality report and entered either into a written log or, preferably, a computerized data base that will allow for epidemiologic tracking, comparison, and trend analysis.

An institution's or system's annual census, number of admissions, age and racial demographics, and gender statistics must also be accurately maintained so that death rates can be determined.

AUTOPSY

"Hic locus est ubi mors gaudet succurrere vitae" (This is where death rejoices to come to the aid of life). This inscription is in the amphitheater where dissections were performed at the University of Bologna.

A thorough autopsy is an essential tool in determining cause of death. The majority of studies comparing postmortem diagnoses with postmortem findings have disclosed a number of inaccuracies in clinical diagnostic decision-making, a portion of which were judged to have resulted in inappropriate care.[20]

Discrepancies between clinical and autopsy diagnoses have varied from 5%–40%, but on the average remain around 10% even when the clinicians were absolutely "certain" of the premortem diagnosis.[21–24]

In addition to the establishment of the cause of death, autopsies are invaluable in identifying the pathology that caused a patient's symptoms or signs, in confirming the patient's clinical diagnosis, and in determining the extent of the pathologic process and tumor spread.[20] Autopsy data also have the potential for contributing to medical and epidemiologic research and the enactment of data-based clinical and health preventive measures.

In most jurisdictions in the USA, each and every death of an individual who is in the custody of local, city, county, state, or federal authorities is automatically designated as a case for the medical examiner or coroner. Autopsies performed for forensic purposes are instrumental in establishing the cause, time, and manner of death and the circumstances preceding and surrounding death.[23] However, it is the decision of the medical examiner as to whether an autopsy will be performed.

Due to the decline in the number of autopsies being performed in United States and worldwide,[23] medicolegal autopsies have became a leading, if not the main, component of autopsy practice in teaching centers and in certain geographical regions.[25] Forensic autopsies performed on arrested, detained, and incarcerated men and women comprise a not insignificant portion of these medicolegal autopsies.

The availability of autopsy reports in a significant percentage of correctional deaths is an invaluable resource in evaluating the medical care delivered, the causes of death, and in formulating morbidity and mortality prevention programs for incarcerated populations. Mortality reviews and reports in correctional health facilities and systems are only final when the results of the autopsy reports are incorporated into the findings and recommendations of the Mortality Review Committee.

Statistical Reporting

The comparison of mortality rates between incarcerated populations and the general non-incarcerated populations of society requires numerical and statistical measurements that allow for equitable reporting and valid comparison. Mortality rates are reported throughout the world as number of deaths per one hundred thousand population. This must also be the numerical vehicle used to report death rates in prisons and jails. It is also important that deaths are stratified into standardized age groupings (16-24, 25-34, 35-44, 45-54, 55-64, 65-74, and > 75). However, the dynamic census of prisons, and more so of jails, complicate the identification of an acceptable denominator. Correctional censuses are in constant flux. Jail populations turn over from ten to twenty times per year. Some are detained or incarcerated for less than a day, some for the remainder of their lives. The lack of a stable population base in correctional systems must be remembered when trying to compare mortality data and rates of the incarcerated with the non-incarcerated populations.

The accepted method for determining mortality rates in prisons and jails is to divide a facility's or system's average daily census for a year into 100,000, and then multiply the product by the number of deaths for that year. The result will be the annual death rate for the correctional population being studied.

Example: Prison M, a correctional facility with 5,000 inmates on an average day, had 12 deaths in the year being evaluated. 100,000 divided by 5,000 = 20. 20 times 12 deaths = 240. The mortality rate for Prison M for the period being evaluated is 240 deaths per 100,000 population. ($y/100,000 = 12/5,000$. $y = 12 \times 20$. $y = 240$).

Another commonly used comparative tool is the standardized mortality ratio (SMR), which compares the actual number deaths in a facility or system with the number of deaths that would have been predicted based on established age and ethnicity mortality rates. Using established mortality rates, the number of anticipated deaths is determined in a facility or system. This anticipated number of deaths is divided by the actual number of observed deaths. The quotient is a numerical value less than, equal to, or greater than 1.0.

Example: Prison M with its 5,000 average daily census had 12 deaths in the year being monitored. The USA mortality rate for an age-matched population was 160 deaths per 100,000 population. The anticipated number of deaths in Prison M would be 100,000 divided by 5,000 (M's average daily census) = 20. The expected 160 mortality rate divided by 20 = 8 anticipated deaths in Prison M per year. 12 actual deaths divided by 8 anticipated deaths = 1.5 standardized mortality ratio (SMR).

An alternate method of calculating the SMR is to divide the actual mortality rate by the age-matched USA rate. 240 (actual) rate divided by 160 (USA) rate = 1.5 SMR. In short-term facilities (jails and police lockups), a useful additional method of measuring and comparing mortalities with other similar institutions is to report the number of deaths per the number of admissions and the number of deaths calculated for 100,000 admissions.

Example: Jail W had 50,000 annual admissions and had 5 deaths in the year being evaluated. The death incidence would be 50,000 admissions divided by 5 deaths = 1 death per 10,000 admissions. Extrapolated to 100,000 admissions, the incidence would be 100,000 divided by 50,000 admissions = 2. 2 times 5 deaths = 10 deaths for every 100,000 admissions. This alternate method is of value in measuring the mortality in jails with rapid population turnover.

Policy and Procedures

Each correctional institution and system must have written policies and procedures to guide the process by which deaths are evaluated and reviewed. The prison and jail standards for accreditation promulgated by the National Commission on Correctional Health Care (NCCHC) contain policies (P-09 and J-10) that mandate that correctional facilities have "written policyand defined procedures that, in the event of the death of an inmate, the medical examiner ... is notified immediately, a mortality review is conducted, and a postmortem examination is requested."[26] The NCCHC advise that mortality reviews be performed by multidisciplinary correctional health staff and that mortality data be tracked so that each inmate death can be compared to detect emerging patterns.

Each institution's mortality policy should detail the steps by which deaths are investigated, evaluated, and reviewed. The policy should mandate the collection, tracking, and reporting of mortality data. If not directed by legislative act, the policy should designate that all deaths in correctional facilities be reported to the office of the medical examiner. All correctional facilities should have standing mortality committees, the membership of which is determined by policy, which are convened to analyze all deaths in police lockups, jails, and prisons.

Mortality Review Committee

The mortality review committee should always be included under the auspices of the institution's quality assurance and improvement committee. It must be established so that its investigations, discussions, findings, and recommendations are considered confidential. The ability of the internal mortality review committee to formulate objective reports will be severely comprised if its proceedings were not confidential.

Depending on the size of the institution and the incidence of detainee and inmate deaths, mortality review committees will either be formed adhoc or will be ongoing established committees. Smaller facilities will generally form adhoc committees to investigate infrequent deaths or will assign the death review functions to its quality improvement committee. Larger facilities and all systems require established mortality review committees.

The composition of the mortality review committee should be defined in the facility's policy and procedure and should include representatives from the medical and correctional administration, a medical physician, a member of the mental health team, a nurse, and a member of the quality assurance support staff. Other members (pharmacist, mid-level provider, paramedic, correctional technician) can be substituted or added as deemed necessary or as is appropriate to the institution. Although in smaller facilities it may be difficult, health care providers not involved in the direct care of the decedent would ideally have the responsibility of reviewing the health care provided. In certain settings and circumstances, the inclusion of an expert or a health provider who is not on the staff of the correctional institution may be appropriate.

The committee has the duty to review all aspects of the care provided to the deceased inmate. It must have at its disposal the individual's medical chart, the medication records and logs, the emergency room and hospital summaries, all incident reports that were generated by the death, and the final autopsy report including toxicology screenings. The committee must have the right to interview health care and correctional employees that it deems appropriate to its review.

The inclusion of correctional staff on the mortality review committee is logical and adds a necessary expertise to the assessment of the circumstances of the death in a jail or a prison. This may, however, be difficult to accomplish.

Historically in many facilities, correctional health and correctional teams have conducted their own mortality reviews and rarely have shared their confidential reports except to point out deficiencies in the other staff's actions. This is especially true when reviews of suicides, homicides, accidental deaths, and deaths due to the use of correctional force were investigated. The cooperation and support of both the health care and the correctional leaderships are essential for a multidisciplinary correctional health and correctional mortality review committee to effectively function in an atmosphere that is objective and confidential and focused on identifying areas of improvement in the correctional facility.

IMPLEMENTATION OF MORTALITY REVIEW COMMITTEE RECOMMENDATIONS AND PREVENTION PROGRAMS

The benefit of a comprehensive mortality audit and report is limited if the facility and the correctional health system do not implement the recommendations of its mortality review committee. The recommendations should be logged, responsibility assigned for action, and timelines established. It is obvious that the recommendations will require the imprimatur of the correctional health and the correctional directors if they are to have the opportunity to impact on the delivery of care in an institution.

Correctional health services can have significant impact on decreasing the mortality rates in prisons and jails by the institution of select and well-planned preventive measures. The initiation of suicide screening at high-risk time frames of incarceration and the elimination of horizontal bars in inmate housing units have been shown to have the potential of decreasing suicide rates by 40%.[1]

Housing units with enhanced nursing observation and monitoring for inmates with medical conditions (e.g., early alcohol withdrawal, insulin requiring diabetes, recent severe asthma attacks) or receiving complicated medications or regimens (e.g., warfarin, chemotherapy) have been established pursuant to the recommendations of mortality committees.[1]

All recommendations must be tracked and regularly monitored for compliance. As with any quality improvement process, mortality review recommendations require ongoing surveillance and reassessment. The status of system modifications and mortality prevention processes must be reported to both the mortality review committee and the quality improvement committee at pre-defined intervals.

SUMMARY

Correctional medical experts previously have noted that "one of the major inadequacies of health services in correctional institutions is failure to recognize the need for and to systematically collect epidemiologic information concerning health needs of the population."[4] The gathering and evaluation of data on the causes, circumstances, at-risk populations, and trends of mortality in correctional facilities will assist the development of policies, programmatic enhancements, and even physical plant modifications that address mortality prevention significantly. Each and every correctional institution, no matter how small or large or whether part of a larger system, must have in place a defined process to investigate and review all mortalities of detainees and prisoners. The absence of an established mortality review process could be considered institutional negligence.

REFERENCES

1. Raba JM: Mortality at the Cook County Department of Corrections, 1981-1990. Presentation at the Third International Conference on Correctional Health Care, Anchorage, Alaska; May 7, 1991.
2. Smith R: Deaths in prison. *Br Med* J 288:208-212, 1984.
3. Aks S, Mansour M, Hyhorczuk D, et al: Barium sulfide ingestion in an urban correctional facility population. *J Prison Jail Health* 12(1):3-12, 1993.
4. King LN, Whitman S: Morbidity and mortality among prisoners: An epidemiological review. *J Prison Health* 1:7-28, 1981.
5. Jones D: Health Risks of Imprisonment. Lexington, MA, DC Heath, 1976.
6. Clavel F, Benhamou S, Flamant R: Decreased mortality among male prisoners. *Lancet* 2:1012-1014, 1987.
7. Faiver KL: Epidemiologic Review of Deaths in a Prison Setting: A Review of Mortality Occurring in the Institutional Population of Michigan Department of Corrections from January 1, 1977 to June 30, 1983.
8. Salive ME, Smith GS, Brewer TF: Death in prison: Changing mortality patterns among male prisoners in Maryland, 1970-1987. *Am J Prison Health* 80:1479-1480, 1990.
9. Salive ME, Brewer TF: Suicide mortality in the Maryland state prison system, 1979-80. *JAMA* 262(3):365-369, 1989.
10. Kamara SG, Concannon KW, Butler JF, Bet al: The descriptive epidemiology of unnatural deaths in Oregon's state institutions: A 25-year (1963-1987) study, IV. The reduction of unnatural death rates during 1988-1992 in three facilities as a result of planned changes. *J Forensic Sci* 39(6):1432-1444, 1994.
11. Murphy GP: Mortality for leading causes of death, United States, 1992. Cancer statistics 1996. *CA Cancer J Clin* 46(11):18, 1996.
12. City of Chicago, Department of Public Health: A Comparison of Chicago Health Measures with United States Year 2000 Goals. *Epidemiology Program Report,* March 1997.
13. Paris JE: Mortality Review: Learning From Inmate Death to Improve Health Care in Corrections. Presentation at the Nineteenth National Conference on Correctional Health Care, Washington, D.C.; November 14, 1995.
14. Amankwaa A: Causes of deaths in Florida prisons: The dominance of AIDS (letter). *Am J Public Health* 85(12):1710-1711, 1995.
15. Novick LF, Remmlinger E: A study of 128 deaths in New York City correctional facilities (1971-76). Implications for prisoner health care. *Med Care* 16:749-756, 1978.
16. King LN: Morbidity and Mortality Among Prisoners: Imperatives for the Future of Correctional Health Care. Opening Remarks at the Eleventh National Conference on Correctional Health Care, Chicago, November 5, 1987.
17. Smialek JE, Spitz WU: Death behind bars. *JAMA* 240:2563-2564, 1978.
18. McDonald D, Thomson NJ: Australian deaths in custody, 1980-89. ed. 2. Causes. *Med J Aust* 159:581-585, 1993.
19. Raba JM, Barrett-Obis C: Male intake screening at a large urban jail. *J Prison Health* 1982.
20. Saladino AJ: The efficacy of the autopsy in medical quality assurance. *Clin Lab Med* 4(1):165-184, 1984.
21. Charlton R: Autopsy and medical education: A review. *J R Soc Med* 87:232-235, 1994.
22. Gambino SR: The autopsy: The ultimate audit. *Arch Pathol Lab Med* 108:444-445, 1984.
23. McPhee SJ, Bottles K: Autopsy: Moribund art of vital science? *Am J Med* 78:107-113, 1985.
24. Pelletier LL, Klutzow F, Lancester H: The autopsy: Its role in the evaluation of patient care. *J Intern Med* 4:300-303, 1989.
25. Research after death. Editorial. Lancet 344(8936):1517-1518, 1994.
26. Standards for Accreditation: National Commission of Correctional Health Care, Prisons 1992, Jails 1996.

Section Seven

Special Issues in Corrections

26

Quality Improvement Through Care Management

Robert B. Greifinger, M.D.
Martin Horn, M.A., B.A.

DEFINING CARE MANAGEMENT

Managing care is a systematized effort to improve quality, avert morbidity and mortality, and reduce waste and rework. This is done through a linked series of activities, each of whose successes depends on the others. An underlying principle is that quality of care and service are to be enhanced and never compromised. The components of a managed care program attend to prevention, acute care, and the management of chronic disease. These are viewed from both the quality perspective and that of resource use, called utilization management. The latter component includes systematic attention to access to care and the assessment of potential underuse, overuse, and mishaps of medical care.

IS MANAGED CARE COST-CONTAINMENT?

Managed care is not a synonym for cost-containment, and the two terms should not be confused. Generally, high-quality care (regardless of whether it is "managed") is most cost-effective in the aggregate. Individual care, however, is not the aggregate and may not be the least costly for the

payer. This apparent contradiction is because the payer's responsibility may be limited. For example, a prison health unit may seek to delay care until the inmate is transferred or released to the community, where there is a different payer.

Inappropriate restrictions on care or service do not belong in the sphere of care management, and they should not be disguised under the rubric of care management.

Managed care has a variety of meanings to different audiences; these include:

- A population-based approach to quality improvement
- A method for cost-containment
- The aggregation of health care delivery
- The structured management of health care delivery

This is a guide for the management of health care using a quality improvement approach. Quality has been an elusive concept in health care. Although it is hard enough for physicians to evaluate the care of others, it is especially difficult for nonphysicians to assess how health care programs are working. This guide will present some of the tools developed in the managed care industry and will discuss some of the pitfalls of these programs.

The methods described are tools to improve accountability. They are less than perfect, but should be useful in tracking the progress of programs and evaluating the process of care in the facility. These tools should be used in conjunction with common sense and traditional supervision, or, if the system is privatized, they may be used through the contract management process.

High-quality health care is valuable for the inmates themselves, for the protection of the work force, and for the public health in the communities to which inmates return. Personal health interests do not lie in a vacuum. The prevention of communicable disease, for example, reduces risk to others. The reduction in unnecessary care reduces the expense to the payer, who is often the taxpayer. Improving quality through care management requires, among other things:

1. Mechanisms to assure and enhance the quality of all health care delivered to inmates;
2. Coordination with other facility and agency functions;
3. Formal methods to conserve resources.

Prison and jail health programs are managed care programs. They are prepaid and have a defined network of practitioners and structured benefit packages. Nonetheless, health care needs to be actively managed in this model.

CORE VALUES

Most correctional systems face annual budget constraints, that is, there are many inmates and precious little public funding support for their medical services. As a result of the successful cost-containment programs in commercially insured managed care organizations, there has been a widespread expectation that managed care can achieve similar cost savings behind bars.

This is correct, to a point. However, managing care can achieve savings without compromising quality. Commercial managed care has a few underlying values that must be incorporated into correctional health care. Translated for corrections, these mean that every inmate has rights to:

1. Appropriate access and availability of a wide range of services, both preventive and nonpreventive;
2. Complain and appeal decisions;
3. Physician participation in the adoption of all clinical guidelines and utilization management guidelines;
4. Physician review of all potential denials;
5. Properly credentialed staff with performance evaluations that consider quality of care, quality of service, patient complaints, and appropriate use of resources;
6. Good medical records;
7. Participation in treatment decisions, including knowledge of all of the options and their potential effects;
8. Quality management systems to improve care and service and to prevent under-utilization and disruption of continuity of care.

Managed care is about managing the system of care and providing professional guidance by a primary care physician. Managing care does not mean:

1. Managing physicians (this is another matter);
2. Increasing co-payments to reduce use;
3. Restructuring formularies to avoid expensive medication;
4. Denying appropriate referrals, elective surgery, and consultation;
5. Delaying care, with hopes of avoiding it, or dumping on the next payer;
6. Forgetting prevention, early detection, and management of acute and chronic disease.

WHY HIGH QUALITY?

One piece of the mission of any department of corrections is to provide needed health care to inmates, in a clinically appropriate manner. This simple statement has complex implications. It requires that we devise mechanisms to assure and enhance the quality of all health care delivered to inmates and to conserve system resources as much as possible. This applies to all needed inmate health care services, even those provided by vendors, community physicians, nurses, dentists, and hospitals.

The question of managing care is not whether to do it, but how to do it. High-quality care is:

- The most efficient and effective way to deliver care. It saves departmental and taxpayer dollars in the short- and long-term.
- Aimed to reduce rework and waste and minimize error.
- A good risk management tool. High-quality care and service reduce complaints, grievances, and litigation.
- Measurable, so that performance can be tracked and trended over time.
- A service to our workforce and the community by protecting them from occupational exposure to communicable disease.
- A way of assuring accountability to the agency, the government, and the public.

UTILIZATION MANAGEMENT TECHNIQUES

Until 1995, health care costs had been rising faster than any segment of the economy. As this had been true for several decades nationally, it is no surprise that correctional health costs, likewise, had increased. Part of the increase in corrections is because of the use of new technologies and new, expensive medications. Another part of the increase is because of the aging inmate population and the decade-long increase in communicable diseases, especially HIV infection and viral hepatitis.[1] Managed care strategies can be applied to correctional health systems to reduce cost without compromising care.[2]

Managed care organizations have been especially helpful in minimizing the annual increases in health care costs during the past few years. However, gaining control requires an understanding of the factors that inflate health care costs and identification of those that are amenable to intervention. The key components of a utilization management program address overuse, underuse, and misuse of medical care.

Overuse can cause injury. This occurs when the risk of a procedure or treatment exceeds the benefit for that individual patient. Examples of overuse include some prostate surgeries, hysterectomies, and tonsillectomies. Underuse is common in areas in which proven, effective interventions are not applied, for example, with immunizations and selected medication after myocardial infarction. Misuse is the category applied to negligence that causes adverse outcomes, such as pharmaceutical misadventures.

Benefit Packages and Medical Necessity Guidelines

A well-functioning utilization management program coordinates the use of limited resources to optimize effectiveness. A sound utilization management program addresses potential overuse, underuse, and misuse. It begins with the definition of the range of services available (normally called a benefit package outside the correctional system) and a process for assessing the use of new and emerging technologies. The utilization management program provides for fair and consistent application of medical necessity decision rules and evaluates medical appropriateness, so that the consequences of overutilization or underutilization are avoided.

In addition to the application of medical necessity guidelines, classic case management can be used to reduce medical service readmissions. This involves frequent contacts for education and care by nurse case managers who follow protocols and communicate frequently with the primary care physician.[3] Readmissions of identified high-risk patients are potentially preventable in more than one third of cases.[4]

Unnecessary medical care is expensive and can be dangerous. It taxes medical, security, and fiscal resources, and makes us less able to provide needed services. Underuse of referral resources has a similar impact. Use of services must be managed, yet excessively restricted access to appropriate care is equally expensive and dangerous. Underuse and overuse of referral resources are caused by:

- Legitimate medical disagreement on appropriateness of care;
- Imperfect policies and procedures for utilization management;
- Insufficient continuing education for primary care physicians;
- Defensive medicine or requirements of court orders;
- Careless medical practice or inappropriate response to patient demand;
- Inappropriate decisions or conclusions by outside resources;
- System problems outside the scope of facility physicians, such as inadequate control of trip scheduling, timing, and staffing.

All but the first are fixable. The remedies for the others lie in consistent policies, managed access, and support for the clinician. The clinician may be undereducated, responding solely to patient demand, or practicing defensively. There are nationally recognized guidelines for medical-necessity decision making, such as those published by Milliman & Robertson[5] and InterQual.[6] The use of nationally recognized guidelines should help assure that costs are being controlled without compromise of care. Their use will also help in mitigating litigation.

A prospective review can be used for elective hospital admissions, ambulatory surgery, selected diagnostic procedures, and off-site referrals. Such a review should be selective and not universal. It should be reserved for diagnoses and procedures with wide variation in use, and for instances for which there are accepted guidelines.

Using Guidelines

Acute low back pain is a good example of opportunity with guidelines. There is an evidence-based, nationally accepted guideline for the evaluation and treatment of low back pain.[7] Low back pain is highly prevalent, ranks high on reasons for a physician visit, and can be costly. Without signs of potentially dangerous underlying conditions, however, there is no need for special studies because 90% of patients will recover spontaneously within 4 weeks. A focused medical history and physical examination are sufficient to assess the patient with an acute or recurrent limitation caused by symptoms whose duration is less than 4 weeks. For these 90%, nonsteroidal anti-inflammatory medication will suffice.

Medical necessity criteria are useful for common problems such as hernia repair. A correctional system can take a nationally accepted guideline and modify it to use in prisons and jails. Using herniorrhaphy as an example, the InterQual indications are either (1) "physical examination reveals presence of … inguinal hernia, or (2) presence of nonreducible strangulated hernia evidenced by pain, cramping and nausea and vomiting." This would allow repair on an asymptomatic hernia. The correctional system could make a decision that these criteria apply, but only if there is discomfort or another functional disability.

The InterQual guideline for septoplasty requires (1) a nasal airway obstruction by septal deviation, (2) a nasal deformity, with or without persistent bleeding, (3) the need for a pituitary surgery approach, or (4) a cosmetic/psychological reason. Correctional systems can choose the first and third indications and reject the second and fourth. As long as these rules are applied consistently and are well documented, they can provide much assistance to clinical staff in the field. Similar indications can be developed for other common problems, such as knee surgery.

There are other clinical conditions that do not have nationally accepted guidelines, but are frequent confounders for correctional health staff. The use of interferon

---

Box 26-1 Criteria for the Treatment of Chronic Hepatitis with Recombinant Interferon-α2b

1. Older than 18 years of age
2. Chronic hepatitis proved by biopsy
3. Disease must be compensated, with
   - No history of hepatic encephalopathy, variceal bleeding, ascites, or other signs of decompensation
   - Bilirubin level less than 2 mg/dL
   - Stable and normal albumin level
   - Prothrombin time less than 3 sec prolonged
   - White blood cell count > 4,000/mm^3
   - Platelet count > 100,000/mm^3
   - Serum creatinine level normal or near normal
   - Elevated serum alanine aminotransferase level
4. No other causes of hepatitis, such as autoimmune disease
5. For hepatitis C, must have
   - History of blood or blood product exposure
   - Anti-HCV positive status
   - HIV-negative status
6. For hepatitis B only, must have HBsAg-positive status for more than 6 months AND demonstrate HBV replication as indicated by serum HBeAg-positive status
7. Cooperation with therapy and availability to receive the full course of therapy

---

Abbreviations: HCV, hepatitis C virus; *HBsAg*, hepatitis B surface antigen; *HBV*, hepatitis B virus; *HBeAg*, hepatitis B early antigen.
*National Committee for Quality Assurance (NCQA), 2000 L Street NW, Suite 500, Washington, D.C. 20036, (202) 955-3500.

for hepatitis B or C is an example. In this situation, the Quality Management Committee or the Pharmacy and therapeutics Committee can research the literature and make an affirmative statement as to indications for this sometimes useful and always expensive therapy. There are excellent review articles to help develop policy.[8] Each policy should have sections on background, treatment options, outcome expectations, and recommended criteria for treatment. Box 26-1 demonstrates an example of a Criteria for Treatment section for treating chronic hepatitis with recombinant interferon-α2b (all must be met).

As new medications become available for prevalent conditions, the system can adopt or develop guidelines. This is fair, consistent, and very helpful for the practicing physician. The use of protease inhibitors for HIV infection is a current example.

If an inmate complains that he has been denied access to a specialist medical service, the practitioner or vendor can be asked what medical necessity guideline was followed to make the decision. The inmate is entitled to a copy of it. If the decision cannot be justified with a guideline, the central office might be consulted for another opinion.

Likewise, there are published benefit packages that clarify what may or may not be covered. These include those developed by the Oregon Health Services Commission for

the Oregon Medicaid program, as implemented by the Oregon Department of Corrections.[9] They use an evidence-based approach to decide what will and will not be covered. Anyone with health insurance has received a benefit package, often called a subscriber contract. The scope of coverage, as well as terms and conditions, are described. Any of these can be used as a prototype for a corrections version. The Oregon program, however, is the most specific and is more limited than typical indemnity or managed care benefits packages.

Any of these national guidelines can be adopted or modified for use in the correctional setting. They are very helpful in taking the emotional charge out of medical necessity and benefit package decision making.

Methods for Checking for Underuse

There are a variety of methods available for checking for potential overuse or underuse of care. The first method is to listen to the patient and analyze the nature of unhappy responses. Well-organized facilities will keep logs of complaints, grievances, and litigation with a categorization of the nature of each. These can be sorted to look for problems with access, such as complaints about delays to see a physician, delays in getting diagnostics, or delays in getting to referral resources. If there is a pattern, a small work group can analyze the data, suggest system barriers that may be causing the problem, and identify interventions to solve the problem.

Another useful method is to look for proxy measures of underuse, such as rates of immunization, mammograms, Pap smears for women, and administration of influenza or pneumococcal vaccine to the elderly and those with chronic diseases. A focus group with nonusers can reveal much about why these valuable services are not being accessed.

A third, and critical, type of review is the careful consideration of all unexpected hospitalizations and deaths, rehospitalizations within 30 days, and adverse surgical outcomes. These can be reviewed for preventable occurrences.

MUST WE REINVENT THE WHEEL?

The standards of the American Correctional Association (ACA) and the National Commission for Correctional Health Care provide a sound basis for health care programs.[10, 11] They focus on structural issues, such as the existence of policies and procedures. The model presented in this paper, however, moves beyond structure to clinical process and begins to address the more important topic—the outcome of care.

One useful method is used by the National Committee for Quality Assurance (NCQA), the leading accreditation body for managed care organizations. It has surveyed more than half of the nation's HMOs, comparing the HMOs' standards with accepted standards, and is currently developing adapted standards for preferred provider organizations, medical groups, credentialing verification organizations, and managed behavioral health care organizations.[12] The NCQA standards for accreditation are divided into six categories: (1) quality management and improvement, (2) utilization management, (3) credentialing, (4) member rights and responsibilities, (5) preventive health services, and (6) medical records. The NCQA uses a dynamic model, one that weaves expectations for structure, processes, and outcome into a quality improvement program.

The dynamic model is consistent with most continuous quality improvement programs that use a sequential approach, such as Plan—Do—Study—Act. The planning phase involves selecting topics for study that reflect the population served and are amenable to change. This is followed by a measurement process to quantify the problem, a study process to analyze potential interventions, and an intervention phase designed to solve the problem. These processes are followed with remeasurement and analysis of the effectiveness of the actions taken.

The structural elements provide the tools and framework for improving quality, including a clear definition of the authority of the program, its relationships to nonmedical functions, and its accountability. The structure should clearly answer such questions as, how is the program organized? who is expected to act? when are the results deliverable? and how is the program evaluated? A written program describes the methods and reasons for topic selection, performance monitoring, utilization decision making, and credentialing activities.

Process elements are defined in the annual work plan; they set the expectations for action. The work plan answers questions such as, what measures will be monitored and analyzed? who is involved in the development? how will we use the information to make changes? and how do we evaluate our progress?

Constructive changes in health status are the ultimate objectives. This is the outcome. Here we ask, can we demonstrate meaningful improvement from our efforts? have we saved money without compromising access or quality? and is our mortality rate reduced, or have we been able to measurably reduce the risk of transmission of communicable disease?

In the criminal justice system, we modify traditional quality improvement measures with those that are unique to the correctional environment. These include matters of privacy, coercion, civil rights litigation, communicable disease control, and selected ethical issues.

QUALITY MANAGEMENT TECHNIQUES
Organization

A well-structured program defines a scope of activities that are a direct reflection of the inmate population served. The emphasis here is to study and report on topics that are relevant to the population, with the potential for constructive change. Such a population-based approach is much more effective in driving change than a case-by-case retrospec-

tive review of care. It involves a work plan and methods for study and evaluation and links health care activities with security functions, and all of these are aimed at having a smooth facility operation.

Quality management works best on three levels, with accountability beginning at the top. The commissioner or director approves a quality management plan and delegates the responsibility for its operation to the Quality Improvement Committee (QIC). This committee is typically chaired by the chief medical officer and includes the physician leadership of the contracted vendors, if any.

This department-wide committee addresses areas of broad concern for the staff and inmates, including such domains as credentialing of health practitioners, communicable disease, intake, transfer, access to emergency and urgent care, continuity of care, the formulary, preventive health services, and disease management for common chronic diseases. The QIC drives the broad range of activities that concern the agency. This is the working engine. It is the conduit for input from central office staff, regional medical directors, vendors, and other staff. The QIC advises the commissioner and chief medical officer on policy and designs specific performance monitors and interventions for identified problems.

Regional and local QIC activities can be formalized with individual committees or, better yet, with focused task forces, which have a dual role. The first is to implement QIC and regional QIC activities aimed at improving performance as compared with statewide standards. The second is to solve local problems specific to the institution. Sometimes, these activities can be used as pilots for broader-scale action once the processes are streamlined.

Facilities can be compared by the use of defined, valid, and measurable performance indicators. These can be activities, events, occurrences, or outcomes for which data can be collected to allow for comparison with other facilities, an objective, or prior performance. They can be process indicators (derived from practice guidelines or clinical pathways) or outcome indicators, such as prevalence rates of desirable or undesirable health states.

Measurement of Performance

Most performance indicators will be designed centrally, but the data are collected either through administrative systems (for example, automated data on tuberculin skin tests) or through periodic review of medical records against specific criteria. The indicators selected must be responsive to the following questions:

- What do we really want to know?
- Is it amenable to change?
- Will improvements in the delivery system actually affect this change?
- Is it practical or realistic to believe that the organization can affect this change?
- Do we have the resources lined up?

Chronic Disease

Here is an example of how to use data for managing care through quality improvement. The Pennsylvania Department of Corrections identified performance indicators for six chronic diseases that are common in its population,[13] diseases for which there was so much variation in patterns of care that the QIC believed clinical guidelines would be appropriate. The guidelines are descriptions of nationally accepted practices, ones that are often not followed well enough inside or outside prisons and jails. They include algorithms and flow sheets, among other things. The indicators were selected to be proxy measurements for use of the guidelines. The conditions selected include:

1. HIV infection
   - Is a flow sheet used?
   - Is there an interim evaluation at least every 6 months?
   - Are baseline and interim laboratory tests performed for CD4+ cells or RNA viral load?
   - Are vaccines given appropriately?
   - Is a Pap smear done according to protocol?
2. Diabetes mellitus
   - Is a flow sheet used?
   - Has there been a dilated retinal examination within 12 months?
   - Are vaccines given appropriately?
3. Hypertension
   - Is a flow sheet used?
   - Is there an interim evaluation at least every 6 months with blood pressure and laboratory tests?
4. Convulsive disorders
   - Is a flow sheet used?
   - At least every 6 months, are drug levels and medication monitored and is a physical examination performed?
5. Asthma
   - Is a flow sheet used?
   - Is a peak expiratory flow rate documented?
   - Are oral corticosteroids used?
   - Are vaccines given appropriately?
6. Inmates receiving neuroleptic medication who are at risk for tardive dystonia and tardive dyskinesia
   - Is a flow sheet used?
   - Is there a documented test for abnormal involuntary movement done every 6 months?

Patients with these conditions are identified by lists kept at each facility. Charts are selected by the central office to review and increase confidence that the sample will not be biased. The review itself is performed by facility health staff. This "self-reporting" is validated periodically by external review teams who audit the results. Thus far, the self-reported data have been demonstrably valid and reliable.

Continuity of Care and Access

In addition to chronic disease management, the Pennsylvania Department of Corrections tracks and trends performance indicators for:

1. Diagnostic reports—Are they initialed by a physician or physicians' assistant?
2. Clearance for transfer—Is every transferred inmate cleared medically?
3. Emergency response—Is the ambulance timely?
4. Specialty referrals—Do they occur within 30 days of referral?
5. Annual health appraisals for inmates older than 50 years—Do they follow the guideline?
6. Access—Is the sick call for inmates in restricted housing following the guideline?
7. Tuberculosis skin testing—What proportion of inmates had timely testing?

Data are then reported back to facilities on charts. There is a line graph for each performance indicator to track the facility's performance over time. This is compared with a similar line for the region and the department as a whole.

It is important to remember that this kind of activity is not clinical research; rather, it is a tool for quality improvement. Data are to be analyzed and decisions made as to whether an intervention is appropriate. Some facilities are expected to vary. For example, expectations might be different for intake and reception centers or facilities with chronic disease units.

The indicators generally address processes involved in the provision of patient care (e.g., access to clinic visits, medication administration), treatment of specific diseases (mostly related to practice guidelines), administrative tasks (e.g., discharge planning), use of resources (e.g., pharmacy expenses, emergency department trips, use of isolation rooms), and patient satisfaction (e.g., inmate grievances regarding health services).

The use of performance measures based on standards or clinical guidelines is helpful for improving quality. The comparative display of information may be helpful in changing practice patterns.

Where performance continues to fall short of expectations, focused studies can help identify barriers to improvement. A focus group can be assigned the task of outlining the range of barriers that might be influencing this particular measure. It should not be limited to health staff; there should be input from security and program staff. In some cases, it is expeditious to ask a group of inmates, especially when cooperation with therapy poses a problem, or where certain system problems seem to impede access.

Once barriers are identified, the local task force can decide on interventions for improvement. It is important here not to jump to conclusions or to be simplistic. For example, difficulties in cooperation with recommendations should not be written off as "noncompliant inmates." Inmates do not cooperate for a variety of reasons. Perhaps they have competing activities, such as family visits or opportunities to earn wages. They may not understand the reason for the request, or may be acting out some anger regarding an unrelated individual or event. As with the process of identifying barriers, focus groups can be helpful in identifying solutions. Likewise, wide variations between physician practice patterns should not be written off simplistically. There may be valid reasons for such variation, perhaps as simple as difficulties with the formulary or a special program at a facility (such as a hospice or a unit for the physically disabled).

REASONS AND REMEDIES

Utilization of services in prisons and jails is high, but there are underlying reasons.[14] It is important to consider the differences in circumstances between inmates and patients on the outside. These include:

1. Increased need: the health care an inmate received before incarceration was often scanty. The lifestyles of many inmates were stressful. Their bodies are older than their chronological age, and there is often a high prevalence of communicable disease existent among inmates.[15]
2. Crowding: crowding brings a new set of stresses on health status, not the least of which is the opportunity for rapid contagion.
3. Institutional rules: the rules for diets, mattresses, bed boards, shoes, medication administration, and use of over-the-counter medications are different in the extreme from those in the outside world. They generate visits that would not occur anywhere else but in a prison.
4. Institutional policies: intake histories and physicals, tuberculin tests, hepatitis B vaccination, clearances for work, and screening for transfer each impose visit burdens that exceed those outside. Although these impose rework, they are important functions unique to the correctional setting.
5. Institutional inefficiencies: medication administration schedules and the inability to use the telephone to call the physician create unusual tensions. This is compounded by screening by a nurse when a sick call is made, which imposes an extra step in getting to a physician or physician assistant.
6. Psychological factors: the stress of incarceration is high. There is a lot of anxiety and depression, each of which can lead to illness behavior, for either coping or manipulation for secondary gain.

There are generic remedies to some of these aggravating conditions, each of which can help control unnecessary utilization.[14] Together, they can conserve resources for more appropriate medical use. These include:

1. Letting inmates carry their own medication and letting them take it as they see fit. The only exceptions to this policy would be psychotherapeutic agents and controlled substances that are often abused or traded, tuberculosis medications that should be directly observed, and medications for inmates who have proved themselves irresponsible as patients.
2. Keeping the health staff out of the shoe and mattress business. All people need shoes that fit and firm mattresses or bed boards. If shoes are available in a sufficient range of sizes and widths, there should be minimal need for physician authority for special shoes. A few common orthotic devices, such as arches and metatarsal pads, can be available in the commissary. These will largely reduce the podiatry referrals. Most adults have low back pain at some point in their lives. Although this ranges from occasional stiffness to a serious disability, the prescription in all cases includes, at a minimum, either a firm mattress or a bed board. If cots had a solid foundation for the mattress, medical visits and much complaining would be reduced.
3. Teaching the health staff the difference between secondary gain and cries for help. Not all inmates are "gaming" the system. This is an important distinction. Legitimate cries for help are often couched in physical complaints. The mental health staff can be especially helpful as trainers in this area. Once cries for help are recognized for what they are, the real problem can be addressed. Visits will be fewer, and the risk of litigation will be reduced.
4. Teaching physicians how to say no, when appropriate. Too often, busy physicians give in to what they know is not going to address the problem. It might be a bed board, a pass, a prescription, a referral to a specialist, or an allowance for a special diet, any of which might not be appropriate for that patient at that time. Giving in, in this circumstance, sets an expectation for this inmate and all of his colleagues for unreasonable requests. It compounds the problem and results in unhappy health staff.
5. Working on the diets. Prison food is often less than tasty. If the general diet was modest in fat and salt, the need for special diets would be reduced. Because special diets are for chronic diseases, they are for life. They do not need to be reviewed every 30 days; this is a waste of physician time. If inmates do not want to stay on special diets, that is their prerogative, just as it would be on the outside. If an inmate abuses the privilege of a special diet, it is not a medical matter and should be solved administratively in the facility. This particular piece of advice appears on the surface to be contrary to ACA Standard 3-4299. It is not. To comply with the standard, the inmate does not need to be seen monthly, nor does the physician have to write individual monthly renewal orders. The standard can be met by a physician's signature on a list of inmates requiring renewal of their special diets; one signature per month is adequate for the facility.
6. Defining a benefit package to save a lot of medical-necessity decision making. Each system should have one, or at least a list of, exclusions in policy known to the health staff. This includes, at a minimum, statements about:

Cosmetic surgery	Transsexual surgery
Clinical research	Experimental therapies (defined)
Hernia repair	Fertility evaluation and treatment
Hospice	Do-not-resuscitate policy
Breast reduction	Prosthetics, orthotics, custom shoes
Vaccines	Contact lenses
Optometric services	Nicotine patches
Nutritional supplements	Braces and other appliances
Preventive services	Vitamins
Impotence treatment	Contraception
Condoms	Dental exclusions

7. Sharing health information on transfer, to reduce duplication of effort.

8. Discontinuing the compilation of useless statistics. Individuals in correctional settings are good at counting, and well they should be. However, many logs, reports, and other counts have lost their connection to some value. In health care, each log and count should be reviewed for relevance and utility. Many can be discontinued, which will save valuable staff time.

9. Assigning a primary care physician (PCP) to each inmate with a chronic disease and, perhaps, to each inmate regardless of health status. The PCP can manage the medical care for the patient and can be held accountable for the care. This assignment will often lead to better continuity and coordination of care, which will reduce the need for off-site referrals and some hospitalizations.

WHAT ARE SOME OF THE PITFALLS IN QUALITY IMPROVEMENT?

1. Random chart review is one of the most common so-called quality assurance activities performed. It is an inspection process that seeks to find faults that have already occurred and is rarely productive. It is much more productive to focus on preventing defects than on identifying them.

   Selective chart review is helpful if it is done for a purpose. Looking at sentinel events, for example, has a higher yield than random chart review. Typically, this would involve review of medical records in instances in which there have been deaths, suicide attempts, hospitalizations, or major complications. Is the review done with an eye toward what might have prevented this occurrence? How can we make sure that this is prevented in the future?

2. Practitioners must be involved in the design and analysis of policies, standards, guidelines, and almost any quality improvement activity. Notwithstanding the command–control culture of prisons, health professionals resent such intrusions by nature. When they are involved, two things occur: (1) the program is assured of

hitting the mark, and (2) the practitioners will feel ownership in it.

3. Too often, nurses are given the task of finding faults with the physicians. This pits health professionals against each other and assures that multidisciplinary activities will fail. Likewise, pitting nurses or central office administrative staff against individual facilities or vendors is counterproductive. Quality improvement activities succeed only when there is a staff alliance to improve things for the greater good.

4. Not using multidisciplinary teams is a pitfall. Whatever problem is identified, it surely cannot be solved by individuals in a single discipline. Particularly in the correction setting, it is too easy to neglect the role of security and program staff in solving problems, and they surely appreciate the sense of ownership when a problem is solved.

5. Do not make assumptions that either inmates or staff are unable to change. Although there may be some political issues to address in problem solving, it is shortsighted to issue glib answers like "They will never get it," and "they don't want to take care of themselves." Getting individuals to buy into your agenda is a difficult but manageable task. It requires attention to the basic principles of marketing.

6. Although they do not stand on pedestals and are not more entitled than the rest of the staff, physicians are key to health care quality improvement. Excluding physicians makes quality improvement virtually impossible, because they control the gates to care. They write the prescriptions, generate the orders, and approve or deny the referrals. The resources flow through their heads and their hands. They must be involved in all quality improvement activities and decisions about resource use. For example, a physician must issue any denial of care by reason of medical necessity.

CONCLUSION

The objectives of managing care through quality improvement are to improve the health of the population served, fairly, and with efficient use of resources. It must not detract from security interests; in fact, good quality management in correctional health care should contribute to security interests by reducing unnecessary stress among inmates. There is much unnecessary use of services, which allows ample opportunity for cost savings with appropriate utilization and quality management techniques.

The creative solutions to budgetary pressures should follow national guidelines. There must be physician input into the adoption of these guidelines at the local level, and the final determination of medical necessity should lie with physicians practicing in the correctional system. Correctional health care staff must remain vigilant to prevent unnecessary delays or denials of medically necessary care for inmates in their practices.

REFERENCES

1. Hammett TM, Widom R, Epstein J, et al: *Issues and Practices 1994 Update: HIV/AIDS and STDs in Correctional Facilities.* Washington, D.C., National Institute of Justice, December 1995.
2. McDonald DC: *Managing Prison Health Care and Costs.* Washington, D.C., National Institute of Justice, May 1995.
3. Fitzgerald JF, Smith DM, Martin DK, et al: A case manager intervention to reduce readmissions. *Arch Intern Med* 154:1721–1729, 1994.
4. Weinberger M, Oddone E: Strategies to reduce hospital readmissions: A review. *Qual Rev Bull* 15:255–260, 1989.
5. *Healthcare Management Guidelines.* Seattle, Milliman and Robertson.
6. *Surgical Indications Monitoring for Appropriateness: Adult Version.* Northampton, NH, InterQual, 1995.
7. Agency for Health Care Policy and Research: *Acute Low Back Problems in Adults: Assessment and Treatment.* Rockville, Md, U.S. Department of Health and Human Services, DHHS Publication No 95-0643, December 1994.
8. The Institute for Medical Studies: Current concepts in the diagnosis and management of chronic viral hepatitis. *Clin Courier* 14:16, 1996.
9. *Medical Necessity Guidelines.* Salem, Ore, Oregon Department of Corrections.
10. *Standards for Adult Correctional Institutions.* Laurel, Md, American Correctional Association, 1990.
11. *Standards for Health Services in Prisons.* Chicago, National Commission on Correctional Health Care, 1992.
12. *1997 Standards for Accreditation.* Washington, D.C., National Committee for Quality Assurance, 1996.
13. *Quality Improvement Plans 1995 & 1996.* Camp Hill, Pa, Commonwealth of Pennsylvania Department of Corrections.
14. Anno BJ: Keynote remarks (summary). Presented at the National Commission on Correctional Health Care Meeting, Nashville, Tenn, 1996.
15. Glaser JB, Greifinger RB: Correctional health care: A public health opportunity. *Ann Intern Med* 118: 1993.

27

Care of the Impaired and Disabled

Joseph E. Paris, M.D., Ph.D., C.C.H.P.

Persons with physical and mental impairments and disabilities are sometimes incarcerated. Hearing, vision, and speech impairments, as well as mobility impairments requiring special medical devices, are examples of disabilities that present problems for physicians practicing in correctional settings. Private practitioners are not responsible for the living accommodations of their handicapped patients; however, correctional physicians may have to intervene to protect impaired inmates who are unable to fend for themselves in the correctional environment. In addition, correctional physicians are often asked to assess individuals with impairments relative to their work or housing assignments. Appropriate judgement protects the safety of the inmate and reduces risk-management issues for the facility authority.

DEFINITIONS OF IMPAIRMENT AND DISABILITY

Conventional definitions of impairment and disability are only partly useful in a correctional environment. These definitions are often associated with work-related injury and subsequent compensatory awards. For civilians, impairment for this purpose is defined as an abnormality in a body part or organ system and its functioning that interferes with an individual's activity of daily living.[1] Disability is, consequently, an impairment that impairs the ability to work. Not all impairments lead to disability. For example, loss of a fifth digit may not lead to inability to work. These definitions are the basis of disability evaluations used in workmen's compensation, social security disability evaluations, and other work-related disability evaluations.

Using these definitions of disability, it is estimated that about 7.1 million persons in the U.S. have disabilities affecting their ability to perform activities of daily living (ADL).[1] The scope of disability was considerably widened, however, with the passage of the Americans with Disabilities Act (ADA). The findings of that act state that 43 million Americans have one or more physical or mental disabilities. Disabilities are defined as a physical or mental impairment that substantially limits one or more major life activities.[2] The ADA may have a significant effect on structural and health care delivery problems within correctional facilities.

LITIGATION AND DISABILITY

One concern of correctional officials is whether they can be sued by inmates using the ADA. The National Prison Project, an offshoot of the Americans For Civil Liberties Union (ACLU), has stated that inmates with disabilities are protected by both constitutional claims and federal statutes.[3] Circuit courts have ruled both for and against the applicability of the ADA in correctional facilities. The fundamental question of whether the ADA applies to state prisons has not been entirely settled.

Box 27-1. Health Conditions Covered by NCCHC Special Needs Treatment Plan Standard

1. Chronic illness (asthma, heart disease, diabetes, hypertension, chronic obstructive lung disease, etc.)
2. Communicable disease (HIV, syphilis, tuberculosis, etc.)
3. Physical handicaps (blind, mute, deaf, paraplegics, etc.)
4. Frail elderly
5. Terminally ill (life expectancy less than 1 year)
6. Inmates with special mental health needs (self-mutilators, aggressive mentally ill, sex offenders, and suicidal inmates)
7. Developmentally disabled

Box 27-2. Specifics of NCCHC Treatment Plans

1. Series of written plans specifying course of therapy
2. Indicates roles of health care staff
3. Individualized by patient
4. Multidisciplinary
5. Based on patient need
6. Includes short- and long-term goals
7. Includes methods to pursue goals
8. Lists supportive or rehabilitative services
9. Suggests chronic clinic follow-up as indicated
10. Includes problem in master problem list

Legal rights organizations may be involved in pursuing ADA litigation. The National Prison Project is one such organization that actively litigates to pursue ADA claims for disabled inmates. When complaints regarding the ADA are sent to the Department of Justice, they are currently referred to the Disability Rights Section of the Justice Department for evaluation. Under the ADA, all individuals have a right to have their complaint reviewed. If the ADA applies to correctional settings, structural and functional deficiencies in accommodating the disabled may lead to significant legal entanglement. For correctional physicians, it is important to recognize the problems associated with impairment and disability and provide the correctional authority with humane and reasonable advice to address those problems.

Complaints lodged with the National Prison Project principally center around hygiene issues (personal communication, NPP). Individuals with disabilities complain that routine daily hygiene is difficult to achieve in a correctional setting. This often involves structural deficits in accommodating paraplegics, as well as accommodating the cleaning and supply needs of inmates with special devices such as colostomies or urostomies.

NATIONAL COMMISSION ON CORRECTIONAL HEALTH CARE STANDARDS

Legally unenforceable standards have been promulgated by the National Commission on Correctional Health Care (NCCHC) regarding patients with "special needs."[4, 5] Most of these individuals would qualify as disabled under the ADA. These standards (Special Needs Treatment Plans) attempt to encourage health care staff to develop treatment plans for individuals who are impaired, disabled, or have other special needs (e.g., the terminally ill), and who may or may not have medical conditions that warrant treatment. For example, the standard suggests that individual written treatment plans be developed for developmentally disabled inmates to ensure their safety. While this is not considered a medical treatment ordinarily provided by medical staff, it has become accepted that medical staff provide a protective role

for persons unable to endure the harsh correctional environment.

The NCCHC standard suggests a multidisciplinary written treatment plan be developed by a physician or other qualified health care person, which includes instructions about diet, exercise, adaptation to the correctional environment, medication, diagnostic testing, and follow-up medical care[4] (Box 27-1). These treatment plans are not meant to be written only once, but should be modified over time as indicated by the treatment needs of the patient (Box 27-2).

Based on the author's NCCHC accreditation reviews of several selected states, treatment plans are often in place for mental health patients and patients with chronic diseases (personal communication, Joe Paris). Patients with impairments or disabilities may have their impairment/disability included on the problem list, but generally do not have a written treatment plan evident in the medical record. The accreditation process, by revealing these deficits, can serve as an educational tool for correctional health care staff.

Other NCCHC standards[6, 7] require that prostheses be provided when the health of the inmate would otherwise be adversely affected. This determination is made by a physician or dentist.

PREVALENCE OF DISABILITY IN INCARCERATED SETTINGS

There are little published data on the prevalence of impaired inmates in jails or prisons. Based on classification data in 1996, the Georgia Department of Corrections had an impairment prevalence of 2.4% (Table 27-1) (unpublished data, Joe Paris). Impairment in this classification system was defined as a deficiency that required some type of institutional or programmatic support in assistance with activities of daily living.[8] Of the 32,887 inmates at the time these data were collected, there were 81 wheelchair-bound inmates (0.2%). As of May 1997, the Florida Department of Corrections listed 1,003 of 73,000 inmates as impaired (1.4%) (personal communication, Jerry Ellsworth).

These data are only partially useful in describing the extent of impairments in correctional settings. Definitions of impairment and disability in correctional settings are not

Table 27-1. Impairment in the Georgia Department of Corrections, May 1997

Total number of inmates	32,887
Impaired males	670
Impaired females	5
Transportation impaired, male	99
Transportation impaired, female	2
Total impaired	776

standardized and are often determined by the needs of the system to define an individual's ability to function in that system. Standardized prevalence rates of various impairments would facilitate facility and health care planning and development of policies for compassionate release.

CLASSIFICATION SYSTEMS AND FITNESS FOR WORK

An institutional definition of impairment is imprecise in correctional settings, because impairment is often arbitrarily defined. There are no national standards for disability determination for correctional facilities despite the fact that many states require inmates to work. Physicians in correctional settings are often asked to make a determination if an inmate is fit to work and to set limits on the types of work an inmate can perform.

Practicality and safety should guide correctional physicians in making a judgement on whether an inmate can work. There is a mentality on the part of some of the public, some correctional officials, and some public officials that inmates should be punished by hard labor (e.g., chain gangs, breaking rocks, etc). Work may assume a punitive function rather than being functional or rewarding. In addition, some inmates would prefer not to work despite administrative mandates that they must work. This places the physician in a position of not being an agent of the patient, which may create ethical concerns. However, the Hippocratic oath binds physicians to be compassionate and to act in the best interest of their patients. To avoid these conflicts, the physician must try to base his assessment on objective findings that are reproducible, maintain concern for the safety of the inmate, and involve the patient in the evaluation.

Because of the large numbers of inmates who need assessment for work, it is not practical or desirable to perform a comprehensive disability evaluation on all inmates prior to work assignments. Fitness evaluations that help assess functional abilities are more appropriate for screening purposes. Inmates who claim impairments can be selected out and receive more in-depth evaluations.

Disability is both perceived and objectively defined. More people consider themselves disabled than are actually unable to work.[9] The gap between what the inmate can do and what they want to do is difficult to determine, due to sub-

jective factors that may be difficult to measure. The American Medical Association and others have published guidelines on evaluations for impairment and disability.[1, 9, 10] These guidelines are intended for workmen's compensation-type evaluations, and are not completely applicable to correctional settings. They do, however, offer guidelines on defining the degree of impairment that may result in disability. These types of evaluations may be useful as objective criteria for complicated cases, or when there is disagreement with the inmate about ability to work.

The state correctional systems of Georgia and Florida use a classification system (PULHES) that evolved from a military fitness classification system.[8] This system is useful in describing functional classification, which then permits correctional administrative officials to make safe work assignments. The PULHES system numerically grades inmates on their functional work capacity, level of impairment, and mobility, and includes categories for mental health and dental health. Grading an individual automatically determines that inmate's ability to perform work. Grades are assigned subjectively by health care personnel. Some grades are assigned on the ability of an inmate to lift certain amounts of weight. There are mechanisms to temporarily restrict an inmate from work during episodes of disability due to sickness or injury.

When physicians are asked to determine fitness for work, hard labor, or housing assignment, it is important for them to understand what the inmate may be asked to do and where they may be housed. For this reason, physicians should become familiar with the facilities and the prison work environment. This can be done by touring work facilities and observing the types of work inmates may be assigned to. While touring, it is useful for physicians to discover how paralyzed inmates or inmates with special devices will be caring for themselves. Toilets and showers should be checked periodically for grab bars, wheelchair accessibility, appropriate hygiene facilities, etc. It may be useful to tour the facility with an impaired inmate (e.g., paraplegic) to assess their difficulties with structural impediments. Physicians may have little control over these items, but they can inform the correctional officials about the needs of the impaired.

STRUCTURAL ISSUES AND MOBILITY IMPAIRMENTS

Significant problems occur when inmates have mobility impairments. Legal and medical problems may arise when paraplegics, for example, do not have appropriate equipment, or face structural barriers to carry on activities of daily living. While these issues are the responsibility of the correctional administrator, they may become medical in nature when inmates are harmed as a result of improper transfer equipment, structural impediments to appropriate hygiene, fecal contamination of housing units as a result of inability to access a commode or shower, etc. When no handicap accessible facilities are available, mobility impaired inmates are sometimes housed on infirmary units. These are generally inappropriate housing decisions and, in the long run, are costly. Physicians need to bring these issues to the attention of the correctional authority.

Inmates who need aids, such as crutches, canes, walkers, etc., present difficult challenges in correctional environments. Ordinarily, civilian inmates can buy a cane or crutch whenever they want. In correctional environments, these devices are viewed as potential weapons and correctional officials are very concerned when inmates have access to devices that can be taken apart (such as a walker) or used as a weapon (canes). Physicians need to be deliberate in making a safe and objective assessment of an inmate's impairment. It is unethical not to prescribe a device simply because the correctional officials refuse to allow inmates to have them. Occasionally, these problems can be resolved by working with correctional administrative staff. Special housing is sometimes designated for inmates who use these devices. It is useful to document use of these devices and have them returned when the inmate no longer needs them, because, if devices remain unused in housing units, other inmates may use them as weapons. This makes correctional staff wary of permitting their use for other inmates.

Special passes or "exemptions" are granted to inmates that allow them privileges due to mobility problems or other impairment. For example, an inmate may need extra time to ambulate between their housing unit and the dining hall to eat. This may require a medical pass. These exemptions should never be granted casually or as favors, because of the potential of inmate abuse and because inappropriate assignment of an exemption may lead to cynicism toward medical staff by correctional staff. Physicians should always make objective physical assessments and recommendations based on physical findings.

MEDICAL DEVICES

Inmates may need medical devices on a permanent or temporary basis. Colostomy bags, urostomy bags, and other devices acting as a receptacle for human waste are problems in correctional environments. Lack of replacement bags and lack of facilities to change bags are among the most frequent complaints lodged with the ACLU.

Physicians should become familiar with the types of devices required by their patients. Maintenance and replacement of medical devices may require physician intervention in correctional settings. Urinary catheter maintenance should be part of the treatment plan when a patient has one of these devices.

Indwelling Foley catheters made of latex should be changed every 2 weeks; silicone catheters should be changed every 4 to 6 weeks. Patients performing self-catheterization can re-use catheters. Catheters can be cleaned by running tap water through the catheter after use. Once a week, the catheter should be sterilized or a new catheter provided.

> ### Box 27-3. Equipment Required for Intermittent Catheterization
>
> 1. Soft, pliable #12 or #14 (French) catheter
> 2. Waterproof pads for lap
> 3. Antiseptic wipes or soap and water for hand washing
> 4. Antiseptic solution or saline to clean perineum (females)
> 5. Antiseptic solution or soap and water to clean penis (males)
> 6. Water-soluble lubricant to lubricate catheter
> 7. Clean, self-sealing storage bag to store catheter

Adapted from Zejdlik C: *Management of Spinal Cord Injury.* Jones and Bartlett, 1992.

Deteriorating or brittle catheters should be discarded.[11] Appropriate hand washing facilities and soap should be available in the vicinity of the urinal, or the inmate can have a container to receive the urine that can be placed near the sink (Box 27-3).

Colostomy bags are a frequent source of problems in correctional environments. Ostomy care has progressed considerably in the past few decades. However, containing stomal output and protecting periostomal skin are challenges for patients and caregivers.

Patients who undergo colostomy should not leave the hospital until appropriate training for maintaining the ostomy has been provided. While inservice education on ostomy care should be provided to correctional health care staff, consultation arrangements with enterostomal therapists may be useful for difficult cases or for inservice education efforts.

Key elements for proper stomal care include appropriate choice of equipment and preparation and maintenance of the skin surrounding the stomal site. Adherence of ostomy bags to the skin surrounding the stoma is highly brand- and individual-dependent. This is related to the variety of adhesives and skin structures. In some facilities, only one brand is available. Physicians may need to intervene to assist the patient in obtaining supplies that lead to a satisfactory result.

Stomal sizes may vary and, when pouches do not fit the stoma, the patient needs scissors to cut the pouch opening to fit. Because scissors are contraband in most facilities, the patient may need to perform all pouch changes in the health care unit.

Nurses and physicians should familiarize themselves with stoma care, including choosing the appropriate pouch and adhesive, ensuring proper fit and adherence, preparing and applying the pouch, teaching the patient proper pouch emptying, cleaning the pouch and surrounding skin, and helping the patient to adapt to activities of daily living with a pouch.[12] Special diets and instruction may be necessary for individuals who produce flatus from particular foods.

Care must be taken to avoid skin deterioration around ostomy sites. Common skin complications surrounding an ostomy include denuded skin, periostomy hyperplasia, contact dermatitis, psoriasis, folliculitis, and candidiasis, as well as other inflammatory processes.

Colostomy bags are reusable until the adhesive attaching the bag to the surrounding skin fails. This occurs after 2 to 3 days of use in many cases, and the bag must then be changed. If the bag is not changed when the adhesive fails, the unit will leak. Box 27-4 lists equipment normally associated with changing colostomy bags. Normally, scissors are included as standard equipment but are not provided in correctional settings, because they are contraband. Bags are emptied in a toilet and used bags are placed in a plastic bag for disposal.

Continuous positive airway pressure (CPAP) devices and oxygen delivery systems usually cause distress to correctional staff because of an assumed potential for explosion and the possibility that other inmates may tamper with the equipment while the patient is asleep. For this reason, it may be prudent to advocate single-cell occupancy for inmates who require oxygen or CPAP equipment. Continuous positive airway pressure equipment and some oxygen equipment require an electrical outlet that may not be available in cells. This may limit the housing choices for these patients. Some correctional institutions use infirmary-type settings for these patients. Although this is a poor use of an infirmary bed because it requires long-term use, it may be the only alternative in certain settings.

The use of insulin pumps is not practical in correctional settings. However, on rare occasions, a person requiring one of these devices will be incarcerated. Only one inmate who needed an insulin pump was incarcerated in the Florida Department of Corrections over a 10-year period (an incidence rate of 1/150,000). This individual misused the pump by injecting intravenous drugs and allowed other inmates to use the pump for that purpose as well. Because the individual was not highly motivated, erratic blood sugar control was obtained. These pumps should not be used in correctional settings, except in highly motivated individuals who can live in a housing setting conducive to appropriate use of the device.

Demand pacemakers and implantable defibrillators do not usually pose major problems in correctional environments. Certain devices that are unshielded may malfunction when exposed to microwave radiation. However, these types of devices have not been implanted for many years. Newer implanted pacemakers and defibrillators do not pose a risk to patients exposed to microwave radiation. Demand pacemakers have batteries that may need replacement. Cardiology consultation is suggested for evaluation of inmates with these devices. Demand pacemakers should be tested monthly to ascertain whether sensing and capturing is accurate. This can usually be performed by phone link-up with consultants.

PLACEMENT OF DISABLED INMATES

The correctional authority is expected to make a reasonable accommodation to house disabled inmates appropriately. Physicians may be asked to assist in this process by classifying or describing the type of disability. Placement refers both to finding the most suitable institution and the most appropriate housing unit within a facility. Most prisons and many jails have separate housing for mentally ill patients. Persons with severe intellectual impairments, deafness, and blindness need protection from the harshness of the correctional environment. They may or may not specifically need medical care for their condition, but they may gravitate toward infirmaries as last-resort housing. When this occurs, the medical functioning of the infirmary unit is disrupted. This type of placement is acceptable for the short term, but long-term infirmary housing reduces bed availability for the acutely ill. In addition, disabled inmates housed in infirmaries are frequently cut off from certain activities, jobs, and programs available to general population inmates. An additional burden is placed on infirmary health care staff because ordinary activities, such as eating or taking medication, are "medicalized," which increases work for staff. To avoid these problems, some state correctional departments develop chronic care units that use nursing staff to assist in caring for these individuals.

Patients who have terminal illness should be medically cared for in the most humane manner possible (see chapter on Infirmaries). Patients with senile dementia, advanced parkinsonism, multiple sclerosis, and other similar conditions need frequent medical care. While infirmary housing may not always be indicated, it is best to house these patients near a health care unit. The patients should have interdisciplinary rounds or treatment plans that involve all staff in addressing their situation. Special attention should be placed on medication delivery to cognitively impaired patients. It is advisable to administer medication dose by dose to any inmate who has decreased cognitive functioning, and it is prudent to occasionally update the warden or correctional authority about their status. Frequently, correctional authorities will assist in application for parole for individuals who by virtue of their condition are deteriorating cognitively. In some states, physicians can initiate this process. When parole is expected for a cognitively impaired inmate, the health care staff should assist in appropriate civilian placement. Sometimes, severely mentally impaired individuals are not eligible for or permitted parole. These patients should then be treated as nursing home patients. Unfortunately, many have to be housed on infirmary units.

SPINAL CORD INJURY PATIENTS

Jails occasionally assume custody of quadraplegics or paraplegics who are hospitalized after gunshot wounds to the spine. It is important to assess whether the inmate has received an appropriate level of rehabilitation before returning to the correctional facility. Rehabilitation is vitally important in obtaining an optimal functional status. Patients should not be accepted into a jail or prison after a recent spinal cord injury until their rehabilitation has been completed. Few correctional facilities have the ability to provide appropriate rehabilitative services. Bladder and bowel training, optimal motor and ambulatory functioning, transfer techniques, and optimal education in activity of daily living therapies should be provided before an inmate is released to a correctional facility. Physical therapy once or twice a week is usually never an acceptable alternative to appropriate rehabilitation services.

Wheelchairs are a frequent problem in correctional settings. This is particularly true for paraplegics who come into the facility with no wheelchair or one that is broken. National Commission of Health Care standards require that wheelchairs be provided to inmates when the health of the inmate would otherwise be adversely affected. Often, a standard wheelchair is provided to the inmate. However, a person's neurologic status and level of spinal cord injury should be determining factors in the individualized choice of wheelchair. Wheelchairs should be provided that allow independent mobility.[11] In short-term facilities, it is often impractical to issue personalized wheelchairs for patients who may only have short lengths of stays. In prisons, however, where long-term use is expected, universal-fit wheelchairs may lead to functional impairments or injuries. Rehabilitation consultation may be sought in choosing an appropriate wheelchair.

The skin is an important element of care for spinal cord-injured patients. Pressure on anesthetic skin creates a high potential for skin breakdown and decubitus ulcers. Regular bathing, followed by application of lanolin or ointment, help protect the skin. Wheelchair cushions and special mattresses are useful in preventing compressive forces that may result in ulcerations. Disposable absorbent pads (chucks) should be available to function as diapers in the event of spontaneous bowel or bladder emptying. These events should be followed by cleaning the skin to reduce the risk of breakdown and infection.

Toilet seats, shower seats, and beds should be at a height that permits easy transfer from a wheelchair. This is often difficult, because there may be more than one patient with paraplegia on a unit. Because paraplegic patients may require suppositories or digital stimulation, the seat should have arm and body supports (armrests) to prevent loss of balance.

Spasticity is a common problem in paraplegics. Diazepam is a poor choice of medication for any individual with a history of substance abuse. Frequently, paraplegics who have been on diazepam, for extended periods are incarcerated. There are also patients who have not been on diazepam but say they are. In these cases, consultation with the prior treating physiatrist should be obtained to provide a verifiable medication history. Patients should not be abruptly withdrawn from diazepam because of the potential for an acute withdrawal syndrome (see chapter on Withdrawal). If a medication change is contemplated, withdrawal syndromes should be taken into consideration and the medication dosage should be appropriately tapered. Baclofen is a drug of choice in both civilian and correctional settings for spasticity of paraplegia, because of equivalent potency and fewer side effects. Dantrolene is another acceptable alternative, but does have risk of liver toxicity in dosages greater than 300 mg.[11]

There are many management issues surrounding the care of paraplegics, which are beyond the scope of this chapter. Excellent texts are available and should be present on infirmary units where paraplegics are cared for.[11]

REFERENCES

1. *Guides to the Evaluation of Permanent Impairment*, American Medical Association, ed 4. Chicago, AMA, 1993.
2. Americans with Disabilities Act Section 3; 42 USC 12102.
3. Boston J, Manville D: *Prisoners' Self Help Litigation Manual.* 3rd ed. Dobbs Ferry, NY, 1995. Oceana Publications,
4. National Commission on Correctional Health Care. Standard J-49; Standards for Health Care in Jails, 1996.
5. National Commission on Correctional Health Care. Standard P-50; Standards for Health Care in Prisons, 1992.
6. National Commission on Correctional Health Care. Standard J-57; Standards for Health Services in Jails, 1996.
7. National Commission on Correctional Health Care. Standard P-58; Standards for Health Services in Prisons, NCCHC 1992.
8. Paris JE, Davis DE, Ellsworth GP: Medical classification of inmates: The key for successful managed health care in corrections. Presented at the 18th National Conference on Correctional Health Care, San Diego, CA, September 26-28, 1994.
9. Demeter (ed.): *Disability Evaluation*. St Louis, Mosby, 1996.
10. *The Medical Disability Advisor*, ed 2. Presley Reed, 1994.
11. Zejdlik C: *Management of Spinal Cord Injury*, ed 2. Jones and Bartlett, 1992.
12. Paulford-Lecher N: Teaching your patient stoma care. *Nursing* 23: 47-49, 1993.

28

Special Problems of Health Services for Juvenile Justice Programs

Michael D. Cohen M.D., F.A.A.P.

R esidents in juvenile justice programs are not only lawbreakers, but also children. Because they are children, they have certain special rights and social standing. In general, the upbringing and support of a child is the responsibility of the parents. When the courts place children outside the home, then the state is responsible to satisfy those broad parental responsibilities. In response, delinquency programs have traditionally emphasized education and rehabilitation. While corrections systems may deprive an adult of liberty without providing any special programs, juvenile facilities must have programs to address the special needs of the confined children.[1]

Health programs must treat the acute needs of sick and injured residents, provide periodic assessments and preven-tive services for all residents, and special services for those with chronic or disabling health problems. Health services are not merely a necessity like food, shelter, and clothing, but can also be an integral part of the rehabilitation program for youth. Like health services in adult prisons and jails, juvenile programs must have organized systems of care with adequate administrative support, budget, staff, space, and equipment. This chapter will focus on the health needs of incarcerated youth.

Adolescents have a particular variety of health problems and unique attitudes about health and disease. Health staff must be able to work with physically mature youth who, like other children, are developmentally immature and in many ways unable to deal with their health needs in a responsible way. It is not uncommon for a youngster to be resistant and refuse care at one time, and a very short time later choose to cooperate fully.

The particular health needs of young adults are largely related to the physical, emotional, cognitive, and behavioral consequences of puberty. Impulsive behavior results in high incidence of trauma, sexually transmitted diseases, unintended pregnancy, and suicide among adolescents. Asthma is the most common chronic medical condition, but there are a wide variety of childhood chronic illnesses with a prevalence of one per thousand or less, which may be regularly found in youth served by juvenile justice programs. In addition, chronic problems often begin in adolescence, and health staff must be alert to the onset of a significant symptom to facilitate an early diagnosis and initiate treatment.

Juvenile facilities tend to be much smaller than adult prisons. Small facilities do not readily support a large health program. A 25-bed facility may have a half-time registered nurse, who works solo, and a contracted physician, physician assistant, or nurse practitioner who comes on-site every 2 weeks for a few hours. How to provide comprehensive services to small populations is one of the key administrative problems of these programs.

Juvenile justice is undergoing dramatic changes. Larger proportions of young people are being tried as adults in criminal courts and sentenced to adult corrections systems. Traditional juvenile delinquency programs are expensive, and there is increasing pressure to demonstrate that they are effective. As the principal goal of incarceration shifts from positive youth development to punishment, prisons become more cost-effective than special juvenile programs. There is a risk that special programs for youth development will not be continued in the new juvenile prisons that are being built to house youth committed to adult corrections agencies under new criminal procedures.

Health services for juvenile justice programs are also undergoing significant changes. Reduction of the state workforce has resulted in contracting for health services with private health care organizations. A shift from fee-for-service to capitated care is also occurring. This provides an opportunity for expansion of preventive services, but also the risk of reductions in other needed services, especially for chronically ill and disabled residents.

STANDARDS OF CARE

Juvenile justice programs should meet the standards that are recommended for adolescent programs that serve the general public. The American Academy of Pediatrics and the Maternal and Child Health Bureau of the U.S. Public Health Service collaborated on recommendations for child and adolescent primary care.[2] The Medicaid Early and Periodic Screening, Diagnosis and Treatment program (EPSDT) in each state has standards for adolescent screening and follow-up.[3] The American Medical Association has

published Guidelines for Adolescent Preventive Services.[4] Some of the U.S. Public Health Service's Year 2000 National Health Objectives concern the health of adolescents and should be addressed by all health programs for young people.[5]

The Standards for the Administration of Juvenile Justice of the National Advisory Committee presented a best practices model, circa 1980. These standards emphasized youth development, including the role of health services as part of the individual rehabilitation program.[6]

Both the American Correctional Association and the National Commission on Correctional Health Care have specific standards for juvenile facilities and certification programs.[7, 8] These standards provide a systematic approach to development and maintenance of an adequate health program.

The American Public Health Association Standards place greater emphasis on the quality and completeness of health services, and provide more specific guidelines for certain aspects of clinical care.[9]

The Juvenile Detention Centers' Association of Pennsylvania published detailed standards that provide small detention centers with explicit guidelines for implementation of a comprehensive health program.[10]

Models for public health collaboration with juvenile justice were developed in detail in Thompson and Farrow's *Hard Time, Healing Hands. Developing Primary Health Care Services for Incarcerated Youth.*[11]

CONDITIONS OF CONFINEMENT

A recent study by the National Institute of Justice surveyed conditions in juvenile facilities throughout the United States.[12] Six basic health services were examined: initial health screening, health appraisal, explaining how to gain access to health services, sick call, written arrangements for emergency care, and staff training in first aid and cardiopulmonary resuscitation. Important findings included lack of routine screening on admission in 56% of training schools and absence of minimal health appraisal in 20% of detention centers, 18% of training schools, and 44% of ranches. Only 26% of the facilities surveyed conformed fully to all six basic health services that were assessed.

SPECIAL ROLE OF THE NURSE IN JUVENILE JUSTICE HEALTH PROGRAMS

Nurses are the principal health care providers in juvenile justice health programs. The nurse organizes and manages all aspects of the health program in small facilities. Nurses assess ill or injured residents and treat the vast majority with supportive care. When health problems are beyond the scope of nursing interventions and local standing orders, the nurse refers to the facility physician for further diagnosis and treatment.[13]

There must be an effective system to train staff nurses and ongoing support and supervision of the advanced clinical practice performed by nurses in correctional settings. This is especially important in small programs, where a single registered nurse may be the only health professional on site.

QUALITY ASSURANCE

In the author's experience evaluating health services programs for juveniles in eight states, it was repeatedly found that health problems are lost to follow-up, needed physician referrals are not made, diagnostic evaluation is not ordered, recurrent or chronic health problems are assessed as isolated single events, and regular follow-up of the chronically ill does not occur. These omissions often arise from complete reliance on the clinical judgment of isolated individual health professionals who practice without supervision, clinical guidelines, or ongoing monitoring of the quality and completeness of their work.

Explicit standards for management of commonly occurring problems may be established through problem-oriented clinical protocols for nursing and medical staff. Clinical protocols should define a logical approach to assessment and management of health problems, including specific time frames and expected outcomes. Clinical care can then be monitored for compliance with established protocols.

A formal quality assurance program brings improvements in health programs by monitoring services, identifying problems, analyzing the causes, developing and implementing corrective interventions, and subsequently monitoring again to determine if the problems have been resolved.[14] The purpose of quality assurance is to improve health services, not produce audits that show compliance with a narrow set of process indicators.

Sentinel events are occurrences that signify a possible failure of the health program, such as true emergencies, emergency room visits, hospitalizations, deaths, unusual incidents, and resident grievances. Monitoring sentinel events can provide information about how a health program is responding to special health needs.

Monitoring routine components of the health program assures that they are well implemented. Completeness of initial health evaluation, staff and youth tuberculosis screening, sick call assessments, medication administration, outstanding dental needs, and outstanding requests for specialty consultations reflect the access, evaluation, and treatment functions of the health program.

HEALTH RECORDS

There must be a separate health record for each youth. The layout and contents of the record should be defined and consistent throughout a system. A single common set of forms should be used to document the initial screening and health appraisal at entry into the system. There should be a problem list and a written management plan for every problem.

Criminal charges must be completely absent from the health record. Knowledge of criminal history may preju-

dice the health staff and inappropriately influence their approach to the patient. There is no general need for health staff to know a youth's criminal history. If truly needed in special circumstances, this information is available in the case record.

Combining the separate medical, dental, and mental health charts into a single health record supports coordination of care among the different disciplines.

HEALTH APPRAISAL

Initial screening and comprehensive health evaluation should be completed at admission. Admission screening occurs at entry into each facility. The goal of initial screening is to identify active medical, dental, mental health, or communicable disease problems before the youth enters the general population. Medications, including birth control pills, should be continued without interruption.

A comprehensive medical history, physical examination, screening tests for specific diseases, as well as vision and hearing screening should be obtained promptly for every youth.

A complete unclothed physical examination, including careful examination of the skin, feet, teeth, and genitalia, is required. Sexual maturation should be assessed using the stages defined by Tanner.[15] Delayed growth and physical maturation is a health problem that should be noted and evaluated.

Formal screening tests of vision and hearing should be used to identify youth who need further evaluation by hearing and vision professionals.

Youth should be screened for tuberculosis using the Mantoux intradermal skin test.

Blood tests should include syphilis serology; a complete blood cell count to identify youth with anemia and other abnormalities of the red blood cells, white cells and platelets; and an automated chemistry panel to identify youth with abnormalities of major organs, such as the kidney and liver.

Urine should be screened for blood and protein to assist in identification of chronic kidney disease. Urine screening for leukocytes in males identifies youth with symptomatic and asymptomatic urethritis.[16, 17] Treatment of chlamydia, gonorrhea, and non-specific pathogens can prevent individual complications and reduce community transmission after release.

For sexually active females, a pregnancy test should be performed and the physical examination should include a pelvic examination with cervical cytology and tests for gonorrhea and chlamydia. Cervical cytologic study results help identify young women with human papillomavirus infection who are at risk for early cervical cancer. Follow-up evaluation with colposcopy and aggressive treatment of significant lesions can prevent progression of disease. Gynecologic services should include initiation or continuation of contraception.

Documentation of childhood immunizations should be obtained. Sources for this information include parents, public schools, and past providers of primary care. Residents should be brought fully up to date for their age in compliance with current recommendations for adolescent immunization.[18] Mere compliance with narrow school entry requirements misses an opportunity to fully immunize these high risk youth. Many youth in juvenile justice programs have not received the adolescent dT booster, the second MMR, or the hepatitis B series. Varicella vaccine may be given to youth whose parents cannot confirm a history of chickenpox earlier in childhood. Confirmation of chickenpox history and vaccination of susceptible youth on admission to program simplifies subsequent management if chickenpox exposure should occur. Vaccines are available free from the federally funded Vaccines for Children program for high-risk children up to age 18.[19]

After gathering all the health appraisal information, it must be reviewed carefully to make a complete list of the youth's health problems and a management plan for each problem. The problem list and management plan are the expected products of the health appraisal and form the basis for each youth's health program. Needed services cannot be provided, unless the problem is identified and care is planned. Approval of the problem list and management plan is an essential supervisory function of the facility physician.

REHABILITATION PLAN

Health concerns should be included in the development of each youth's individual program and in periodic reviews of performance.[20] General health goals related to personal hygiene, exercise, injury prevention, and health education are appropriate for every youth and provide an opportunity for early achievement of some program goals.

Residents with chronic health needs may be given specific goals that address the knowledge and behaviors young people need to manage their care effectively. Residents with diabetes, asthma, seizures, tuberculosis exposure, and HIV infection, for example, must learn how to care for themselves to live healthy and independent lives in the future.

HEALTH PROMOTION AND DISEASE PREVENTION

Young people have the most to gain from health promotion and disease prevention programs. Disease prevention includes efforts to reduce smoking, drinking, drug abuse, obesity, dietary fat, and higher-risk sexual behaviors. Health promotion includes physical exercise; a diet rich in whole grains, fresh fruits, and vegetables; personal hygiene; universal precautions to avoid contact with body fluids; handling anger; conflict resolution; and other healthy behaviors. A structured health education program to achieve sound health practices, habits, attitudes, and behaviors should be part of an adolescent health program.

Health education should be integrated into the daily activities of the facility in the school, in residential group activities, in recreation, or at meals. Personal hygiene practices, such as handwashing after using the toilet and before every meal, should be required. Staff should model healthy behaviors, such as handwashing, universal precautions for all body fluid contacts, and nonviolent conflict resolution.

Programs that participate in the USDA school breakfast and lunch programs are reimbursed for meals that meet the Surgeon General's dietary recommendations for all Americans, including a maximum of 30% of calories from fat, and 10% from saturated fat.[21]

ACCESS TO CARE

Youth should be permitted to request sick call directly from health staff. This may be accomplished through a signup sheet or box in housing units or dining rooms, which are collected and reviewed daily by nursing staff.

Small facilities must rely on the training and judgment of nursing and child care staff to decide when to seek medical care from a physician. Staff should be trained to recognize and describe significant health problems, with a clear chain of command and established sources of acute or emergency care.

Unlicensed health staff, such as a correctional health aide or medical assistant, may have only a limited clinical role that supports the licensed professional staff. Substitution of an unlicensed non-professional for a nurse denies patients access to appropriate professional care. In addition, substitution of line staff for health staff compromises confidentiality of health services.

When there is a separate disciplinary unit, health staff should make daily rounds there to assess the physical and mental condition of the youth, as well as the general conditions of confinement.

Health staff should not be isolated in a medical unit all day. They should be out and about the facility to administer medications; attend meals; make rounds in special housing units; instruct staff; and collect sick call signup sheets.

SICK CALL

Routine sick call should occur at a regularly scheduled time, not continuously throughout the day. It should not conflict with other important programs, such as meals or school. Afternoons when school is over works well in many juvenile justice programs.

Residents must be examined at sick call. Collection of complete vital signs (temperature, pulse, respiratory rate, and blood pressure) is an essential component of the assessment of a sick patient. Height and weight meaurements should be obtained every 3 months in growing children, and the measurements plotted on standard growth charts to assess the pattern of growth.

Sick call assessments must be recorded on the youth's health record. When a log book is used instead, clinical information about the youth's care, particularly patterns of illness such as chronic headaches, persistent cough, or seasonal asthma, is lost to the health record.

The health record should be reviewed at sick call to consider other health problems that may be present. Review of the problem list and management plan provides an opportunity to assure that no other problems have been lost to follow-up.

FOLLOW-UP SERVICES

There must be follow-up for every health problem identified in the initial health appraisal, or subsequent sick call visit. Management protocols for common problems will help assure that problems are managed consistently and completely. Routine periodic review of health records to assure that all problems are being addressed will assure none are lost to follow-up.

SPECIALTY CONSULTATION SERVICES

Specialists who are willing to evaluate and treat youth from juvenile justice programs should be identified in advance. Commonly needed specialty services include orthopedics for injuries; optometry for glasses; oral surgery for wisdom teeth; general surgery for abdominal pain; cardiology for significant murmurs, palpitations, and chest pain; ophthalmology for eye trauma; neurology for seizures; pulmonary medicine or allergy for asthma; otolaryngology for hearing loss; obstetrics for pregnancy; gynecology for abnormal cervical cytologic results; and psychiatry for management of mental illness.

The facility physician is responsible for coordination of workups, assessing the results of diagnostic tests, and assuring that the whole patient is cared for. He makes referrals to specialists, providing necessary background information and the reason for the consultation. The consultant should respond in writing with a summary of the evaluation and recommendations for treatment. Reports of all diagnostic tests should always be obtained for the facility health record.

All states provide consultant services to children with special health care needs under Title V of the Social Security Act. These programs are a resource for support of specialty care for delinquent youth, both while in residential programs and to continue needed services after release.

CHRONIC ILLNESS

Chronic health problems in adolescents tend to be less advanced than those in adults. The need for medical attention is still substantial, as early diagnosis and intervention may prevent continuing damage and disability as the patient grows older. Recurrent or persistent symptoms in an apparently healthy youth may be the initial presentation of a serious chronic illness.

The facility physician is responsible for monitoring the condition of youth with chronic illness and overall coordi-

nation of their care. They should be seen at least every 3 months to assess disease activity and adequacy of management. Consultation with a specialist is necessary when chronically ill youth do not respond to the facility physician's routine approach to management of that particular illness. It is also important to plan ahead for continuing care of youth with chronic illness after release.

Several studies have examined the prevalence of chronic conditions in adolescents and delinquents. An analysis of the 1984 National Health Interview Survey showed a prevalence of 6.2% for all types of disability.[22] The four most common disabling conditions among U.S. adolescents were: mental disorders; respiratory conditions, principally asthma; nervous system disorders, principally seizures; and disorders of the ear and mastoid, principally hearing impairments. An older study of chronic health problems of inner-city adolescents found a high prevalence of headache, heart, obesity, and blood pressure problems.[23]

There have been only a few studies of chronic illness among youth in juvenile justice programs. A review of health histories of 156 residents in the Washington state system found 12% gave a history of asthma, 7% had peptic ulcer disease, 1.3% had juvenile diabetes, and 1.3% had seizures.[24] Another study compared 53 white Massachusetts delinquents with 51 matched, non-delinquent youth.[25] Delinquents were more likely to have suffered adverse health events such as hospitalization, unconsciousness, and accidents; and less likely to have regular medical care. The delinquents were more likely to have a history of hearing problems, asthma, head injury, and seizures. They were also more likely to demonstrate abnormalities of the spine, knee, vision, and hearing on physical examination.

Health programs must also consider the variability of special health needs of delinquents. Table 28-1 presents significant chronic health problems that were identified among youth placed in the custody of the New York State Division for Youth over 2 years (1995-1996).

Asthma

While 10%–12% of youth give a history of asthma, only 1%–2% have active disease. Management of active asthma requires a continuous care approach to control symptoms, prevent exacerbations, and reduce chronic airway inflammation. Important components of asthma treatment include patient education, environmental control, medicine tailored to the patient's needs and objective measures of airway narrowing, such as the peak expiratory flow rate. This approach optimizes the patient's condition, teaches how to recognize early signs of an attack, and provides the tools to control the disease.[26] Nebulizers and peak flow meters should be available in every facility to treat asthma.

Some youth use metered dose inhalers excessively. These residents should be educated concerning the risks of excessive medication. Frequent unneeded use of inhalers can be controlled by requiring objective evidence of disease

Table 28-1. Significant chronic medical problems encountered in New York State delinquency program 1995-1996

System	Problem
Nutrition	Morbid obesity
Skin	Severe acne
Head	Seizures, migraine, post-concussion headaches
Eyes	Myopic amblyopia, enucleation with prosthetic eye
Ears	Moderate and severe hearing loss, congenital malformation of the ear with deafness
Throat	Post-traumatic tracheostomy
Teeth	Impacted third molars, missing teeth due to decay, orthodenture in progress
Immunity	Anaphylaxis to peanuts, anaphylaxis to bee stings, post-splenectomy
Chest	Scoliosis, pectus excavatum with shortness of breath and fainting
Heart	Hypertrophic cardiomyopathy presenting as harsh murmur, supraventricular tachycardia presenting as palpitations and dizziness, aortic insufficiency and mitral regurgitation due to rheumatic heart disease, first degree heart block with fainting, congenital bicuspid aortic valve
Blood vessels	Coarctation of the aorta, Marfan syndrome with dilated aortic root, hypertension, elevated cholesterol with type IIA familial hyperlipoproteinemia pattern
Blood	Iron deficiency anemia, sickle cell trait, hereditary persistence of hemoglobin F, hemoglobin C trait, beta-thalassemia trait presenting with mild anemia and significant microcytosis
Coagulation	Immune thrombocytopenic purpura, previously undiagnosed Factor IX deficiency presenting with prolonged bleeding after extraction,
Malignancy	Post-leukemia, Post-Wilms tumor, rhabdomyosarcoma presenting with a lump behind the ear,leukemia with chemotherapy in progress
Lungs	Asthma; sarcoid presenting with chronic cough, shortness of breath and hilar lymphadenopathy
Digestive	Peptic ulcer disease, esophagitis and gastritis due to H. pylori infection, post-traumatic colostomy ready for closure
Urinary	Proteinuria, hematuria, IgA nephropathy presenting with proteinuria, rapidly progressive IgA nephropathy presenting with hypertension, post-nephrectomy in infancy, proteinuria with focal glomerulosclerosis,
Male reproductive	Foreskin adhesions, undescended testicle
Female reproductive	Venereal warts, abnormal cervical cytology due to human papillomavirus infection, ovarian cyst
Endocrine	Diabetes mellitus;hypothyroid presenting with weight loss, right upper quadrant pain, and constipation; delayed onset of puberty; Klinefelter syndrome with delayed puberty
Spine	Scoliosis due to uneven leg length
Extremities	Chronic disability after major trauma, knee trauma with cruciate ligament tear, hand amputee outgrew prosthesis, painful osteochondroma involving the knee
Feet	Severe onychomycosis, severe pes planus
Infections	Positive TB skin test, recurrent meningitis with congenital CSF leak, HIV infection

activity, such as wheezes or diminished peak flow, before each dose. On the other hand, persistent shortness of breath with wheezes or reduced peak flow indicates active chronic asthma in need of more aggressive treatment. Inhaled steroids, cromolyn, or other anti-inflammatory agents are used to control persistent airway narrowing to prevent more severe attacks.

Line staff should be trained to recognize wheezes, tachypnea, retractions, and use of accessory muscles for breathing as signs of a severe asthma attack in need of immediate treatment.

Health programs should monitor asthma hospitalizations and review outpatient care of these patients to assure that asthmatics receive early and aggressive treatment of chronic disease and acute exacerbations to prevent future asthma admissions.

Diabetes Mellitus

Diabetes mellitus is a complex chronic illness with disabling, long-term complications. Standards for care of diabetes have been established by the American Diabetes Association.[27] Adolescents with diabetes are sometimes resistant to care, angry about their chronic illness, and tired of the daily demands of the disease.

The facility physician should be well informed regarding current approaches to the care of diabetes. Referral to a hospital diabetes program may provide access to other members of the diabetes treatment team: an endocrinologist, a nutritionist, and a certified diabetes educator.

Patient education about diabetes and self-management skills are essential components of diabetes care. Diabetics need to understand how to choose foods to adhere to an individual diet plan tailored to the facility menu.

Prevention, recognition, and management of low blood sugar and ketoacidosis are important skills. Hypoglycemia is common, especially in the middle of the night. Nutritious snacks must be available to supplement regular meals, including at bedtime. Glucose tablets and a protein-starch snack, such as peanut butter crackers, should be immediately available when a diabetic feels the symptoms of low blood sugar.

The chronic kidney, eye, and nerve complications of diabetes begin in adolescence. The Diabetes Control and Complications Trial demonstrated that control of blood glucose within the normal physiologic range prevents or slows some of these chronic complications.[28] Optimal diabetic care seeks tight control of blood sugar through adjustment of insulin, diet, and activity each day based on frequent blood sugar monitoring. A correctional facility, by virtue of its highly structured daily program and diet, provides a special opportunity to teach and practice diabetes self-management skills. However, developing a health program to implement tight blood sugar control for an adolescent in an institutional setting is a challenge. The fundamental requirements for tight control are trained professional education and scrupulous patient cooperation with the program. Clearly it is not for everyone, but some individuals with the ability and commitment should be encouraged and supported to try.

Patients must understand their diet plan, how many choices of each food type they have for each meal, and how to select and count portions from the regular facility diet. They must understand that changes in daily activities, such as more exercise for acute illness, may have significant impact on the blood sugar level, and be able to modify their diet accordingly. Health staff must be trained to adjust insulin doses properly in response to blood sugar results.

HIV Infection

While there are relatively few adolescents with AIDS, the natural history of the disease suggests that most people with onset of AIDS in their twenties were originally infected during their teens. An HIV seroprevalence survey of teenage applicants for U.S. military service (1985-1989) showed a rate of 0.34 per thousand overall, but 1.06 per thousand among blacks.[29] A survey of Job Corps applicants (1987-1990) showed an HIV infection rate of 3.6 per thousand overall, with higher rates in the south and among women.[30]

A 1994 survey of juvenile justice agencies by the National Institute of Justice reported that blinded seroprevalence surveys of residents of juvenile facilities in Texas, Colorado, New Mexico and San Bernardino, California identified no seropositive youth. A survey in Alabama found 0.7% and another in Illinois found only 0.1% seropositive.[31] With such low HIV infection rates, juvenile justice programs should focus resources on HIV prevention.

To monitor behaviors that affect health, the Centers for Disease Control and Prevention established the Youth Risk Behavior Survey program in 1989.[32] Recent studies of risky behaviors among high school students have shown high levels of sexual activity, including 19% with four or more lifetime sexual partners, and only 46% used a condom during their most recent sexual encounter. In addition, 2% had used injected drugs.[31] The National Commission on Correctional Health Care conducted a similar health risk behavior survey in 39 juvenile facilities, which showed earlier onset of sexual activity and lower condom use at last intercourse, compared with high school students.[33]

Most prevention education programs teach facts regarding transmission of HIV and inform youth how to avoid exposure and limit risks. There is little evidence, however, that knowledge alone reduces risky behaviors or HIV infection rates. Evaluations of intervention programs have suggested that young people are more likely to change behavior when they perceive there is a substantial risk to themselves, when they believe that others like them are taking the same precautions, when they have the necessary skills, and when they believe that what they do makes a difference.[34–37] Programs led by other teens are more likely to influence perceived risk and peer norms, while role-playing the negotiation of condom use will support the self-efficacy of youth to reduce unprotected sex.[38]

Infection with HIV is a chronic disease that requires a multidisciplinary approach to management. Implementation of a comprehensive treatment program for infected youth requires collaboration with a clinical center for adolescents with HIV. The facility health staff provide primary care. The clinical center provides current management of HIV infection.

Short Stature and Delayed Puberty

In children with short stature, the growth pattern should be investigated by obtaining records of height and weight from parents, schools, or past health care providers, and plotting the measurements on standard growth curves. History of growth and development of parents and siblings may be informative regarding familial short stature and constitutional delay in growth or maturation. Initial laboratory evaluation should include thyroid studies and gonadotropin levels to rule out possible endocrine disorders.

Overweight and Obesity

The National Health and Nutrition Examination Surveys have shown that the prevalence of overweight among U.S. adolescents has increased from 5.7% in 1976-1980, to 10.8% in 1988-1991 and 11.5% in 1988-1994.[39] Management of obese youth includes diet, exercise, and individual or group counseling. Initial efforts to limit calories should be very modest, perhaps focusing primarily on reducing calories from snack foods and fat. Cessation of rapid weight gain is a significant achievement in an adolescent and is an appropriate initial goal, rather than weight loss. Modest success with a less restricted diet that is well tolerated by the youth may be followed by further reductions in total daily calories, sometimes even with enthusiastic support of the youth.

PREGNANCY AND CONTRACEPTION

Juvenile justice health programs should assure early diagnosis of pregnancy through screening on admission and attention to missed menstrual periods. Pregnant youth must have access to counseling regarding options to terminate a pregnancy, or continue with a choice to keep or place the child for adoption. Those opting to terminate a pregnancy must have timely access to abortion. Health and administrative staff must assure the confidentiality of an early pregnancy and of the youth's plans.

Those choosing to continue a pregnancy must have timely access to comprehensive prenatal care designed for high-risk teens. An appropriate diet and exercise program must be provided at the facility. Pregnant teens should be provided with education concerning healthy pregnancy, infant care, and parenting. Staff must be trained and alert to the common signs of complications of pregnancy. Efforts must be made to assure continuing prenatal care is available when a youth is released before term. The juvenile justice program should assist in the enrollment of pregnant youth and their infants in the state Medicaid program.

Reproductive health services should include continuation or initiation of a reliable form of contraception. Contraception is important because sexual exposure occurs following unexpected early release, illicit sexual intercourse, and unsupervised home visits.

MEDICATIONS

During hours that health staff are on site, medications should be administered by a nurse. At other times, medication administration must be supervised by other staff. When line staff are trained and reliable to supervise medication administration, small facilities can readily comply with evening and weekend doses as well as more frequent dose schedules, which some medications require.

Administration of medication by line staff requires an organized system of training, documentation, and monitoring. Complete and accurate documentation of medication administration must occur. Unit dose dispensing of prescriptions eliminates dosage errors and facilitates monitoring for missed doses. Health staff should monitor medication administration records to assure drugs are administered on the schedule that was prescribed.

Sometimes angry youth refuse to take prescribed medications. Refusal of medication is a behavior that is amenable to change. Efforts to communicate with youth to understand their reasons for refusing will identify the causes of this behavior and indicate an approach to changing it.

VISION SERVICES

Youth with decreased visual acuity need glasses to participate effectively in school. Visual acuity is commonly screened using a Snellen wall chart. Rolling E charts may occasionally be needed for mentally retarded or illiterate youth. Those with visual acuity screen of 20/40 or worse should be referred to an optometrist for examination with refraction.

Eye trauma often occurs in juvenile facilities. Examination of the injured eye and screening visual acuity are important components of the nursing assessment. Emergency evaluation by an eye specialist is indicated when there is obvious injury to the eye, such as hyphema; when there is diminished visual acuity; when the eyes cannot move normally; and when the eyelids are so swollen that the eye cannot be examined adequately at the facility. When such findings are present, an ophthalmologist should evaluate the eye for blowout fracture, retinal injuries, and other serious complications of eye trauma.

HEARING SERVICES

Youth with hearing disability need treatment to succeed in school and in the workplace. Hearing screening should use a pure-tone device over a range of frequencies and loudness. The so-called "whisper" test or tuning forks are not effective methods to screen hearing. There should be well-defined criteria for referral to an audiologist; these criteria should include youth with partial or unilateral deafness. When a youth requests a hearing evaluation because he has difficulty hearing in school, evaluation of speech reception by an audiologist is needed.

Standards of hearing loss that were established for management of workers' compensation claims are really not applicable to children and adolescents. School and health staff must be certain that residents with mild hearing loss can truly hear and understand their teachers and counselors in classroom and group sessions.

Residents with severe hearing loss should be referred to a comprehensive program specializing in care of hearing impairments. Referral for speech therapy or instruction in signing may be an important part of a particular individual's program.

COMMUNICABLE DISEASES

Prompt identification of youth with communicable diseases allows for timely treatment and appropriate isolation from the general population to limit spread of disease. Large open dormitories are similar to daycare centers, providing an environment where respiratory, hand to mouth, and dermatologic pathogens may easily spread among residents. Daily populations that are significantly greater than planned capacity promote communicable disease transmission due to overcrowding.[40, 41] Crowded older facilities that do not meet current ventilation standards are particularly problematic.

Tuberculosis is of concern, because many residents come from communities where tuberculosis is more common.[42] Skin test screening for tuberculosis exposure of 4,851 admissions to New York State residential delinquency programs between 1991 and 1995 showed 5.39% positive results from New York City; 3.69% from the surrounding metropolitan region, including Long Island; 2.04% from the Upstate urban counties, including Buffalo,

Rochester, Syracuse, and Albany; and 1.38% from the remaining upstate rural counties. Black residents had 4.61% positive results, while all other races combined were 2.81%.[43] Only one case of suspect active tuberculosis occurred in the New York system over the past 3 years, from a population in excess of 6,000 youth. The central office health bureau tracks staff and youth TB tests to assure statewide compliance with TB screening and follow-up policies. Positive TB skin test results occur more frequently among adult staff than among youth in New York.

Full immunization of residents will prevent outbreaks of measles, rubella, and chickenpox. Exclusion of staff with communicable disease from work is also important. An adult staff person can be the source of chickenpox and cause an outbreak among susceptible residents.

Influenza vaccination for certain youth and staff with chronic illness is indicated to prevent severe disease and complications. Some systems provide routine immunization to all staff or residents to prevent large outbreaks that occur in institutions during influenza epidemics.

EMERGENCIES

True emergencies are relatively unusual occurrences in juvenile justice programs. For this reason, there is little opportunity to use emergency care skills, and preparedness training is most important for health staff as well as line staff. All staff should be trained and certified in CPR. Staff must initiate CPR rather than await the arrival of a nurse or ambulance crew. There should be periodic emergency drills to be certain that staff are prepared to take appropriate action when a real emergency situation arises.

In facilities with health staff, emergency equipment should be available to provide more than basic life support, including portable oxygen, bag-valve-mask for ventilation, oral airways, and portable suction. Health staff should be trained to use the equipment effectively. Other equipment for stabilization and transportation of youth with fractures or head or neck injuries is also important.

BED REST AND INFIRMARY CARE

An overnight infirmary may be needed for isolation of communicable diseases, to provide for bed rest and nursing care during acute illness, for close clinical observation such as after head trauma, or during recovery from surgery or orthopedic injuries when a resident cannot engage in full daily activities. When there is no infirmary for 24-hour care of youth who are sick or disabled, alternatives must be developed that meet their needs. Some facilities allow for bed rest in the medical unit during the hours it is staffed. Many small facilities simply allow bed rest in the room or dormitory. In those circumstances, staff should provide supportive care, such as meals, analgesics, and fluids, to help the resident stay comfortable and rest.

Early hospital discharge, particularly after surgery, is common. Even patients with limited ability and extensive supportive care requirements are released with the expectation that family can provide necessary care at home. Facilities that have no infirmary are usually not suitable to accept back residents after surgery or major trauma until the patient can ambulate comfortably and take care of all personal hygiene needs. Another few days of physical therapy and full nursing care may be what the patient needs before he is ready for discharge to a small juvenile justice program. After femur fracture transfer, to a residential rehabilitation program for 1 to 2 weeks may be more appropriate than returning directly from the acute care hospital to a small facility.

DENTAL CARE

A study of dental needs at the time of admission was conducted at two New York State residential programs in 1994-1995 and findings were compared to adolescent samples from 1971–1973, 1979–1980, and 1986–1987.[44–46] The national samples showed that total dental disease in children, as measured by the index of decayed, missing, and filled surfaces (DMFS), has been declining steadily over time. The total DMFS of the 1994–1995 juvenile program residents was the same as the 1986–1987 sample. However, the New York delinquents had significantly more decayed surfaces, and fewer filled surfaces, indicating reduced access or use of dental care in the home community prior to placement. Nevertheless, 39.6% had no restorative needs on admission and 17% were caries free in their permanent dentition.

An adequate dental program restores normal function, prevents deterioration, and maintains oral health. This is done by assessing restorative, preventive, and oral hygiene needs on admission, and providing dental services to treat those needs. Timely care for acute dental problems, such as toothache or avulsed teeth, is also needed. Adolescence is the time of greatest incidence of decay in the permanent teeth. Placement of sealants on occlusal surfaces in early adolescence prevents cavities during this vulnerable period.

Repair and replacement of missing and damaged teeth, especially the front four, may be an important part of a youth's rehabilitation plan. Success in employment and personal relationships may be significantly affected by defects in appearance. Young people are very aware of their appearance and grateful for efforts to help them improve themselves. Cooperating in a dental treatment program may be an important first step forward for a youth.

Pain is commonly associated with eruption of wisdom teeth in middle and late adolescence. A practical approach to relief of this type of pain involves local gum massage, topical anesthetics, and over-the-counter analgesics. Dentist evaluation is needed to diagnose impacted teeth.

Health programs must plan ahead for proper management of avulsed teeth. Staff must be aware that this emergency requires urgent treatment. Special transport media are available that help preserve the tooth until it is replanted. Prompt access to a dentist or oral surgeon is needed to replant avulsed teeth.

CRISIS MANAGEMENT AND PHYSICAL RESTRAINT

Staff in juvenile programs should be trained to recognize emotional crises and prevent escalation into a violent confrontation. Staff are generally permitted to physically restrain residents to prevent injury to the youth or to others, and to prevent substantial damage to property. The purpose of physical restraint is to allow the child to regain control of his behavior and calm down. For this reason, some agencies have adopted specific techniques that hold the resident without inflicting pain. Physical punishment is not permitted and should be reported to the state child abuse hotline for immediate investigation by an outside agency, as should any significant injuries that occur during physical restraint.

All youth who are restrained should be evaluated by a health professional immediately if they are injured, and at the earliest time health staff are available in all other cases. The purpose of this evaluation is to determine if the youth has been hurt, to observe and inquire concerning his mental status, and to provide for immediate intervention by mental health or medical staff when indicated. It also provides an opportunity for cooling off and separation of youth from staff involved in the incident.

Because staff are often significantly larger and heavier than juveniles, there is a risk of injury during physical restraint. When heavier staff lay on the chest of smaller youth, there is a risk of asphyxia due to restriction of chest movement.[47] Under such circumstances a child may still exhale and protest, with his last breath, that he cannot breathe. Staff may mistakenly believe that speech indicates adequate breathing. Immediately thereafter, hypoxia due to poor ventilation stimulates intense struggle to breathe, which staff may mistakenly believe indicates a need to apply greater pressure to maintain the restraint. Restraint training should inform line staff of the risk of restraint asphyxia and teach safe restraint techniques.[48]

Some juvenile justice programs permit the use of tear gas or pepper spray in certain circumstances. All respiratory irritants pose a substantial risk to youth with active asthma. Skin and eye injuries have also occurred with pepper spray and CS tear gas. None of the gases has been adequately studied to determine the full range of harmful human effects.[49, 50]

Analysis of one state's experience with mandatory correctional officer exposure to pepper spray showed that symptoms requiring medical attention occurred in 5% and included shortness of breath, hypertension, chest pain, severe headache, or loss of consciousness. Symptoms persisted for a week or more in some cases.[51] Juvenile justice programs should use alternative crisis control techniques, rather than expose staff and residents to known and as yet undefined health hazards associated with tear gases and pepper spray.

SUICIDE PREVENTION

Every facility should have a suicide prevention program. The National Center for Institutions and Alternatives publishes a newsletter on suicide prevention programs in corrections.[52] Effective suicide prevention requires written policies and procedures, screening for suicide risk on admission, training of front line staff to recognize subtle changes in behavior early in the course of an emotional crisis, prompt access to mental health evaluation for those suspected of suicide risk, and effective emergency medical care on-site.[53]

Placement of an immature adolescent in an adult jail or prison can precipitate suicidal behavior. One study demonstrated an increased rate of suicide among youth placed in adult facilities, compared with the rate in those in juvenile facilities.[54]

A substantial intention to die may be present, even when a non-lethal suicide attempt is made. Conversely, even youth with other goals may inadvertently cause their own death.[55] Therefore, all self-injury behavior requires mental health assessment.

Hanging is the most common method of suicide. Staff must understand that apparently lifeless hanging victims can sometimes recover fully with aggressive resuscitation after the ligature has been removed.

Placement in an isolation room, often in a disciplinary unit, is a common administrative response to a suicidal resident. Forced isolation in a hostile environment can exacerbate a young person's emotional crisis.[56] A system of levels of close observation by trained staff, up to and including staff within arms reach of youth at all times, can be an effective alternative to isolation. Youth who cannot be managed with a close watch belong in a crisis mental health unit, not a juvenile facility.

MENTAL HEALTH

Mentally ill youth need a comprehensive treatment plan that includes individual or group therapy, behavioral interventions, and medication in selected cases. Psychotropic medications should only be used for diagnosed mental illness, under the care of a psychiatrist, with appropriate monitoring for intended and adverse effects.[7, 8]

Special housing units and programs for the mentally ill have been developed in response to increasing numbers of mentally ill youth committed by the courts to juvenile justice programs instead of mental hospitals. In such units, residents are observed closely by mental health professionals who are on the unit every day, and child care staff receive special training to support a therapeutic environment.

LEGAL ISSUES

When providing health services to minors, informed consent must be obtained from the parent or legal guardian for significant procedures, such as removal of teeth, surgery, and, in some jurisdictions, for use of psychotropic medications. Although most parents are accessible, some can be difficult to reach. The resident may know how to reach them promptly. Minors are emancipated and provide consent for their own care when the youth is married; is the parent of a child; or for the purpose of obtaining care for a sexually transmitted disease, contraception, pregnancy, or HIV testing. The rights of older adolescents to consent for their own care varies from state to state.

General consent for routine health care for detained or adjudicated youth should be provided by statute to permit timely health appraisal in the best interests of youth and disease control in residential facilities. In New York, for example, the court order remanding or committing the youth is deemed sufficient consent for routine health services. "Routine" would include the necessary components of the health appraisal, such as physical examination, diagnostic tests, and primary care, such as immunizations. Youth should not be denied health appraisal and preventive care simply because a parent cannot be located or does not appear.

Juveniles have a right to refuse treatment. Use of force to impose treatment must be limited to situations when the resident is legally incompetent, or when lack of treatment is life threatening. Those who refuse tests for communicable diseases may be isolated until they comply with the required tests.

STAFFING FOR HEALTH SERVICES

A health program cannot operate without professional health staff. Staffing requirements depend on the size of the facility, the rate of admission and discharge, and the nature of any special programs. A rapid turnover detention center or reception program requires more health staff than a stable residential program of the same bed capacity. Also, experience has shown that programs for girls require more health staff and services than programs for boys.

The medical, dental, and mental health programs need to be supported by sufficient direct care staff to accomplish movement of youth to and from the professional staff. Timely movement is particularly important when specialists are brought in to provide services on site.

FUNDING JUVENILE JUSTICE HEALTH PROGRAMS

While state and local governments bear the primary responsibility for funding juvenile justice health services, a number of public health resources are also available. Residents of non-secure facilities with 25 beds or less are eligible for Medicaid under Title IV-E of the Social Security Act. Medicaid eligibility for all children in correctional or juvenile justice residential facilities is a much-needed federal reform that would more adequately fund the health programs.

State programs for children with special health care needs are provided under Title V of the Social Security Act. These public health programs may provide chronically ill or disabled youth access to subspecialty services that are not available from private practitioners in the community.

The state Vaccines for Children programs make federally subsidized immunizations available to poor and high-risk children and youth. Children in correctional institutions are eligible for free vaccines.

Special education must be provided to eligible children through age 21. For residents with physical disabilities who are eligible for special education services. Special education funds may help support needed diagnostic evaluation and treatment, including speech and language services, occupational therapy, physical therapy, and management of hearing and vision impairments.

CONCLUSION

This chapter presents the special health needs of adolescents in juvenile justice programs. Neither still children nor yet adults, adolescents require health services that encompass pediatric and adult medical expertise. As more youth are tried and sentenced as adults, state prison systems will have to learn to provide appropriate and comprehensive health programs for this population. With the trend toward longer obligatory sentences for young offenders, health promotion and disease prevention programs become more important from both a humane and a cost-savings point of view.

REFERENCES

1. Costello JC, Jameson EJ: Legal and ethical duties of health care professionals to incarcerated children. *J Legal Med* 1987;8:191-263.
2. Green M (ed): *Bright Futures. Guidelines for Health Supervision of Infants, Children and Adolescents.* Arlington, VA, National Center for Education in Maternal and Child Health, 1994.
3. *Medicaid Management Information System Provider Manual-Physician*, Child/Teen Health Plan. Albany, NY: Computer Science Corporation, 1997, pp 4-1 to 4-60.
4. *AMA Guidelines for Adolescent Preventive Services.* Chicago, American Medical Association, 1992.
5. *Healthy Communities 2000 Model Standards.* Washington, D.C., American Public Health Association, 1991.
6. *Standards for the Administration of Juvenile Justice.* Washington, D.C., Office of Juvenile Justice and Delinquency Prevention, 1980.
7. *Standards for Juvenile Training Schools,* ed 3. Laurel, MD, American Correctional Association, 1991.
8. *Standards for Health services in Juvenile Detention and Confinement Facilities.* Chicago, National Commission on Correctional Health Care, 1995.
9. Dubler N (ed): *Standards for Health services in Correctional Institutions*, ed 2. Washington, D.C., American Public Health Association, 1986.
10. *Juvenile Detention Program Standards.* Harrisburg, PA, Juvenile Detention Centers' Association of Pennsylvania, 1993.
11. Thompson LS, Farrow JA (eds): *Hard Time, Healing Hands. Developing Primary Health Care Services for Incarcerated Youth.* Arlington, VA, National Center for Education in Maternal and Child Health, 1993.
12. Parent DG, Lieter V, Kennedy S, et al: *Conditions of Confinement:*

Juvenile Detention and Corrections Facilities. Washington, D.C., Office of Juvenile Justice and Delinquency Prevention, 1994.

13. *Scope and Standards of Nursing Practice in Correctional Facilities.* Washington, D.C., American Nurses Association, 1995.

14. Evaluation of health services (quality assurance). In Dubler N, (ed): *Standards for Health Services in Correctional Institutions.* Washington, D.C., American Public Health Association, 1986.

15. Tanner JM: *Growth at Adolescence,* 2d ed. Oxford, Great Britain, Blackwell Scientific, 1962.

16. O'Brien SF, Bell TA, Farrow JA: Use of a leukocyte esterase dipstick to detect chlamydia trachomatous and neisseria gonorrhea urethritis in asymptomatic adolescent male detainees. *Am J Public Health* 1988;78:1583-1584.

17. Braslow CA, Safyer SM, Cohen MD: Screening adolescent male detainees. *Am J Public Health* 1989;79:902.

18. Immunization of Adolescents. *MMWR* 1996;45:Supplement RR-13.

19. Vaccines for Children, Childhood Immunization Initiative created under the Omnibus Budget Reconciliation Act of 1993 as Section 1928 of the SSA.

20. 4.214 Development and Implementation of an Individual Program Plan; 4.217 Health and Mental Health Services; 4.2171 Initial Health Examination and Assessment. In *Standards for the Administration of Juvenile Justice.* Washington, D.C., Office of Juvenile Justice and Delinquency Prevention, 1980.

21. Public Law 103-448 re-authorized the child nutrition programs.

22. Newacheck PW: Adolescents with special needs: Prevalence, severity, and access to health services. *Pediatrics* 1989;84:872-881.

23. Brunswick AF, Josephson E: Adolescent health in Harlem. *Am J Public Health* 1972;62(10)Supplement:S1-S62.

24. Farrow JA: Health issues among juvenile delinquents. In Thompson LS (ed): *The Forgotten Child in Health Care: Children in the Juvenile Justice System.* Washington, D.C., National Center for Education in Maternal and Child Health, 1991.

25. Palfrey JS: Health profiles of early adolescent delinquents. *Public Health Rep* 1983;98:449-457.

26. National Asthma Education Program: *Guidelines for the Diagnosis and Management of Asthma.* Bethesda, MD, National Institutes of Health, 1991.

27. American Diabetes Association: Clinical Practice Recommendations 1996. *Diabetes Care* 1996;19(1)Supplement 1:S1-S118.

28. The Diabetes Control and Complications Trial Research Group: The effect of intensive treatment of diabetes on the development and progression of long-term complications in insulin-dependent diabetes mellitus. *New Engl J Med* 1993;329:977-986.

29. Burke DS, Brundage JF, Goldenbaum M, et al: Human immunodeficiency virus infections in teenagers. Seroprevalence among applicants for U.S. military service. *JAMA* 1990;263:2074-2077.

30. St Louis ME, Conway GA, Hayman CR, et al: Human immunodeficiency virus infection in disadvantaged adolescents. Findings from the U.S. Job Corps. *JAMA* 1991;266:2387-2391.

31. Widom R, Hammett TM: HIV/AIDS and STDs in juvenile facilities. *National Inst Justice Res Brief* April 1996, pp 1-11.

32. Kann L, Kolbe LJ, Collins JL (eds): Measuring the health behavior of adolescents: The youth risk behavior surveillance system. *Public Health Rep* 1993;108:Supplement 1, 2-67.

33. Morris RE, Harrison EA, Knox GW, et al: Health risk behavioral survey from 39 juvenile correctional facilities in the United States. *J Adolesc Health* 1995;17:334-344.

34. D'Angelo LJ, Getson PR, Luban NLC, et al: Human immunodeficiency virus infection in urban adolescents: Can we predict who is at risk? *Pediatrics* 88:982–986, 1991.

35. Diclemente RJ: Predictors of HIV-preventive sexual behavior in a high risk adolescent population: The influence of perceived peer norms and sexual communication in incarcerated adolescents' consistent use of condoms. *J Adolesc Health* 1991;12:385-390.

36. Belgrave FZ, Randolph SM, Carter C, et al: The impact of knowledge, norms, and self-efficacy on intentions to engage in AIDS preventive behaviors among young incarcerated African American males. *J Black Psychol* 1993;19:155-168.

37. Rotheram-Borus MJ, Mahler KA, Rosario M: AIDS prevention with adolescents. *AIDS Education Prevention* 1995;7:320-336.

38. Middlestadt S, Hoffman C, D'Andrea EM, et al: What Intervention Studies Say About Effectiveness. A Resource Guide for HIV Prevention Community Planning Groups. Academy for Educational Development, 1996.

39. Update: Prevalence of overweight among children, adolescents, and adults—United States, 1988–1994. *MMWR* 46:199-202, 1997.

40. Bellin EY, Fletcher DD, Safyer SM: Association of tuberculosis infection with increased time in or admission to the New York city jail system. *JAMA* 269:2228-2231, 1993.

41. Tappero JW, Reporter R, Wenger JD, et al: Meningococcal disease in Los Angeles county, California, and among men in the county jails. *New Engl J Med* 335:833-840, 1996.

42. Controlling TB in Correctional Facilities. Atlanta, Centers for Disease Control and Prevention, 1995.

43. Situ JH, Cohen MD: TB Screening Analysis. MS Project, Department of Biometry and Statistics. SUNY Albany School of Public Health, Spring 1996.

44. Hsu JW, Cohen MD, Kumar J: Dental Needs Assessment for Delinquent Youth in a New York State Facility. Presented at the 124th Annual Meeting of the American Public Health Association, New York, 1996.

45. The Prevalence of Dental Caries in United States Children 1979–1980. Washington, D.C., National Institute of Dental Research, 1981.

46. The Prevalence of Dental Caries in United States Children 1986–1987. Washington, D.C., National Institute of Dental Research, 1995.

47. O'Halloran RL, Lewman, LV: Restraint asphyxiation in excited delirium. Am J Forensic Med Pathol 14:289-295, 1993.

48. Brattan WJ, Hirsch C, Julian M: Preventing In-Custody Deaths (training video). New York, New York City Police Department, 1995.

49. Hu H, Fine J, Epstein P, et al: Tear gas: Harassing agent or toxic chemical weapon? JAMA 262(5):660-663, 1989.

50. Cohen MD: The human health effects of pepper spray. J Correctional Health Care, in press.

51. Stopford W: Statement of Dr. Woodhall Stopford, M.D., M.S.P.H., concerning the pathophysiology of capsaicin and risks associated with oleoresin capsicum exposure. Statement submitted by plaintiff to the U.S. District Court for the Western District of North Carolina in *Ryder v. Freeman.* Docket Number 1;95-CV-67.

52. Hayes LM, (ed): Jail Suicide/ Mental Health Update. Mansfield, MA, National Center for Institutions and Alternatives. Quarterly.

53. Sherman LG, Morschauser PC: Screening for suicide risk in inmates. Psychiatric Q 60:119-138, 1989.

54. Community Research Center: Juvenile Suicides in Adult Jails. Champaign, IL, University of Illinois, 1983.

55. Haycock J: Manipulation and suicide attempts in jails and prisons. Psychiatric Q 60:85-98, 1989.

56. Room confinement. In: Standards for the Administration of Juvenile Justice, 1980. Op. cit.

29

Legal Considerations in the Delivery of Health Care Services in Prisons and Jails*

William J. Rold, J.D., C.C.H.P.-A.

SUMMARY

The obligation of government officials who incarcerate inmates to provide for their medical, psychiatric, and dental care is well established. The more than 20 years that have passed since the United States Supreme Court ruled that prisoners had a right to be free of "deliberate indifference to their serious health care needs" has resulted in the development of both case law and national standards regarding correctional health care.

As the courts have sought to protect inmates from unnecessary medical suffering and to restore bodily func-

tion where this is possible, three basic rights have emerged: the right to access to care, the right to care that is ordered, and the right to a professional medical judgment. The failure of correctional officials to honor these rights has resulted in protracted litigation, the awarding of damages and attorneys' fees, and the issuance of injunctions regarding the delivery of health care services.

*This chapter, reprinted with permission, is an updated version of an article orignally written under a contract with the Agency for Health Care Policy and Research of the U.S. Department of Health and Human Services.

To provide for constitutional care and to protect themselves from litigation, correctional administrators must adopt procedures to protect inmates' basic rights, including a functioning sick call system that uses properly trained health care staff, a means of addressing medical emergencies, a priority system so that those most in need of care receive it first, the development and maintenance of adequate medical records, liaison with outside resources for specialist and hospital care when needed, a system for staff development and training, and an ongoing effort at quality control. Jail wardens and prison superintendents and their chief medical officers must development policies and procedures for meeting the special needs of disabled, elderly, and mentally ill inmates, as well as those with HIV infection and AIDS, and to preserve the confidentiality of medical information.

Because litigation is so expensive, all efforts should be made to achieve voluntary compliance with national standards of care and to gain accreditation. Facilities that meet community standards of care are much less likely to face class action or even individual lawsuits.

INTRODUCTION

During 1980–1990 in the United States, the number of prison inmates increased by 134%,[1] and the average daily census of jail inmates rose by more than 200%.[2] Between 1990 and 1995, 213 new federal and state prisons were built.[3] The more than 1.3 million adults now behind bars on any given day collectively comprise one of the largest public health challenges in the world.

Drawn largely from disadvantaged segments of society, for whom regular health care is often unavailable, ignored, or haphazard, inmates have health care needs more complex than their youthful demographics would suggest. In addition to chronic diseases, such as diabetes mellitus, hypertension, and asthma, incarcerated patients bring to prisons and jails the ravages of substance abuse, the debilitating effects of AIDS and HIV infection, and the challenge of multiple-drug-resistant tuberculosis.

Inmates also disproportionately require mental health services. According to the National Alliance of the Mentally Ill, of 250,000 people in the United States with serious mental illness, 100,000 are in jails and prisons, and 68,000 are in mental hospitals.[4] One study found that at least 25% of prison inmates were suffering from a significant psychiatric or functional disability that required mental health intervention.[5] Moreover, in jails, virtually all estimates of mental disability among inmates exceed those for prison populations.[6]

In addition to the mentally ill, correctional institutions confine inmates drawn from the estimated 3% of the United States population who are mentally retarded,[7] or developmentally disabled[8]; and seizure disorders comprise one of the most common chronic illnesses in prisons and jails, where the prevalence of epilepsy may be three times that found in the general population.[9, 10]

In general, since inmates have little money and no health insurance and are ineligible for welfare, the cost of their health care is borne at public expense. When increasing numbers of inmates requiring health care meets a scarcity of resources appropriated to meet their needs, litigation is a frequent result.

INMATE LAWSUITS

Although the perception is widespread that massive numbers of inmates are abusive litigants filing frivolous cases, the data do not support this view. While prisoner filings, especially civil rights suits, have increased substantially over the past 25 years, prisoner filings have not kept pace with the explosion of civilian filings, and have actually grown more slowly than has the increase in the numbers of persons incarcerated.[11] Moreover, the vast majority of inmate filings concern their criminal cases, not their conditions of confinement, and are raised as petitions for habeas corpus; and, while a few prisoners file multiple court cases, most inmates litigate but a single suit (Table 29-1).[11]   Although inmate lawsuits concerning conditions of confinement such as health care are a small part of the volume of federal litigation filed by inmates, substantial damages have been awarded in such cases. In a 2-year summary of lawsuits against 34 state departments of corrections that resulted in settlement or recovery of damages for denial of proper medical care, the awards ranged from $200 to $640,000, with a mean of $133,931.[12] Attorneys' fees were also awarded in many of these cases.

In addition to individual lawsuits concerning the conditions of confinement of a particular individual, class action lawsuits, where an entire population of a prison or jail, or even all the inmates in a correctional system, are challenging the delivery of services. Such litigation can last for years and cost hundreds of thousands, or even millions, of dollars. At least 40 states plus the District of Columbia, Puerto Rico, and the Virgin Islands are or were under court order or consent decree to limit population and/or improve conditions in either the entire system or its major facilities.[13, 14] This compares with 25 states under court order in 1981.[15] Scores of county jails have also been, and continue to be, the subject of class action litigation.

Health care is a primary issue in most class action suits alleging unconstitutional conditions. In eight of the 11 jurisdictions, where the entire prison system is under court order or consent decree, the adequacy of health care services was a major focus of the litigation.

Remedies ordered by the courts in class action cases have included increased funding for staffing, equipment, and services. Time deadlines for provision of care, detailed record-keeping requirements, and the adoption of quality control and other supervisory mechanisms have also been imposed. Where unconstitutional conditions are the result of antiquated facilities, courts have prompted, and sometimes ordered, the closing of prisons or jails and the construction of new ones.

Table 29-1. Inmate lawsuits: The data.

(Jim Thomas, an associate professor of sociology at Northern Illinois University, compiled numerous statistics concerning inmate filings, from which the following are drawn:)

Annual percent increase of civilian and prisoner filings, 1973–1986:

1986 increase over	All civilian	All prisoner
1972	176.7%	107.6%
1976	99.5%	70.5%
1981	44.6%	21.8%

Increase of state and federal prison populations and filings, 1970–1986:

% change state prisoners	174.7%
% change state prisoner's filings	148.3%
% change federal prisoners	121.2%
% change federal prisoner's filings	5.9%

Grounds of prisoner cases in Northern District of Illinois, 1980–1986:

Section 1983 (Civil Rights)	19.7%
Habeas Corpus	64.4%

Single and repeat filings in Northern District of Illinois, 1980–1986:

Civil rights		Habeas corpus	
1 filing	864	1 filing	789
2 filings	128	2 filings	68
3 filings	41	3 filings	11
4 filings	11	4 filings	1
5 or more filings	30	5 filings	0

(Excludes 14 multiple filers, with 273 filings, or 8.3% of all suits.)

Commonly, class action lawsuits involve both the court and the attorneys for the inmates in a long-term, continuing effort to monitor compliance with the court's orders or consent decree. Frequently, the court appoints a special master with full quasi-judicial powers or substantial authority to interpret the judgment or independently to order actions to be taken to effectuate compliance. Such appointments have occurred in over half of the jurisdictions currently involved in major litigation on crowding and/or conditions of confinement.[14] In the most extreme cases of noncompliance, the court may appoint a receiver to supersede or replace the defendant officials, as occurred, for example, in the past in Alabama and Georgia, and recently in the District of Columbia. All of these compliance costs are also usually borne by the government.

In short, there is not a jurisdiction unaffected by the role of the courts in enforcing the requirement of the Eighth Amendment that prisoners be free of cruel and unusual punishment. It was not always so.

THE EIGHTH AMENDMENT

The antecedents of the law's prohibition of excessive punishment date from the time of the Magna Carta. Under the rule of Edward I, however, misdemeanors were still punishable by whipping, by mutilation, or by removal of a hand or an ear; felonies, by decapitation. Treason carried particularly harsh punishment, and, as late as 1782, the unfortunate David Tyree was sentenced to be drawn, hanged, castrated, disemboweled, burnt, beheaded, quartered, and then "disposed of where His Majesty shall think fit."[16] In his Commentaries, Blackstone wrote that, although some punishments, such as "banishment ... to the American colonies," did not involve physical injury, most were "mixed with some degree of corporal pain."[17]

It was in light of this history that the drafters of the American Bill of Rights sought in 1791 to prohibit "cruel and unusual punishment." Early applications of the Eighth Amendment interpreted it to forbid torture or wanton infliction of suffering, but the courts rarely interfered with prison administration. In 1871, for example, the Virginia Supreme Court of Appeals wrote: "[the prisoner] is for the time being a slave, in a condition of penal servitude to the State, and subject to such laws and regulations as the State may choose to prescribe."[18] The Eighth Amendment would lay largely dormant for a century.

THE EVOLUTION OF JUDICIAL INVOLVEMENT IN CORRECTIONAL HEALTH CARE

One of the earliest cases to recognize the right of incarcerated persons to health care arose in North Carolina in 1926. An inmate, wounded in the course of his arrest, required emergency surgery, and the sheriff took him to a physician. Requiring the county to pay the surgeon's bill, the North Carolina Supreme Court ruled that "[i]t is but just that the public be required to care for the prisoner, who cannot, by reason of the deprivation of his liberty, care for himself."[19] Fifty years later, this standard would be adopted by the United States Supreme Court.

In the 1960s, the judiciary began to scrutinize conditions in prisons and jails more assiduously and to enforce more strictly the precepts of the Eighth Amendment. With respect to health care, judges applied the amendment to prohibit not only the infliction of pain and suffering, but also the failure to relieve pain and the failure to restore function. Recognizing that prison and jail inmates are restrained by the arm of the state from securing care on their own, the federal courts became increasingly involved in reviewing complaints from inmates in state and local facilities.

One of the first federal cases concerned conditions in the prisons of Alabama. The evidence detailed serious shortages of staff, equipment, and supplies; the use of inmates to

---

Box 29-1. The Eighth Amendment and "State of Mind"

A violation of the Eighth Amendment requires a "subjective" showing of "deliberate indifference." It is not enough that the defendant should have known or ought to have understood the danger to the inmate. The defendant must *know of* and disregard a substantial risk *(Farmer v. Brennan)*. Such knowledge, however, can be inferred from the surrounding facts where the failure to respond to a clear risk constitutes "recklessness." In *Farmer,* a frail, transsexual inmate was raped by other inmates after placement by prison officials in general population at a maximum security prison. The Supreme Court found that the obviousness of the risk could establish a defendant's "deliberate indifference."

In health care, failure to provide access to care, denial of care that is ordered, or the absence of professional medical judgement in the delivery of medical services, will usually satisfy the "subjective test" of *Farmer,* where the unaddressed medical needs are serious.

Box 29-2. Breakdown in Access to Care: A Prison Dental Clinic's Experience

In June 1987, a federal court placed New York's Bedford Hills Correctional Facility for Women under a comprehensive court order after it found a "total breakdown in the administration of the dental clinic," resulting in the inmates "suffering from pain, loss of teeth, discomfort, weight loss, and infection." *Dean v. Coughlin.* At trial, the prison's dentist testified that it often took him three days to see all the patients on one day's emergency list and that he was still working on February's emergency list in May. With respect to routine care, the evidence showed that more than 300 requests for appointments had been submitted to the dental clinic over the last year, but nothing had been done with them. They were kept, unacknowledged, in a gauze box. The court's order required same-day evaluation of emergency requests and routine dental appointments within one week.

---

administer treatment, dispense medication, and perform minor surgery; absent or incomplete medical records; and emergency conditions left unattended for extended periods. Individual cases of maggot-infested wounds, unnecessary amputations, and deaths because of medical neglect convinced the court that the practices were "so bad as to be shocking to the conscious of a reasonably civilized people."[20]

In the landmark Texas case, *Estelle v. Gamble,*[21] the United States Supreme Court affirmed federal court jurisdiction over prison and jail health care systems and ruled that, where constitutional rights are jeopardized, the courts have not only the right but the duty to intervene. According to Estelle, the Eighth Amendment is violated when correctional officials are "deliberately indifferent" to an inmate's "serious medical needs."

DELIBERATE INDIFFERENCE

In the more than 20 years since Estelle, the notion of "deliberate indifference" has been articulated in various ways by the courts, but at least three categories of "deliberate indifference" have emerged: denied or unreasonably delayed access to a physician for diagnosis and treatment; failure to administer treatment prescribed by a physician; and the denial of a professional medical judgment.

The constitutional standard does not require that an express intent to inflict pain be shown,[22] but the test is relatively narrow. See Box 29-1 for discussion of the Eighth Amendment's "state of mind" requirement. The Eighth Amendment does not render prison officials or staff liable in federal cases for malpractice or accidents, nor does it resolve professional disputes about the best choice of treatment. It does require, however, that sufficient resources be made available to protect the three basic rights.

The Right to Access to Care

The right to access to care is fundamental: when access is denied or delayed, the health staff does not know which patients need immediate attention and which patients need care that can wait. Indeed, "[a] well-monitored and well-run access system is the best way to protect prisoners from unnecessary harm and suffering and, concomitantly, to protect prison officials from liability for denying access to needed medical care."[24]

The right to access to care includes access to both emergency and routine care. All institutions, of whatever size, must have the capacity to cope with emergencies and to provide for sick call. Access to specialists and to in-patient hospital treatment, where warranted by the patient's condition, are also guaranteed by the Eighth Amendment. Access to care must be provided for any condition (medical, dental, or psychological) if denial of care may result in pain, continued suffering, deterioration, less likelihood of a favorable outcome, or degeneration.[20] For an account of a breakdown in access and the remedies ordered by the court, see Box 29-2.[25]

The Right to Care That Is Ordered

Generally, courts assume that care would not have been ordered if it were not needed. Thus, once a health care professional orders treatment for a serious condition, the courts will protect, as a matter of constitutional law, the patient's right to receive that treatment without undue delay.

A failure to provide ordered care for a serious medical need violates the Eighth Amendment.[26] In *Martinez v. Mancusi,*[27] which was cited with approval by the Supreme Court in *Estelle v. Gamble,*[21] a constitutional claim was recognized where a prisoner was refused his prescribed medication and his leg surgery was rendered unsuccessful

---

Box 29-3. The Severed Ear Case and Other Examples of Failure to Exercise Medical Judgment

In *Williams v. Vincent*, cited with approval by the Supreme Court in *Estelle v. Gamble*, an inmate whose ear had been severed presented himself for medical treatment. The physician's choice of the "easier and less efficacious treatment" of throwing away the prisoner's ear and stitching the stump was attributed to "deliberate indifference" rather than the exercise of professional judgment.

Numerous other examples are found in the case law: *Thomas v. Pate* (injection of penicillin with knowledge that prisoner was allergic, and refusal of doctor to treat the allergic reaction); *Rogers v. Evans* (psychiatrist avoided prisoner after complaints were made about treatment); *Wells v. Franzen* (deprivation of a shackled inmate of exercise, clothing, and showers, and requirement that he eat with his fingers next to his two-day old urine); *Jones v. Johnson* (denial of treatment for painful condition for budgetary rather than medical reason).

---

by requiring him to stand, despite contrary instructions from his surgeon.

To ensure that care that is ordered is, in fact, delivered, courts have required the treating physician to specify the time for a test or examination or within which a specialist consultation or hospital admission must occur. In turn, once the doctor has determined the appropriate time limits, the court will direct that the order be honored by other medical and correctional staff.

The Right to a Professional Medical Judgment

In general, the courts will not determine which of two equally efficacious treatment modalities should be chosen. The adjudication of constitutional claims is not the business of "second guessing" health care professionals. Rather, the courts seek to:

> *... ensure that decisions concerning the nature and timing of medical care are made by medical personnel, using equipment designed for medical use, in locations conducive to medical functions, and for reasons that are purely medical.*[28]

The actual decisions of prison medical personnel are at issue under *Estelle v. Gamble*[21] only when they are not actually medical in nature, or are so extreme or abusive as to be completely outside the range of professional medical judgment. See Box 29-3 for the severed ear case and other examples of failure to exercise medical judgment.[29–33]

By ensuring professional judgment, the federal courts have not only protected the sphere of discretion surrounding medical practitioners' treatment and diagnostic decisions, but have often enhanced it. At issue in a typical injunctive case are such matters as staffing, physical facili-

ties, transportation, sick call, and follow-up procedures. When a court orders relief in these areas, it is assuring that the raw materials from which responsible professional judgment is formed are available to practitioners.

SERIOUS MEDICAL NEEDS

The Constitution requires that correctional officials provide medical care only for "serious medical needs." Generally, a medical need is "serious" if it "has been diagnosed by a physician as mandating treatment or ... is so obvious that even a lay person would easily recognize the necessity for a doctor's attention."[34, 35] Conditions are also considered to be "serious" if they "cause pain, discomfort, or threat to good health."[25] A condition need not be life-threatening to be deemed "serious," and many treatment plans that are labelled "elective," nevertheless, are deemed "serious" within the meaning of *Estelle v. Gamble.*[21]

In general, courts consider three factors in determining whether correctional officials are being deliberately indifferent to "serious medical needs": 1) the amenability of the patient's condition to treatment; 2) the consequences to the patient if treatment does not occur; and 3) the likelihood of a favorable outcome. Within this mix, the court may also consider the length of the patient's anticipated incarceration. It is one thing to decline the provision of dentures or an artificial limb to an inmate with a 3-day jail sentence. It is quite another to withhold such adjuncts to an inmate serving 20 years to life.

THE CONSTITUTIONAL CLASS ACTION CHALLENGE

Class action challenges to correctional health care delivery are put together in two ways, either of which is "independently sufficient."[26] First, numerous examples of individual cases of deliberate indifference closely related in time can establish a pattern of unconstitutional care. Alternatively, evidence of systemic deficiencies in staffing, facilities, record-keeping, supervision, and procedures can show that unnecessary suffering is inevitable unless the deficiencies are remedied.[36]

The best preventive medicine against a successful class action challenge is adequate funding, sound procedures, adherence to standards, staff training, and quality control. Where these safeguards are in place, numerous examples of inmate suffering and systemic deficiencies will be much less likely to occur.

COMPONENTS OF A CONSTITUTIONAL SYSTEM

A constitutional system of health care delivery combines a number of critical elements, each of which serves to reinforce the others; among these are the following.

A Communications and Sick Call System

Prisoners must be permitted to communicate their health care needs to the medical staff, and sick call must be available to all inmates regardless of security classification.[37] National standards (Table 29-2) vary as to the frequency of sick call, generally according to the size of the facility; but all standards agree that inmates in segregation must be visited daily.[38–41]

Adequate sick call requires a professional evaluation by trained personnel. Uniform or lay staff may convey sick call requests, but they cannot be allowed to decide which prisoners will receive medical attention.[42–44]

In one system of nurses' screening found unconstitutional, nurses allotted inmates 15-20 seconds to present their complaints through a cashier's window. No physical examination was performed, and only "cryptic notes" (e.g., "stomach," "headache") were made. Later, the patients were assigned priorities on the basis of the notes. The court ordered the keeping of detailed records and the individual examination of each patient by a nurse trained in triage.[26] Indeed, the smooth functioning of a priority system in any facility is dependent on adequate examination and triage.

A Priority System

A correctional health system with generous funding can simply let the patients' demands determine ordered care. A system with scarcer resources, however, must set priorities calculated to relieve pain and to restore function in accordance with the seriousness of the patients' conditions. A priority system for care is not only more equitable for the patients,[45] but it is also one that parallels the concerns of the courts in evaluating the constitutional sufficiency of systems under review.

When assessing the adequacy of a priority system, the courts recognize that no correctional clinic can provide complete state-of-the-art health care or the full range of health services available to unincarcerated persons. Decisions about the scope of care, necessarily turn in part on the length of the inmates' incarceration, and a scaled-down program sufficient to relieve suffering in a jail may be inappropriate in a maximum security prison. Where such issues are resolved in accordance with a reasonable priority system, however, courts are likely to defer to it in determining what care is appropriate.

Personnel

Most cases in which courts have found constitutional violations of inmates' rights to health care were fostered by the exigencies of an over-burdened staff coping with too few resources. No amount of concern or good faith effort by medical staff can overcome inadequate financing, and it is perhaps in this area that the courts have made their greatest contribution by prompting, and, if necessary, forcing governmental decision-makers to appropriate the funds necessary to maintain humane health care. While most courts are reluctant to mandate staffing and equipment levels (preferring instead to set constitutional standards and to leave the means to achieve them to the institution to fashion), the

Table 29-2. Frequency of sick call.

American Correctional Association:	
Population < 100	1 x week
Population 100–300	3 x week
Population > 300	4 x week

National Commission on Correctional Health Care:	
Population < 200	3 x week
Population 200–500	4 x week
Population > 500	5 x week

American Public Health Association:	
5 days per week, regardless of size	

courts will impose specific requirements when circumstances warrant.

A large institution, such as a state prison, may be required to have full-time health professionals, including physicians, on site; the largest facilities may need 24-hour coverage.[35] Even the smallest county jails, however, must have a means (such as an on-call system and officers trained in first aid) to deal with medical emergencies when no health care staff is present.[46]

The use of unqualified "medical technicians" and inmate assistants to provide care can pose a problem of constitutional magnitude. Use of untrained or unqualified staff to meet shortages in licensed physicians, nurses, and other personnel has led to findings of unconstitutional care in Louisiana, Texas, Oklahoma, and Illinois, to name a few.

Many facilities have turned to contractual providers in their search for personnel. Some state systems have contracted out their entire health care delivery system. The use of independent contractors, however, while often a solution of choice, does not relieve the institution (or the contractors) of legal responsibility for health care (Box 29-4).[47] However the employees are supplied, staffing health care delivery systems with sufficient and sufficiently qualified staff is key to a successful operation.

The National Commission on Correctional Health Care now offers certification as a "Correctional Health Professional" to health care employees in corrections and others, based on credentials, experience, and a written examination. Hundreds of correctional nurses, doctors, dentists, and others have become certified as a result of this program.

Medical Records

Maintenance of adequate medical records is "a necessity,"[48] and numerous courts have condemned the failure to main-

---

Box 29-4. *West v. Atkins* **and Contractual Care**

Samuel Atkins, M.D., was an orthopedist under contract with the State of North Carolina to conduct a clinic twice monthly and to provide necessary surgery. Quincey West was a dissatisfied inmate patient who sued Dr. Atkins, alleging deliberate indifference in the doctor's treatment of his Achilles tendon. Reversing a lower court decision that Dr. Atkins, as a physician merely under contract, could not be sued in federal court, the Supreme Court ruled that independent contractors who provide medical care to inmates are held to the same Eighth Amendment standards as state civil service employees.

---

tain an organized and complete system of health care records. At a minimum, records should be kept separately for each patient and include a medical history and problem list; notations of patient complaints; treatment progress notes; and laboratory, radiographic, and specialist findings. Not only do proper medical records promote continuity of care and protect the health and safety of the inmate population, but they also provide correctional administrators with evidence of the course of treatment when individual inmates sue them asserting that care was not provided.[49]

Outside Care

No correctional facility can provide complete medical care within its confines. If an inmate requires a specialist evaluation, a sophisticated diagnostic test, or in-patient care that is not available in the prison system, the failure to provide it may constitute deliberate indifference. In such cases, security and administrative considerations concerning transportation and cost must yield to medical determinations when a particular patient is in need of prompt treatment.[50, 51]

Facilities and Resources

Space and supplies must be adequate to meet the health care needs of the institutional population.[52] Dangerous or unsanitary physical conditions, inadequate or defective space or equipment, or unavailability of medications or other ordered items, such as eyeglasses, dentures, braces, prostheses, or special diets, can all lead to violations of the Constitution.

Federal courts ordered officials in Louisiana to build a new infirmary in *Hamilton v. Landrieu*,[53] and New York City was recently compelled to construct appropriate facilities for respiratory isolation of tuberculosis patients on Rikers Island. Once constitutional violations are shown, courts have "broad discretion to frame equitable remedies" to alleviate them.[26]

Quality Assurance and Accreditation

Quality assurance has been defined as "[a] process of ongoing monitoring and evaluation to assess the adequacy and

appropriateness of the care provided and to institute corrective action as needed."[20] It is an essential aspect of any well-run system; in its absence, courts have often imposed external audits or appointed monitors over health care services as part of a remedy for constitutional violations and to ensure compliance with court orders.[54, 55]

In the free world, accreditation of health care facilities is encouraged by at least three factors: participation in the Medicare program; eligibility for intern and resident training; and lower liability insurance premiums. None of these community incentives directly affects corrections; and, in fact, the development of national standards relating to correctional health care did not occur until 1976.[56] The first accreditation of a prison (the Georgia State Prison in Reidsville) did not occur until 1982.[20]

Currently, three national bodies offer accreditation to correctional facilities: the American Correctional Association, which accredits the entire operation of an institution, including health care services; the Joint Commission on Accreditation of Health Organizations, a free-world oriented organization that has accredited a handful of health care facilities serving prisoners exclusively; and the National Commission on Correctional Health Care, an interdisciplinary organization focusing exclusively on health care delivery in corrections that has accredited several hundred prisons, jails, and juvenile facilities in the United States. Unlike the standards of the other two bodies, the National Commission's standards address only health care delivery for correctional facilities.

Much of the impetus for development of standards and the move toward accreditation has come from litigation. According to Vincent M. Nathan, who has served as a special master for federal district courts in Ohio, Georgia, Texas, New Mexico, and Puerto Rico:

> [T]he standards of medical care in jails and prisons ... have, to a large extent, translated the vague legal rulings of the courts into practical and viable tests for measuring the legal adequacy of institutional health care programs.[57]

Litigation has been a factor in achieving accreditation, for example, in Georgia and Texas, largely due to Mr. Nathan's efforts.[20, 58, 59]

Faced with court allegations of unconstitutional care, and in the absence of legislative or other incentives to accreditation of correctional health care delivery, voluntary compliance with national standards is not only a hedge against liability but also a sound investment in quality of care. The cost, generally a few thousands dollars,[20] is a fraction of the resource drain that occurs with litigation.

SPECIAL NEEDS AND POPULATIONS

Reflecting society, prisons, and jails have many inmates who have special health care needs. Medical and mental health services must adjust to provide the individualized care the patient requires.

Disabled Inmates

That fact that unusual accommodations may be necessary, in light of their special needs, to accomplish the provision of minimal conditions of incarceration does not absolve correctional officials of their duty toward handicapped inmates.[59] Thus, inmates who cannot walk are entitled to wheelchairs or necessary prostheses and braces, and patients with impaired hearing or vision are entitled to assistance.[59–61]

The protections afforded disabled inmates have been expanded by the American with Disabilities Act (ADA).[62] Although there is contrary authority, the prevailing view (and that of the U.S. Department of Justice — see 28 C.F.R. 35.190) is that the ADA applies to prisons and jails (Box 29-5).[63] It, therefore, appears that correctional officials will have to make substantial efforts to make their services, programs, and activities available to inmates suffering from paralysis, deafness, blindness, and other actual and perceived physical or mental handicaps.

Mental Health Care

Denial of adequate mental health care for serious mental health needs may violate the Eighth Amendment under the same "deliberate indifference" standard applied to other medical needs. A mental health need is "serious" if it "has caused significant disruption in an inmate's everyday life and ... prevents his functioning in the general population without disturbing or endangering others or himself."[64]

Prisons and jails must provide mental health screening intake to identify serious problems, including potential suicides[65]; treatment for serious conditions by mental health professionals[66]; and training of officers to deal with mentally ill inmates.[52] Additionally, there must be some means of separating severely mentally ill inmates from the mentally healthy. Mixing mentally ill inmates with those who are not mentally ill may violate the rights of both groups.[67] Finally, failure to provide treatment for mentally retarded inmates may also violate the constitution, if regression occurs.[7]

Except in cases of short transfers for evaluation purposes, inmates are entitled to notice and a hearing before being committed to a mental hospital because the stigmatizing consequences of a psychiatric commitment and the possible involuntary subjection to psychiatric treatment constitute a deprivation of liberty requiring due process.[68] Psychiatric treatment may not be used for disciplinary purposes,[69] and use of seclusion and restraint must be based on professional judgment reasonably related to its purpose.[32]

Inmates have the right to avoid the involuntary administration of antipsychotic medication, but correctional officials may force the patient to submit to them if he has a serious mental illness, if the inmate is dangerous to self or others, and if the treatment is in the inmate's medical interest (Box 29-6).[70]

Inmates with mental problems frequently find themselves in trouble in prisons and jails for violating institutional rules. The administrative punishment of inmates who are not mentally responsible for their actions has been of concern to the courts (Box 29-7).[72]

Training of correctional staff and hearing officers in recognition of mental health issues in misbehavior can assist in avoiding litigation. Conditions that lead to psychiatrically based misbehavior can also be addressed in part by development of intermediate and chronic care capability for mental health services, by closely monitoring the mental health condition of inmates in solitary confinement, and by reviewing the disciplinary and administrative classification of inmates who are returned to facilities after psychiatric hospitalization, especially if a return to solitary confinement is being considered.[73]

Pregnancy and Abortion

The number of pregnant inmates in prisons and jails is substantial. In one federal prison housing 1,300 women, the government estimates that about fifty are pregnant at any one time.[74] Treatment for the complications of pregnancy (or to avoid them) constitutes a serious health care need within the meaning of the Eighth Amendment.[42]

Babies born to incarcerated women, however, can be separated from their mothers, because there is no constitutional right to keep a child in prison. One federal court, however, has required prison officials to permit a prisoner to breast feed her newborn child during visiting hours.[74]

The termination of an unwanted pregnancy is also considered a serious medical need, and the denial of an abortion constitutes deliberate indifference. Jail or prison officials must provide for abortions, regardless of the prisoner's ability to pay.[75]

AIDS and HIV Infection

In general, claims of inadequate medical care for AIDS and HIV infection are evaluated under the same deliberate indifference standard as other medical care claims. The AIDS crisis, however, has generated several troublesome legal issues for corrections; and, for the most part, courts

---

Box 29-5. The Americans with Disabilities Act

The ADA provides that "no qualified individual with a disability shall, by reason of such disability, be excluded from participation in or be denied the benefits of the services, programs, or activities of a public entity, or be subject to discrimination by any such entity."

"Public entity" includes any state or local government or any department or agency therof. (Federal agencies are covered by a separate statute). The ADA makes no exceptions for prisons or jails. The accommodations required to avoid discrimination include modifications to architectural, communication, or transportation barriers; and the provision of auxiliary aids and services (see *Tucker*, 1989).

Box 29-6. Involuntary Administration of Anti-Psychotic Drugs

In *Washington v. Harper,* the Supreme Court ruled that inmates have a "significant liberty interest" in avoiding the unwanted administration of anti-psychotic drugs. The court approved such use only where certain procedural protections were available, such as those in the Washington State case before it:

1. Only a psychiatrist may order the drugs.
2. Patients who object are entitled to an administrative hearing before professional staff not currently involved in their treatment.
3. The patient may attend the hearing, present and cross-examine witnesses, and have the assistance of a lay advisor with psychiatric knowledge.
4. Minutes must be kept with judicial review available.
5. Continuation of the medication is subject to periodic review.

Note: Additional protections may exist under state law—see *Rivers v. Katz.*[71]

have largely deferred to the decisions of correctional administrators. For example, mandatory testing for HIV accompanied by segregation of HIV-positive inmates and the refusal to do mandatory testing have both been upheld.[76–78]

LEGAL-ETHICAL CONSIDERATIONS

Correctional facilities impose unusual constrictions on the delivery of medical services. They are "inherently coercive institutions that for security reasons must exercise nearly total control over their residents lives and the activities within their confines."[47] Schedules regulate work, exercise, and diet. Inmates cannot self-treat even minor ailments, and must seek medical assistance even if all they need is an over-the-counter remedy or a day in bed. Additionally, health care professionals are frequently involved in the custodial functions of the prison or jail; and institutional security, productivity, discipline, and administrative convenience all affect the exercise of medical judgment.

The Provider-Patient Relationship

The provider-patient relationship in corrections is imposed by the state, and neither the dissatisfied patient nor the sometimes frustrated provider are at liberty to change it. This situation can be destructive of the professional relationship between the provider and the patient and can engender distrust. As one commentator put it:

> *No individual, however skilled and compassionate a doctor, can maintain a normal doctor-patient relationship with a man who the next day he may acquiesce in subjection to solitary confinement.*[79]

Box 29-7. Punishment of the Voodoo-Cursed Inmate

A prisoner was serving a sentence for manslaughter for the stabbing death of his wife, which he believed was compelled by evil spirits that inhabited his body as a result of a voodoo curse. In prison, he killed another inmate, for which he was found not guilty by reason of insanity. Nevertheless, prison disciplinary charges were brought for assaulting the second victim, and the inmate was given seven years' solitary confinement and four years' loss of good time. The court vacated the punishment, ruling that the inmate could not be punished for acts for which he had already been found insane. The court also ordered a new hearing at which the inmate would be represented by a "counsel substitute." *People ex rel. Reed v. Scully.*

Confidentiality

Inmates have a constitutional right to privacy in their medical diagnoses and other health care records and information.[80, 81] That right is not violated by the reporting of medical findings in the ordinary course of prison medical care operations, or probably even to prison and jail executives with a reason to know, but the "[c]asual, unjustified dissemination of confidential medical information to nonmedical staff and other prisoners" is unconstitutional.[80]

Maintaining confidentiality in corrections is a "monumentally difficult task."[20] Medical information may be surmised from things as simple as an inmate's movement, a cell search, or a pattern of scheduled visits.[20] Nevertheless, health care encounters should be performed in medical settings, out of earshot of other inmates and officers; health staff should not discuss one patient in front of another; medical records should be stored securely and transported in sealed containers; and inmates should not be assigned duties where they have access to confidential information.

The Right to Refuse Treatment

A mentally competent adult has a constitutional right to refuse medical treatment, including the direction that life-saving or other extraordinary measures be withdrawn in terminal cases.[82] As Judge Cardozo stated almost 80 years ago: "Every human being of adult years and sound mind has a right to determine what shall be done with his own body."[83] This right extends to prisoners as well.[84]

The right has never been regarded as absolute, however, and it may be overridden if there are strong public health reasons to administer treatment, as when the Supreme Court upheld mandatory smallpox vaccination in 1905, despite the patient's religious objections.[85] Inmates have been required, for example, to submit to blood and tuberculosis tests and to diphtheria and tetanus injections.[86–88]

The right to refuse is based on the concept of informed consent. As one court stated:

A prisoner's right to refuse treatment is useless without knowledge of the proposed treatment. Prisoners have a right to such information as is reasonably necessary to make an informed decision to accept or reject proposed treatment, as well as a reasonable explanation of the viable alternative treatments that can be made available in a prison setting.[84]

There are "reason[s] to be leery of refusals of care in prisons,"[20] and care must be taken in corrections to determine if a refusal of care is genuine. Some investigation of an inmate who does not appear for treatment should occur to determine if the patient was too ill to report; was prevented from doing so by a cellblock lockdown or other impediment; or had a genuine conflict with a school examination, a family visit, or another program.

Finally, as society in general increasingly plans for terminal illness with advanced directives and living wills, and as the numbers of deaths increase in corrections due to AIDS, and the proportion of elderly inmates grows, correctional administrators will face requests to terminate treatment. If advanced directives are appropriate for use in corrections, they must be truly voluntary and not be permitted to mask denials of care. A multidisciplinary committee of health providers from the prison and the community, as well as clergy and public officials, may help to ensure oversight and fairness.[20]

FUTURE TRENDS

In addition to privatization, which has already been discussed, the past few years have witnessed the advent of other developments that are influencing the course of correctional health care and the law, including fee-for-service plans and the Congressional passage of the Prison Litigation Reform Act. As of this writing, the legal ramifications of such events are still emerging.

Charging Inmates for Health Care

A growing number of states and localities have adopted policies that charge inmates for various types of health care encounters.[89] Although there are practical and ethical questions regarding implementation of a fee-for-service system,[90] the courts have tended to uphold carefully crafted systems (Box 29-8). To date, there are very little data on the efficacy of fee-for-service in terms of statistically valid studies. More sophisticated analysis is expected as experience with such programs continues.

The Prison Litigation Reform Act

The Prison Litigation Reform Act (PLRA),[91] passed in 1996, restricts the ability of the federal courts to issue injunctive relief and approve consent decrees by requiring a specific finding of constitutional violations prior to entry of

---

> **Box 29-8. Fee-for-Service and the Courts**
>
> While some early efforts at fee-for-service faced court hostility, most newer plans have passed muster. The courts tend to scrutinize the following factors in evaluating such systems:
>
> 1. Is medical care provided first with assessment of costs to follow?
> 2. Are inmates who cannot pay nevertheless provided with necessary care?
> 3. Is emergency care being provided regardless of payment?
> 4. Is the payment amount so severe relative to the inmate's resources or earnings that it effectively denies care?
> 5. Are chronically ill inmates effectively being denied access to follow-up care by the charges?
> 6. Is there a fair system for applying the charges and granting exceptions?

---

such orders. The PLRA also places restrictions on the appointment and responsibilities of special masters and provides a means for reopening and/or terminating existing court orders. There has been considerable activity in courts following the passage of the PLRA, and its scope — and even whether it is constitutional, about which the courts are divided — remains to be determined in future litigation. If the PLRA is sustained, it may well have a profound impact on the ability of the courts to enforce the Eighth Amendment's prohibition against "deliberate indifference" to serious medical needs.

CONCLUSION

"No serious student of American correctional history can deny that litigation has provided the impetus for reform of medical practice in prisons and jails."[57] Yet, as resources become increasingly scarce, government officials are constantly faced with doing more with less, and the expense of litigation should not absorb funds that are available to upgrade delivery of services. Voluntary adoption of community standards and accreditation are a less tortuous road to reform, and, in the long run, are likely to be more successful and less divisive.

The protection of basic rights to access, to ordered care, and to professional judgment can be achieved without litigation where correctional administrators and health care professionals work together from within to promote excellence and strive continually to upgrade the quality of the care that is delivered.

REFERENCES

1. Prisoners in 1990, Bureau of Justice Statistics Bulletin, U.S. Dept of Justice, May 1991.
2. Jail Inmates, 1990, Bureau of Justice Statistics Bulletin, U.S. Dept of Justice, June 1991.

3. In 90s Prison Building, The New York Times, August 8, 1997, p A-14.

4. Fuller: Care of the Seriously Mentally Ill. Washington, D.C., Public Research Group, National Alliance of the Mentally Ill, 1990.

5. Steadman, et al: A survey of mental disability among state prison inmates. Hosp Commun Psychiatry 38: 1987.

6. Teplin, Schwartz: The prevalence of severe mental disorder among male urban jail detainees. *Am J Publ Health* 80:663–669, 1990.

7. Ellis, Luckasson: Mentally retarded criminal defendants. George Washington Law Rev 414:53, 1985.

8. Inmates with Developmental Disabilities in New York State Correctional Facilities. New York State Commission on Quality of Care for the Mentally Disabled, 1991.

9. The Legal Rights of Persons with Epilepsy, ed 6. Epilepsy Foundation of America, Landover, Md. 1992.

10. King, Young: Increased prevalence of seizure disorders among prisoners. JAMA 239:2674, 1978.

11. Thomas: The 'reality' of prison litigation: Repackaging the data. Crim Civil Confinement 15:27, 1989.

12. Inmate Lawsuits. Contact Center, 1985.

13. American Civil Liberties Union: Status Report. Washington, D.C., ACLU, 1995.

14. Koren: Status report: State prisons and the courts. National Prison Project J 8:1, 1993.

15. Twenty Five States Now Under Prison Court Orders, Criminal Justice Newsletter, February 16, 1981.

16. Howell: A Complete Collection of State Trials. 844, 1814.

17. Blackstone: Commentaries on the Laws of England. 377, 1769.

18. *Ruffin v Commonwealth,* 62 Va (21 Gratt) 790 (1871).

19. *Spicer v Williamson,* 132 SE 291 (NC 1926).

20. Anno: Prison Health Care: Guidelines for the Management of an Adequate Delivery System. Washington, D.C.: U.S. Dept of Justice, National Institute of Corrections, 1991.

21. *Estelle v Gamble,* 429 US 97, 97 SCt 285 (1976).

22. *Wilson v Seiter,* 501 US 294, 111 SCt 2321 (1991).

23. *Farmer v Brennan,* 511 U.S. 825, 114 SCt 1970 (1994).

24. Winner: An Introduction to the Constitutional Law of Prison Medical Care. J Prison Health 1:67, 1981.

25. *Dean v Coughlin,* 623 FSupp 392 (SDNY 1985).

26. *Todaro v Ward,* 431 FSupp 1129 (SDNY), aff'd, 565 F2d 48 (2d Cir 1977).

27. *Martinez v Mancusi,* 443 F2d 1192 (2d Cir 1970).

28. Neisser: Is there a doctor in the joint? The search for constitutional standards for prison health care. Va Law Rev 63:921, 1977.

29. *Williams v Vincent,* 508 F2d 541 (2d Cir 1974).

30. *Thomas v Pate,* 493 F2d 151 (7th Cir 1974).

31. *Rogers v Evans,* 792 F2d 1052 (11th Cir 1986).

32. *Wells v Franzen,* 777 F2d 1258, 1264-65 (7th Cir 1985).

33. *Jones v Johnson.* 781 F2d 769 (9th Cir. 1986).

34. *Duran v Anaya,* 642 FSupp 510 (DNM 1986).

35. *Ramos v Lamm,* 639 F2d 559 (10th Cir 1980).

36. *Bishop v Stoneman,* 508 F2d 1224 (2d Cir 1974).

37. *Hoptowit v Ray,* 682 F2d 1237 (9th Cir 1982).

38. American Correctional Association: Standards, 1990.

39. National Commission on Correctional Health Care: Standards for Health Services in Jails, 1992.

40. National Commission on Correctional Health Care: Standards for Health Services in Prisons, 1997.

41. American Public Health Association: Standards for Health Services in Correctional Institutions, ed 2. 1986.

42. *Boswell v Sherburne County,* 849 F2d 1117 (10th Cir 1988).

43. *Kelley v McGinnis,* 899 F2d 612 (7th Cir 1990).

44. *Mitchell v Aluisi,* 872 F2d 577 (4th Cir 1989).

45. Conte: Dental treatment for incarcerated individuals: For whom? How much?" J Prison Jail Health 3:25, 1983.

46. *Green v Carlson,* 581 F2d 669 (2d Cir 1978), aff'd, 446 US 14 1980.

47. *West v Atkins,* 487 US 42, 108 SCt 2250 (1988).

48. *Johnson-El v Schoemehl,* 878 F2d 1043 (8th Cir 1989).

49. Kay: The Constitutional Dimensions of an Inmate's Right to Health Care. Washington, D.C., National Commission on Correctional Health Care, 1991.

50. *United States v State of Michigan,* 680 FSupp 928 (WD Mich 1987).

51. *Ancata v Prison Health Services,* 769 FSupp 700 (11th Cir 1985).

52. *Langley v Coughlin,* 888 F2d 252 (2d Cir 1989).

53. *Hamilton v Landrieu,* 351 FSupp 549 (ED La 1972).

54. Byland: Dental Care in Prisons: Quality Assurance of Dental Programs, Address to Second World Congress on Prison Health Care, Ottawa, 1983.

55. *Lightfoot v Walker,* 486 FSupp 504 (SD Ill 1980).

56. American Public Health Association: Standards for Health Services in Correctional Institutions, 1976.

57. Nathan: Guest editorial. J Prison Health 5:1, 1985.

58. *Guthrie v Evans,* Civ Act No 3068 (SD Ga) (First Report of the Special Master).

59. *Ruiz v Estelle,* 503 FSupp 1265 (SD Tex 1980), aff'd in part and rev'd in part, 679 F2d 1115 (1982).

60. *Johnson v Hardin County,* Ky, 908 F2d 1280 (6th Cir 1990).

61. *Cummings v Roberts,* 628 F2d 1065 (8th Cir 1980).

62. American with Disabilities Act of 1990, 42 USC §12101, et seq.

63. Tucker: The Americans with Disabilities Act: An Overview. Univ Ill Law Rev 923, 1989.

64. *Tillary v Owens,* 719 FSupp 1256 (WD Pa 1989), aff'd, 907 F2d 418 (3d Cir 1990).

65. *Balla v Idaho State Board of Corrections,* 595 FSupp 1558 (D Idaho 1984).

66. *Smith v Jenkins,* 919 F2d 90 (8th Cir 1990).

67. *DeMallory v Cullen,* 855 F2d 442 (7th Cir 1988).

68. *Vitek v Jones,* 445 US 480 (1980).

69. *Knecht v Gillman,* 488 F2d 1136 (8th Cir 1973).

70. *Washington v Harper,* 494 US 210, 110 SCt 1028 (1990).

71. *Rivers v Katz,* 67 NY 2d 485, 504 NY S2d 74 (NY 1986).

72. *People ex rel Reed v Scully,* 140 Misc2d 379, 531 NY S2d 196 (Sup Ct, Oneida Co 1988).

73. *Eng v Kelly,* Civ 80-0385T (WD NY, January 27, 1987).

74. *Berrios-Berrios v Thornburg,* 716 FSupp 987 (ED Ky 1989).

75. *Monmouth County Correction Institutional Inmates v Lanzaro,* 834 F2d 326 (3d Cir 1987).

76. *Dunn v White,* 880 F2d 1188 (10th Cir 1989).

77. *Harris v Thigpen,* 727 FSupp 1564 (MD Ala 1990).

78. *Glick v Henderson,* 885 F2d 536 (8th Cir 1988).

79. Brazier: Prison Doctors and Their Involuntary Patients. Publication Law 282, 1982.

80. *Woods v White,* 689 FSupp 874 (WD Wisc 1988).

81. *Doe v Coughlin,* 697 FSupp 1234 (ND NY 1988).

82. *Cruzan v Missouri Department of Health,* 497 US 261, 110 SCt 2841 (1990).

83. *Schloendorff v Society of New York Hospitals,* 211 NY 125 (1914).

84. *White v Napoleon,* 897 F2d 103 (3d Cir 1990).

85. *Jacobson v Massachusetts,* 197 US 11 (1905).

86. *Thompson v City of Los Angeles,* 885 F2d 1439 (9th Cir 1989).

87. *Zaire v Dalsheim,* 698 FSupp 57 (SD NY 1988).

88. *Ballard v Woodard,* 641 FSupp 432 (WD NC 1986).

89. Weiland: Fee-for-service programs: A literature review and results of a national survey. J Correctional Health Care 3:145, 1996.

90. Rold WJ: Charging inmates for medical care: A legal, practical, and ethical critique. J Correctional Health Care 3:129, 1996.

91. Prison Litigation Reform Act. Pub L No 104-134 (April 24, 1996).

30

End-of-Life Care in Prisons and Jails

Nancy Neveloff Dubler, L.L.B.
Budd Heyman, M.D.

INTRODUCTION

Death is not the worst possible outcome of medical care. Death is not even the worst possible outcome of incarceration. Dying alone, in pain, without social, familial, and spiritual supports is the terrifying end that many prisoners and, indeed, most people fear. Unfortunately, it is too often the reality they experience.

In the community, the past decade has seen substantial progress in accommodating the needs and wants of dying patients, their families, and other loved ones. Physicians, nurses, and social workers have enhanced their communication skills, permitting them to discuss diagnoses and prognoses openly and honestly, even when the choices are difficult and the future dim. The use of advance directives has permitted decisionally capacitated patients to make choices in the present that will control their care in the future when they are no longer able to participate in decision making. The appointment of health care agents ("proxies") permits the patient to designate a person, ideally one who knows the patient's values and the preferences, to make decisions for the patient when he is no longer capable of considering the risks and benefits of alternative treatments. When patients are dying, their needs for analgesia, spiritual support, and physical comfort care are most effectively met by evolving

practices that reflect the growth of hospice and palliative care. Protocols for addressing pain and suffering are proliferating. Research on the dying process provides increasingly specific guidance on the least invasive and most supportive techniques that promote death with dignity.[1]

Despite this progress, however, studies indicate that, even in the most advanced academic medical centers, many patients still die in pain.[2] Sobering data indicate that concerted efforts to encourage patients to execute advance directives is only partially successful. Indeed, despite the best efforts of clinicians and advocates, it is rare to find any patient population where more than 25% actually sign either a living will or a health care proxy appointment.[3] Directly relevant to a discussion of prisons and jails, many of those who decline to sign advance directives see them not as a support for care, but as part of a systemic denial of care. Patients who are old, of color, infected with HIV, or IV drug users, are suspicious of the systems in which they receive care. Many of these patients are not interested in limiting care; they are interested in accessing care.

This complex picture becomes increasingly convoluted when the care is delivered in a correctional institution or in a medical facility related to the prison or jail system. Inmates, in contrast to non-incarcerated patients, do not assume that correctional institutions are acting in their best interests. If decisions are made to limit care and permit death, prisoners may not be convinced that everything has been done to extend and support life. In the nonincarcerated community, over-treatment and inappropriately aggressive care required harnessing medical technology to the needs of the dying. In correctional institutions, strides are still necessary to ensure that every inmate-patient receives the most aggressive care to extend life when that is medically appropriate. Decent end-of-life care requires a trusting alliance between the care providers and the patient. Forging an honest and supportive relationship is a prerequisite for a good death in any setting.

DYING IN PRISONS—INCREASING PREVALENCE

Death is increasingly the last stage of a prison sentence. Acquired immunodeficiency syndrome (AIDS) is intimately associated with injection drug behavior, and American criminal policy has made determined efforts to incarcerate drug users. As a not-surprising result, AIDS has become the single largest cause of death in prisons and jails.[4] As one inmate stated, "Somehow they should not have to get the death sentence just because they have the habit."[5]

The actual number of inmates with HIV and those with AIDS is difficult to identify. Most prison systems neither perform mandatory testing for HIV disease nor conduct anonymous serologic surveys. The national survey conducted by the Bureau of Justice Statistics for the U.S. Department of Justice indicates 22,713 inmates infected with HIV in 1994, the most recent date for which the data have been compiled. Consequently, the numbers reported —4,849 cases of AIDS for 47 state and federal prison systems in 1994—are clearly inaccurate, as they largely reflect the disease for those inmates who have already become symptomatic. Because the definition of the disease also encompasses a T-cell count below 200, many more inmates qualify as having AIDS, although they may not yet exhibit the opportunistic infections that would bring them to the attention of the health services.

A more accurate picture is provided by a blinded anonymous 1996 serology survey done in New York State that showed approximately 9,500 infected inmates.[6] Because many inmates do not volunteer for confidential testing, fearing the discrimination or segregation that may result if the disease were revealed, only anonymous surveys can correctly reveal the numbers of infected persons. Unfortunately, as treatment for AIDS becomes more sophisticated and preventive interventions more effective, the reluctance to submit to testing consigns many inmates to substandard care that may actually shorten their lives. This suspicion of the correctional health care system is precisely what works against the therapeutic alliance that is demanded for high quality end-of-life care.

But inmates with AIDS are not the only segment of the prison population whose deaths may occur within correctional walls. In 1994, there were 2,888 male deaths and 123 female deaths in federal and state correctional systems. Of those totals, 888 men and 35 women died of AIDS. The remainder died of other illness or natural causes, suicide, injury, execution, attack by another inmate, or unspecified causes. These numbers identify an epidemic in the corrections system—close to 3,000 deaths a year.[7]

The trend toward increased sentences and the proliferation of "three strikes and you're out" laws, determinate sentences and mandatory minimums have combined with AIDS to begin the "graying" of the prisons. Prisoners also tend to be physiologically older than their years would indicate. A prisoner aged 50 may be classified by society as middle-aged; he may, in fact, already be an aged person if many of his years have been spent in the prison system. Socioeconomic status and lack of access to preventive and acute medical and dental care may create as much as a 10-year aging differential to the prisoner.[8] Nationally, the number of inmates 55 and older more than doubled from 1981 to 1990.[9] Estimates are that the number of prisoners over age 50 will reach 125,000 by the year 2000, with 40,000 to 50,000 being over age 65.[10] Given the hyperaging phenomenon of the inmate population, many of these prisoners will be aged and infirm with multiple medical problems. These problems, if they mirror the general population, will include kidney failure, diabetes, cancer, heart disease, dementias, and the other degenerative diseases that fill geriatric practices and long-term care facilities.

Were these abstractions not sufficiently troubling, caring for geriatric inmates is likely to be extremely expensive. Estimates for the care of an elderly inmate range from $60,000–$69,000 per year, in contrast to about $20,000 per year for non-elderly inmates without AIDS.[11] The majority of these monies cover the costs of medical treatments and medications, special equipment for the handicapped, special education, recreation and work programs, prison hospital beds, and special facilities needed to protect the frail and elderly in the violent prison world.[12]

CARE FOR THE DYING IN PRISON

Absent effective and publicly accepted compassionate release programs, many prisoners will die in correctional hospitals and long-term care facilities. For these prisoners, the judicial sentence they received has been automatically converted to a sentence of death. For inmates, as for most people, terminal illness is a time of great sorrow, loneliness, suspicion, pain, and suffering. The good death—an acceptance of the inevitable and reconciliation with family and friends, supported by spiritual counselors in a comfortable surrounding—is rarely available inside prison walls. The problems with implementing a plan for a good death often run afoul of prison rules and regulations, the structure of medical care organization, the distance of families, and the barriers to communication and affection that exist in the punitive correctional environment.

In jails and prisons, death is always suspect as an event that will upset the inmate population or undermine security. As articulated in the 1979 case of *Commissioner of Corrections v. Myers,*[13] a case involving an inmate's attempt to refuse dialysis, the court overruled the right of the prisoner to refuse treatment and stated that the interests of the state, as represented by the department of corrections, included "the preservation of internal order and discipline, the maintenance of institutional security, and the rehabilitation of prisoners." These, the court held, permit the corrections officials to administer life-saving treatment without consent and over the specific refusal of the inmate. This case and others have consistently put the requirements of corrections administration over the rights of inmates to consent to or refuse treatment. Nevertheless, this case, although often cited, has little applicability to general issues of terminal care. With frail elderly inmates, those with cancer and AIDS, the issue is rarely that an inmate chooses to refuse care, but rather that care has not been provided to meet his needs for support and comfort. Despite the fact that decent prison and jail health care should come as close as possible to the standard of care in the community, end-of-life care for the incarcerated almost always fails to reach that goal.

Where Should Care Be Delivered?

In an effort to streamline care, gather trained staff and meet the needs of inmates, many systems are developing special care units for dying patients. At the start of the AIDS epidemic, many correctional medical personnel and officers were afraid to treat patients with AIDS. As the epidemic has progressed, the absolute neglect of patients has given way to decent treatment in some facilities and barely acceptable treatment in others. Many systems are experimenting with Designated Death Units (DDU), to which terminally ill prisoners can be transferred at the end of life. Although a dedicated unit might seem reasonable because staff can be trained in end-of-life care and materials and equipment procured to meet individual needs, these units often turn out to be a problem rather than an innovation.

Many correctional physicians come to see the DDU as an alternative to aggressive treatment for possibly correctable medical problems. Patients with complex oncologic problems or infectious disease syndromes, including AIDS, can be transferred to this unit rather than receiving specialty care from a fully trained expert. Prisoners come to see transfer to the unit as a death sentence, which it very well may be. As a consequence of a centralized facility, many of the inmates will find themselves further away from their families and less likely to have the frequent visits that a dying person craves. These special terminal units are also likely to have special security classifications and to be less likely to offer educational and rehabilitation programs, congregate religious services, or access to the law library, all

activities that enrich life no matter what stage of dying has been reached.

Good medical practice dictates that there should be no assignment to a DDU unless the patient has been examined and his care reviewed by a specialist in the field. This sort of review, which should precede classification as a person with a terminal illness for whom comfort care is the appropriate plan, should help to ensure that aggressive acute care is not discontinued prematurely (personal communication, Robert Cohen, 1997).

What Sorts of Care Should Be Provided?

Inmates, no less than other persons, should be provided with diagnostic and treatment interventions to meet their needs. In the event that cure is no longer the goal of care, palliation, comfort, and spiritual support need to be part of the care offered.

- Palliative care protocols should be in place to assure that the care team can accurately assess the level of physical discomfort and provide effective response. The fact that an inmate has a history of drug use does not disqualify this patient from receiving adequate analgesia and even opioids when required for pain control.
- The prison formulary should have adequate pharmaceutical interventions available to support pain management;
- Family members and other loved ones should be permitted increased access to the patient;
- Chaplains and other spiritual advisors, including inmates, should be permitted enhanced access to the inmate;
- Family members who are not particularly involved should be sought out to support the inmate, if they can, or to make some provisions for the burial. As much as the death, the prospect of a burial in a "Potters field" is an additional horror for an inmate;
- Rituals to commemorate those who have died should be part of the prison culture for terminal care. Other inmates and staff need to have some way of remembering and commemorating those who have died. It can be especially numbing for staff to dispatch an ever-increasing number of inmates to the morgue.

How Is Care at the End of Life Affected by the Americans With Disabilities Act?

It is clear that, outside of prisons, persons with AIDS and the elderly disabled are protected under the provisions of this federal law. However, it is not so clear whether the ADA requires certain special accommodations to the needs of these persons when they are incarcerated. Not surprisingly, given increasing judicial support for correctional administrative discretion, it is likely that some or even most courts will "elevate the penological interests of security and efficiency above the statutory rights"[14] of inmates. This is especially true because it is far from clear that prisoners would be considered qualified individuals under the terms and definitions of the act.[15]

What Sorts of Supportive Care Should Be in Place for End-of-Life Care?

The philosophy of medicine—to diagnose, comfort, and cure—and the approach of corrections—to confine and punish[16]—clash most directly in end-of-life care. Should the visiting rules be relaxed to permit greater family involvement? Should more available comfort measures, such as access to food and fluid on request, be made available and staffed for those who cannot provide for themselves? Should inmates be shackled when moved outside of the facility for some sort of consultation? These questions illustrate the sorts of quality-of-life issues that must be confronted if the care delivered to the dying is to be morally adequate.

These questions also identify some of the issues that make care at the end of life so hard to manage in a correctional facility dedicated to punishment and retribution. A prisoner who is dying is about to face the ultimate sentence, not as a matter of judicial decree, but rather as a result of reality. The antagonism, suspicion, anger, opposition, and fear that have governed the relationship between the inmate and the authorities prior to this stage of illness will continue to define and constrain the relationship during the inmate's dying. For this reason, among others, compassionate release of dying inmates is such an important part of planning for terminal care.

How can Advance Directives Be Used to Improve End-of-Life Care?

Do-not-resuscitate orders, living wills, and health care proxy agent appointments are increasingly part of advance planning to support decent end-of-life care. They can also be important in the correctional setting with one major caveat: It is very difficult and, in some settings, nearly impossible to distinguish between a refusal of care and a denial of care. If the inmate fails to arrive for a particular treatment, has he decided not to come, or has the corrections officer at the gate denied him access to the medical units? Has the inmate decided to see a visitor instead, or has he been sent off, unexpectedly, for a court appointment? The secluded nature of movement and the disparities of the power relationships combine to exclude inmates from care when they have not chosen to refuse care. This reality must accompany the creation of documents that are used to prospectively refuse care. These documents, and the powers they represent, are only appropriate if they truly reflect the values and preferences of the inmate, and are in no way coerced or imposed on the inmate by others.

With these warnings, advance directives can be important to the dying inmate and his family. They provide the basis for discussion of terminal care, including an outline of the issues that need to be addressed. They represent perhaps the final way for the inmate to exercise control in the present and for the future. They also provide important guidance for the correctional authorities and should be used to permit the inmate to die in the facility, rather than being transferred at the end of life to another strange location where, once again, he has no friends or known care providers. Continuity of care at the end of life is one of the most important elements that decent terminal care can provide. Remaining in the prison to die also avoids one of the greatest injustices of transfer—shackling the terminally ill inmate.

A living will is a document, executed when the patient is capable of making health care decisions, that can be invoked when the patient is no longer able to participate in health care decisions. Philosophically, the living will is a valuable neutral instrument and can be used prospectively to request or refuse care. Practically, however, it is almost always used to refuse care, reflecting its origins as a mechanism to guard against unwanted over treatment at the end of life.[17] A living will has a classic structure, including a trigger event—"If I am ever terminally ill and my doctors say that I will not recover, then . . ." or "If I cannot recognize and relate to family, friends, and loved ones and my doctors say that I will not recover, then . . ." And it proceeds to state a series of care interventions that the person wished to accept or refuse. Traditionally, the list of treatments to be accepted or refused includes dialysis, surgery, antibiotics, or respiratory restrictions, or exclusions that apply in the particular jurisdiction.[18]

Health care agents or proxy appointments are, like living wills, now also permitted in every state. These documents allow the patient to designate a specific person, and if that person is unavailable, an alternate, who has the legal authority to make health care decisions on the patient's behalf. Outside of prisons, these appointments are generally preferable to a living will. They provide for a person who can discuss the options with the care team and can weigh the risks and benefits in the real time of the moment. They allow for questions and discussion, which a living will does not. They assume, however, that there will be a person on the spot to discuss the issues and participate in the decision making. As such, they are only useful if the correctional administration permits the proxy agent to be at the site of care to participate in the discussion of alternatives. This will almost always require flexibility in visiting rules and administrative protocols that preclude non-correctional personnel from being in the medical facility, except for small periods at regular visiting hours. Absent flexibility, proxy appointments are hardly useful. It is extremely difficult for a surrogate to make decisions that permit the death of a loved one. If the person is in a correctional facility and can see the situation of the patient and hear the suggestions of the care staff, these anguishing decisions become a possibility. Without this sort of support and connection, the decisions become nearly impossible to effect, imposing a terrible burden on the proxy.

Orders not to resuscitate have also become part of the ethical armamentarium of providers of terminal care. These orders state that, if the patient's heart or lungs fail, attempts to provide cardiopulmonary resuscitation (CPR) will not be made. They are appropriate for a terminally ill patient whose chances of surviving the resuscitation attempt are slight and whose quality of life, if the resuscitation were to be successful, would likely be severely compromised. When the patient decides to authorize this sort of withholding of treatment, the danger is that some member of the care team or the administration has convinced him to refuse CPR when that would not be the inmate's real choice. The issue of imposed care plans, rather than freely chosen care options, is inherent in the power disparity of the correctional setting. On the other hand, it should be of equal concern if inmates are not being offered the option to refuse resuscitation and are, thus, suffering the indignity and possibly the pain of an aggressive and futile intervention.

One way to address the concerns about freely chosen care plans for the terminally ill is to involve someone outside of the prison structure in the process of discussion and deciding. The most helpful person in managing these issues is likely to be the prison chaplain or a spiritual leader from the community. All of these instruments, if used correctly to inform and empower the inmate, can help to structure end-of-life care in a fashion that the inmate finds most comfortable. If used oppressively only to smooth administration, they can further erode the dignity to which the inmate and his family are entitled.

COMPASSIONATE RELEASE

On January 31, 1997, The Press Association Limited reported that the Director General of the English Prison Service had "apologized publicly for the treatment of a terminally ill prisoner who was shackled to a bed until just 3 hours before he died." The report could have come as easily from the many correctional facilities in the United States now housing the terminally ill. For dying prisoners, there will inevitably be substantial barriers to the humane care that their situations demand. The inherent disjunction between the goals of medicine and the goals of correctional facilities will continue to require a fundamental reworking of correctional policies and procedures to accommodate the needs of the dying. Compassionate care for the terminally ill is a difficult paradigm to create in a prison environment, and it requires constant tending to ensure that it does not revert to a more retributive and punitive model.

There are many Compassionate Release programs in the United States (Box 30-1). While some correctional systems frequently and successfully use the compassionate release option, others rarely do. Effective use of the compassionate release program would require 1) early identification of potential candidates; 2) creation of a mechanism for family members to request consideration; 3) appointment of an advocate for each applicant with powers to negotiate the process through the correctional, criminal, and judicial administrations; and 4) an appeal procedure available to

prisoners and their families if the application were denied at any point in the process (personal communication, Robert Cohen, 1997).

In the California state prison system, with an average daily census of approximately 150,000 inmates, there has been an average of 78 inmates per year submitted for compassionate release since 1991. In this period, an average of 28 inmates have been granted compassionate release (personal communication, Joy Hirai). In Florida, where the average population of the Department of Corrections (DOC) is approximately 64,000 inmates, prisoners must be incapacitated so that they will not be a danger to themselves or others (personal communication, Emile Baudoin d'Ajoux). In 1995 and 1996, 170 inmates were referred for compassionate release, and 42 were approved. Compassionate release is almost never approved for prisoners in Illinois, since no formal system exists for medical parole. Instead, prisoners are placed in hospices and they die in prison (personal communication, Harry Shuman, MD).

With an average daily census of 41,000 inmates in Michigan, 12 patient-prisoners have been submitted for compassionate release since 1994, and only 3 have been approved for release. The Michigan DOC will recommend medical parole only for those prisoners who are physically or mentally incapacitated (personal communication, Gayle Lafferty). In 1997, there have not been any requests for compassionate release in Michigan.

In New Mexico, the state corrections department will consider any inmate who has not been convicted of first-degree murder, and who is either elderly or permanently incapacitated or terminally ill.[19] With an average daily population of approximately 4,700 inmates, the New Mexico DOC has referred 21 patients for medical parole over the past 18 months. Six have been released.

In Vermont, inmates who have been certified as being terminally ill by a qualified, licensed physician may be released by the parole board. The condition of these individuals must be so debilitating that it is unlikely they will harm themselves or others.[20] According to Tom Powell, Ph.D., Director of Clinical Services for the Vermont Department of Corrections, if the patient-prisoner is critically ill and expected to die soon, "I can directly order the release of the patient via administrative medical furlough and in this manner the patient-prisoner can be released within 1 day." The average daily population of inmates in the Vermont DOC is 1,200, and the average yearly number of patient-prisoner releases on medical parole is seven. Ninety percent of the medical parole requests are successful.

In Utah, the Board of Pardons can approve compassionate release for those patient-prisoners who are unlikely to recover and incapable of repeat offenses. Once their incapacitation is known, they can be released in as little as 24 hours. The most common reason for compassionate release referral is end-stage cancer. Patient-prisoners appropriate for compassionate release are given the option of either

---

Box 30-1. Compassionate Release—A Comparison of Programs

California
Contact person: Joy Hirai (916-322-2544)
    Classification Analyst
    Classification Services Unit
    California Department of Corrections
Average number of prisoners - 150,000
Average number of referrals per year - 78 (1991-1997)
Average number of releases per year - 28 (1991-1997)

Florida
Contact person: Emile Baudoin d'Ajoux (907-487-4702)
    Impaired Inmate Service Coordinator
    Office of Health Services
    Florida Department of Corrections
Average number of prisoners - 64,000

1995
Referred - 86
Approved - 19
1996
Referred - 84
Approved - 23

Illinois
Contact person: Harry Shuman, M.D. (312-814-3233)
    Medical Director
    Illinois Department of Corrections

Michigan
Contact person: Gayle Lafferty (517-373-3629)
    Administrator
    Bureau of Health Care Services
    Michigan Department of Corrections
Average number of prisoners - 41,500
Number of prisoners recommended for medical parole in
   1994 - 0

Number of prisoners recommended for medical parole in
   1995 - 8; 3 were paroled
Number of prisoners recommended for medical parole in
   1996 - 4; none were paroled
Number of prisoners recommended for medical parole in
   1997 - none submitted to this date

New Mexico
Contact person - John Robertson, M.D. (505-827-8533/8762)
    Medical Director
    State of New Mexico Corrections Department
Average number of prisoners - 4700
Referrals - 21 (note: over an 18-month period)
Approvals - 6
(Note: Some patients applied for release through methods other
than the formal process.)

Vermont
Contact person - Tom Powell, Ph.D. (802-241-2380/2295)
    Director of Clinical Services
    Vermont Department of Corrections
Average number of prisoners - 1200
Referrals - 21 (note: over an 18-month period)
Approvals - 6
(Note: Some patients applied for release through methods other
than the formal process.)

Utah
    Bureau of Clinical Services
    Utah Department of Corrections
Average number of prisoners - 4700
Average number of referrals per year - 4 (approximately 100%
success rate)

---

being transferred to an incarcerated hospice setting, or of being released. Although there are three prisons in Utah, the Utah State Prison Draper houses most of the terminally ill patients, since this facility has an infirmary. The Utah DOC has an average daily census of 4,700 inmates. Approximately four patients are given compassionate release annually; the success rate is 100% (personal communication, Robert Jones, MD).

The compassionate release program at the 40-bed Bellevue Hospital Prison Ward in New York is run as a cooperative effort by Bellevue Hospital, a member of the New York City Health and Hospitals Corporation (HHC) and the New York City DOC. Since 1993, 196 of 307 patients submitted for release have been granted their freedom, a 64% rate of success. In the last 2 years, the rate of success has risen to 78% due to refinements in the process. The remainder of this chapter will describe how this has been accom-

plished, and in doing so will provide a blueprint for the creation of an effective compassionate release program.

The Bellevue Hospital compassionate release program relies on the cooperation of physicians, nurses, social workers, administrators, judges, defense attorneys, district attorneys, correctional staff, parole and/or probation personnel, and the patient. The Medical Director of the Bellevue Hospital Prison Health Service serves as the coordinator of this program. In this system, the coordinator is a general internist experienced in correctional medicine who possesses a sophisticated knowledge of the criminal justice system. In addition, the coordinator must have excellent interpersonal skills, great determination, and be willing ***and*** able to make firm judgments concerning a patient's functional capacity and survival time. Most important, the coordinator should be dedicated to doing whatever can be done to prevent a patient from dying in custody.

Identifying Candidates for Compassionate Release

Determine the patient's medical condition. The first step in the compassionate release process in the identification of appropriate candidates. Eligible candidates usually fall under one or more of the following categories:

- Terminally ill patients with a survival time of days to months (e.g., AIDS, cancer)
- Significant physical disability (e.g., hemiplegia, quadriplegia)
- Significant mental illness (eg, Alzheimer's disease)

Referrals for compassionate release are made by clinical staff (physicians, physician assistants, nurse practitioners, nurses) through their knowledge of patients. It is important that clinical staff understand how to refer and what the criteria are. The nursing opinion is a critical step in the process; patients with terminal illness can deteriorate suddenly and nurses are frequently the first to notice. Early identification of appropriate candidates permits additional time in which to attain compassionate release.

Not all decisions concerning compassionate release submission are obvious from the outset. Frequently, a patient must be observed for days to weeks before a decision can be made as to whether he is an appropriate candidate for release. Frivolous applications for compassionate release to the court and/or parole system would quickly lose credibility and with it the ability to obtain compassionate release. At the other extreme, the patient near death must have the release process handled expeditiously.

Determine the patient's current medical status and medical history. In some systems, the defined role for physicians in obtaining compassionate release is quite limited, and may only include writing a letter to correctional authorities or the parole board that documents the patient's medical condition. In other systems, significant medical involvement may be permitted. The medical leadership must understand the intricacies of the process of obtaining compassionate release for their system. Prisons and jails may have different processes for obtaining compassionate release largely related to the fact that inmates in jails are not yet convicted, but inmates in prisons are convicted. It may be easier to obtain compassionate release for someone who has not yet been found guilty. On the other hand, prison inmates are sentenced and it may be assumed by the public that they are sent to prison for punishment. This makes compassionate release more difficult, even when it is practical and reasonable for the correctional authority to release a dying inmate. It is useful to advocate with correctional officials for a formalized process because standardization of the process can expedite release.

After a patient is deemed appropriate for compassionate release, the medical director should attempt to discover why a patient has been incarcerated. This is an important step for the following reasons:

- The patient's current charges and criminal history will have a large impact on the likelihood and the rapidity of the patient being granted compassionate release, and,

- It determines which authorities will be involved in the compassionate release process.

For example, in New York City, if the patient has been detained on a criminal charge, the defense attorney, assistant defense attorney, and presiding judge all play a role. A patient sentenced to state time (a term greater than 1 year) will either be presented to the sentencing judge or the state parole board for compassionate release consideration. If the patient has been sentenced to city time (a term of 1 year or less), the Conditional Release Board of New York City makes the decision concerning release. Finally, a patient whose parole has been revoked must have a request for compassionate release submitted to the New York City Division of Parole. A patient with new criminal charges while on parole generally will have his parole revoked. If this patient becomes a candidate for compassionate release, both the court and parole board division will be required to agree to release before the patient can be freed from custody.

A patient's current criminal charges and criminal history largely determine if and how quickly a patient will be freed from custody by the criminal justice system. Patients who have committed crimes that have resulted in personal injury, or have a history that demonstrates a propensity for violence are unlikely to be released if they are still functional. In general, these patients must be unable to commit further criminal acts before they will be considered for release (e.g., the terminally ill, bed-bound patient). Patients with lesser charges and fewer past criminal events may be candidates for release before they reach the terminal stage of illness. Earlier discharge permits the patient more extended time with family members and an opportunity to arrange emotional and economic accounts.

The Medical Summary Letter

The patient may not want compassionate release. Some inmates have no homes or anyone to care for them. Dying in prison or jail may be a better choice than release. In addition, the release process most always involves documenting medical information to correctional authorities. This requires patient permission to release information concerning his medical condition to the authorities involved in the compassionate release process. A medical summary letter is often required (Box 30-2). It should contain the following information:

- patient's name and relevant identification numbers
- diagnosis
- functional capacity
- chances for recovery (and to what extent)
- prognosis

The Medical Director is the appropriate person to compose the medical summary letter; other medical staff have neither the time nor experience to write such a letter in a timely and appropriate manner. The object of the letter is to paint a clear picture of the patient's deteriorated medical

---

Box 30-2. Compassionate Release Worksheet

Patient Name: _____ , _____

Book and Case Number: _____ - _____

New York State I.D. Number: _____

Legal Status: -Detainee   -Sentenced (< 1 year; > 1 year)   -Parole Violator

Criminal history (if any):

Medical History

Primary diagnosis: _____

Secondary diagnosis: _____

Functional capacity: _____

Prognosis: _____

Contact People

	Name	**Telephone #**
Defense Attorney:		
Presiding Judge:		
Assistant District Attorney:		
Parole Supervisor:		
Condition Release Supervisor:		

Telephone number of court room: (   )   -

---

condition. With this in mind, the letter should state the diagnosis and prognosis, the patient's physical and mental limitations, and the chances for recovery. Most important, it should give a concrete survival estimate, which should be written in bold and italicized type in the following manner: ***"Mr. Jones has 3–6 months to live and will need 24–hour nursing care to attend to his daily activities for the remainder of his life."*** A letter that does not document estimated survival time minimizes the patient's chances of being freed from custody.

Speaking With the Right People

In the course of working in a correctional system, physicians often develop a circle of influence with correctional officials. In addition to formal processes, it may be helpful to call the warden or other key correctional officials to expedite this process. It may also be useful to contact defense attorneys, assistant defense attorneys, and presiding judges. If an inmate is incarcerated for parole violation, the parole board may need to be contacted. A patient with a sentence of 1 year or less may require special application. For example, in New York City, inmates serving less than 1 year must gain approval of the conditional release program to be contacted. Also, in New York City, a patient with a sentence of greater than 1 year has two options: either the sentencing judge or the state parole board may be contacted. At Bellevue, asking the sentencing judge to reduce a dying patient's sentence to "time served" has been far more successful than submitting the request to the state parole board, because the judge can make a quick, unilateral decision. On the other hand, the state parole board must agree to a compassionate release request, and it is not possible to speak directly with Board members.

How to Speak to the Right People

The defense attorney. Jailed inmates often have court-appointed attorneys. These attorneys are either employed by the state Legal Aid Society (public defender), or are private practitioners appointed by the court to represent the client at a predetermined hourly fee. Defense attorneys may not have experience in the compassionate release process. In New York City, if the patient is critically ill, the Medical Director will request the defense attorney to petition to advance the court date to the earliest possible date. In many instances, the court date has been moved up to the following day. A copy of the medical summary letter is then faxed to the defense attorney. In New York City, it is helpful when the Medical Director requests that the defense attorney contact him promptly if any obstacles arise (e.g., opposition from the assistant district attorney concerning the patient's release).

The assistant district attorney. In some systems, petitions for compassionate release may require interface with the state's attorney or the district attorney. In New York City, the Medical Director contacts the ADA if there is opposition to releasing the patient. The goal of the conversation is to assure the ADA of the patient's stage of illness. This may require more than one telephone call as the ADA must then speak with his supervisor for his approval to release the patient from custody. On rare instances, the Medical Director may find it necessary to speak directly with the DA to have the prosecutor's office drop its opposition. When speaking with the ADA, the Medical Director should emphasize the patient's poor condition, the inability of the patient to commit further criminal acts, and his willingness to put this in writing. This assumption of responsibility is critical. He should also inform the ADA of the emotional stress to patients and staff that occurs when dealing with terminally ill patients in custody. Finally, the ADA should be made aware of the plans for the patient should he be freed from custody. In most instances, the patient will be transferred to a hospital bed on the civilian units. Immediately after speaking with the ADA, the medical summary letter with updated information (if necessary) should be faxed to the ADA.

The judge. In certain situations, medical staff may need to speak with a presiding judge to obtain compassionate release. In New York City, this occurs in the following situations:
- If the patient has days to live and immediate release is necessary
- If the ADA opposes the patient's release
- If the judge opposes the patient's release

While no two judges are alike, most have one thing in common: they do not want to free a man who may commit further criminal acts. Thus, as with the ADA, the Medical Director must convey to the judge the patient's deteriorated status and his inability to commit further criminal acts. It is usually possible to have the judge agree to having the court date advanced if the patient is expected to expire shortly (as long as the defense attorney and the ADA can agree on a date and time). Matters become difficult when the ADA opposes the patient's release. In these cases, the Medical Director may find it necessary and productive to telephone the judge and inform him of the patient's condition. Once the patient's condition and prognosis are made clear, the judge will usually agree to free the patient from custody despite the ADA's opposition. The most difficult scenario arises if the judge opposes the patient's release. The only avenue available to the Medical Director and the defense attorney at this point is to appeal to the judge on the facts and the prognosis as the basis for a compassionate decision.

The parole supervisor. In New York City, patients who have had their parole revoked must have it restored before they can be released in custody. This may be similar to other systems. The people to contact are those assigned to the parole revocation and restoration unit and their supervisors with whom the Medical Director needs a good working relationship. The Medical Director should speak with the supervisor to determine the patient's history, as this will determine to a large extent whether "parole" will opt in favor of restoration. As with other areas of the criminal justice system, the sicker and more debilitated the patient, the more likely it is the patient will be released; if the patient is a candidate for restoration, the parole supervisor will expedite the release. In some systems, compassionate release is decided without public hearings. In some jails, compassionate release is offered simply by the sheriff releasing the inmate on recognizant bond. In New York City, compassionate release is obtained in the context of a hearing. When hearings are required, medical staff can further the process by providing up-to-date medical information to those concerned. If the patient has been granted release, he must make certain that the release papers are received by the prison ward that day. Without scrupulous oversight, these papers may take days to arrive, and in some instances, have been lost. To avoid this, the Medical Director should devise a system in conjunction with the DOC where a faxed copy of the release papers will be accepted at the prison ward pending arrival of the hard copy. At the very least, this expedites the patient's release by hours. To get the copy faxed to the prison ward, the DOC liaison for compassionate release is informed of the release by the Medical Director. He then telephones the courtroom and instructs that the release papers be delivered to the DOC office located in the courthouse. At that point, the liaison has the correctional staff fax the papers to the prison ward after he informs the prison ward staff of their impending arrival.

While this is occurring, the Medical Director informs the nursing staff of the decision, so they may call the admitting department to designate a bed for the patient on a civilian ward. He then instructs the house staff caring for the patient to write orders to transfer the patient to the civilian unit. Once the faxed copy of the release papers arrives, the Medical Director informs the patient of his release from custody and its ramifications.

Patients who have their parole restored are freed in a different manner. The parole officer must come to the prison ward and "lift" the parole warrant in person. In the case of the critically ill patient, it is essential that the parole officer come to the prison ward on the day the decision is made to restore parole. This can be a problem, as the parole officer may not be close to the prison ward or may be busy attending to other matters. In these situations, the parole supervisor in charge of revocation and restoration has seen to it that another parole officer is sent to lift the warrant. In a few instances, his assistance has meant the difference between a patient dying in custody or as a free civilian.

Epilogue

Once the patient has been freed from custody, the Medical Director should visit the patient the following day to see if there is anything the patient needs. The most common request from the patient is for the retrieval of his property being held by the correctional authority. The Medical Director will ask the DOC to deliver this property. The Medical Director also contacts family members, where available, to inform them of the patient's release. Lastly, the social worker is informed of the patient's change of status so that appropriate planning, discharge, and otherwise, may be begun.

CONCLUSION

Although a compassionate release process with real integrity would be expensive, it would cost many thousands of dollars less than providing adequate end-of-life care in the prison setting.[21] Cost savings need not be one of the factors necessarily considered in evaluating any particular inmate for compassionate release, but should surely be taken into account in creating the program itself.

Punishment and caring are generally incompatible. The best illustration of this fact can be seen in end-of-life care in prisons. But, even if retribution is justifiable, dying alone, in pain, without comfort, exceeds the boundaries of the permissible for the vast majority of inmates. For these, simple humanity and primitive justice demand compassion.

REFERENCES

1. American Board of Internal Medicine: Caring for the Dying: Identification and Promotion of Physician Competency. Project of the American Board of Internal Medicine, 1996; 11-18; Dubuwitz V: Withdrawing intensive life-sustaining treatment-recommendations for compassionate clinical management, *New Engl J Med* 336:652-657, 1997; Cassel CK, Vladeck BC: ICD-9 Code for palliative or terminal care. *New Engl J Med* 335:1232-1234, 1996; Wanzer S, et al: The physician's responsibility toward hopelessly ill patients. *New Engl J Med* 320:844-849, 1989; Zerwekh J: Do dying patients really need IV fluids? *Am J Nurs* 97:26-30, 1997; Council on Ethical and Judicial Affairs, American Medical Association, Council Report: Decisions near the end of life. *JAMA* 267:2229-2233, 1992.

2. SUPPORT Principal Investigators: A controlled trial to improve care for seriously ill hospitalized patients. *JAMA* 274: 1591-1598, 1995.

3. Gamble ER, McDonald PJ, Lichstein PR: Knowledge, attitudes, and behavior of elderly persons regarding living wills. *Arch Intern Med* 151:277-280, 1991.

4. Pagliaro LA, Pagliaro AM: Sentenced to death? HIV infection and AIDS in prisons—Current and future concerns. *Can J Criminol* 34:201-214, 1992.

5. Braithwaite RL, Hammett TM, Mayberry RM: *Prisons and AIDS: A Public Health Challenge,* Jossey-Bass, 1996, 116.

6. Purdey M: As AIDS Increases Behind Bars, Costs Dim Promise of New Drugs. New York Times, May 26, 1997, A1.

7. Brown JM, Gilliard DK, Snell TL, et al: Correctional populations in the United States, 1994. Washington, D.C., Department of Justice, 1996, p 85.

8. Morton JB: An Administrative Overview of the Older Inmate. Washington, D.C., U.S. Department of Justice, 1992, p 4.

9. Youth and Special Needs Program Office, Florida Department of Corrections: Status Report on Elderly Inmates. 1993, p5 cited by Adams WE, Jr: The Incarceration of Older Criminals: Balancing Safety, Cost, and Humanitarian Concerns. 19 Nova Law Review, 465 1995; p 12.

10. Chaneless S: Growing old behind bars. *Psychology Today* 47:49, 1987.

11. Ornduff JS: Releasing the elderly inmate: A solution to prison overcrowding. *Elder Law J* 173:26, 1966.

12. Wright JH Jr: Life without parole: An alternative to death or not much of a life at all? *Vand Law Rev* 529:563, 1990.

13. Commissioner of *Corrections v. Myers,* 379 Mass 255; 399 NW 2d 452 (1979).

14. Robbins IP: George Bush's America Meets Dante's Inferno: The Americans with Disabilities Act in Prison. *Yale Law Policy Rev* 49: 49-112, 1996.

15. Robbins at 49.

16. Dubler N, Anno, BJ: *Ethical Considerations and the Interface with Custody. Prison Health Care: Guidelines for the Management of an Adequate Delivery System.* Chicago, National Commission on Correctional Health Care, 1991, p 54.

17. Dubler N, Nimmons D: *Ethics on Call: A Medical Ethicist Shows How to Take Charge of Life-and-Death Choices.* New York, Harmony Books, 1992, p 350.

18. Sabatino C: Health Care Power of Attorney Legislation as of January 1, 1995. American Bar Association, Commission on Legal Problems of the Elderly, pp 1-8.

19. New Mexico State policy.

20. Vermont Parole Board policy.

21. Russell, MP: Too little, too late, too slow: Compassionate release of terminally ill prisoners—Is the cure worse than the disease? Widner J Pub Law 799:804.

Index

Note: Page numbers in *italics* indicate illustrations; "t" indicates tables.